£135·00

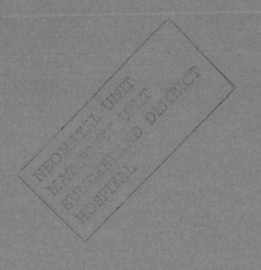

Neonatal Surgery
Third edition

Dedication

The first and second editions of this book were dedicated to the paediatricians who referred cases to us. We remain grateful to them.

The present edition is dedicated to the memory of Isabella Forshall, who contributed so much to the establishment of the paediatric surgical service in Liverpool.

Neonatal Surgery

Third edition

James Lister MD, FRCS(Ed.), FRCS(Glas.), FRCS(Eng.), FAAP(Hon.)
Professor Emeritus, University of Liverpool; Formerly Professor of Paediatric Surgery, University of Liverpool and Consultant Surgeon, Royal Liverpool Children's Hospital (Alder Hey), Liverpool, UK

Irene M. Irving BSc, MB, ChM, FRCS(Eng.)
Formerly Senior Lecturer in Paediatric Surgery, University of Liverpool and Consultant Paediatric Surgeon, Royal Liverpool Children's Hospital (Alder Hey), Liverpool, UK

Butterworths
London Boston Singapore Sydney Toronto Wellington

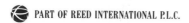 PART OF REED INTERNATIONAL P.L.C.

First published 1969
Reprinted 1970
Second edition 1978
Reprinted 1980
Third edition 1990

© Butterworth & Co. (Publishers) Ltd, 1990

British Library Cataloguing in Publication Data

Neonatal surgery. – 3rd ed.
1. Newborn babies. Surgery
I. Lister, James II. Irving, Irene M. III. Rickham,
P.P. (Peter Paul). Neonatal surgery.
617'.98
ISBN 0–407–01490–X

Library of Congress Cataloging-in-Publication Data

Neonatal surgery/edited by James Lister, Irene M.
Irving. – 3rd ed.
    p.   cm.
    Rev. ed. of: Neonatal surgery/P.P. Rickham,
James Lister, Irene M. Irving. 2nd ed. 1978.
    Includes bibliographical references.
    ISBN 0–407–01490–X :
    1. Infants (Newborn) – Surgery. I. Lister, James.
II. Irving, Irene M. III. Rickham, P. P. (Peter Paul)
Neonatal surgery.
    [DNLM: 1. Surgery – in infancy & childhood.
WO 925 N4381]
RD137.5.R53   1990
617.9'8–dc20

Photoset by Scribe Design, Gillingham, Kent
Printed and bound in Great Britain by Hartnolls Ltd, Bodmin, Cornwall

Foreword

Publication of the third edition of *Neonatal Surgery* coincides with the 75th anniversary of the opening of what was then the Alder Hey Infirmary, later to become Alder Hey Children's Hospital, and more recently, the Royal Liverpool Children's Hospital, Alder Hey. The pioneering contributions made by members of the surgical staff, notably Isabella Forshall, Peter Rickham and Herbert Johnston, during the two decades following the Second World War are landmarks in the evolution of paediatric surgery as a specialty. Not to be overlooked is the essential complementary role played by Jackson Rees in the development of paediatric anaesthesia. Two major events during this era were first, the establishment in 1953 of the world's first purpose-built neonatal surgical unit, the Liverpool Neonatal Surgical Centre at Alder Hey Children's Hospital. The second event was the publication in 1969 of *Neonatal Surgery*, the first major textbook devoted entirely to the management of the newborn surgical patient. It is pleasing to note that in the third edition, 20 years later, the first chapter is by the senior founding editor. Publication of this edition also coincides with a sad event, the death in August 1989 of Isabella Forshall at the age of 89.

Remarkably in this age of disseminated multiple authorship, the editors of this edition, James Lister and Irene Irving, have again been able to draw their contributors from the Alder Hey family. The result is an invaluable insight into the experiences of the team of committed, thoughtful clinicians involved with the Regional Neonatal Surgical Unit. To maintain vitality it is essential not to live in the past, but to build on experience and move forwards, refining established methods and seeking new frontiers of knowledge and understanding. This is very much a living textbook which has adapted to the changing newborn population and encompasses a wide range of developments in neonatal surgical care. The third edition of *Neonatal Surgery* stands not only as a tribute to the past but also as a symbol of the vitality of neonatal surgery.

David A. Lloyd, MChir, FRCS
Professor of Paediatric Surgery, University of Liverpool; Consultant Paediatric Surgeon, Royal Liverpool Children's Hospital (Alder Hey)

v

Preface to the third edition

It is now 36 years since the Regional Neonatal Surgical Unit in Alder Hey Children's Hospital was opened, and 20 years since the publication of the first edition of this textbook. Neonatal surgery is no longer a specialty confined to a few specialist centres in wealthy countries; indeed, in many developing countries where the persistently high infant mortality rate clearly demands improved social conditions as the first step towards its reduction there is a widespread demand for the concurrent provision of specialist services for the surgical correction of life-threatening conditions in the newborn. Much of the demand has come from paediatricians, notably from the specialist neonatologists amongst them, and the enormous advances in neonatology in the past few years have changed the scene for paediatric surgical units. The special units set up for the care of sick newly born infants, particularly those of low birth-weight, demand environmental conditions, equipment and experienced specialist staff similar to those required for neonatal surgical units. Some of the larger centres may still be able to justify the provision of an independent neonatal surgical unit but there is a widespread trend towards sharing of facilities between such units and special care baby units. It may well be that the neonatologists will have administrative charge of such units, but the surgeon must maintain his responsibilities in the pre- and postoperative care of his patients wherever they may be nursed. Because of these developments we felt that the chapters on the organization, structural and staffing requirements and equipment of a regional neonatal surgical unit are no longer required, although those chapters in the first two editions of the book are of considerable historical interest.

Neonatologists have also been instrumental in changing the workload of the neonatal surgical unit. Not only have they increased to a significant extent the survival of low birthweight babies with multiple anomalies (and hence their subsequent referral for surgical correction), but they have also produced a new population of survivors of early neonatal care suffering from diseases of survival which may require surgical treatment; necrotizing enterocolitis is one of these and, less obviously, post-haemorrhagic hydrocephalus.

In this constantly changing scene it is not surprising that there have been many changes in detail and emphasis in the book. Five new chapters have been included in Part 1, covering the topics of fluid and electrolyte management and nutritional support, antenatal diagnosis, X-rays and imaging, the low birthweight infant, and antibiotics and infections. There have also been changes in editors and authors. Professor Rickham retired several years ago but many of his original contributions remain in the book. His chapter on ethics sums up a lifetime's experience and provides wise advice for young consultants. The two current editors, James Lister and Irene Irving, have also retired during the preparation of the book and a number of the younger consultants in the Royal Liverpool Children's Hospital at Alder Hey have joined the team of contributors.

We do not present our experience because we believe our methods are the only valid ones but the Regional Neonatal Service at Alder Hey still drains a population of around 3 million and the workload is that which might be expected from such a drainage area. The paediatric surgeons serving the unit work closely together and in most conditions the case material is more than sufficient to allow for analysis and the drawing of valid conclusions. Furthermore, although the authors may emphasize their personal experience, wide coverage is also given to the work of other specialists in the field of neonatal surgery and there is an extensive bibliography.

We are indebted to many people for a great deal of help. Dr Agnes Pierce has meticulously recorded and retrieved the neonatal surgical statistics which form the basis of many of the chapters. Many surgeons in training both from the UK and overseas have reviewed our experience with specific problems: their published works are referred to throughout the text. Mrs D. Bolger, Mrs J. Bowen, Mrs P. Chegwin, Mrs F. Hesketh, Mrs C. Ireland, Mrs S. Longworth and other secretarial staff in Liverpool, and Ms J. Edmundson, Miss F. Sinclair and Mrs C. Forsyth in Edinburgh have devoted much time and effort to typing the manuscripts. Mrs S. Curbishley, Mrs M.F. Samuels and Miss S. Grey at the Liverpool Medical Institution and Mrs M. Smith at the Royal College of Surgeons in Edinburgh have provided invaluable help with reference checking. Mr C.T. FitzSimon, Chief Medical Photographer at Alder Hey Hospital and Mr K. Walters, Department of Medical Illustration, Institute of Child Health, Liverpool University, have again provided excellent photographic material. Most of the drawings in this edition are those prepared by Mrs H. Blundell and Miss J. Weston for the previous editions, but for the extra artwork required we have had the expert help of Mrs Angela Christie.

To all these people and to any whom we have failed to name we extend our sincere thanks.

Finally, we would like to thank the editorial staff of Butterworths for their patient help during the preparation and publication of this volume.

JAMES LISTER
IRENE M. IRVING

Preface to the second edition

The surprisingly rapid sale of the first and second printing of the first edition of this book made a new edition mandatory. Since the first edition was published in 1969 there has been great progress in the management of the surgical neonate. This necessitated a complete revision of the various chapters. The writing of this book was delayed by a number of changes in the staff of Alder Hey Children's Hospital. The senior Editor (P.P.R.) moved to Zürich from Liverpool in 1971 and J.L. moved to Liverpool from Sheffield in 1974, taking administrative charge of the Regional Neonatal Surgical Centre at Alder Hey Children's Hospital. I.M.I., who did so much for the first edition, joined us as co-Editor. Mr J.H. Johnston has concentrated his efforts to paediatric urology and has therefore given up the general editorship.

A number of contributors to the first edition have left Alder Hey Children's Hospital since 1969 and new appointments have been made, and this is reflected in the list of contributors to the second edition. Furthermore, members of the staff of the University Children's Hospital, Zürich, have joined as contributors and the book thus reflects the close collaboration of the surgical staff of the Liverpool and Zürich Children's Hospitals.

The steady fall in the birth rate in the Western world, with a consequent reduction in the annual admissions of newborn children for surgery, has posed a question for the survival of neonatal surgical units. In many smaller areas neonatal intensive care centres treating both medical and surgical patients have been found to be the solution to the problem. This fact detracts nothing from the desirability of neonatal surgical units in centres accepting infants from a sufficiently large population. Further changes in the frequency of admissions of surgical neonates have been brought about by the change in the climate of opinion with regard to the treatment of myelomeningoceles with a consequent reduction in the number of children undergoing aggressive treatment for spina bifida and hence less pressure on the neonatal surgical centre. In some areas, prenatal screening and pregnancy terminations have significantly reduced the number of liveborn children with myelomeningocele. On the other hand, there has been a considerable increase in the surgical treatment of congenital heart disease in the first few weeks of life during the last 10 years. A section on cardiac surgery is therefore included in this volume.

The editing of this book would have been impossible without the splendid help we received from a number of people. Mrs M.L. Cantlay, Miss C. Tedford, Mrs M. Bratherton and other surgical seretaries in Liverpool and Miss R. Vaisanen in Zürich were responsible for typing the manuscripts and have done a splendid job. Miss B. Gill, FRCS, and Miss J. Robson, FRCS, have collected and classified the case material and have given us much valuable information, and a succession of visiting Fellows in Alder Hey have given great help in analysing material, particularly Dr T.K. Subramanian and Dr R.R. Rios. Mr C.T. FitzSimon, Head of District Photography Unit, Liverpool Area Health Authority (Teaching) Eastern District (Teaching), Mr K. Walters, AIMBI, Department of

Medical Illustration, Institute of Child Health, Liverpool University, and Mr O. Brunner, clinical photographer at the University Children's Hospital, Zürich, have helped to add many excellent new photographs, thus greatly enriching the book and making it easier to understand. Mrs H. Blundell (née Carline) whose artistic work appeared in the first edition has produced many fine new drawings for this edition; we are also indebted to Miss Jacqueline Weston, medical artist in Liverpool, and Mr W. Adank, clinical artist at the Zürich Children's Hospital, for contributions to the illustrations of chapters newly written or revised by both Liverpool and Zürich authors. To all these we extend our sincere thanks.

Some of the research necessary to produce this book has been financed by grants made by the Liverpool Neonatal Surgical Research Fund.

We hope that this edition, like the first, will help paediatric surgeons, paediatricians and all other physicians who come into contact with surgical neonates.

P.P. RICKHAM
JAMES LISTER
IRENE M. IRVING

Preface to the first edition

Since World War II a number of excellent textbooks on paediatric surgery, at both undergraduate and postgraduate levels, have been published on both sides of the Atlantic. In the early 1950s it was still possible for such men as Robert Gross of Boston and Max Grob of Zürich to write, single-handed, comprehensive volumes on the subject. Progress in paediatric surgery has, however, been so rapid and there have been so many new developments in the field that it has become virtually impossible for one man to master the whole of the subject and consequently a number of large, multi-author, multi-volume works on children's surgery have appeared. Since these tend to ever-increasing bulk, it appears to us that the time has come for their replacement by concise monographs on selected subjects within the specialty.

In this volume we have concentrated entirely on the surgery of the newborn since we believe that this subject has become so extensive as to merit separate treatment in a book. Originally we had intended to include the whole range of neonatal surgery, but it was soon apparent that this would make the book too large. We therefore excluded such subjects as cardiac and orthopaedic surgery and concentrated on those conditions which we have treated in the Liverpool Neonatal Surgical Centre. This Centre was founded by Isabella Forshall and one of us (P.P.R.) in 1953. One of us (J.H.J.) joined in 1957 and has concentrated mainly on the urological problems. Since Miss Forshall, who operated on many of the infants mentioned in this volume, has retired Mr N.V. Freeman, who also contributes some chapters to this volume, has joined us.

We felt it would be of more value to the reader if we would concentrate on those less rare surgical conditions of the newborn of which we have had extensive experience, and exclude rarities, conditions of teratologic but of little therapeutic interest and conditions, which although they may be present during the first few weeks of life, are more commonly encountered in older infants and children. During the 14½ years of its existence, over 2800 infants have been admitted to the Neonatal Surgical Centre. In addition, many neonates suffering from such conditions as pyloric stenosis, strangulated hernia, obstructive jaundice, some urological conditions, etc., could not, in the past, be admitted to the Centre because of lack of space. This book is therefore based on our experience with over 3500 newborn infants with surgical lesions whom we have treated since 1953.

The rapid advances in neonatal surgery during the last two decades have been brought about by two developments. Firstly, there was the development of paediatric surgery as a specialty in its own right. Unless a surgeon is trained to deal with and is experienced in the many special problems of infancy and is aware of the embryological, metabolic, physiological and medical problems involved, his chances of obtaining consistently satisfactory results in this branch of surgery are small. The second major development has been the recognition that, unless these infants are dealt with by a team of surgeons, physicians, anaesthetists, biochemists, pathologists, radiologists and, especially, nurses who are interested and trained in this type of work, little can be achieved. We have stressed this fact by including in the book chapters by the nursing staff and by our colleagues in the departments of anaesthesia, paediatrics, otorhinolaryngology and orthodontics who, having taken a particular interest in this type of work, have been of the greatest help to us. We also thought that this book would be incomplete without a lengthy section on all the various aspects of general management of newborn infants undergoing surgery.

x   Preface to the first edition

We have not written this volume because we believe that our methods are better or our results superior to those achieved elsewhere. We are very well aware that equally good and often better results have been obtained by other surgeons in other centres. Our main aim has been to show what can be done when a regional neonatal surgical service drains a circumscribed area virtually completely. When discussing treatment we have given preference to those methods which we have found most useful but, where relevant, we have taken pains to point out that alternative techniques exist and have been found valuable by other surgeons working in this field.

The organization of a neonatal surgical service on a regional basis and the standardization of diagnostic procedures, emergency management and matters of transport would have been quite impossible without the active and enthusiastic co-operation and help which we have received at all times from the paediatricians attached to the large maternity hospitals in the north-west of England and North Wales. Their constant encouragement and wise counsel has helped us to overcome the many administrative and technical difficulties which we have encountered. We are very much in their debt and as an inadequate token of our gratitude we have dedicated this volume to them.

The preparation and writing of this book would have been impossible without the great help we have received from many people. Miss Irene M. Irving, FRCS, working as a Research Fellow with the aid of a grant by the Research Fund of the United Liverpool Hospitals and the Liverpool Regional Hospital Board, has been responsible for the collection, sifting, classification and coding of the clinical material which forms the basis of the book. Her meticulous accuracy and conscientious dedication to this enormous task are beyond praise. We gratefully acknowledge the devoted help we have received from Miss M.M. Barlow, Miss H. Valentine and Miss J.E. Rome, who have typed and re-typed these chapters. Mr R.R. Green, Mr C.T. FitzSimon and Mr K. Walters have been responsible for the photographic illustrations; no effort has been too much for them and they have helped us whenever we needed their services, regardless of the difficulties involved or of the time of the day or night when we needed them. Our Medical Artist, Miss H. Carline has been responsible for almost all the drawings in this volume. We believe that the supreme skill of this young artist has done much to enhance the value of our efforts. Finally we should like to thank the editorial staff of Butterworths for their help during the preparation and publication of this volume.

P.P. RICKHAM
J.H. JOHNSTON
Liverpool

List of contributors

Robert Arnold MB, ChB, FRCPE, FRCP
Consultant Paediatric Cardiologist, Royal Liverpool
Children's Hospital, Liverpool, UK

P.D. Booker MB, BS, FFARCS
Consultant Paediatric Anaesthetist, Royal
Liverpool Children's Hospital, Liverpool, UK

Gordon H. Bush MA, DM, FFARCS, DA
Consultant Paediatric Anaesthetist, Royal
Liverpool Children's Hospital (Alder Hey),
Liverpool, UK

Helen M.L. Carty MB, FRCPI, FRCR
Consultant Radiologist, Royal Liverpool Children's
Hospital (Alder Hey), Liverpool, UK

R.C.M. Cook MA, BM, FRCS
Consultant Paediatric Surgeon, Royal Liverpool
Children's Hospital (Alder Hey), Liverpool, UK

Richard W.I. Cooke MD, FRCP, DCH
Professor of Neonatal Medicine, University of
Liverpool, Liverpool, UK

R.E. Cudmore DCH, FRCS
Consultant Paediatric Surgeon, Royal Liverpool
Children's Hospital (Alder Hey), Liverpool, UK

A. Roger Green FRCS
Consultant Plastic Surgeon, Mersey Regional
Health Authority; Clinical Lecturer in Plastic
Surgery, University of Liverpool, Liverpool, UK

David I. Hamilton MB, BS, FRCS(Eng.),
FRCS(Ed.)
Professor of Cardiac Surgery, University of
Edinburgh, Royal Infirmary and Royal Hospital for
Sick Children, Edinburgh, UK; Formerly Senior
Cardiothoracic Surgeon, Royal Liverpool
Children's Hospital, Liverpool, UK

C. Anthony Hart MB, BS, BSc, PhD, MRCPath
Professor of Medical Microbiology, University of
Liverpool; Honorary Consultant Microbiologist,
Royal Liverpool Children's Hospitals, Liverpool, UK

Irene M. Irving BSc, MB, ChM, FRCS(Eng.)
Formerly Senior Lecturer in Paediatric Surgery,
University of Liverpool and Consultant Paediatric
Surgeon, Royal Liverpool Children's Hospital
(Alder Hey), Liverpool, UK

James Lister MD, FRCS(Ed.), FRCS(Glas.),
FRCS(Eng.), FAAP(Hon.)
Professor Emeritus, University of Liverpool;
Formerly Professor of Paediatric Surgery,
University of Liverpool and Consultant Surgeon,
Royal Liverpool Children's Hospital (Alder Hey),
Liverpool, UK

D.O. Maisels MB, ChB, FRCS(Ed.), FRCS(Eng.)
Formerly Consultant Plastic Surgeon, Mersey
Regional Health Authority, Liverpool, UK

Roxane McKay MD, FRCS
Senior Consultant Paediatric Cardiothoracic
Surgeon and Clinical Lecturer in Cardiothoracic
Surgery, The Royal Liverpool Children's Hospital,
Liverpool, UK

Thomas McKendrick MB, FRCP
Consultant Paediatrician and Nephrologist, Royal
Liverpool Children's Hospital (Alder Hey),
Liverpool, UK

Margaretha Lehner Dr med.
Chefärztin der Kinderchirurgischen Klinik des
Olgahospitals, Pädiatrisches Zentrum, Stuttgart,
Federal Republic of Germany

J.R. Owens MB, ChB, MRCP, DCH
Consultant Paediatrician, Macclesfield District
General Hospital, Macclesfield, UK

David W. Pilling MB, DCH, FRCR
Consultant Radiologist, Royal Liverpool Children's
Hospital (Alder Hey) and Liverpool Maternity
Hospital, Liverpool, UK

Peter P. Rickham MD, MS, FRCS, FRCS(I),
FRACS, DCH, FAAP
Professor Emeritus of Paediatric Surgery,
University of Zürich, Switzerland; Formerly Senior
Surgeon, Royal Liverpool Children's Hospital
(Alder Hey), Liverpool and Director of Paediatric
Surgical Studies, University of Liverpool, UK

A.M.K. Rickwood MA, FRCS
Consultant Paediatric Urological Surgeon, Royal
Liverpool Children's Hospital (Alder Hey),
Liverpool, UK

J.H. Rogers MA, BM, BCh, FRCS
Consultant Otolaryngologist, Royal Liverpool
Children's Hospital (Alder Hey), Liverpool, UK

U.G. Stauffer MD
Professor of Paediatric Surgery, University of
Zürich, Switzerland; Director of Department of
Paediatric Surgery, University Children's Hospital,
Zürich, Switzerland

Paul K.H. Tam MB, BS, ChM, FRCS(Ed.),
FRCS(Glas.)
Senior Lecturer in Paediatric Surgery, University of
Liverpool; Consultant Paediatric Surgeon, Mersey
Regional Health Authority, Liverpool, UK

C.J. Taylor MD, MRCP, DCH
Senior Lecturer in Paediatrics and Paediatric
Gastroenterology, University of Sheffield;
Honorary Consultant Paediatrician, Sheffield
Children's Hospital, Sheffield, UK

Jenny Walker ChM, FRCS
Senior Registrar in Paediatric Surgery, Royal
Liverpool Children's Hospital (Alder Hey),
Liverpool, UK

Contents

Part 1

General

Part I

1

The ethics of surgery in newborn infants

P.P. Rickham

Introduction and historical considerations

As science and medicine progress and the community develops and becomes more and more complex, ethical standards will change as well, and whether they like it or not, doctors will have to ensure that the development of the ethics of their profession keeps in step with scientific development.

In former times the problems posed by the management of deformed children were relatively simple. In antiquity most states headed by the Greeks, whom we believe to be the fathers as well as the shining example of European civilization, practised infanticide for deformed children [28]. One would think that the advent of Christianity would radically change the attitude towards this problem, but this was not so.

The ancient legal enactment of the Norsemen was that:

'Every child which is born into this world shall be reared, baptized and carried to the church except that only which is born so deformed that the mother cannot give strength to it. . . It shall be carried to the beach and buried where neither men nor cattle go; that is the beach of the evil one.' [2]

In the nineteenth as well as at the beginning of this century surgeons were hardly ever faced with the problem of whether they should withhold treatment. If a decision about life or death of the patient had to be made, it was the surgeon who did it and the patient and/or the family were perfectly happy for him to do so. For the surgeon of those days medical ethics were not concerned with the management of the patient, but with the surgeon's relationship with his colleagues [13].

The spectacular development of neonatology in general and neonatal surgery in particular after the Second World War has enabled us to save an ever-increasing number of newborn infants suffering from severe congenital malformations. To cite one example from neonatology: between 1970 and 1980 the neonatal mortality of otherwise normal infants was almost halved [30], whilst to cite an example from neonatal surgery, the mortality in Zürich for infants with gastroschisis has decreased from 80% before 1968 to 9%. The enormous expenditure on highly specialized personnel and sophisticated medical equipment on the one hand and on the other hand the fact that at the same time many children die all over the world because of lack of rudimentary care, raises a number of moral problems. Already in the 1960s we had to reconcile ourselves to the fact that numbers of neonatal surgical patients would grow up suffering from a greater or lesser physical handicap [25]. We had simply become too good at saving these infants and were left with a residue of surviving children experiencing some difficulties [26].

Thus medicine's and surgery's increased ability to forestall death in seriously ill newborn infants made the task of assessment more difficult. It is usually stated that the first debates about the ethics of life-sustaining treatment for newborns appeared in the professional journals of the early 1970s [3,17], but in fact neonatal surgeons had been forced to consider these questions during the preceding decade. When the first edition of this book was being written during 1966/67, it became clear that a chapter on the ethics of surgery in newborn infants had to be included, but it was soon found that virtually nothing had been written about this subject. The only guide then available was Pope Pius XII's [22] discourse on 'ordinary' and 'extraordinary' means of treatment.

Since then there has been a veritable explosion of recognition of the ethical issues involved and hundreds upon hundreds of articles on this subject have been published in medical, philosophical, theological and legal journals. The literature has become so complex and bewildering that it is hardly possible for a practising surgeon to keep himself up to date in these matters, especially as a plethora of radically opposing views has been expressed. It is interesting to speculate on why this development has occurred. There are probably two main reasons. One was the emergence of the concept of selection of infants for operation, which became pertinent when paediatricians were dissatisfied with the long-term results of some neonatal operations [14,15]. The other was the ever increasing number of legal proceedings, sometimes instituted by the state, sometimes by the parents involved, which because of their emotive nature were widely reported and discussed in the mass media which viewed them as another opportunity to sow distrust of the medical profession amongst the general population.

In the face of this excess of conflicting information it appears a formidable, if not impossible, task to express a considered view on these matters. The writer believes that certain very tentative suggestions may be of value, always provided that some factors are clearly recognized.

1. The decisions of whether to operate or not and how to manage infants and parents when an operation is not carried out are highly personal matters and will in the final analysis have to be decided between the surgeon and his conscience. Others may help, but they will never be able to interfere drastically with the patient/doctor relationship.
2. Any attempt by the state to interfere and to legislate in these matters will, in most cases, make the situation worse, not better. It is, of course, inevitable that the state will attempt to fill a vacuum produced by the inability of the medical profession to come to a more or less unanimous conclusion. As long as doctors do not agree amongst themselves, it will be impossible to attempt to educate the general public in these matters. In the absence of authoritative and informed medical opinion the public is wide open to the misinformation and emotional halftruths beloved of the mass media.
3. We have to recognize that there exists a definite generation gap between the attitude of paediatric surgeons who pioneered neonatal surgery after the Second World War and those who started to practise in the 1970s and 1980s. The older generation of paediatric surgeons felt that they were in some way bound by the Hippocratic oath and that they would try to do their best towards their patients and certainly would never do them any harm. The contract was between doctor and patient and nobody else. The next generation is much more aware of the familial and social implications

involved. The question of how to operate on these infants has somehow been replaced by the question of whether to operate at all. This is a natural and understandable development and has to be taken into account.

Types of cases for selection

If it is agreed that some selection for operation on newborn infants has to be carried out, difficulties arise when considering which classes of patients should be selected for treatment and who should be left to die. If surgery is clearly not going to benefit the patient, it should not be carried out, but those for whom it is at least theoretically beneficial can be classified on medical grounds. Since the original classification was published in the first edition of this book, numerous much more elaborate classifications have appeared. These seem to have complicated matters unnecessarily and we believe that for practical purposes the original classification may still be of value. This was as follows:

Class 1: Infants who are likely to be completely cured by surgery.
Class 2: Infants who, after treatment, will be handicapped to some extent but may still be able to lead a relatively normal life.
Class 3: Infants who, after treatment, will have severe physical handicaps and will have to lead a more or less sheltered life.
Class 4: Infants in classes 1 to 3 who, in addition, are of subnormal intelligence but can be trained up to a point.
Class 5: Infants in classes 1 to 3 who, in addition, are severely mentally defective and leading a 'vegetable' existence.

It may be added that these different classes denote different degrees of living as human beings, but we must take care not to project our own feelings into these problems. There is considerable danger that in assessing the quality of outcome, we attempt to make judgements about the quality of life, a judgement which is virtually impossible [29]. It must also be added that it is often difficult, even impossible, to predict at birth the class to which a particular infant belongs – it is easiest in classes 1 and 5. No surgeon in the western world would be likely to withhold operation on another wise normal, full-term infant with oesophageal atresia, regardless of the family and social background, although we are all aware of the fact that even such a child may cause the gravest complications in a labile family situation or in bad social surroundings. However, in such a situation we suddenly realize that we cannot look into the future. Conversely nobody in his senses would operate upon a newborn with an urgent surgical condition as well as anencephaly, although even anencephalic children may occasionally live for months or even years.

When it comes to classes 2 to 4, in many children the exact degree of future physical or mental disability is impossible to foretell. To cite two examples: first, there is the ever-recurring difficulty with Down's syndrome children, where mental defect may vary from very slight to very severe and where we have as yet no reliable method of predicting the degree of involvement at birth; second there is the child with meconium ileus. The majority of these children will grow up suffering from cystic fibrosis, but here too the severity of the condition may vary considerably. Even more important is the fact that a small minority will show no evidence of cystic fibrosis in later life for, as yet, unexplained reasons.

The problem of antenatal prediction

Recent advances in the diagnosis of some malformations by amniocentesis, maternal blood investigations and maternal ultrasound screening and the resulting selective abortions have raised new problems which, although they usually do not concern the paediatric surgeon directly, should be discussed briefly.

Maternal blood and amniocentesis examination of alpha-fetoprotein can detect anencephaly and open myelomeningocele [11]. Cytological investigation of the amniotic fluid can establish the diagnosis of Down's syndrome and other chromosomal abnormalities. Ultrasound screening now enables us to discover an ever increasing number of fetal abnormalities. If it is accepted that some of the fetal malformations provide moral and legal reasons for killing the fetus by abortion, it may well be argued that similar considerations should pertain to the treatment of neonates with the same malformations. In this connection the question of whether the child is different because he still is connected to the mother by an umbilical cord seems somewhat artificial. Consideration of the size and gestational age of the fetus is certainly not pertinent, as modern neonatal surgery has increasingly concerned itself with the management of smaller and smaller infants and a whole new science has sprung up dealing with the management of surgical neonates below 1500 g and even below 1000 g [13]. If we accept abortion because of a malformation in a fetus weighing 1000 g, we seem to suffer from some sort of schizophrenia when operating on a child of similar weight and with a similar condition after birth. Certainly abortions for malformations of the fetus do not eliminate the feelings of guilt in at least some of the parents. It is quite possible, as Fletcher [6] has suggested, that the feedback from amniocentesis may be more negative than positive where defective children are concerned.

The problem of operation

The first question which needs answering is whether we are justified in operating on any of these infants. Most, if not all, will agree that every conscientious doctor will try to effect a cure as long as there is a reasonable hope of doing so, and will try to preserve life as long as the patient himself can reap any tangible benefit from the prolongation of his life. If these criteria are accepted, then all infants should theoretically be operated upon, because however badly handicapped the child and however much social and economic factors will make subsequent progress doubtful and risky, it is at least theoretically not impossible that the patient will derive some benefit from the operation. Furthermore, although operation in classes 3, 4 and 5 will not produce a normal child, it often prevents unnecessary painful or debilitating complications.

In practice, however, two difficulties will be encountered: One is the term 'quality of human life' and what it really means. Reading through the relevant literature it appears to mean widely different things to various people. At one end of the spectrum we have the traditional Catholic and Protestant fundamentalistic view that all types of human life are valuable and sacrosanct [24]; at the other end there is the notion that a severely defective human infant may be inferior to a non-human animal, such as a dog or a pig [28]. To many an intermediate definition would be preferable, but this is a highly personal matter and each surgeon will finally have to decide which sort of life should be preserved and which should not. Care must be taken, however, not to succumb to outside familial and social influences and to give them too much weight when deciding on the child's future, because we cannot see into the future and, at least theoretically, extraneous conditions can be changed. There is also a great danger that in attempting to judge the future quality of life of an infant, medical attendants will invariably project their own feelings on to their patients. For many adults, life with a severe mental or physical handicap would be so burdensome as to offer no benefits. This reflection is, however, based on the adult's existing hopes and aspirations and does not take account of the feelings of the infant who grows up with such a handicap, who never knew anything else and may with help still lead a more or less useful and happy existence without undue frustrations [19]. People who have little experience with the upbringing and training of handicapped infants will find evaluation of their future hopes and happiness extremely difficult. It has been suggested that the assessment of 'quality of life' of an infant should be based on his 'potential for human relationship' [16]. This sounds very good, but in the case of a newborn infant there must always be some doubt as to whether this potential for human relationship exists [9]. Furthermore, there is little doubt that even children with a severe mental handicap can have feelings of happiness, fear, gratitude and love and that caring for them can be a rewarding occupation [12].

The second difficulty arises in connection with Pope Pius XII's attempt to solve the problem by distinguishing between 'ordinary' and 'extraordinary' means of preserving life. These terms are highly relative to time, locale and the circumstances of the patient [18]. 'Ordinary' methods of preserving life would in this context mean treatment which in that particular locality is standard treatment carried out with a reasonable degree of success, which can be done without affecting too deeply the interests and wellbeing of other members of the community and for which there exists a possibility, either actual or potential, of satisfactory aftercare. To carry out a complicated operation on a newborn infant in a developing country where it would be absolutely impossible to give him the prolonged aftercare he may need and where the undue expenditure of highly specialized medical and nursing care could be better used to save the lives of numerous infants suffering from comparatively simple and easily curable complaints is 'extraordinary' and problematic.

Only the doctor actually concerned with the treatment of the infant can be the judge of whether the necessary operation can be classified as 'ordinary' or 'extraordinary' treatment and it is obvious that every case has to be judged on its own merits. The operation must be viewed in its setting of medical care in general and, more specifically, in its setting of medical care for infants at this particular time and in this particular place. Some may argue that even in the highly industrialized and rich countries of western Europe and North America the money and staff devoted to this type of surgery should be directed to other spheres of comparatively simpler medical care, but before designating an operation as 'extraordinary' on these grounds it would have to be shown clearly that other types of medical care are being neglected and that other patients would greatly benefit if this particular operation were not carried out. Strictly speaking we are not dealing here with moral standards or ethics but with deontology, the science of duty (after the Greek 'deón' or 'what must be done'). Whilst moral standards are more or less consistent, deontology differs from locality to locality [8].

It must also be added that assessment of the good effect of neonatal operations cannot simply be a matter of counting the numbers of useful lives saved, as the perfection of this type of surgery must advance the mastery of paediatric care. This does not imply that so-called hopeless cases should be subjected to experimental surgery. Surgery should never be advised unless it gives us at least a modicum of hope that it may be successful and of benefit to the patient.

An argument that is sometimes raised by those worried about eugenics is that operation on these infants is wrong because many malformations are genetically determined. However, few of these malformations are unequivocally recessive diseases. Even in recessive diseases, in which most of the abnormal genes are latent in the population, if treatment was universally effective and if all cured patients subsequently beget children, it would only increase the gene frequency per generation by the square root of the number of abnormal gene carriers in the population. This is hardly a matter for immediate concern in neonatal surgery [4]. In this connection it is interesting to note that the incidence of pyloric stenosis, which has a genetic element in its aetiology, is apparently declining in spite of successful surgical treatment in the vast majority of patients for three generations.

The problem of selection for operation

Once it is agreed that operation on at least some of the classes outlined above is 'ordinary' medical treatment and justified and that 'extraordinary' medical treatment may also occasionally be justified for some special reasons, the question arises of how infants should be selected for operation.

In localities where it is clearly impossible to operate on all neonates and to give them adequate aftercare, a method of selection – distasteful as it will be to many medical minds – will have to be instituted. Under these circumstances it may appear reasonable to give priority to those patients who are likely to derive the greatest benefit from an operation. Although, as stated previously, every case has to be judged on its own particular merits, by and large the higher the infant can be placed in the classification outlined earlier, the greater may be his ultimate benefit. The possibility of ultimate overall success will have to be evaluated, which is extremely difficult. Social factors, for instance home conditions and parental dedication, have to be examined in the same light, but it must be freely admitted that it may be virtually impossible to come to a correct assessment of these factors. These arguments are not universally accepted. Many authorities on ethics doubt the validity of the argument that if resources are limited, the fittest must of necessity be selected for the best treatment.

It may well be that in some localities, even in the western world, provision for satisfactory aftercare (for example training and schooling of physically and/or mentally handicapped children) does not exist, but it should be within the realms of possibility to put these matters right. The aim should be to improve our social services rather than making their deficiencies the reason for refusing operation. With regard to social factors, unsatisfactory home conditions, etc., it is usually possible as a last resort to commit these children to institutional care. As in cases of child abuse, doctors as well as magistrates rightly shrink from such a step, but it may be the only solution and again in every industrialized country it should be possible to develop the quality of institutional care to a generally satisfactory level.

In the final analysis it is the population of the locality concerned who will have to decide how much of the available resources in terms of finance and manpower should be set aside for dealing with this problem. This, after all, is one of the functions of a democracy. Doctors can and should advise, but they can only work in the framework of the community in which they live.

Once again it must be emphasized that, in the opinion of the author, the patient's doctor bears the ultimate responsibility of making up his mind as to whether an operation is justified or not. He may want the advice of medical or nursing colleagues or of an ethical committee. In fact the law of the land may require it and in any case with possible future legal complications, he is well advised to do so. Finally, however, it will be his judgement, his common sense and his humanity that must decide the issue. If he does not like to accept this sort of responsibility, it would be wiser if he ceased practising neonatology or neonatal surgery.

The problem of the doctor–parent relationship

It is in this sector that most difficulties have arisen during the last dozen years. The fact that the newborn infant cannot express an opinion and that his future is so closely connected with his parents makes their views obviously of the greatest importance. It must, however, be realized that the neonate is an individual human being and does not belong to his parents like a domestic pet. Unfortunately, in the writer's opinion, many legal complications have arisen in the past because well-intentioned outsiders, be they individuals or associations, have attempted to interfere and have thereby tended to disturb the doctor–parent relationship. It is difficult to believe that all the legal complications which have arisen in the past [7,10], and which are the delight of the popular press, would have occurred had the trust between doctor and parents not been undermined.

If the parents want the infant to be operated upon and the surgeon agrees, there is no problem. If the parents want an operation however bad the prognosis (which has been carefully explained to them), some surgeons may feel that they have to comply with the parents' wishes, but some may still feel that a major operation with little hope of permanent benefit should not be carried out. This state of affairs should, however, be very rare indeed because, in practice, it is unlikely that after full explanation the parents will not agree with the surgeon. If they do not, the surgeon should insist that a second opinion is sought.

A more common and much more difficult situation is where the parents refuse permission for operation, regardless of what the surgeon advises. It may be asked why parents arrive at such a decision. Some, no doubt, are unwilling to look after a temporarily ill and/or permanently handicapped child or fear that their social surroundings are unsuitable for the upbringing of such a child. The future of the child must therefore be carefully explained, care being taken to point out all the help that the authorities of the locality can provide. In order to do so, the surgeon must either acquaint himself with these facilities or enlist the help of an expert in such matters, such as a social worker in this field.

Very few parents are unwilling to give permission for operation because of doctrinal reasons. In such cases there exist legal possibilities in most western countries allowing for the child to be placed under the temporary jurisdiction of the local authority [20].

In a surprisingly large percentage of cases the parents' refusal of permission for operation is based on gross misinformation which they may have received prior to talking to the surgeon. This misinformation may have come from a lay person, often an elderly relative, but it frequently comes from another doctor, be it the family doctor, the obstetrician or a geneticist. Undoubtedly these doctors try their best to help the family involved but unfortunately their factual knowledge is insufficient or more correctly not up to date. The writer has had many experiences of doctors quoting to him some piece of book knowledge which was totally out of date and related to a quite different locality. Many of these self-appointed experts have no idea about the results which are routinely obtained in the hospital involved. If the surgeon meets this state of affairs, he should not only ask for a second expert opinion but insist on discussing the matter in the presence of the parents with the person who gave the first negative opinion.

In some cases the decision not to operate does not mean that the child will die immediately, as the parents often believe. This must therefore be explained to them as must be the fact that the death may be far from pleasant. Should the child survive, his condition will usually deteriorate and any chance of improvement by surgery may then be lost. The surgeon's attitude will to a certain extent depend on the infant's medical category outlined above. The lower the category, the more ready the surgeon may be to comply with the parents' wishes, bearing in mind that the parents' rejection of the infant might greatly decrease his chances of satisfactory rehabilitation and might thus change an otherwise 'ordinary' means of treatment to an 'extraordinary' one.

Although privately the surgeon may not agree with the parents, he should attempt to make their decision officially his own in the hope of alleviating their possible future feelings of guilt [27]. In every case, however, the surgeon should discuss the whole issue not only with another experienced surgeon but also with his juniors and the nurses on the ward concerned. Not only is it absolutely essential that all involved in the management of the infant agree amongst themselves and express the same opinion to the parents, but it must always be remembered that it is the junior doctors and the nursing staff who will bear the brunt of looking after the child and who are in constant contact with the parents. Many of the spectacular law suits in recent years would probably not have taken place had this precaution been observed.

In some cases where permission for operation is refused, the surgeon may be convinced in his own mind that the operation should be carried out and that even under unfavourable external conditions the ultimate prognosis will be reasonably good. In former editions of this book the writer held the opinion that if, in spite of the surgeon's explanation, the parents persisted in what seemed to be an unreasonable attitude, one's moral duty was to operate without consent. Although this action possibly did not conform with the law of the land, it was believed that nobody would prosecute a doctor because he had attempted to save the life of a child who had a reasonable chance of leading a relatively normal existence later on. Subsequent developments have proved this to be wrong. A surgeon behaving like this might risk the most severe legal proceedings. Present conditions would demand from the surgeon that he enlists the help of colleagues, ethical committees, local authorities and judiciary in an attempt to convince the parents, or even to override their wishes, with all the delays and unfortunate publicity that this would involve. Personally I think that this solution is a bad one as has been frequently shown by events reported in the press.

In the vast majority of cases the parents will not demand or refuse an operation outright but will seek guidance from the surgeon. It must be remembered that the mother is recovering from the after-effects of labour and is often not in an emotionally fit state to make a grave decision of this kind, so that the responsibility lies mainly with the father. Every conscientious doctor will, of course, give as correct a prognosis and as impartial an opinion about the possible future of the child as he can, but he will not be able to be wholly impartial and, whether he wants it or not, his opinion will influence the parents to a remarkable degree. As was said earlier, in the final analysis it is usually the surgeon who has to decide the issue in his own mind and it is quite wrong to try to shift the responsibility by asking the parents to decide. It is not only cruel to ask parents whether they want their child to live or die, it is dishonest because in many cases the parents are consciously or unconsciously influenced by the surgeon's opinion.

In recent years there has been a marked move to shift the responsibility for these decisions from the surgeon's shoulders to those of a so-called ethical committee [13]. Although we live in times of 'team management', the author is somewhat doubtful about this development. An ethical committee for cases such as these must be composed at least of a neonatologist, geneticist, neonatal surgeon, psychiatrist and intensive-care nurse. If possible, a paediatrician working outside the hospital, a lawyer, a clergyman, a social worker and a lay person should also belong to this committee. Such a team is very large and unwieldy; it is difficult to convene and much valuable time will be lost before even some of the members can get together. Moreover, the very large number of members carries the danger of such a committee turning into a debating society. Finally, it usually falls to the surgeon to carry out the committee's decision, if any. 'Many have noticed that diffusion of responsibility often acts to make no one feel responsible' [31]. Having worked in a hospital where an ethical committee has been in existence since 1971, the author is not convinced that it has done much to help in these difficult decisions although it is of course of value as legal protection.

Problems of management if operation is not carried out

If, for one reason or another, operation is not carried out and if the infant does not succumb immediately, the problems associated with the management of these patients are very great indeed.

Although the care of such a child is primarily the parents' moral responsibility, it is often cruel to return him to his home, especially when there are other children in the family. It is usually possible to keep him in hospital for a limited period of time, but finally the question of institutional care will arise, unless of course the parents express the wish to look after the child themselves. Unfortunately there are very few cots available for nursing these hopeless cases, and the emotional stress that these infants cause is very great, not only to their families but also to the medical and nursing personnel looking after them.

If it is agreed that these patients should not be killed, they have to be given proper treatment, including all natural means of preserving life (food and drink, etc.), good nursing care and appropriate measures to relieve distress and pain. These basic nursing methods have been called 'minimal means' by some authorities, implying that they must always be used irrespective of the condition of the patient [21]. The doctor will have to decide in his own mind whether the provision of artificial life-sustainers, such as antibiotics in cases of intercurrent infection, should be withheld. It is advisable that the doctor discusses his decision with his medical colleagues and with the nursing staff involved and possibly an ethical committee. The writer is of the opinion that usually the doctor has no moral obligation to use antibiotics provided he explains his reasons in detail to the parents and the other medical and nursing staff. As always, every case has to be treated individually; it seems impossible to lay down rules of behaviour in these instances.

It is in connection with these cases that the possibility of euthanasia has to be discussed. This question has been debated extensively during recent years [1,5]. This issue tends to raise immediately all kinds of emotional, moral and religious objections. There has been the widest discussion of this subject in parliaments, in the mass media and amongst the judiciary all over the world and it must be realized that active killing of a patient, such as by giving him poisonous overdoses of drugs – although secretly widely practised – is still a criminal offence in most civilized countries. If the doctor concerned is willing to kill the child in question and if society condones this, it is his responsibility and on his conscience alone, but he must not involve others. Killing these children by starving them to death or by giving them unsuitable feeds or prescribing overdoses of drugs, shifts the responsibility for the actual execution to the junior medical or nursing staff and this is quite indefensible. Furthermore, the fine differences now often made between 'active' killing and killing by omission are at best very doubtful.

Conclusion

An attempt has been made to deal briefly with this difficult subject in as practical a manner as possible. It is realized that the surgeon who hopes to find cut-and-dried rules for the ethical basis of the management of these children will be disappointed. The writer is of the opinion that those who try to produce such dogmatic rules, be they philosophers, religious

functionaries or lawyers, are in danger of at least sometimes promoting injustice. In 1984 the Surgeon General of the United States, a paediatric surgeon of distinction, in a lecture to the Medical College of Wisconsin stated that 'no answer' to these questions is unacceptable. Whilst one sympathizes with this view, it must be added that these problems depend on many individual factors and are such a personal matter between the surgeon and his patient and the parents that definite answers on hypothetical questions can often not be given. Moral pluralism is characteristic of our democratic society and we therefore have to accept widely different views and still come to terms with each other and live amicably together. It all depends on our view of how such a society should work and which values should be looked for. In this connection one can do no better than to quote the view expressed to us ten years ago by Fr K.T. Kelly, Professor of Moral Theology, who was one of the original members of our working party discussing the issues described in the first edition of this volume:

'I would think that a good indication of the moral calibre of a society is the amount of attention and care it gives to its sick, especially those who have nothing to contribute directly to society, the aged, the mentally ill, the severely handicapped and the very young. As long as man's dignity is not based simply on his usefulness to society, this must hold true.'

References

1. Downing, A.B. (1969) *Euthanasia and the Right to Death*, Peter Owen, London
2. Du Chaillu, quoted by Ballantyne, J.W. (1902) *Manual of Antenatal Pathology and Hygiene*, William Green and Sons, Edinburgh
3. Duff, R.S. and Campbell, A.G. (1973) Moral and ethical dilemmas in special-care nursery. *New Engl. J. Med.*, **289**, 890–894
4. Edwards, J.H. (1965) The application of knowledge. *Birth Defects*, **1**, 75
5. Eibach, V. (1974) *Recht auf Leben – Recht auf Sterben*, Theologischer Verlag Brockhaus, Wuppertal
6. Fletcher, J. (1974) Attitudes towards defective newborns. *Studies*, **2**, 37
7. Gillon, R. (1985) An introduction to philosophical medical ethics: the Arthur case. *Br. Med. J.*, **290**, 1117–1119
8. Hamburger, J. (1966) In *Ethics and Medical Progress* (ed. G.E.W. Wolstenholme and M. O'Connor), Churchill, London
9. Hellegers, A. (1974) Relating is the criterion for life. *Obstet. Gynec. News*, Oct. 15
10. Johnson, D.E. and Thompson, T.R. (1984) The 'baby Doe' rule: is it all bad? *Pediatrics*, **73**, 729–730

11. Laurence, K.M. (1974) Clinical and ethical considerations of alpha-fetoprotein estimation for early prenatal diagnosis of neural tube malformations. *Dev. Med. child. Neurol.*, **16**, (Suppl. 32), 117–121
12. Leuenberger, A. (1975) Personal communication
13. Lister, J. (1984) Lecture to the Scandinavian Paediatric Surgical Association
14. Lorber, J. (1971) Results of treatment of myelomeningocele. *Dev. Med. Child. Neurol.*, **13**, 279–288
15. Lorber, J. (1972) Spina bifida cystica. *Arch. Dis. Child.*, **47**, 854–873
16. Lowe, J.F. (1966) Abortion Law Reform. *Ampleforth J.* 174
17. McCormick, R.A. (1974) To save or let die. *J. Am. Med. Ass.*, **229**, 172–176
18. McCormick, R.A. (1975) Theological studies. *Studies*, **3**, 121
19. Metzler, K.M. (1976) Human and handicapped. In *Moral Problems in Medicine* (ed. S. Gorrovitz) Prentice Hall, New Jersey p. 358
20. *Ministry of Health Circular No. CMO 23/66* (1968) Refusal of parental consent to a life-saving blood transfusion or operation for a child
21. O'Donnell, T.J. (1974) Medical morals. *Newsletter*, **11**, 5
22. Pius XII (1954) *Discori al Medici*, Orissorte Medico, Rome
23. Puri, P. (1985) *Surgery and Support of the Premature Infant*. Karger, New York
24. Report of a working party of the Linacre Centre (1982) *Euthanasia and Clinical Practice*, The Linacre Centre, London
25. Rickham, P.P. (1960) Vesico-intestinal fissure. *Arch. Dis. Child.*, **35**, 97–102
26. Rickham, P.P., Stauffer, U.G. and Cheng, S.K. (1977) Oesophageal atresia: triumph and tragedy. *Aust. N. Z. Surg.*, **47**, 138–143
27. Ringeling, H. (1975) Kriterien und Maximen für die genetischen Leidensindikationen. *Gesellschaft und Entwicklung*, **2**, 36
28. Singer, P. (1983) Sanctity of life or quality of life? *Pediatrics*, **72**, 128–129
29. Smith, D.H. (1974) On letting some babies die. *Studies*, **2**, 37
30. Wegman, M.E. (1981) Annual summary of vital statistics – 1980. *Pediatrics*, **68**, 755–762
31. Zachary, R.B. (1981) Commentary. Stinson, R. and Stinson, P. (1981) On the death of a baby. *J. Med. Ethics*, **7**, 5–18

2

Incidence and causation of congenital defects

J.R. Owens

Introduction

To all intents and purposes neonatal surgery is the surgery of congenital malformations. It is therefore important for paediatric surgeons to know something about the frequency of malformations, their aetiology, and the risk of the same defect occurring in subsequent pregnancies. During this century congenital malformations have gradually increased in importance as a cause of perinatal and neonatal mortality. This is not because malformations have increased in frequency but because other causes of infant death such as infection, poor nutrition and birth asphyxia have been controlled. Thus, in 1920 approximately 1 in 30 infant deaths were due to a malformation, whereas now about 1 in 4 are [18].

A *congenital anomaly* is defined as any departure from normality, whether structural, chemical or functional. A *congenital malformation* is a structural abnormality. It will be obvious that all congenital malformations are also anomalies but that the reverse is not true. In this chapter we shall be examining three aspects. Firstly, the frequency of some of the malformations of interest to the paediatric surgeon; secondly, their aetiology and causation; and lastly, what can be done to prevent their occurrence or recurrence.

Birth prevalence

The *incidence* of a disease is the number of new cases per unit time per unit population (usually annual cases per 1000). The *prevalence* is the number of cases of a disease at any one time per unit population (usually per 1000). Prevalence will be influenced by the mortality of the particular disease studied. The frequency of congenital malformations at birth has commonly been termed incidence. However, the true incidence of a malformation, i.e. the number of new cases, is theoretically the number of malformed conceptions. By the time of birth this number will have diminished considerably because of spontaneous and therapeutic abortions. It is therefore more correct to talk of *birth prevalence*, and this term will be used in the discussion that follows.

Two to three per cent of all babies are born with a major malformation. The eight conditions listed in Table 2.1 make up about 60% of the total. Surgery

Table 2.1 Most common congenital malformations

Neural tube defect
Facial clefts
Down's syndrome
Clubfoot
Congenital dislocation of the hip
Ventricular septal defects
Hypospadias
Polydactyly/syndactyly

will be required for most of these defects. The body system most commonly affected by malformations is the cardiovascular system with a birth prevalence of 5–7 per 1000. The neonatal surgeon has a special interest in malformations of the gastrointestinal and genitourinary systems. Birth prevalences for some of the conditions are given in Table 2.2. The epidemiology of a few of the most important malformations is given below.

Table 2.2 Birth prevalence of some surgical malformations, Liverpool and environs, 1979–83 (per 1000 live and still births)[a]

Oesophageal atresia	0.27
Duodenal stenosis	0.11
Jejunal atresia	0.03
Ileal atresia	0.01
Hirschsprung's disease	0.06
Anorectal atresia	0.36
Diaphragmatic hernia	0.22
Exomphalos	0.26
Gastroschisis	0.10
Hydronephrosis	0.12
Ectopia vesicae	0.05
Urethral valves	0.01

*There were 101 816 total births over this time in the geographical area under surveillance

Neural tube defects (NTD)

These include anencephalus, spina bifida, and encephalocele. There has been a dramatic fall in birth prevalence in NTD over the last ten years (Figure 2.1). Although this has been partly due to prenatal screening and selective abortion there must be other factors as well because, when one adds on the number of abortions to the number going to term, the frequency of NTD is still seen to be falling [20]. It is not clear what this factor is. However, the birth prevalence of NTD has risen and fallen before

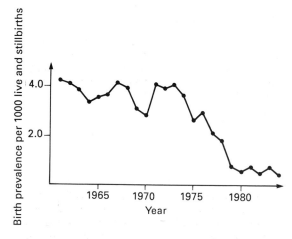

Figure 2.1 Birth prevalence of spina bifida per 1000 live and stillbirths, Liverpool and environs 1961–84. (Figures for 1961–78 are for Liverpool and Bootle, and for 1979–84 are for the health districts of Liverpool St Helens and Knowsley, Southport and Formby, South Sefton and Wirral)

over the last century with an epidemic in the 1930s [7] and this may be a recurring cycle. At present the birth prevalence of spina bifida and encephalocele is about 1.0 per 1000 live and stillbirths in Liverpool and its environs. Because of this low frequency and the trend towards conservative management of babies born with NTD these conditions will be dealt with by the neonatal surgeon considerably less frequently than when this textbook was last published.

Down's syndrome

Down's syndrome is of interest to the paediatric surgeon because of its commonly associated gastro-intestinal malformations, particularly duodenal obstruction which occurs in 8% of cases. In Liverpool there has been a gradual decrease in birth prevalence over the last 25 years [21] to reach a basal level which has remained fairly constant recently. This decrease is thought to be due to the decline in the proportion of mothers over 35 years old who are having babies. Antenatal screening of older mothers by amniocentesis and selective abortion has very little effect on the overall birth prevalence of Down's syndrome.

Facial clefts

The birth prevalence of 'pure' facial clefts (i.e. associated with no more than one other malformation in a different body system) shows no consistent trends with time, although there are occasional peaks and troughs [22]. Approximately 1.5 per 1000 live births are born with a facial cleft, about one-third of this number having cleft lip alone, one-third cleft lip and palate and one-third cleft palate alone. It is likely that cleft lip, with or without cleft palate, has a different aetiology from isolated cleft palate. For instance, the male:female ratio in the former is about 2:1, whereas in the latter it is slightly more common in females. In spite of this, the peaks and troughs in birth prevalence of the two conditions tend to follow each other.

Hypospadias

Hypospadias is a common congenital malformation, although 85% of cases are the minor glandular or coronal forms. Over the last 10–15 years increases in birth prevalence have been reported from the UK [13], Europe [3], Sweden [9], and the USA [29].

In Liverpool there are now between 2.5 and 3.0 cases of hypospadias per 1000 live births. Imbalance in sex hormones during pregnancy is thought to be the most likely cause. Therapeutic progestins given in early pregnancy for threatened abortion, hormonal pregnancy tests, and continuation of oral contraceptives into early pregnancy have all been suggested as possible reasons for the observed increase in birth prevalence [1]. Another possible cause is greater ascertainment of milder cases.

Gastrointestinal malformations (see Table 2.2)

Diaphragmatic hernia showed a rise in birth prevalence in the 1970s according to OPCS data for England and Wales [19]. Although increased paediatric skill in recognizing this condition is a possible reason for this rise the rates for oesophageal atresia/tracheo-oesophageal fistula, another condition difficult to diagnose, have remained fairly constant over the same period. On the other hand, exomphalos began to decrease in birth prevalence in the late 1970s; it has been suggested that this might be due to increased prenatal diagnosis by alpha-fetoprotein screening leading to therapeutic abortion [19]. The rates for rectal and anal atresia and stenosis did not show any significant change over the 1970s. Alimentary malformations appear to be especially common in Indians [28].

Aetiology (see Table 2.3)

Genetic

Although genetic defects are individually rare about 7.5% of all malformations have a monogenic basis. The commonest autosomal recessive condition in Caucasians is cystic fibrosis, with a birth prevalence of about 0.6 per 1000 in the UK [24]. About 1 in 20 individuals carry the abnormal gene. Cystic fibrosis is of importance to the paediatric surgeon mainly because 6–25% of cases present at birth with

Table 2.3 Aetiology of congenital malformations [10]

	(%)
Genetic	7.5
Chromosomal	6
Environmental	5
Genetic/environmental interaction	20
Unknown	>60

meconium ileus. However, meconium ileus equivalent, rectal prolapse, intussusception and bleeding oesophageal varices will also require surgical involvement. Recently, the abnormal gene responsible for the clinical effects has been located on the long arm of chromosome 7. Genetic markers have been discovered which will aid in the prenatal diagnosis of this handicapping condition (see below) [30].

Chromosomal

About 6% of malformations are caused by chromosomal anomalies. Down's syndrome is the commonest of these. In the European Congenital Malformations Registry for 1980–83 the birth prevalence for all chromosomal anomalies was just under 2 per 1000 [5]. However, conditions such as Turner's and Klinefelter's syndromes may not be recognized for some time after birth. The prevalence of chromosomal defects in aborted fetuses of 5–12 weeks' gestation is about ten times the rate in full-term babies [32].

The commonest chromosomal abnormalities are due to non-disjunction. This is the failure of one or more pairs of homologous chromosomes to separate during cell division. Trisomy results when a gamete which has received both of a set of homologous chromosomes fuses with a haploid gamete from the other parent. Monosomy is due to the fusion of a gamete containing neither homologous chromosome and a haploid gamete from the other parent. In some individuals two or more cell lines are present (mosaicism). Breaks in chromatids during meiosis are quite common but usually correct themselves. If persistent, the detached piece of chromosomal material may be lost (deletion) or fuse with part of a non-homologous chromosome (translocation). Just over 90% of cases of Down's syndrome are due to trisomy of chromosome 21 secondary to non-disjunction [21]. The latter increases in frequency after a maternal age of 35 years and explains the greater risk of chromosomal anomaly in this group. About 5% of Down's syndrome are due to translocation of material from chromosome 21; the remaining 1% are mosaics.

Discrete environmental causes

Although this group only makes up about 5% of all causes of malformations [10] it is in many ways the most important as the causative factors should be amenable to change leading to prevention. The group falls under two main headings:

1. Maternal infections and other illnesses.
2. Drugs and environmental teratogens.

Maternal illness

Cytomegalovirus, rubella and toxoplasmosis unquestionably cause congenital malformations. However, the evidence that other infections, such as herpes simplex and herpes zoster, are teratogenic is more circumstantial. Cytomegalovirus is the commonest cause of congenital infection in the UK with a prevalence of 3 per 1000 [23]. Fortunately, less than one-tenth of this number have a major handicap at birth although a proportion will develop deafness in the first year or two of life. Congenital rubella was first recognized in Australia in the early 1940s. Its effects are widespread, with congenital heart disease, cataracts, deafness and mental retardation as frequent manifestations. In the USA, where both sexes are immunized against rubella as children, the birth prevalence had fallen to 1.33 per 100 000 live births in the years 1970–80 [17]. In the UK there has been no such change [2].

Maternal insulin-dependent diabetes increases the risks of congenital malformations about threefold [31]. Congenital heart disease, neural tube defects and sacrofemoral agenesis are over-represented. There is increasing evidence that the better the control of blood sugar in early pregnancy the less the risk of malformations [15].

Dietary control in phenylketonuria is essential in the early years of extrauterine life, but can subsequently be relaxed. However, the diet must be resumed during pregnancy as there is an increased risk of microcephaly, congenital heart disease and mental retardation. Other maternal conditions associated with malformations include iodine deficiency and virilizing tumours.

Drugs and other teratogens

Organic mercury is the only environmental substance for which there is indisputable evidence of an effect on prenatal development [10]. Outbreaks of disease have occurred in Japan caused by eating contaminated fish or shellfish (Minamata disease) and in Iraq after ingestion of bread produced from contaminated grain. Non-specific neurological effects on the exposed infant have been described.

Maternal smoking does not appear to be teratogenic. As regards alcohol the evidence is conflicting. A specific fetal alcohol syndrome has been described, although there has been discussion as to whether this constitutes a separate entity [27]. The features of this syndrome include failure to thrive in spite of adequate calorific intake, microcephaly, narrow palpebral fissures, midfacial hypoplasia, thin upper vermilion border and developmental delay. Mothers who take the equivalent of more than 80 g of absolute alcohol per day are at risk of producing an affected infant.

In spite of all the publicity regarding drug teratogenicity since the thalidomide disaster of the early 1960s, drug prescription during pregnancy has increased gradually over the years [4]. Fortunately thalidomide has so far proved unique in its capacity to produce major birth defects. Female sex hormones can cause masculinization of female external genitalia. Cytotoxics such as aminopterin (which is a folate antagonist) can cause malformations. Warfarin given in the first trimester can cause hypoplasia of the nasal skeleton, epiphyseal stippling, hypoplasia of the skeleton and eye abnormalities. Anticonvulsants, particularly phenytoin, may increase the

risk of malformations two or threefold [14]. Congenital heart disease, facial clefts, nail and digital hypoplasia, abnormal midfacial characteristics, and microcephaly have been described. The role of anticonvulsants in teratogenesis is not a straightforward one, however, as it appears that patients with epilepsy are at a higher risk than the general population of having certain malformations themselves [8]. Sodium valproate taken in pregnancy has been associated with a possible increase in spina bifida in France [25].

Interaction of genes and environment

Whilst a proportion of malformations have their origin in single gene or chromosome defects on the one hand and a specific environmental effect on the other, in the majority a combination of inheritance and intrauterine nurture gives rise to an abnormality. Neural tube defects and facial clefting are good examples of malformations where this interaction occurs, environmental influences being more prominent in the former, genetic ones in the latter [11].

There are some racial differences in the birth prevalence of neural tube defect, this malformation being less common in Negroes and Mongoloids than it is in Caucasoids. A map of the birth prevalence of neural tube defects in the UK shows a gradual increase as one moves northwards and westwards from the south-east. This may be partly due to racial differences (the Celts versus the Anglo-Saxons) but the greater mobility and mixing of racial subgroups these days makes environmental influences a more likely reason for these geographical variations. Interestingly, the Irish American population has a lower birth prevalence of neural tube defects than the Irish in Ireland but a higher one than their other American neighbours [16].

Two other epidemiological factors associated with neural tube defects suggest environmental factors are active. Firstly, the birth prevalence of anencephaly and spina bifida increases as one descends the socioeconomic scale. This might be explained by some nutritional factor which is lacking in the diets of poorer mothers. Secondly, births of babies with neural tube defects show a seasonal trend with a winter excess. Climate, diet or infections are all possible causes of this pattern.

Facial clefting is a little more complex as it appears that the aetiology of cleft lip (CL) with or without cleft palate (P) (CL ±P) differs from that of solitary cleft palate (CP). There is some geographical variation in the birth prevalence of CL±P but it seems that this is mostly due to ethnic differences [11]. Thus the condition is commonest among Mongoloids and least common amongst Negroids – Caucasoids are somewhere in between. Ethnic differences show no consistent trends in CP. Some studies have shown seasonal trends in facial clefts but most have not. There is no effect of social class. Several studies have shown an association with anticonvulsant medication. On the other hand, family studies have shown a very strong genetic aetiology, CL±P and CP being inherited separately.

Unknown

Unfortunately the aetiology of the majority of congenital malformations is unknown. For most the teratogenic insult will have occurred in the first trimester of pregnancy. However, this is not always the case. For instance, congenital jejunoileal atresia, which is rarely associated with other malformations, is probably due to impairment of the blood supply to the fetal intestine some time after embryogenesis [12]. Congenital clubfoot may be secondary to intrauterine pressure effects after the first trimester [6]. Thus the study of the causation of malformations is a highly complex one.

Prevention of malformations

Control of genetic disease

Most regional health authorities now have a department of clinical genetics where advice about recurrence risks can be given to parents whose child has been born with a malformation. If the condition is due to a single gene defect the risk factor is straightforward. If the malformation is due to a chromosomal anomaly parental chromosomal analysis is essential in order to predict the chance of future offspring being affected. Empirical risks are known for malformations of more complex aetiology, e.g. the recurrence risk for neural tube defects in an area of high prevalence is in the order of 5%. There must, of course, be no pressure brought to bear on the parents as to whether or not they should go ahead with further pregnancies. The job of the genetic counsellor is to explain in a clear and simple way the risks of bearing a similarly affected child.

Nowadays, an increasing number of malformations can be diagnosed *in utero* early enough for the pregnancy to be terminated. Before prenatal diagnosis is attempted it must be ascertained whether or not the parents are willing to agree to an abortion if an affected fetus is discovered. A significant minority will object to this on ethical or religious grounds and prenatal diagnosis will cause them avoidable anxiety. Techniques used in prenatal diagnosis include amniocentesis, ultrasound, fetoscopy and chorionic villus biopsy [17].

Amniocentesis has been used for more than 50 years but has only been used for *in utero* diagnosis for just over a decade. Amniotic fluid analysis on both the supernatant and cells is performed. The fluid is examined in the diagnosis of neural tube defects as well as certain enzyme deficiencies. Examination of the cells yields information on chromosomal anomalies, enzyme deficiencies and some inherited haemolytic anaemias. In the best units there is an increased spontaneous abortion rate of well under 1%. The main disadvantage of amniocentesis is that it cannot be performed until 16 weeks' gestation, so that subsequent termination of the pregnancy at a late stage carries increased risks of physical and emotional trauma for the mother.

Ultrasound examination can be used in prenatal diagnosis in one of three ways. Some defects, such as encephalocele, can be seen directly. Disproportionate growth of a particular fetal part, e.g. the limbs in achondroplasia, can be demonstrated. Finally, one can sometimes see the effect of the anomaly on other structures, e.g. the dilated urinary tract in posterior urethral valves. A large number of malformations can be diagnosed before 26 weeks' gestation.

Chorionic villus biopsy is a very promising technique, one of its advantages being that it can be performed between 8–11 weeks' gestation. It is too early to be sure, but the risk of spontaneous abortion seems to be low.

Control of maternal disease

Rubella is a well-defined cause of congenital malformations and is readily preventable by immunization. Thus, it is a great pity that the vaccination programme in the UK has had such a poor uptake. Unfortunately, there is no vaccine against cytomegalovirus or toxoplasma. Mothers who suffer from insulin-dependent diabetes should be monitored closely during pregnancy as fetal outcome is dependent on adequacy of blood sugar control. Unfortunately embryogenesis is complete by the time of antenatal booking. It is thus important that the diabetic physician encourages his female patients of childbearing age to inform him when they plan to start a family so that blood sugar surveillance can be stepped up.

Control of environmental hazards and drugs

So little is known of the effect of environmental toxins on the developing human embryo that it is difficult to suggest any preventive measures. Alcohol abuse is theoretically preventable but extremely resistant to treatment in practice. Education of children in the dangers of excess alcohol intake is important here. Testing of drugs for teratogenicity in experimental animals has been of very limited value in predicting their effects on the developing human embryo. The best advice to pregnant women is that they should not take any drug, particularly in the first trimester, unless absolutely necessary.

Periconceptional vitamin therapy

Prenatal diagnosis has had the greatest impact of all these preventive measures on lowering the birth prevalence of malformations. However, no-one would consider the killing of an affected fetus an ideal method of 'prevention'. Recently a multicentre trial has demonstrated that if a multivitamin preparation is taken periconceptionally by mothers who have previously given birth to a baby with a neural tube defect the recurrence risk is significantly reduced [26]. An MRC study is currently being conducted to confirm or refute this. If confirmed, this will be a great advance in the prevention of a common, serious and incapacitating condition.

Conclusion

Two to three per cent of births give rise to babies with congenital malformations. Many of these defects will be of interest to the paediatric surgeon. For the majority of malformations the cause is unknown. Further advances in aetiology will require the combined resources of the paediatrician, paediatric surgeon, epidemiologist, embryologist and experimental teratologist, as well as the parents of these unfortunate children.

References

 1. Aarskog, D. (1979) Current concepts: hypospadias. *New Engl. J. Med.*, **300**, 75–78
 2. Banatvala, J.E. (1982) Rubella vaccination: remaining problems. *Br. Med. J.*, **284**, 1285–1286
 3. Czeizel, A. (1985) Increasing trends in congenital malformations of male external genitalia. *Lancet*, **i**, 462–463
 4. David, T.J. (1983) Pathogenesis of congenital malformations. In *Perinatal Medicine* (eds R. Boyd and F.C. Battaglia) Butterworths, London, pp. 264–285
 5. De Wals, P. and Lechat, M.F. (eds) (1986) *Surveillance of Congenital Anomalies Years 1980–1983*. Department of Epidemiology, Catholic University of Louvain, Brussels
 6. Dunn, P.M. (1976) Congenital postural deformities. *Br. Med. Bull.*, **32**, 71–76
 7. Elwood, J.M. and Elwood, J.H. (1980) *Secular Trends in Epidemiology of Anencephalus and Spina Bifida*. Oxford University Press, Oxford, pp. 107–119
 8. Friis, M.L., Broeng-Nielsen, B., Sindrup, E.H., Lund, M., Fogh-Andersen, P. and Hauge, M. (1981) Facial clefts among epileptic patients. *Arch. Neurol.*, **38**, 227–229
 9. Kallen, B. and Winberg, J. (1982) An epidemiological study of hypospadias in Sweden. *Acta Paediat. Scand.* (Suppl. 293), 1–21
10. Kalter, H. and Warkany, J. (1983) Congenital malformations: etiologic factors and their role in prevention. *New Engl. J. Med.*, **308**, 424–431, 491–497
11. Leck, I. (1984) Neural tube defects and oral clefts. *Br. Med. Bull.*, **40**, 390–395
12. Louw, J.H., Cywes, S., Davies, M.R.Q. and Rode, H. (1981) Congenital jejunoileal atresia: observations on its pathogenicity and treatment. *Z. Kinderchir.*, **33**, 3–17
13. Matlai, P. and Beral, V. (1985) Trends in congenital malformations of external genitalia. *Lancet*, **i**, 108
14. Meadow, S.R. (1979) Congenital malformations and seizure disorders in offspring of parents with epilepsy. *Dev. Med. Child. Neurol.*, **21**, 536–538
15. Miller, E., Hare, J.W., Cloherty, J.P. *et al.* (1981) Elevated maternal hemoglobin A_{1C} in early pregnancy and major congenital abnormalities in infants of diabetic mothers. *New Engl. J. Med.*, **304**, 1331–1334
16. Naggan, L. and MacMahon, B. (1967) Ethnic differences in the prevalence of anencephaly and spina bifida in Boston, Massachusetts. *New Engl. J. Med.*, **277**, 1119–1123
17. Nicolaides, K., Rodeck, C.H., Whitfield, C.R., McNay, M.B., Loeffler, F.E. and Smith, P.A. (1984) Prenatal diagnosis. *Br. J. Hosp. Med.*, **31**, 396–426
18. Office of Health Economics, *Birth Impairments*, London, (1978)
19. Office of Population Censuses and Surveys (1983) *Congenital Malformation Statistics 1971–80*, HMSO, London
20. Owens, J.R., Harris, F., McAllister, E. and West, L. (1981) 19-year incidence of neural tube defects in area under constant surveillance. *Lancet*, **ii**, 1032–1034
21. Owens, J.R., Harris, F., Walker, S., McAllister, E. and West, L. (1983) The incidence of Down's syndrome over a 19-year period with special reference to maternal age. *J. Med. Genet.*, **20**, 90–93
22. Owens, J.R., Jones, J.W. and Harris, F. (1985) Epidemiology of facial clefting. *Arch. Dis. Child.*, **60**, 521–524
23. Peckham, C.S., Chin, K.S., Coleman, J.C. *et al.* (1983) Cytomegalovirus infection in pregnancy: preliminary findings from a prospective study. *Lancet*, **i**, 1352–1355
24. Prosser, R. (1976) Screening for cystic fibrosis in the newborn. In *Proceedings of the VII International Cystic Fibrosis Congress*
25. Robert, E. and Guibaud, P. (1982) Maternal valproic acid and congenital neural tube defects. *Lancet*, **ii**, 937
26. Smithells, R.W., Sheppard, S., Schorah, C.J., Seller, M.J., Nevin, N.C., Harris, R., Read, A.P. and Fielding, D.W. (1981) Apparent prevention of neural tube defects by periconceptional vitamin supplementation. *Arch. Dis. Child.*, **56**, 911–918
27. Smithells, R.W. and Smith, I.J. (1984) Alcohol and the fetus. *Arch. Dis. Child.*, **59**, 1113–1114
28. Terry, P.B., Condie, R.G., Mathew, P.M. and Bissenden, J.G. (1983) Ethnic differences in the distribution of congenital malformations. *Postgrad. Med. J.*, **59**, 657–658
29. US Department of Health, Education and Welfare (1976) *Congenital Malformation Surveillance Report:*

April 1975–March 1976, DHEW Publication No. [DC] 77-8262, Center for Disease Control, Atlanta

30. Wainwright, B.J., Scambler, P.J., Schmidtke, J. *et al.* (1985) Localization of cystic fibrosis locus to human chromosome 7cen-q22, *Nature*, **318**, 384–385

31. Watkins, P.J. (1982) Congenital malformations and blood glucose control in diabetic pregnancy. *Br. Med. J.*, **284**, 1357–1358

32. Yamamoto, M. and Watanabe, G. (1979) Epidemiology of gross chromosome anomalies at the early stage of pregnancy. *Contrib. Epidemiol. Biostat.*, **1**, 101–106

3

Neonatal physiology and its effect on pre- and postoperative management

P.D. Booker and G. H. Bush

The great advances that have been made in reducing the morbidity and mortality following neonatal surgery are attributable to a number of factors. Apart from improved techniques of anaesthesia and intraoperative care, better obstetric management and the development of specialized units and improved surgical techniques, a better appreciation of neonatal physiology and the application of this knowledge have all undoubtedly played a decisive role. The newborn infant undergoing surgery has to contend not only with the problems associated with the transition from intra- to extrauterine life, but also with all the hazards consequent upon the surgical correction of the operable lesion. A thorough understanding of neonatal physiology is therefore essential so that the optimum conditions are provided to encourage extrauterine adaptation.

Adaptation to extrauterine life

Classification of newborn infants

Infants can be classified according to their weight as well as their gestational age. The estimation of gestational age from the obstetric history is often unreliable but a method of assessing gestational age based on neurological evaluation and physical characteristics has made it possible to assess the gestational age of any newborn infant irrespective of birth weight. When available, ultrasound scanning antenatally will give an accurate estimate of gestational age. Newborn infants can now be categorized as appropriate weight for the gestational age (AGA), small for gestational age (SGA) and large for gestational age (LGA). They can also be identified as preterm (less than 37 weeks' gestation), term (37–

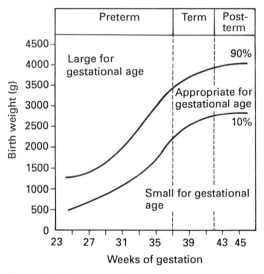

Figure 3.1 The relationship between gestational age and birth weight, showing the expected distribution curve

42 weeks' gestation) or post-term (greater than 42 weeks' gestation) (Figure 3.1).

The causes of early delivery of SGA infants include maternal toxaemia, malnutrition, infection, congenital anomalies, cigarette smoking and drug addiction. LGA babies are commonly born to diabetic mothers. The importance of distinguishing between the SGA term baby and the AGA preterm baby lies in the fact that the clinical problems encountered differ. Both SGA and LGA babies have a higher mortality rate than AGA babies at all gestational ages and thus assessment of gestational age has important therapeutic and prognostic implications (Table 3.1).

Table 3.1 Clinical problems encountered in babies small for gestational age and preterm appropriate for gestational age

	Small for gestational age (24–44 weeks)	*Preterm (less than 37 weeks)*
Pulmonary Problems	Aspiration syndrome Pneumothorax Pulmonary haemorrhage	Hyaline membrane disease
Apnoeic attacks	+	+ + +
Hyperbilirubinaemia	+	+ + +
Hypocalcaemia	+	+ + +
Mortality	+	+ +
Hypoglycaemia	+ + +	
Blood volume	Polycythaemia	Normal
Feeding capacity of stomach	+ + +	+
Congenital malformations	+ + +	+

Adaptation of respiratory system

During vaginal delivery the baby's chest is squeezed as it passes through the birth canal and up to 35 ml of amniotic fluid can drain out of the mouth. As the thorax re-expands at birth, this volume of fluid is replaced by the entry of an equivalent volume of air into the trachea and bronchi.

Although birth asphyxia is probably the strongest stimulus for the newborn to breathe, experimental evidence indicates that sensory stimulation such as cooling or pain can initiate breathing in the term fetus [25]. Stimuli such as touch, proprioception and audiovisual input may also play an important role in initiating and maintaining breathing. It has been suggested that these peripheral stimuli recruit central neurons and thus increase central arousal [4]. Animal experiments suggest that fetal carotid chemoreceptors are not essential for spontaneous intrauterine breathing, nor for the establishment of effective breathing at birth [21].

The first few breaths may require large transpulmonary pressures of 30–70 cmH$_2$O, but within a few minutes a normal functional residual capacity of 30 ml/kg is usually established and much lower pressures are then needed. Remaining lung fluid is removed by the pulmonary lymphatics and lung capillaries which open up with lung expansion. For further discussion of neonatal respiratory physiology the reader is referred to Chapter 4.

Adaptation of the cardiovascular system

The circulation of blood undergoes a remarkable re-routing during the change from fetal to neonatal life. Right atrial pressure falls at birth following the cessation of umbilical blood flow. The simultaneous decrease in pulmonary vascular resistance (PVR) which follows the onset of respiration and opening of the pulmonary vascular bed results in an increase in pulmonary blood flow and consequently left atrial pressure. This left to right pressure difference between the two atria results in the functional closure of the foramen ovale. PVR continues to fall under the influence of increasing P_{ao_2}, decreasing P_{aco_2} and rising pH.

Closure of the ductus arteriosus by contraction of its spirally arranged smooth muscle begins at birth under the stimulus of increasing P_{ao_2} levels, possibly prostaglandin mediated. This physiological closure is complete in 10–15 h, but anatomical closure by fibrosis needs 2–3 weeks [19]. During this latter period there are a number of stimuli which can cause the duct to remain open or actually to re-open. These include hypoxia, acidosis, hypoglycaemia, hypocalcaemia, pulmonary hypertension and prostaglandins E$_1$ and E$_2$ [26]. This leads to the possibility of shunting in either direction, depending on the relative resistances of the pulmonary and systemic vascular beds. A left to right shunt leads to increased pulmonary blood flow and the possibility of pulmonary oedema. On the other hand, a right to left shunt produced by an increase in pulmonary vascular resistance (e.g. secondary to the hypoxia due to hyaline membrane disease), causes a further fall in P_{ao_2} which further inhibits ductal closure and raises PVR, so that a vicious spiral is produced. Despite pharmacological manipulation of PVR and ductal muscle tone, the patent ductus arteriosus has to be ligated at operation before some preterm infants with hyaline membrane disease can be weaned successfully from intermittent positive pressure ventilation. Conversely, for some babies with congenital heart disease an open ductus is necessary to maintain life. Babies with pulmonary atresia or coarctation of the aorta, for example, are now given prostaglandin E_1 or E_2 therapeutically to maintain ductal patency until the definitive operation can be performed.

Another vascular bed which undergoes important changes in the first few days of life is the renal vasculature. After birth, all babies have low rates of tubular reabsorption and a tendency to produce high urine flow rates in the first few hours of life, the magnitude of which is related to the extent of placental transfusion. Urine production then falls for the next 48 h, to rise again by the end of the first week. This secondary rise is related to the increase in renal perfusion pressures, and more importantly, to a dramatic decrease in renal vascular resistance. This decrease in renal vascular resistance is probably related to a reduction in the initially high levels of circulating catecholamines found in the newborn [9] as the renal vasculature of these babies is highly sensitive to catecholamines, their vessel walls having a preponderance of alpha-adrenergic receptors [13].

Blood volumes

The blood volume of the newborn infant is dependent on the gestational age and on the degree of placental transfusion. The average value for a term infant with a normal haemoglobin level is about 85 ml/kg. The preterm baby often has a higher level, sometimes as much as 100 ml/kg. The blood volume may be calculated by adding the more constant plasma volume (50 ml/kg) to the haematocrit, since this will take into account normal variations in haemoglobin values and allow a more rational approach to blood transfusion when indicated.

The haemoglobin level of the normal term newborn is 17.1 ± 1.8 g/dl and the haematocrit 53%. The value of the haemoglobin level declines progressively due to slow replacement of fetal haemoglobin (HbF) with adult haemoglobin (HbA) after the first week; the physiological anaemia of infancy. This fall in Hb levels is most pronounced in preterm babies – the average level being 8 g/dl at 4–8 weeks of life in babies weighing less than 1.5 kg at birth, compared with an average level at their age of 11.4 g/dl in full-term babies. This haemoglobin level decrease is partly due to the short red blood cell survival; about 65 days in the term infant and only about 35 days in preterm infants.

The use of blood peroperatively is guided by the amount lost, the pre-operative haemoglobin and haematocrit levels, any associated clinical condition such as septicaemia (which may depress erythropoeitin production and increase oxygen consumption), and the anticipated loss postoperatively. For losses of between 5 and 20% of the estimated blood volume (EBV), the blood volume should be maintained by the use of human albumin solution. A blood transfusion is usually indicated when the blood loss at operation exceeds 20% of the EBV.

Adaptation of thermal control

The change from the constant, insulated environment of the uterus to the unprotected extrauterine environment following birth makes considerable demands upon the newborn infant. It is many years since the disastrous effect on survival of infants nursed in low incubator temperatures was first noted [29]. There are now known to be several reasons why newborns can be seriously affected by environmental temperature. Certainly their ability to shiver in response to cold is poorly developed, particularly in the preterm infant. The main mechanism for maintaining a normal body temperature in the newborn is chemical. Exposure to cold results in a release of noradrenaline at sympathetic nerve endings and subsequently in an increase in the circulating levels of cyclic adenosine monophosphate [18]. This in turn activates protein kinases which promote the lipase hydrolysis of triglycerides in brown fat stores. The oxidation of triglycerides, together with liver glycogenolysis can cause a marked increase in metabolic rate. Thus the ideal or 'neutral' thermal environment will be that in which oxygen consumption and metabolic rate are minimal.

However, despite this good metabolic response, neonates cannot maintain body temperatures outside a narrow range of environmental temperatures because of the rapid rate of heat loss. Heat transfer from the body core to the surface occurs due to changes in skin blood flow, the large surface area/weight ratio, the paucity of subcutaneous fat and, hence, poor insulation. Heat loss occurs from the body surface to the environment by radiation, conduction, convection and evaporation of water. A warm surface, minimal air flow and high ambient humidity will counter most losses by the latter three components. Loss by radiation presents a much greater challenge since this loss is partially independent of the surrounding air temperature and is related to the temperature of the solid surroundings such as the incubator walls. This in turn is related to room temperature. Radiant heat loss can be minimized by using either a double-walled incubator or a plastic heat shield placed over the baby inside the incubator. Alternatively, particularly where greater access to the patient is required, overhead radiant heaters may be used. Since the initial response of the infant when nursed in a lower than neutral thermal environment is to lower skin blood flow with a consequent fall in the skin temperature, advantage can be taken of this response by arranging a servo device so that the temperature of the abdominal skin controls the heat output of the incubator or radiant heater so as to maintain the abdominal skin temperature at 36.5°C.

The incubator or heater should be in a warm room and a baby who is relatively well should be clothed

Table 3.2 Incubator temperatures (°C) according to age and birth weight

Birth weight	Hours				Days		Weeks		
	0–2	*2–6*	*6–12*	*12–24*	*1–7*	*7–14*	*2–4*	*4–6*	*6–8*
<1500 g	36	35 —————————————————————————→ 34					33 —————————→ 32		
1500–2000 g	36	35 ———————————→ 34			33 ——————————————→ 32		————→		
2000–2500 g	36	35	34	33	————————————————→ 32		————→		
>2500 g	36	35	34	33	32 ——————————————————————————————→				

as much as is practicable. Sick infants should be nursed naked, as any changes in circulatory and respiratory patterns may be detected earlier and observations performed without disturbing the infant. All nursing procedures, blood sampling, setting up of intravenous infusions and radiography should be performed without disturbing the infant's environment. The use of a headbox to control oxygen and humidity therapy is especially useful. Table 3.2 gives an indication of the incubator temperature settings.

Hypothermia, defined as a body core temperature of less than 36°C, produces severe disturbances with depression of respiration, central nervous function, cardiovascular function and considerable metabolic derangements. Sclerema may occur. In the absence of a low thermal environment the possibility of septicaemia, disseminated intravascular coagulation (DIC) and hypoglycaemia should be considered. Hyperthermia arises because of an excessively high environmental temperature, infection, dehydration or cerebral birth trauma.

Adaptation of metabolism

Hypoglycaemia

In normal term infants the average blood glucose level is 2.7–3.3 mmol/l (50–60 mg/100 ml). Low birthweight infants have average levels around 2.2 mmol/l (40 mg/100 ml). Hypoglycaemia is defined as a true blood glucose below 1.6 mmol/l (30 mg/100 ml) in full-term infants and 1.1 mmol/l (20 mg/100 ml) in low birthweight infants during the first 3 days of life. After this period the blood glucose level should always be above 2.2 mmol/l (40 mg/100 ml) [5] and levels below 2.2 mmol/l (40 mg/100 ml) should always be corrected [17].

Hypoglycaemia may be entirely asymptomatic but may be associated with a number of signs, including tremors, apnoea, cyanosis, apathy, hypotonia, hypothermia and convulsions. Hypoglycaemia should be anticipated in any baby with these signs and particularly if the baby is preterm or small for gestational age, or was born to a diabetic mother or has suffered from birth asphyxia or hypothermia. Since Dextrostix estimation may be unreliable in the very low ranges, a true blood glucose should be estimated using capillary blood if hypoglycaemia is suspected.

Transient neonatal hypoglycaemia may occur at 4 h of age, but usually presents between 24 and 72 h. The pathogenesis in the small-for-gestational-age baby is usually associated with inadequate glycogen stores, whilst in the appropriate gestational age preterm baby, glycogen reserves may be exhausted by increased energy consumption caused by lower than neutral thermal environment, hypoxia, acidosis or increased respiratory work. Infants of diabetic mothers have a high incidence of hypoglycaemia 2–4 h after birth, though the blood glucose level is usually stabilized by 6 h. These infants have islet cell hyperplasia and probably hyperinsulinism. Other causes of hypoglycaemia include the exomphalos-macroglossia-gigantism (EMG) syndrome (see Chapter 26), glycogen storage disease, adrenogenital syndrome and islet cell tumours. Symptomatic neonatal hypoglycaemia is associated with a 30–40% incidence of subsequent neurological involvement though asymptomatic infants and hypoglycaemic infants of diabetic mothers have a good prognosis.

Whenever possible, hypoglycaemia should be prevented by early feeding even in the smallest babies. If this is not possible, and in those babies suffering from hypothermia or severe asphyxia, intravenous nutritional support should be given.

Hypoglycaemia should be treated intravenously, maintaining a constant rate of infusion, using 10% dextrose at a rate of 75–120 ml/kg per 24 h for the full-term infant. The concentration of dextrose may be increased to 15% if the hypoglycaemia is not relieved. More urgent correction requires the administration of 1 ml/kg of 50% dextrose, given rapidly, followed by an infusion as outlined above.

Blood glucose levels must be monitored repeatedly to assess the response to therapy, both by Dextrostix and occasionally by laboratory estimation.

Acid-base balance

The neonate has a remarkable ability to maintain acid-base equilibrium. Recognition and treatment of disturbances are dealt with in Chapter 5.

Hypocalcaemia (see also Chapter 5)

The fetus acquires most of its calcium (75%) during the last 12 weeks of gestation. Hence the small-for-gestational-age baby has normal calcium reserves whilst the preterm baby is deficient of calcium stores.

The normal serum calcium is approximately 1.9 mmol/l which may fall slightly immediately following birth but soon regains initial values in the normal infant. Serum calcium is a measure of protein-bound calcium, small-molecule-bound calcium and ionized calcium. Since the signs of hypocalcaemia are due to a lowered ionized calcium fraction, ordinary estimations of total calcium may not demonstrate a significant reduction in the blood level of calcium unless the ionized calcium fraction is measured directly. The normal ionized calcium level is 1–1.1 mmol/l and levels below 0.9 mmol/l should be treated [17].

Hypocalcaemia may occur in the first 48 h of life in sick babies, probably related to a low intake of calcium together with immaturity of the parathyroid glands. Babies fed on cows' milk, which has a high phosphate content, may develop hypocalcaemia at 5–7 days of life.

Hyperbilirubinaemia

Unconjugated bilirubin levels are high even in the normal full-term neonate. This physiological jaundice is characterized by a rise in the serum bilirubin level to a peak of about 120 µmol/l by about 3–4 days of life, gradually falling by the tenth day to reach the adult value of 17 µmol/l. Many factors contribute to this physiological jaundice, including the relatively low activity of liver enzymes, together with a large bilirubin load. This larger load is a result of the shorter life span of red blood cells in the newborn, particularly in preterm infants, and increased enteric reabsorption. Increased reabsorption of red blood cells from haematomas caused by birth trauma may also be a factor in some individuals. The preterm baby has additional problems in that not only may the serum albumin concentration be low [20], but the albumin itself has a reduced binding capacity for bilirubin [27].

Pathological jaundice is due either to overproduction or underexcretion of bilirubin, or both. A rapid rise in bilirubin levels in the first 36 h of life is usually due to overproduction, resulting from a haemolytic process which exceeds the normal hepatic clearance. Increased haemolysis is found in blood group incompatibilities, hereditary spherocytosis, and other haemolytic anaemias. Increased intrahepatic circulation of bilirubin occurs in intestinal obstruction from varying causes. Undersecretion of bilirubin follows metabolic disorders or obstruction of the biliary system. Toxaemia and infection result in both overproduction from haemolysis and undersecretion due to liver cell damage.

The dangers of hyperbilirubinaemia lie in the toxicity of free, unconjugated bilirubin to cellular structures, particularly in the brain, resulting in kernicterus. Signs of central nervous stimulation or depression may be present, but particularly in the preterm infant these may be absent or minimal. Since the amount of free bilirubin is related to the available sites for binding, any reduction in the plasma protein levels due to absolute reduction or occupation of these sites by other substances (e.g. penicillins, sulphonamides, gentamicin, digoxin, frusemide and diazepam), will increase its toxicity. The aim of treatment is to reduce the serum bilirubin level to at least 250 µmol/l, though a lower figure may demand active treatment in the presence of hypoxia, acidosis, hypothermia, low serum protein, prematurity or signs of clinical deterioration.

Phototherapy is now often used to decompose unconjugated bilirubin in the peripheral extravascular tissues and has substantially reduced the need for exchange transfusions. Light with a wavelength of 450 ± 25 nm penetrates the skin and causes photoisomerism of the bilirubin molecules, which then diffuse into the blood to be excreted in the bile, where they again revert to bilirubin [24]. Care must be taken to prevent conjunctival and retinal damage by covering the eyes during therapy and allowance must be made for the significant increases in insensible water loss that will occur. Repeated biochemical monitoring is mandatory.

Sensory stimulation

A number of observations in human infants have stressed the importance of sensory stimuli in neurological and physical development. Hasselmeyer [16] reported that simply fondling the premature infant for 5 min out of every hour for 2 weeks altered bowel motility, crying activity and, possibly, growth. Other authors have found that sensory stimuli increase growth and improve later learning situations. The effects of light, particularly phototherapy, on the subsequent development of the newborn have not been assessed nor have the effects of sounds generated in the immediate area such as those produced by incubators or nebulizers, and other inhalation devices.

It is not generally recognized that, apart from the beneficial effects of sensory stimulation on the developing newborn, maternal responses to separation, with consequent frustration and anxiety, have also to be taken into account when considering the overall pattern of neonatal care.

Fluids and electrolytes

After birth, the infant loses water to the environment by evaporation from the skin and respiratory passages (insensible water loss) and by urine formation and in the stools. Electrolyte losses occur mainly in the urine and faeces.

The volumes of the body water compartments in the newborn are considerably different from those in the older child. The total body water content is higher, due mainly to a large extracellular compartment which accounts for some 35–40% of body weight. This extracellular fluid (ECF)/body weight proportion falls sharply as excess ECF is excreted, and fluid intake is low, in the first few days of life, and then more gradually over the next few months to reach the adult value of 20% by 1 year.

Term newborns can conserve sodium relatively well but preterm babies, particularly those who are critically ill, may have huge urinary sodium losses [10]. Thus term infants are able to maintain a positive sodium balance even when fed on the relatively low sodium intake provided by breast milk, but preterm infants are often hyponatraemic and have a negative sodium balance in the first 2 weeks of life even when given a high sodium intake [30].

Another characteristic of the renal function of newborns is their inability to excrete a sodium and volume load promptly. The renal response to a sodium load improves progressively during infancy, so that by 1 year sodium excretion reaches a level similar to that of older children (16 mmol/h per 1.73 m^2) [2]. However, the development of hypernatraemia is often an indication of the disproportionate loss of water by insensible loss and is not necessarily related to the inability of the kidneys to excrete sodium.

The daily water turnover in the neonate represents 15% of the body weight in the term infant compared with 9% of the body weight in the adult: thus the infant, although possessing a greater reserve of extracellular fluid, nevertheless can more rapidly become dehydrated. The greater volume of extracellular water results in the total amount of sodium and chloride being proportionately greater than that in the older child.

Insensible water loss

Insensible water loss in newborns weighing more than 2 kg is normally about 1 ml/kg per hour. Babies weighing less than this can have values as high as 3 ml/kg per hour [11,31]. Other factors that increase the extent of these losses include the use of infrared radiant heaters [22], phototherapy, pyrexia, tachypnoea and excessively high environmental temperatures. Insensible losses can be decreased by the use of humidity and a radiant heat shield and strict environmental temperature control.

Renal losses

The urine-diluting capacity of the immature kidney is well developed. Preterm infants can decrease the osmolarity of their urine to levels as low as 25 mOsm/l–values below those attained by adults [1]. Despite the production of a maximally dilute urine, however, the ability of the immature kidney to excrete a hypotonic load is limited by low urine flow rates, secondary to low glomerular filtration rates (GFR). The GFR is low at birth and correlates closely with the gestational age. As measured by inulin clearance, the GFR in babies born at 28 weeks' gestation is 5 ml/min per m^2, and is 12 ml/min per m^2 in term infants [12]. Postnatally there is a rapid rise in GFR which doubles by 2 weeks of age and reaches adult values by 2 years. This is largely related to the increase in renal perfusion which occurs over this period.

In contrast to its well developed diluting capacity, the urine-concentrating capacity of the immature kidney is relatively limited. Fluid-deprived newborns can only increase their urine osmolarity to a maximum value of 680 mOsm/l, compared with the 1400 mOsm/l obtained in adults studied under similar conditions [15]. This reduced concentrating capacity is related to several factors. Antidiuretic hormone (ADH) activity is certainly very low in the first 3 months of life and, in addition, there may be some relative insensitivity of the distal tubule to ADH in the neonatal period [28]. Neonates also have limited intrarenal osmotic gradients due to their low urea excretion rates, and this may also contribute to their reduced renal concentrating capacity. Lastly, improvement in the concentrating capacity of the kidney during maturation has been shown to correlate with morphological changes, such as elongation of the loops of Henle and their penetration into the medulla [18].

Most healthy newborns have passed urine within 24 h of birth. Urine volumes begin at about 8 ml/kg per 24 h rising to about 100 ml/kg per 24 h by the end of the first week. The osmolarity normally falls from about 400 mOsm/l to about 100 mOsm/l over the same period.

Transport of the sick neonate

There has been an increasing tendency over the past two decades towards centralization of neonatal surgery and intensive care, not only for economic reasons but also because of the availability in specialized centres of personnel, expensive equipment and the necessary specialized expertise involved. Transport of the sick infant to the surgical centre is therefore necessary. If a properly organized transport system is available, it is now generally accepted that the risks of transport are much less than those of trying to treat a sick neonate in a peripheral hospital without suitable facilities and without adequately trained medical or nursing staff. In fact, various studies and our own experience have shown that babies only rarely deteriorate during the journey, but usually remain stable or even improve [3,6,14].

Many regional centres for neonatal surgery and intensive care send out a team of doctors and a trained nurse to collect sick babies from peripheral hospitals. The baby can then be assessed and prepared for the journey by those more familiar with transport techniques. If this is not possible, then appropriately trained staff should accompany the baby from the referring hospital. In either case it is vitally important that the preparation for the journey is well planned, as it can be extremely difficult to correct disasters that occur during the journey. A pre-packed and regularly checked kit of equipment and drugs for resuscitation is mandatory for all organized transport teams.

Thus, before transport the baby should be warm and have optimal oxygenation and ventilation. If the airway or ventilation are at all suspect then it is much safer to intubate the patient under controlled conditions in the referring hospital, rather than have the risk and difficulty of trying to intubate the baby during transit in the confines of the transport incubator. The endotracheal tube must be extremely well secured to prevent any accidental dislodgement or kinking. Venous access must be assured and any acidosis, hypovolaemia and hypoglycaemia corrected. When gastrointestinal obstruction or diaphragmatic hernia are suspected, a nasogastric tube should be passed and the stomach kept empty by repeated hand aspiration. Abnormal collections of air, such as a pneumothorax, should be drained.

Essential equipment will include a suitable transport incubator, capable of providing a neutral thermal environment, good visibility and easy access (see Figure 3.2). It should be able to be powered by both mains electricity and its own battery. Plasticized aluminium foil wrapped around the baby gives additional protection against heat loss and gauze padding may be used to wedge the baby in the incubator to prevent undesirable movement caused by jolting of the vehicle. In nearly all cases speed is not a particular advantage and a smooth ride with a stable baby is to be preferred. Apparatus for suction together with suitable catheters must be available for endotracheal and nasopharyngeal aspiration. The supply of oxygen together with a battery-driven air compressor, or air cylinders, must be more than adequate for the journey. Spare cylinders should always be carried. The oxygen/air mixture may be given directly into a small headbox within the incubator or by means of a 'T' piece if the baby is intubated. The baby may be ventilated by hand or by means of a portable ventilator which is usually

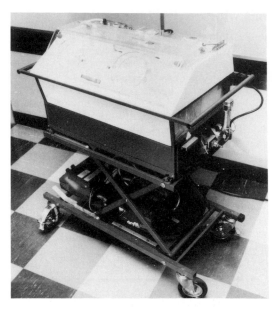

Figure 3.2 Transport incubator with built-in air/oxygen cylinders and ventilator. It can be powered by a mains supply or by batteries (on the bottom shelf)

incorporated into the incubator. We believe that it is preferable to ventilate by hand, as this allows changes in compliance to be detected and any obstruction, leak or disconnection to be noticed at once. All the necessary equipment for endotracheal intubation and ventilation is always carried together with equipment for setting up intravenous and/or intra-arterial infusions.

Maintenance fluids and other drugs may be administered using battery-operated syringe pumps. Fluids should contain glucose, and regular Dextrostix estimations should be performed during the journey. Monitoring of the heart rate and rhythm is best done by using a portable ECG, as auscultation of the heart may be difficult because of the noise and motion of the vehicle. An oximeter may also be a useful aid in these situations as it is relatively unaffected by patient movement. Other monitoring equipment should be available to measure the inspired oxygen concentration and the temperature of the baby and incubator.

The results in many centres throughout the world have shown that all newborns can be safely transported to treatment centres provided a specialized team with the necessary facilities are available. The extra cost of this transportation is more than compensated for by the decrease in mortality and morbidity that results.

Monitoring

The aims of intensive therapy of newborn infants are to recognize dangerous conditions early, before the patient's general condition has deteriorated to such an extent that successful treatment is no longer possible. With good observation as well as surveillance with physical and electronic aids the signs of central nervous, respiratory or circulatory disturbances, as well as early signs of metabolic imbalance or infection, can be recognized even in the smallest neonate. However good and modern the electronic monitoring system may be, however, the attentive and intelligent nurse at the bedside of the patient will remain the most important monitor [7]. The clinical judgement of an attending doctor who is acquainted with the pathophysiology of the newborn cannot be replaced by a computer. The acquisition of monitors will not allow any reduction in the quality of the nursing care, nor compensate for a possible nursing shortage. It is the attending doctor and nurse who will have to recognize the important clinical signs of infection, vomiting, aspiration, convulsions, poor peripheral circulation, cyanosis and excessive gain of weight. Even asymptomatic metabolic disorders such as hypoglycaemia, hypokalaemia, hyperbilirubinaemia, respiratory or metabolic acidosis, can be suspected by careful observation and confirmed by the necessary laboratory investigations. The purchase of monitors can lead to new problems which may increase the workload of the nursing and medical staff since wrong decisions can be taken if too much reliance is placed on information supplied by monitors, and the many cables, electrodes, tubes and transducers undoubtedly add to the problems of nursing care. Careless use of electric appliances may endanger the patient because of electric current or excessive heat. Catheters and cannulas increase the danger of infection. Finally, the cost of patient care is markedly increased by the electronic armamentarium.

At present, the following activities can be monitored with commercially obtainable devices (see Figure 3.3).

Monitoring of body temperature

Thermistor probes can be used to measure rectal, oesophageal, nasopharyngeal or skin temperature accurately and reliably. The skin-core temperature difference which is normally about 2–3°C, can be a most useful guide to the state of the peripheral circulation and, indirectly, cardiac output. Incubators which make use of a servo-controlled mechanism, employing skin temperature to regulate ambient temperature, may therefore deprive the physician of valuable clinical information.

Monitoring of respiration and oxygen therapy

There are various devices which measure respiratory rate and act as apnoea monitors. 'Apnoea mattresses' are used widely and successfully, even though they are not totally reliable. They work on the principle that respiratory movements are transmitted to a segmented, air-filled mattress and detect the shifts of air from one segment to another. Another successful type of respiratory monitor measures changes in transthoracic impedance using ECG leads. Readings of respiratory rate can then be incorporated onto the ECG display. Another type of apnoea monitor, not commonly used, detects changes in the curvature of the abdominal wall.

All mechanical ventilators nowadays have built-in alarm systems of varying complexity which can detect, for example, disconnection in the circuit and excessively high airway pressures. The temptation to switch off these sometimes distracting devices must be resisted.

Whether oxygen is administered into a headbox or from a ventilator, the inspired oxygen concentration must always be measured continuously using an oxygen analyser. The monitoring of respiration and oxygen therapy more indirectly has become easier recently with the introduction of the combined transcutaneous oxygen and carbon dioxide sensors capnography and oximeters. For a fuller discussion of these latter devices the reader is referred to Chapter 4.

Monitoring of circulation

Although the ECG provides a monitor of heart rate and rhythm, it gives no information about blood pressure or cardiac output. Changes in the ECG occur very late in the development of shock states; in the newborn the heart rate may remain relatively constant over long periods despite marked hypovolaemia. Central venous pressure (CVP) can be measured in neonates by percutaneous cannulation of the internal jugular, subclavian or femoral veins. The CVP reflects right heart filling pressure and can provide useful information regarding blood volume status and right heart function. The catheter may also be needed for the administration of drugs or for intravenous feeding.

The blood pressure of neonates can be easily and reliably measured using machines which employ ultrasonic detection of blood flow. Other automated devices which detect arterial pulsations transmitted to a limb-encircling air-filled cuff are also usually reliable, except when the blood pressure is very low or when there is excessive movement. It is important to realize that, whenever indirect methods are used, the accuracy of measurement depends on the use of a cuff wide enough to cover two-thirds of the upper arm. Direct intra-arterial pressure monitoring is

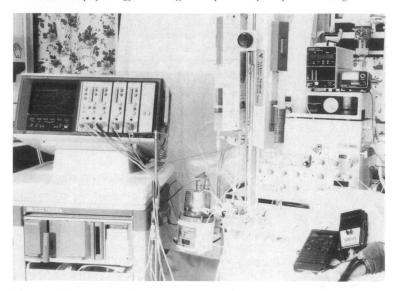

Figure 3.3 Just a few of the available monitoring devices that can be used on small babies. The equipment shown includes a Hewlett-Packard 78534C Clover monitor which has the facility to display six traces simultaneously. Various modules can measure up to seven invasive pressures, cardiac output, two lead ECG, respiration, end tidal CO_2 and two temperatures. A 'Nelcon' oximeter is also being used

advisable if the cardiovascular status is unstable, or when inotropic support or potent vasodilators are being required, or if frequent arterial sampling is envisaged. Although cannulation of the umbilical artery in newborns is technically easy, the risk of thromboembolic complications precludes its continued use for longer than 72 h.

Cannulation of the radial or femoral arteries is to be preferred for infants requiring intra-arterial monitoring for longer than 3 days, though all cannulas should, as a matter of principle, be removed as soon as possible.

The normal blood pressure of neonates will depend on their size and gestational age (see Table 3.3) [23]. However, because an infant's blood pressure is within normal limits for his size, it does not necessarily follow that cardiac output and vital organ perfusion are also normal. Other useful indicators of cardiac output are skin-core temperature differentials and urine output. Indwelling urinary catheters are not usually needed in neonates as light suprapubic pressure will usually suffice to induce micturition. In unconscious or paralysed babies careful expression of the bladder will usually empty it completely. The urine can be collected in

a bag fixed to the skin. The specific gravity, pH, protein and glucose concentrations of the urine can be tested at the bedside and will provide additional information about the hydration status and renal function of the infant.

It must be re-emphasized that electronic monitoring devices are merely aids for the nurse and doctor to use as they see fit. They must not be tempted to treat the figures on the monitor in themselves, but must examine the patient, intelligently interpret *all* information and then act accordingly.

References

1. Aperia, A., Broberger, O., Thodeminus, K. and Zetterström, R. (1974) Developmental study of the renal response to an oral salt load in preterm infants. *Acta Paediat. Scand.*, **63**, 517–524
2. Aperia, A., Broberger, O., Thodeminus, K. and Zetterström, R. (1975) Development of renal control of salt and fluid homeostasis during the first year of life. *Acta Paediat. Scand.*, **64**, 393–398
3. Blake, A.M., McIntosh, N., Reynolds, E.O.R. and St Andrews, D. (1975) Transport of newborn infants for intensive care. *Br. Med. J.*, **4**, 13–17
4. Cordorelli, S. and Carpelli, E.M. (1975) Somatic-respiratory reflex and onset of regular breathing movements in the lamb fetus in utero. *Pediat. Res.*, **9**, 879–889
5. Cornblath, M. and Reisner, S.H. (1965) Blood glucose in the neonate and its clinical significance. *New Engl. J. Med.*, **273**, 378–381
6. Cunningham, M.D. and Smith, F.R. (1973) Stabilization and transport of severely ill infants. *Pediat. Clin. N. Am.*, **20**, 359–367

Table 3.3 Aortic blood pressure in newborn infants [23] (modified)

Birth weight (g)	Systolic (mm Hg)	Diastolic (mm Hg)	Mean (mm Hg)
1000–2000	49	26	35
2000–3000	59	32	43
>3000	70	44	53

7. Duc, G. and Mieth, D. (1973) Clinical requirements for the use of continuous electronic monitoring of the newborn infant. In *Perinatal Medicine, 3rd European Congress of Perinatal Medicine*, April 1972, Hans Huber, Bern, Stuttgart, Wien, pp. 225–229

8. Edwards, B.R., Mendel, D.B., LaRochelle, F.T. Jr, Stern, P. and Valtin, H. (1982) Postnatal development of urinary and neurohypophyseal hormones. In *The Kidney During Development. Morphology Function* (ed. A. Spitzer) Masson Publishing, New York

9. Eliot, R.J., Laur, R., Leake, R.D., Hobel, C.J. and Fisher, D.A. (1980) Plasma catecholamine concentrations in infants at birth and during the first 48 hours of life. *J. Pediat.*, **96**, 311–315

10. Engelke, S.C., Shah, B.L., Vasan, U. and Raye, J.R. (1978) Sodium balance in very low-birth-weight infants. *J. Pediat.*, **93**, 837–841

11. Fanaroff, A.A., Wald, M., Gruber, H.S. and Klans, M.H. (1972) Insensible water loss in low birth weight infants. *Pediatrics*, **50**, 236–245

12. Fawer, C.L., Torrado, A. and Gulgnard, J.P. (1979) Maturation of renal function in full-term and premature neonates. *Helv. Paediat. Acta*, **34**, 11–21

13. Felder, R.A., Eisner, G.M., Montgomery, S.B., Calcagno, P.L. and Jose, P.A. (1980) Renal alpha, adrenergic receptors in canine puppies. *Pediat. Res.*, **14**, 619–627

14. Hackel, A. (1975) A medical transport system for the neonate. *Anesthesiology*, **43**, 258–267

15. Hansen, J.D.L. and Smith, C.A. (1953) Effects of withholding fluid in the immediate postnatal period. *Pediatrics*, **12**, 99–113

16. Hasselmeyer, E. (1964) The premature neonate's response to handling. *Am. Nurs. Ass.*, **11**, 15–18

17. Hatch, D.J. and Sumner, E. (1986) The surgical neonate. In *Neonatal Anaesthesia and Perioperative Care*, 2nd edition (ed. D.J. Hatch and E. Sumner) Edward Arnold, London, pp. 78 and 80

18. Heim, T. (1981) Homeothermy and its metabolic cost. In *Scientific Foundation of Pediatrics*, 2nd edition (ed. J.A. Davis and J. Dobbing) Heinemann Medical, London, pp. 91–128

19. Heymann, M.A. and Rudolph, A.M. (1975) Control of the ductus arteriosus. *Physiol. Rev.*, **55**, 62–78

20. Hyvarinen, M., Zeltzer, P., Oh, W. and Stiehm, R.E. (1973) Influences of gestational age on serum levels of α-1-feto-protein, IgG globulin and albumin in newborn infants. *J. Pediat.*, **82**, 430–437

21. Jansen, A.H., Ioffe, S., Russel, B.J. and Chernick, V. (1981) Effect of carotid chemoreceptor denervation on breathing in utero and after birth. *J. Appl. Physiol.*, **51**, 630–633

22. Jones, R.W.A., Rochefort, M.J. and Baum, J.D. (1976) Increased insensible water loss in newborn infants nursed under radiant heaters. *Br. Med. J.*, **2**, 1347–1350

23. Kitterman, J.A., Phibbs, R.H. and Tooley, W.H. (1969) Aortic blood pressure in normal newborn infants during the first 12 hours of life. *Pediatrics*, **44**, 959–968

24. McDonagh, A.F. (1981) Phototherapy. A new twist to bilirubin. *J. Pediat.*, **99**, 909–911

25. Milner, A.D. and Vargas, H. (1985) Resuscitation of the newborn. In *Neonatal and Paediatric Respiratory Medicine*, (ed. A.D. Milner and R.J. Martin) Butterworths, London, pp. 1–16

26. Mott, J.C. (1980) Patent ductus arteriosus: experimental aspects. *Arch. Dis. Child.*, **55**, 99–105

27. Odell, G.B. (1973) Influence of binding on the toxicity of bilirubin. *Ann. N.Y. Acad. Sci.*, **226**, 225–237

28. Schlondorff, D., Weber, H., Trizna, W. and Frie, L.G. (1978) Vasopressin responsiveness of renal adenylate cyclase in newborn rats and rabbits. *Am. J. Physiol.*, **234**, F16–21

24. Silverman, W., Fertig, J. and Berger, A. (1958) The influence of the thermal environment upon the survival of newly born premature infants. *Pediatrics*, **22**, 876–886

30. Sulyok, E., Nemeth, M., Tenyl, I., Csaba, I., Gyorg, E., Ertl, T. and Vargas, F. (1979) Postnatal development of renin-angiotensin-aldosterone systems, RAAS, in relation to electrolyte balance in premature infants. *Pediat. Res.*, **13**, 817–820

31. Wu, P.V.K. and Hodgman, J.E. (1974) Insensible water loss in pre-term infants: changes with postnatal development and non-ionizing radiant energy. *Pediatrics*, **54**, 704–712

4

Neonatal respiratory physiology and respiratory complications

P.D. Booker and G. H. Bush

Respiratory disorders associated with neonatal surgery form an important group of complications, and indeed 20 years ago Holder *et al.* [19] reported that postoperative pulmonary complications were the cause of death in 218 out of 350 deaths in patients with oesophageal atresia and tracheo-oesophageal fistula, an incidence of 62%. Since then important advances in our knowledge of neonatal respiratory physiology and pathology have been translated into therapeutic measures which have undoubtedly lowered considerably the morbidity and mortality from respiratory complications in newborn infants.

Respiratory complications in the neonatal period of life may arise as a result of the presence of a congenital malformation, either functional or structural in nature, which may be amenable to correction by surgical methods, or may be acquired by the development of pathological processes occurring after birth.

Physiological and pathological considerations

The development of the lung must be taken into consideration if a rational approach to the treatment of respiratory disorders is to be made. By the sixteenth week of human intrauterine life all the conducting airways and preacinar vessels have developed. Subsequent intrauterine and postnatal growth of the conducting airways occurs only in proportional increases in length and diameter and not in the absolute number of airways. The respiratory portion of the lung becomes delineated during the remainder of gestation. The terminal air spaces lined by flattened epithelium branch from the respiratory bronchioles and new vessels develop into

capillary beds. The primitive alveoli are shallow depressions in the saccules but gradually multiply both by segmentation of existing alveoli [9] and by breaking down of the walls of the terminal air passages. The number of saccules and primitive alveoli in a full-term infant are approximately 8% of the total number of alveoli in the adult [18] but these increase at the rate of 100 000 new alveoli formed daily up to the age of 8 years.

The growth of the lung in terms of air/tissue interface is believed to be linearly related to body weight so that there is a twentyfold increase in the respiratory surface from infancy to adulthood. However, since the oxygen requirement of the newborn infant per kilogram body weight is approximately twice that of the adult, it would appear that the neonate is at a considerable disadvantage if the air/tissue interface is reduced, for example by atelectasis, or if oxygen requirement is increased.

These changes during development have important clinical implications when the maturation of the lungs is hindered. External pressure on the lung buds within the thoracic cavity during early intrauterine life will considerably impair lung development. The lungs of infants born with a congenital diaphragmatic hernia are usually hypoplastic, the ipsilateral lung being the more affected [2,31]. Quantitative analysis of the bronchi, arteries and alveoli has confirmed that all are reduced in number in both lungs [2,11,22]. Airway generations are greatly reduced such that interference with lung development is indicated as early as 10–12 weeks' gestation. In both lungs, the alveolar count per acinus is within the normal range. Thus the total number of alveoli is reduced only in relation to the decrease in the number of airway generations.

Another congenital anomaly which may cause respiratory difficulties in early postnatal life is congenital lobar emphysema. Variations in the degree of respiratory embarrassment arise not only because this condition is due to a number of extrinsic and intrinsic causes but also because the age of onset of the congenital pathological factor will influence pulmonary development. Henderson, Hislop and Reid [16], using quantitative methods of examination, have described three anatomical types of emphysematous lobes: those with a normal number of bronchial generations with an increased number of alveoli; a normal number of bronchial generations with a normal number of alveoli; and a reduced number of bronchial generations with a reduced number of alveoli.

By 28 weeks' gestation the lung has reached sufficient maturity to effect adequate gas exchange. The stability of the alveoli, which prevents them from returning to their unaerated state, is due to the presence of the lipoprotein complex called surfactant, which lowers the surface tension in the fluid lining of the alveoli once a fluid/air interface has developed. Without surfactant the alveoli tend to collapse due to surface tension forces which are inversely proportional to their radius. Although specialized type 2 pneumocytes containing inclusion bodies (thought to be the site of surfactant production) can be seen at 24 weeks' gestation, surfactant has only been detected in fetal tracheal fluid at week 28 [15]. After week 32, by estimating the concentrations of various phospholipids in the amniotic fluid, it is possible to predict lung development and maturation. As surfactant production tends to increase with gestational age, it can be appreciated that preterm babies are most at risk from 'hyaline membrane disease', which is due to surfactant deficiency.

Apart from the presence of this stabilizing substance, mechanical forces are also important in maintaining alveolar distension. Recent work has re-emphasized that the distribution of air within the lungs is not uniform and that below a certain lung volume actual closure of airways occurs. Airway closure is believed to occur particularly in children below the age of 6 years [23], so that even at a normal tidal volume some alveoli do not partake in gaseous exchange. The result of this impairment is to increase intrapulmonary shunting of blood and to reduce arterial oxygenation. This mechanism may account for the calculated shunt of 15–20% of the output of the right heart in the normal newborn infant compared with less than 7% in healthy adults [25]. The application of a positive pressure to the airway (positive end-expiratory pressure, PEEP, or continuous positive airway pressure, CPAP) during the respiratory cycle can increase the volume of air in the lungs above the critical closing volume and thus airway closure can be largely prevented. This measure increases arterial oxygenation, stabilizes lung volumes and minimizes the development of

miliary atelectasis, and hence has been largely responsible for the reduced mortality in the treatment of newborn infants suffering from hyaline membrane disease as well as the success achieved in the ventilator treatment of newborn infants with a variety of pulmonary disorders.

Arterial desaturation produced by a right-to-left shunt of blood occurs not only because of intrapulmonary shunting but may also be due to cardiac shunts. Under normal circumstances the ductus arteriosus is functionally closed 10–15 h after birth and anatomically closed around 2–3 weeks later [17], but the muscle of the ductus arteriosus is highly sensitive to oxygen and a fall in arterial P_{O_2} will not only fail to cause contraction of the muscle but may even allow a previously functionally closed ductus to reopen. Surgical closure of the patent ductus arteriosus is often advocated in the newborn infant with persistent respiratory distress associated with cardiac failure [7,21].

Neonates are obligatory nose breathers and about 50% of the resistance to the flow of gases through the airways is accounted for by the nasal passages of the newborn. This resistance can be significantly increased by the presence of a nasogastric tube, or by secretions. The small air passages of the conducting system of the lung also impose a considerable resistance to the flow of gases, and since resistance varies as the fourth power of the radius, a small reduction in calibre causes a disproportionate increase in resistance to gas flow. Thus, retained secretions cause marked increases in respiratory effort and hence oxygen requirements but at the same time produce hypoventilation of the part of the lung supplied by the partially occluded bronchiole. Progression to complete occlusion results in loss of alveolar surface, a fall in arterial oxygenation, and ultimately to the collapse of the lobule or lobe affected. The tracheobronchial tree is normally cleared of secretions by the cough reflex aided by the cilia of the mucosal epithelium. The cough reflex is considerably depressed in the ill infant or may be ineffective because of the increased viscosity of secretions, as in dehydration or mucoviscidosis. Contamination of the air passages by gastric content in infants with a tracheo-oesophageal fistula or following inhalation of vomit can cause considerable mucosal irritation leading to infective purulent bronchitis.

Aetiology of respiratory complications

Respiratory distress

Respiratory distress occurs relatively frequently in the newborn infant and is more commonly due to disease processes inherent in the neonatal period of life than to congenital abnormalities amenable to surgical treatment. The former group of conditions must be considered, however, since they may coexist in infants with surgically correctable lesions and may mimic the signs of intestinal obstruction, with gastric distension and vomiting due to the swallowing of excessive volumes of air. Head retraction, a common sign in an infant with respiratory distress, may be mistaken for meningitis.

The respiratory distress syndrome of the newborn is characterized by an increased respiratory rate, flaring of the nostrils on inspiration, lower chest retraction, intercostal recession and an expiratory grunt. The presence of cyanosis and poor peripheral circulation may also signify respiratory inadequacy. It is important to stress that these clinical signs may be produced by a variety of disorders and detailed investigation will be required for the elucidation of their pathology. The possibility of congenital malformations of other systems must not be overlooked, and cardiac abnormalities can produce identical signs of respiratory distress.

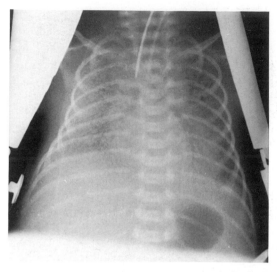

Figure 4.1 Chest X-ray of neonate with hyaline membrane disease showing characteristic ground-glass appearance of lung fields and air bronchograms

Upper airway obstruction

Obstruction of the airway in the nose and mouth may result from a variety of lesions such as postchoanal atresis or stenosis, relative macroglossia which occurs in the Pierre Robin syndrome associated with retrognathia, and absolute macroglossia found in Down's syndrome and in the exomphalos-macroglossia-gigantism (EMG) syndrome [20].

Vocal cord palsy may be due to birth injury or may occur in patients with the Arnold–Chiari malformation with descent of the brain stem through the foramen magnum of the skull causing stretching of the vagus nerve as it passes upwards to reach the jugular foramen [26]. Other obstructive lesions in the larynx include haemangioma, lymphangioma associated with cystic hygroma, congenital cysts of the aryepiglottic folds, laryngeal webs and cartilaginous subglottic stenosis.

The trachea and bronchi may be compressed externally by such lesions as vascular ring, goitre or cysts of the lung or oesophagus, or narrowed as a result of intrinsic lesions such as tracheomalacia or tracheal stenosis.

Retained secretions, particularly if they are purulent secondary to chemical irritation of the tracheobronchial tree in infants with a tracheo-oesophageal fistula, are also an important cause of reversible airway obstruction.

Pulmonary disease

Hyaline membrane disease due to a deficiency of surfactant is the commonest of all causes of respiratory distress in infants, occurring in 1% of live and one-third of premature births [30]. Radiography of

the chest shows a characteristic ground-glass appearance of the lung fields, an air bronchogram and evidence of incomplete expansion of the lung (see Figure 4.1). Considerable success may now be achieved in this condition with the use of intermittent positive pressure ventilation (IPPV) and positive end-expiratory pressure (PEEP). Recent work using exogenous surfactant administered to affected babies is also encouraging [13]. Even so, up to 20% of all neonatal deaths are the result of hyaline membrane disease (HMD) or its complications [12].

Meconium aspiration presents a clinical picture similar to hyaline membrane disease but may be distinguished by a history of respiratory difficulty at birth often preceded by fetal distress *in utero*, and the chest X-ray, which shows coarse mottling of the lung fields (see Figure 4.2).

Atelectasis of the lungs may be either massive or miliary. Segmental collapse of part of the lungs leading to total lung collapse follows obstruction of the air passages associated with either a failure of the cough mechanism or increased viscosity of the tracheobronchial secretions. Miliary atelectasis, on the other hand, occurs without airway obstruction and results from alveolar closure. It is due to a failure of inspiration and can only be diagnosed by measurement of lung volume and compliance and arterial oxygen tension; it cannot be diagnosed by ordinary radiological methods. Stasis of secretions in both massive and miliary atelectasis rapidly leads to infection and the development of bronchopneumonia. The susceptibility to infections and reduced respiratory reserve account for the fact that in infants with oseophageal atresia, deaths from

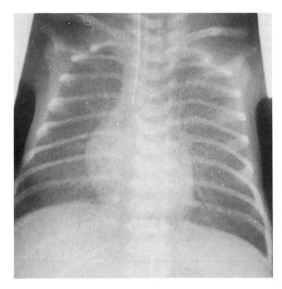

Figure 4.2 Chest X-ray of neonate with meconium aspiration showing coarse mottling of the lung fields

pneumonia occur more frequently in preterm than in term babies [35].

The distinguishing features of the two forms of atelectasis may be compared in Table 4.1.

Collapse of lung tissue must be clearly differentiated from pulmonary hypoplasia since the former is reversible and hence is associated with a more favourable prognosis. These two conditions coexist in infants with congenital diaphragmatic hernia. The effect of artificial pulmonary ventilation on blood gases has been shown to be of value in determining the prognosis in this condition. The ability to raise the P_{ao_2} and reduce the P_{aco_2} values to within the normal range (irrespective of the F_{io_2} values or ventilation parameters), should be associated with a good prognosis [3,14]. Similar considerations apply to infants with congenital lobar emphysema.

Collapse of normal lung tissue may also be found in the absence of pulmonary hypoplasia. The most common cause of extrapulmonary compression is a pneumothorax, which occurs in up to 2% of normal neonates [8], due to their own intense respiratory effort (see also Chapter 22).

The likelihood of alveolar rupture is increased in infants with diaphragmatic hernia and hypoplastic lungs with a tendency to bullae formation, in hyaline membrane disease and in infants with staphylococcal pneumonia with abscess formation. Despite improvements in the survival of infants mechanically ventilated for HMD since 1970, the incidence of pulmonary air leak remains high. In several reports published since 1980, pulmonary air leak occurred in 20–45% of newborn infants receiving IPPV [6,12,27,33]. Pulmonary air leak during IPPV is usually attributed to the use of high peak inspiratory pressure or excessive PEEP. However, a recent report by Tarnow-Mordi *et al.* [33] presented data suggesting that a reduction in ventilator pressure does not decrease the risk of air leak in these babies.

Greenough and Roberton [12] reported that, in their series of 210 infants ventilated for HMD, the development of a pneumothorax caused a significant increase in mortality only in infants of less than 30 weeks' gestation. They also stated that the use of muscle relaxation in those ventilated babies most at risk was associated with a significant reduction in the incidence of air leaks.

A pneumothorax may arise not only from rupture of air-containing lung tissue but also following oesophageal perforation which most commonly results from a breakdown in the anastomosis following primary repair for oesophageal atresia.

The development of a pneumothorax must always be borne in mind when there is sudden deterioration in pulmonary ventilation. The classic signs of diminished air entry, increased percussion note and shift of the mediastinum are often difficult to elicit. Although a chest X-ray is diagnostic, it is not always possible to delay treatment in a critically ill baby who is rapidly deteriorating. If clinically indicated, therefore, it may be necessary to test for a pneumothorax by using a fluid-filled syringe, attached to a 23 G needle, which is inserted into the anterior pleural space with subsequent removal of the plunger. Any significant pneumothorax will be revealed by air bubbling through the water in the syringe. It can then be treated more definitively by insertion of a chest drain connected to an underwater seal drain.

Pulmonary compression is also seen in patients with cystic adenomatoid malformation of the lung,

Table 4.1 The distinguishing features of massive and miliary atelectasis

Massive	*Miliary*
Large localized area	Small diffused lesions
Airway obstruction present	No airway obstruction
Failure of expiration (i.e. cough)	Failure of inspiration (i.e. sigh)
Diagnosis by physical and X-ray examination	Diagnosis only by measurement of lung volume, and
Treatment by removal of obstruction	arterial oxygen tension
	Treatment by increase in depth of inspiration or PEEP

bronchogenic cyst or pulmonary sequestration [4] (see Chapter 22).

Restrictive pulmonary disease is also seen in infants with hydrothorax resulting from excessive drainage of CSF following ventriculopleural shunts. Increased abdominal distension due to intestinal obstruction or following repair of diaphragmatic hernia, exomphalos or staged repair of gastroschisis is of great importance since the respirations in newborn infants are largely diaphragmatic in type. In these latter conditions the abdominal cavity is proportionally reduced in capacity since it has not housed the abdominal contents throughout intrauterine life. Postoperative ventilator therapy may be required in these infants following the return of the abdominal contents to the abdominal cavity, even when it has been enlarged by stretching the abdominal wall during surgery.

Disorders of the central nervous system

About 40% of preterm babies have irregular patterns of breathing, including apnoea, defined as cessation of breathing for more than 20 s. The tendency to apnoeic attacks is increased, even in the term baby, by HMD, septicaemia, intraventricular haemorrhage, hypoglycaemia and hypocalcaemia. Babies of less than 34 weeks' gestation having general anaesthesia are particularly at risk of apnoeic spells and if surgery cannot be postponed, postoperative monitoring for apnoea and its effects is mandatory for at least 18 h. Treatment of apnoeas may include theophylline, continuous positive airway pressure (CPAP) or even IPPV.

Meningitis, cerebral haemorrhage and drug overdose are other important conditions associated with depression of ventilatory activity and should be sought in a newborn infant who develops convulsions, lethargy and apnoeic attacks.

General disorders

Certain general disorders may affect respiration in a number of different ways. Septicaemia, sclerema and metabolic (including electrolytic) disturbances may present with respiratory insufficiency. Hypothermia is a potent respiratory depressant and it is known that the ventilatory response to hypoxia is less in the first weeks of life when the infant is in a cool environment [5]. The importance of nursing the baby in a neutral thermal environment cannot be overstressed.

Assessment of respiratory function

Repeated clinical examination, together with blood gas analysis remains the mainstay of respiratory function assessment in the neonate.

Clinical examination

Babies increase alveolar ventilation by increasing their rate of respiration because of the difficulty they have in increasing their tidal volumes. Thus an increasing respiratory frequency is an early clinical sign of pulmonary pathology. However, probably of more importance are signs of an increase in the work of breathing, such as nasal flaring, grunting, suprasternal, intercostal and subcostal recession. The degree of spontaneous activity should also be noted as restlessness is often a sign of hypoxia. After excluding an inspiratory and/or expiratory stridor, chest auscultation should be performed to assess air entry and the presence of added sounds. Because respiratory and cardiac function are intimately linked, respiratory assessment must always include measurement of heart rate, blood pressure and the state of the peripheral circulation. A chest X-ray may aid in the diagnosis of cardiomegaly, lung collapse, pleural effusion or pneumothorax.

Blood gas analysis

The arterial P_{co_2} is a measure of efficacy of alveolar ventilation and is therefore the ultimate index whereby the extent of pulmonary ventilation can be determined, whether the patient is breathing spontaneously or being artificially ventilated. At least 30 min should be allowed to elapse with a steady level of ventilation before the arterial P_{co_2} is measured, as it is of little value in assessing ventilatory adequacy in the presence of a changing ventilatory pattern. Elevation of the P_{co_2} is indicative of reduced alveolar gas exchange and may be due to either hypoventilation or an increased apparatus dead space or physiological dead space, which may occur in low output states such as haemorrhage or septicaemic shock in which there is a marked alteration in the perfusion/ventilation ratio. The P_{co_2} level must therefore be considered in the light of clinical and other biochemical findings.

The arterial P_{o_2} is primarily a measure of the inspired concentration of oxygen and the evenness of matching of alveolar ventilation and perfusion throughout the lungs. The greater the degree of either relative or absolute circulation of blood through non-ventilated alveoli, the greater the fall in the arterial oxygen tension, and hence estimates of the extent of shunting, which may, of course, not only be intracardiac but also intrapulmonary. Hypoxaemia may also arise in conditions such as incipient pulmonary oedema where the diffusion of oxygen across the alveolar membrane is impaired. Arterial P_{o_2} values can rapidly fluctuate and are only of value if the samples are taken during a steady state.

In the newborn, repeated arterial blood samples may easily be obtained by catheterization of an umbilical artery. Alternatively, there are special catheters with electrodes at their tip which can provide continuous measurement of P_{ao_2} or oxygen saturation. Unfortunately, an umbilical arterial catheter can only safely be left in place for 72 h, as after this time the risk of thromboembolism rises sharply. Great care should be taken to observe the circulation in the lower half of the body, therefore, when an umbilical catheter is in place. The umbilical or lower limb arteries will have lower arterial oxygen tensions than upper limb arteries if there is significant right to left shunting through a patent ductus arteriosus. This difference in P_{ao_2} can be useful in determining changes in shunting secondary to changes in pulmonary vascular resistance.

If the acid-base status and/or P_{aco_2} tension are the most important indicators of change in an infant, then a capillary blood sample provides readings which correlate well with those obtained from an arterial sample, providing that skin perfusion is relatively normal.

In practice, most clinical situations can be managed more than adequately by repeated radial artery sampling together with continuous monitoring of transcutaneous oxygen and carbon dioxide tensions. The new combined sensor provides $T_cP_{o_2}$ and $T_cP_{co_2}$ readings which have a reasonable correlation to arterial gas tensions, providing that skin perfusion is normal [24,36]. Intermittent checking with arterial gas analysis is important to verify that this correlation is maintained, particularly if the haemodynamic status is variable.

An alternative to transcutaneous gas tension monitoring is the measurement of oxygen saturation using an oximeter. This measures accurately the oxygen saturation in the skin and is particularly useful in babies with normal skin perfusion in whom oxygen therapy is expected to give less than 100% saturation. It has the added advantages that the probe is not heated and does not have to be moved at least every 4 h. A pulse rate is also displayed.

Treatment

Because of the likelihood that newborn infants will develop pulmonary complications, particularly following intra-abdominal or intrathoracic surgical procedures, every newborn should have prophylactic measures instituted postoperatively in an attempt to prevent these lesions developing. Whilst it may be argued that repeated handling may lead to exhaustion of the baby and hence defeat its object, there is no doubt that miliary atelectasis occurs more commonly in immobile states and therefore a balance has to be struck between the need for adequate rest periods and for a change in posture. Apart from being effective as a prophylactic measure, frequent changes in posture are even effective in reversing established massive atelectasis [29]. Altering the position of the baby from side to side every 2 h would seem to be an adequate compromise. Chest physiotherapy should be instituted at least 6-hourly to encourage expansion of the lungs and loosening of secretions. In the presence of only a weak cough reflex or copious secretions which are being retained in the trachea the cough reflex should be stimulated by passing a small catheter into the anterior nares each time the baby's position is altered.

Oxygen requirement should be kept to a minimum by ensuring that the baby is nursed in a neutral environmental temperature whether this be provided by an incubator or infrared infant warmer. The latter does allow greater access to the patient for nursing and therapeutic and investigative purposes without removing him from the prescribed environment or disturbing oxygen and/or humidity therapy (Figure 4.3).

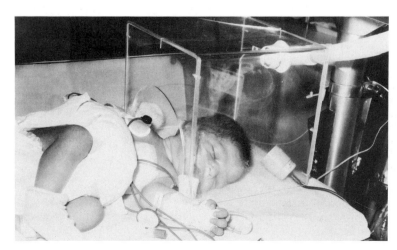

Figure 4.3 Infant nursed under an overhead radiant heater and being administered humidified oxygen into a headbox

Overloading the circulation with excess crystalloid fluids should be strenuously avoided since incipient interstitial or actual intra-alveolar pulmonary oedema will accentuate any previous disturbances of pulmonary exchange or, if severe, will precipitate respiratory failure. Frusemide, 1 mg/kg intravenously, up to 2-hourly and an increase in intravascular oncotic pressure will usually be successful in removing the excess pulmonary fluid. Infants with serious illness frequently have low plasma proteins, in particular the albumin fraction; daily administration of human albumin solution 20–30 ml/kg or 20% salt poor albumin 4–6 ml/kg can be beneficial. On the other hand, deliberate dehydration should be avoided because of the increased viscosity of secretions which result.

Infective lesions such as purulent bronchitis and pneumonia require treatment with the appropriate antibiotic. Aspirated tracheal secretions should be sent for culture and determination of the antibiotic sensitivity. A combination of ampicillin and gentamicin are suitable antibiotics for prophylaxis in those situations where severe pulmonary complications can be anticipated.

Humidification

The presence of tracheal secretions with an increased viscosity (e.g. in dehydration or in mucoviscidosis) which makes their expectoration difficult, or the bypassing of the nasal air passages by an artificial airway, demand the provision of artificially produced ambient humidification to produce 70% relative humidity in the trachea. Hot water humidifiers are commonly used for the intubated patient as the inspiratory limb may be warmed to prevent cooling of the carrier gas and condensation of the water vapour. The temperature of the water in the bowl is usually 'self-pasteurizing'. The gas temperature at the patient end of the inspiratory limb must be monitored continuously to maintain a temperature of 35°C. The equipment must 'cut out' if the temperature of the water in the bowl or gas in the inspiratory limb exceed 70°C or 37°C respectively.

For extubated patients conventional mist nebulizers based on the venturi principle are usually adequate. However, their output is small in terms of volume of water nebulized per unit gas flow, and the density of droplets produced is low, producing a high 'rain out' before reaching the patient's airway. The intermittent addition of ultrasonic nebulization, which produces a cold mist of high density and small particle size, may be necessary. Continuous humidification using ultrasonic nebulization can result in overhydration of small babies. Mist therapy should be given only when definite indications for its use exist and should not be used as a general panacea. The most efficient and effective method of providing humidification is to pass the mist into a headbox which concentrates the water vapour in the head area yet allows the rest of the infant to be observed and nursing care given without interfering with the treatment (see Figure 4.3). Similar considerations also apply to oxygen therapy.

Oxygen

The administration of oxygen to a newborn infant may be necessary to raise the arterial oxygen tension to a normal level of 70–80 mmHg (9.3–10.7 kPa), unless the hypoxia is caused by fixed right to left intracardiac shunting, when much lower levels may have to be accepted. However, in the newborn, oxygen therapy is not without hazard. Preterm babies are at risk from retinopathy of prematurity caused by the vasoconstrictive effects in the retinal vessels of a high P_{ao_2} [10]. High inspired oxygen concentrations have also been implicated in the aetiology of bronchopulmonary dysplasia and the Mikity–Wilson syndrome [34]. Because of these dangers, arterial oxygen tensions have to be monitored frequently in the newborn receiving oxygen therapy, though transcutaneous gas sensors and oximeters have made this task much easier (see above). For the extubated patient a headbox is needed to ensure an accurate and steady concentration of oxygen, whether the baby is in an incubator or a cot. The oxygen concentration should be monitored continuously using an oxygen analyser.

Artificial tracheal airway

An artificial tracheal airway in the form of an endotracheal tube or tracheostomy is indicated when there is upper airway failure as indicated by a P_{aco_2} greater than 70 mmHg (9.3 kPa). It is also indicated when there is retention of tracheal secretions which are not being cleared with physiotherapy, mist therapy and nasopharyngeal suction, and when there is a need for ventilator therapy. Prolonged nasotracheal intubation is now a well established technique, having been originally pioneered by Allen and Steven [1], and Stocks [32]. Provided care is taken to ensure adequate humidification, blockage of the tube should not occur, though if secretions are very viscous, the instillation of 0.5 ml of 0.9% saline down the endotracheal tube prior to suctioning may be beneficial. Catheters with a moulded tip and an end hole have the advantage of causing less tracheobronchial trauma. The other main disadvantage of prolonged intubation is subglottic stenosis, the incidence of which has risen dramatically since the introduction of endotracheal intubation and pulmonary ventilation in very low birthweight infants [28]. The length of the tube should be such that the tip lies in mid-trachea. The position should always be checked radiologically. Tracheostomy is now rarely performed but is still indicated in those patients who have laryngotracheal palsy or tracheal stenosis, in whom an artificial airway is required for a long time.

An artificial airway requires expert care to maintain its patency, and humidification and tracheal suction should have meticulous attention. Because the alveoli of newborn infants readily close, leading to atelectasis and hypoxia, an artificial tracheal airway may need to be connected to a system that allows CPAP to be applied.

Mechanical ventilation

This technique is now a routine method of treatment of any infant suffering from respiratory failure, and together with the application of PEEP, has undoubtedly improved the survival rate. A complete description of this complicated treatment is not within the scope of this chapter and the interested reader is referred to more extensive treatises on this subject [15,37]. This method of intensive therapy has improved very consideraly the prognosis following neonatal surgery over the last 20 years and has been a major advance in neonatal surgical care.

References

1. Allen, T.H. and Steven, I.M. (1965) Prolonged endotracheal intubation in infants and children. *Br. J. Anaesth.*, **37**, 566–573
2. Areechon, W. and Reid, L. (1963) Hypoplasia of lung with congenital diaphragmatic hernia. *Br. Med. J.*, **1**, 230–233
3. Bohn, D.J., James, I., Filler, R.M., Ein, S.H., Wessen, D.E., Shandling, B., Stephens, C. and Barker, G.A. (1984) The relationship between PaCO$_2$ and ventilation parameters in predicting survival in congenital diaphragmatic hernia. *J. Pediat. Surg.*, **19**, 666–671
4. Buntain, W.L., Isaacs, H., Payne, V.C., Lindesmith, G.C. and Rosenkrantz, J.G. (1974) Lobar emphysema, cystic adenomatoid malformation, pulmonary sequestration and bronchogenic cyst in infancy and childhood: a clinical group. *J. Pediat. Surg.*, **9**, 85–93
5. Ceruti, E. (1966) Chemoreceptor reflexes in the newborn infant. Effect of cooling on the response to hypoxia. *Pediatrics*, **37**, 556–564
6. Cooke, R.W.I., Morgan, M.E.I. and Coad, N.A.G. (1981) Pneumothorax, mechanical ventilation and peri-ventricular haemorrhage. *Lancet*, **i**, 555
7. Coran, A.G., Cabal, L., Siassi, B. and Rosenkrantz, J.G. (1975) Surgical closure of patent ductus arteriosus in the premature infant with respiratory distress. *J. Pediat. Surg.*, **10**, 399–404
8. Davis, C.H. and Stevens, G.W. (1930) Value of routine radiographic examination of the newborn on a study of 702 consecutive babies. *Am. J. Obstet. Gynecol.*, **20**, 73–76
9. Emery, J.L. (1970) The postnatal development of the human lung and its implications for lung pathology. *Respiration*, **27**, (Suppl.) 41–50
10. Flynn, J.T. (1984) Oxygen and retrolental fibroplasia; update and challenge. *Anesthesiology*, **60**, 397–399
11. Geggel, R.L., Murphy, J.D., Langleben, D., Crone, R.K., Vacanti, J.P. and Reid, L.M. (1985) Congenital diaphragmatic hernia: arterial hypertension after surgical repair. *J. Pediat.*, **107**, 457–464
12. Greenough, A. and Roberton, N.R.C. (1985) Morbidity and survival in neonates ventilated for the respiratory distress syndrome. *Br. Med. J.*, **290**, 597–600
13. Hallman, M., Merritt, T.A., Harvenpaa, A-L., Boynton, B., Mannino, F., Gluck, L., Moore, T. and Edwards, E. (1985) Exogenous human surfactant for treatment of severe respiratory distress syndrome: A randomized prospective clinical trial. *J. Pediat.*, **106**, 963–969
14. Harrington, J., Raphaely, R.C., Downes, J.J. (1982) Relationship of alveolar-arterial oxygen tension difference in diaphragmatic hernia of the newborn. *Anesthesiology*, **56**, 473–476
15. Hatch, D.J. and Sumner, E. (1986) Perinatal physiology. In *Neonatal Anaesthesia and Perioperative Care*, 2nd Edition, Edward Arnold, London
16. Henderson, R., Hislop, A. and Reid, L. (1971) New pathological findings in emphysema of childhood. 3. Unilateral congenital emphysema with hypoplasia and compensatory emphysema of contralateral lung. *Thorax*, **26**, 195–205
17. Heymann, M.A. and Rudolph, A.M. (1975) Control of the ductus arteriosus. *Physiol. Rev.*, **55**, 62–78
18. Hogg, J.C., Williams, J., Richardson, J.B., Macklem, P.T. and Thurlbeck, W.M. (1970) Age as a factor in the distribution of lower airway conductance and in the pathologic anatomy of obstructive lung disease. *New Engl. J. Med.*, **282**, 1283–1287
19. Holder, T.M., Cloud, D.T., Lewis, J.E. Jr and Pilling, G.D. (1964) Esophageal atresia and tracheo-esophageal fistula. A survey of its members of the surgical section of the American Academy of Pediatrics. *Pediatrics*, **34**, 542–549
20. Irving, I.M. (1967) Exomphalos with macroglossia; a study of 11 cases. *J. Pediat. Surg.*, **2**, 499–507
21. Kilman, J.W., Kakos, G.S., Williams, T.E., Craenen, J. and Hosier, D.M. (1974) Ligation of patent ductus arteriosus for persistent respiratory distress syndrome in premature infants. *J. Pediat. Surg.*, **9**, 277–281
22. Kitagawa, M., Hislop, A., Boyden, E.A. and Reid, L. (1971) Lung hypoplasia in congenital diaphragmatic hernia. A quantitative study of airway, artery and alveolar development. *Br. J. Surg.*, **58**, 342–346
23. Mansell, A., Bryan, A.C. and Levinson, H. (1972) Airway closure in children. *J. Appl. Physiol.*, **33**, 711–714
24. Marsden, D., Chiu, M.C., Paky, F. and Helms, P. (1985) Transcutaneous oxygen and carbon dioxide monitoring in intensive care. *Arch. Dis. Child.*, **60**, 1158–1161

25. Nelson, N.M., Prod'ham, L.S., Cherry, R.B., Lipsitz, P.J. and Smith, C.A. (1963) Pulmonary function in the newborn infant; the alveolar-arterial oxygen gradient. *J. Appl. Physiol.*, **18**, 534–539

26. Pracy, R. (1965) Stridor in children. *Proc. Roy. Soc. Med.*, **58**, 267–270

27. Primak, P.. (1983) Factors associated with pulmonary air leak in premature babies requiring mechanical ventilation. *J. Pediat.*, **102**, 764–768

28. Quirey, R.C., Spencer, M.G., Bailey, C.M., Evans, J.N.G. and Graham, J.M. (1986) Management of subglottic stenosis: experience from two centres. *Arch. Dis. Child.*, **61**, 686–690

29. Rees, G.J. (1958) Neonatal anaesthesia. *Br. Med. Bull.*, **14**, 38–41

30. Roberton, N.R.C. (1979) Management of hyaline membrane disease. *Arch Dis. Child.*, **54**, 838–844

31. Snyder, W.J.H. Jr and Greaney, E.M. Jr (1965) Congenital diaphragmatic hernia: 77 consecutive cases. *Surgery*, **57**, 576–588

32. Stocks, J.G. (1966) Prolonged intubation and subglottic stenosis. *Br. Med. J.*, **2**, 1199–1200

33. Tarnow-Mordi, W.O., Narang, A. and Wilkinson, A.R. (1965) Lack of association between barotrauma and airleak in hyaline membrane disease. *Arch. Dis. Child.*, **60**, 555–560

34. Thibeauet, D.W., Clutario, B. and Auld, D.A.M. (1966) Arterial oxygen tension in premature infants. *J. Pediat.*, **69**, 449–451

35. Waterston, D.J., Bonham-Carter, R.E. and Aberdeen, E. (1962) Oesophageal atresia; tracheo-oesophageal fistula. *Lancet*, **i**, 819–822

36. Whitehead, M.D., Lees, B.V.W., Pagdin, T.M. and Reynolds, E.O.R. (1985) Estimation of arterial oxygen and carbon dioxide tensions by a single transcutaneous sensor. *Arch. Dis. Child.*, **60**, 356–359

37. Friesen, R.H. and McIlvaine, W.B. (1989) Basic techniques of paediatric anaesthesia. In *Textbook of Paediatric Anaesthetic Practice*. Summer, E. and Hatch, D. (eds). Balliere Tindall, London, pp. 113–149

5

Fluid and electrolyte management and nutritional support

C.J. Taylor and Jenny Walker

Over the first days of life rapid changes occur in the neonate's physiology to facilitate adaptation to an extrauterine environment (see Chapter 3). As a result, requirements and tolerance of fluid, calories and nutrients vary on an almost daily basis. Gestational age also has a major influence on the adaptive ability of the neonate with further adverse influences from stress, sepsis and environmental instability.

Low birth weight (<2500 g) alone has a profound effect on neonatal mortality and morbidity. Survival in very low birthweight babies (<1500 g) is 64%, with intact survival falling to less than 50% in such infants [32]. Comparable figures for infants weighing 1500–2500 g is more encouraging with intact survival of 80% being reported in many units offering modern neonatal intensive care. In the UK, approximately 7% of newborns are of low birth weight, one-third of these are dysmature (i.e. weight below the 10th centile for gestational age) and two-thirds are premature (born before 37 weeks of gestation). A successful outcome in these groups following surgical intervention requires input from clinical and nursing staff skilled in neonatal intensive care.

Maintenance of fluid and electrolyte balance (see also Chapter 3)

Physiological differences in the neonate necessitate specific approaches in the management of fluid and electrolyte balance. In a term infant, 75% of the body is water of which 35% is extracellular fluid. In a premature infant of 26 weeks' gestation, 86% of the body weight is water, of which 50% is extracellular. The premature infant will therefore require proportionately more fluid to achieve homeostasis.

Fluid requirements should be assessed individually and modified in the light of the rapid changes in cardiac, renal and hepatic function and skin permeability which occur in the immediate postnatal period. Rapid infusions may result in a symptomatic patent ductus arteriosus [6] and necrotizing enterocolitis [5], but, in contrast, failure to meet fluid needs may quickly precipitate dehydration because of the high insensible losses, particularly in the premature infant [28].

In a small baby fluid balance requires consideration of *all* fluids lost or gained. Frequent blood sampling can lead to both hypovolaemia and anaemia, and antibiotics and other drugs given intravenously (e.g. dopamine infusions) or the use of heparinized infusions to keep arterial lines patent

Table 5.1a Maintenance fluid requirements (ml/kg per 24 h) in normal neonates based on body weight

Day of life	Body weight			
	<1000 g	1000–1500 g	1500–2000 g	>2500 g
Day 1	100–120	80–100	60–80	50–70
Day 2	120–150	110–130	90–110	80–100
Day 3	150–170	140–160	120–140	100–120
Day 4	180–200	160–180	140–160	130–150
Day 5 on	180–200	170–200	150–180	140–160

Table 5.1b Maintenance intravenous electrolyte requirements (all weights)

	mmol/kg per 24 h
Sodium	3–5
Potassium	2–3
Chloride	2–4
Calcium	0.5–1.0
Magnesium	0.25–0.5
Phosphate	0.25–1.0

Table 5.2 Changes in insensible water loss (IWL) with weight and postgestational age [41] (figures for well infants in servo incubators at 35% relative humidity)

Weight (g)	IWL (ml/kg/24 h)	Week 1	Week 2	Week 3	Week 4
<1000	64 ⎫				
1001–1250	56 ⎬	57	50	41	38
1251–1500	38 ⎭				
1501–1750	22 ⎫	20	32	30	30
1751–2000	17 ⎭				

can account for 20–30% of the fluid volume available for supplying nutrition. Maintenance fluid requirements based on body weight are shown in Tables 5.1a and b. Additional losses should be considered in the light of the following factors.

Insensible water loss

Gestational maturity and weight influence the extent of insensible water loss (IWL) so that a wide range of fluid losses have been reported (Table 5.2). Insensible water loss is also increased in infants nursed under radiant heaters and phototherapy lights. Losses can be minimized by nursing infants in humidity with a radiant heat shield. Losses are also decreased by inactivity [30].

Renal water loss

In normal circumstances, the kidney is able to adjust renal water loss to compensate for the discrepancy between intake and output. During the first few days of life however, the infant has a limited ability to excrete a water load. This improves with postgestational age but is still less than the response of an adult [26]. This may be due to the low glomerular filtration rate, but the concentrating ability is also reduced so that the maximum urine osmolality achievable is 600–700 mOsm/kg compared with 1200–1400 mOsm/kg in the adult. This reduced concentrating ability is to some extent caused by a lack of available osmotically active substances since urea excretion rates are low in the anabolic state of the normal infant [22]. Excessive renal sodium losses also occur, particularly in the premature infant, necessitating a relatively high salt intake; but this may not be as high as expected if the bowel is functioning, for compensatory high colonic sodium salvage may also operate. The aim should be to maintain a urine volume of 50–100 ml/kg per 24 h with a urine osmolality between 75 and 300 mOsm/kg.

Loss of gastrointestinal fluid

Stool water loss is normally estimated to be 5–10 ml/kg per 24 h. Large quantities of fluid and electrolytes may be lost from the stomach by vomiting or aspiration (up to 125 ml/kg per 24 h with a sodium concentration of up to 165 mmol/l) or from the intestine (with similar values for water and sodium) as a result of diarrhoea, enterostomy or fistula. Hidden losses into dilated bowel must also be taken into account when estimating total losses. Aspiration of saliva from an upper oesophageal pouch can also result in significant fluid loss.

Normal daily intravenous electrolyte requirements are seen in Table 5.1b. Additional electrolyte requirements may result from abnormal losses through gastric aspiration, aspiration of saliva from upper oesophageal pouches, stoma losses or diarrhoea. Daily losses should be calculated and an allowance made in addition to normal maintenance requirements (see Table 5.3 for the electrolyte composition of secretions).

Table 5.3 Electrolyte composition of secretions (mmol/l)

Secretion	H^+	Na^+	K^+	HCO^{3-}	pH
Saliva	—	15	—	3	6.3–6.8
Gastric	80	50	10	—	1.0–1.5
Pancreatic	—	140	10	70	7.1–8.2
Biliary	—	140	10	30	7.0–7.6
Succus entericus	—	135	15	25	7.0–7.5

Hypocalcaemia (see also Chapter 3)

The fetus acquires most (75%) of its calcium during the last 12 weeks of gestation; hence the term baby has adequate calcium reserves whilst the preterm baby may be deficient.

The normal serum calcium is approximately 2.2–2.5 mmol/l, which may fall slightly immediately following birth but soon regains the initial values in the normal infant. Serum calcium is a measure of protein-bound (inactive) calcium, small-molecule-bound calcium and ionized calcium. Since the signs of hypocalcaemia are due to the lowered ionized calcium fraction which will be influenced by acid/base status, estimations of total calcium may not demonstrate a significant reduction in blood level of calcium unless the ionized calcium fraction is measured directly. A nomogram has been devised for computing ionized calcium from the total calcium level in relation to albumin levels [27].

The signs of hypocalcaemia include apathy, jitteriness and non-specific neurological signs; the diagnosis therefore must be confirmed by chemical analysis whenever it is suspected clinically.

Biochemical hypocalcaemia may be seen in the first few days of life as an accentuation of the normal postnatal fall and is influenced by relative hypoproteinaemia.

The treatment of symptomatic infants is the slow intravenous infusion of 10% calcium gluconate, and then supplements given orally if possible. The infant may also need magnesium, as the symptoms of hypocalcaemia are indistinguishable from those of hypomagnesaemia.

Hypomagnesaemia

Infants with marked loss of intestinal juices may develop hypomagnesaemia with convulsions and tetany [2]. It may also occur following exchange or other massive transfusion where it occurs in combination with hypocalcaemia. Serum levels average 0.7–1.1 mmol/l in the neonate, but the levels can fluctuate rapidly after birth. In the presence of proven hypomagnesaemia, magnesium may be given by intravenous or deep intramuscular injection in the form of magnesium sulphate. The maintenance dose is 0.5 mmol/kg per 24 h but this would be increased for the correction of hypomagnesaemia. Maintenance magnesium can also be given orally, but may induce diarrhoea.

Disturbances of hydration

Assessment

Disturbances of acid-base balance, hydration and electrolyte status must be corrected pre-operatively even if this means delaying operation. The degree of hydration may be assessed by consideration of the following parameters.

Clinical examination

Skin turgor, state of peripheral circulation, depression of fontanelle, lack of sweating and dryness of mouth can all be assessed. Changes in body weight give only a rough indication of fluid loss since rapid catabolism of body protein in infancy can produce marked weight changes.

Blood parameters

Haemoglobin and haematocrit estimations are only of use if serial values are available, owing to the wide variation at birth (haemoglobin 12–24 g/dl). The normal neonate has a haemoglobin of 16–20 g/dl which falls to a nadir of 10 g at 6 months.

Anaemia rapidly develops in sick infants from accelerated red cell breakdown and/or blood sampling. Haemoglobin levels should be maintained above 10 g/dl in neonates, and above 13 g/dl in premature infants.

Plasma sodium levels reflect only the ratio of sodium ions to water, and only if the loss of water has been proportional to that of sodium (isotonic dehydration) will this value be of help in assessing the degree of hydration. Similar consideration applies to the estimation of plasma osmolality. Blood urea may be of value in assessing the degree of hydration but the anabolic and catabolic state of the infant must also be considered. Serum electrolytes should be measured repeatedly and the results interpreted in the light of other investigations.

Urine parameters

Osmolality is the most useful guide to hydration but is not utilized to the extent that it should be, bearing in mind the ease of estimation and the non-invasive method of collection of specimens. It has been shown that the total fluid requirements may be estimated using a formula [12]:

$$\text{total fluid requirements} = \frac{\text{basic fluid requirements} \times \text{urine osmolality}}{228}$$

Urine osmolality is increased with albuminuria and glycosuria.

Urine sodium, urea and creatinine clearances in 24-h specimens may assist not only in assessing the disturbance of electrolytes, but also in estimating renal blood flow and renal function, although normal ranges in the neonate are poorly defined. The urine volume is also an excellent indicator of the degree of hydration and the output should be measured routinely. In sick infants measurements are made hourly, using Paul's tubing in boys, and urine bags in girls, or by weighing nappies. An average of 2–4 ml/kg per h signifies normal hydration in the absence of diuretic factors, disorders of ADH secretion and intrinsic renal disease.

Acid-base balance

The estimation of acid-base balance is an essential part of neonatal monitoring and enables differentiation to be made between respiratory and metabolic disturbances. Alterations in blood pH affect serum potassium, pCO_2 and ionized calcium.

Metabolic acidosis with a pH less than 7.2 and a standard bicarbonate level of less than 22 mmol/l occurs in poor perfusion states such as shock, hypothermia, asphyxia, hypoxia and renal disease. Treatment should be aimed at the primary cause, e.g. hypovolaemia but the metabolic acidosis may be corrected (if the acidosis is severe) by the slow administration of sodium bicarbonate in a 4.2% solution (2 ml = 1 mmol NaHCO₃) using the formula:

amount of $NaHCO_3$ required (mmol) =
  $0.3 \times$ body weight (kg) $\times$ base deficit (mmol)

It is usual to correct only when the base deficit is greater than -10 mmol, and only to correct half the deficit. The sodium bicarbonate must be given slowly (i.e. over 20 min) since this solution has an osmotic concentration of 1000 mOsm/l and can cause a potentially dangerous rise in blood osmolality with the possibility of cellular damage particularly in the brain. It has not been substantiated however, that sodium bicarbonate therapy plays a major role in the pathogenesis of intraventricular haemorrhage [1].

Respiratory acidosis with a pH level less than 7.2 and a pCO_2 above 60 mmHg may indicate the need for controlled pulmonary ventilation.

Metabolic alkalosis with a pH more than 7.5 and a standard bicarbonate more than 26 mmol/l occurs following excessive loss of gastric contents and can be corrected by adequate provision of sodium, chloride and potassium intravenously.

Respiratory alkalosis is frequently seen as a compensatory mechanism in the presence of a metabolic acidosis. It occurs only rarely as a result of a primary respiratory stimulation. The commonest cause is mechanical hyperventilation.

Treatment

The aim of treatment should be:
1. To correct pre-existing deficiencies.
2. To administer normal daily requirements.
3. To replace continuing abnormal losses.

Pre-operative infusions

The presence of hypovolaemic shock as shown by poor peripheral perfusion, a lowered arterial blood pressure, metabolic acidosis and low urinary output should be treated vigorously to restore the initial circulating volume to a normal level. Peripheral oedema can occur even with hypovolaemia.

Hypovolaemic shock should be treated without delay, using 4.3% human albumin solution or plasma protein fraction in sufficient quantity to restore the normal circulatory parameters. The infusion must be closely monitored, ideally by central venous pressure measurements, to determine the degree of response to therapy. The possibility of precipitating cardiac failure in the unstable neonate by over-infusion is a real danger. When hypovolaemic shock is due to acute blood loss, compatible fresh whole blood must be given to replace the volume lost.

Isotonic and hypertonic dehydration should be treated by the infusion of 4% glucose in 0.18% sodium chloride solution. Isotonic dehydration can be treated rapidly (e.g. 150 ml/kg per day) but patients with hypertonic dehydration should have their perfusion restored first if necessary with plasma and then be rehydrated at the slower rate of 100 ml/kg per day plus losses to decrease the risk of convulsions which may occur if the hyperosmolality is corrected too quickly [4]. In hyponatraemic dehydration 0.45% saline in 5% dextrose may be used; in severe hyponatraemic dehydration, additional sodium chloride may be required. Once a urinary flow is established, potassium should be added to the infusion even though the serum potassium may not yet indicate hypokalaemia since loss of potassium from the intestinal tract will have produced a lower intracellular potassium level than the serum level might suggest.

The normal daily requirements of fluid and electrolytes (see Tables 5.1a and 5.1b) must be administered concurrently with the amount required to replace the existing deficiencies. In the presence of fever the fluid requirements are increased by 10% for each degree Celsius rise in body temperature. Allowance (an extra 10%) must also be made for the infant nursed under a radiant heater or receiving phototherapy, or in low humidity, or if he has increased losses through tachypnoea.

Blood sugar levels should be monitored, and hypoglycaemia avoided by administration of intravenous glucose. Hyperglycaemia should also be avoided (renal threshold is a rough guide to sugar tolerance) since each mmol increase in blood glucose produces an increase in serum osmolality of 1 mOsm/l leading to an osmotic diuresis [8].

Intraoperative infusion

It has been shown that fluid is sequestered into a traumatized area [31]. It is current practice to infuse 0.45% sodium chloride with 5% glucose solution at 3–4 ml/kg per h in addition to normal maintenance fluids. Operative blood loss is closely monitored, and is always replaced volume for volume if it is greater than 10% of the total circulating blood volume (of 75–85 ml/kg).

Postoperative infusion

The amount and type of fluid given must depend upon the response of the infant to the pre-operative resuscitation and will be gauged by repeated assessment of the state of hydration, electrolyte balance and gastrointestinal losses as previously described. A volume of isotonic fluid appropriate for the babies' weight and age (4% glucose in 0.18% sodium chloride) is usually used as a basic infusion, with electrolyte supplements if appropriate (see

Tables 5.1a and 5.1b). Nasogastric losses, salivary losses (from blind upper pouches of oesophagus), and excessive stoma losses should be replaced volume for volume, according to the electrolyte content of the fluid (Table 5.3).

Sick infants, or those with pooling of serous fluid in the thoracic or abdominal cavities often have a low serum albumin, and this can be improved with boluses of salt-poor albumin solution (20% human albumin solution) at 10–20 ml/kg per 24 h. Serous losses (e.g. from underwater seal chest drains) can be replaced volume for volume with plasma protein fraction (4.3% human albumin solution).

Nutrition

Having corrected the hydration, electrolyte imbalance and acid-base balance, nutrition must be considered. A term infant can survive 32 days of total starvation, or 80 days of semistarvation. However, a premature infant of 2000 g can only survive 12 days of starvation, and an infant of 1000 g only 4 days [20]. It is therefore very important that nutrition is planned early in the surgical treatment of a neonate. Nutrition is vital for growth (see Table 5.4), brain development, wound healing and for maintenance of immune status.

Experimental evidence suggests that inadequate nutrition when tissues are undergoing rapid cell division results in a reduction in body DNA and also in brain DNA content [14,40]. Since glial proliferation in the human brain is accelerating during the last trimester of pregnancy, preterm infants are likely to be particularly vulnerable to the effects of malnutrition. The resulting cell loss cannot be made up by a 'catch-up' period as is seen following impaired growth in later childhood. Malnutrition

Table 5.4 Basic energy requirements in neonates [9]

	(kcal/kg per day)	
Expenditure		
Resting metabolism	50	
Activity	10	
Thermoregulation	10	
Tissue synthesis	25	} energy cost
Storage	25	} of growth
Total	120	

leads to a reduction in brain DNA synthesis and protein turnover [15] which in turn is related to head growth [39] and developmental outcome [19]. Nutrition therefore needs to provide both the daily maintenance and growth requirements.

The neonatal small bowel measures on average 250–300 cm (along its antimesenteric border) with the premature infant having a slightly shorter

length. Independent survival following resection depends on the length of remaining bowel and the presence or absence of the ileocaecal valve. Wilmore [38] reported no survivors with less than 15 cm of jejunum or ileum and almost 100% survival with more than 38 cm. A 50% survival rate was seen in infants with 15–38 cm of bowel if the ileocaecal valve remained intact.

Following intestinal resection compensatory adaptation of the remaining bowel occurs over a period of approximately 18 months. Ileal adaptation is more efficient than that of the jejunum or colon, and therefore ileal resections are more likely to produce severe metabolic consequences. Changes in intestinal diameter occur subsequent to an increase in mural thickness. Elongation of villi occurs with an increase in cell count and DNA content per unit length. This hyperplasia correlates with an enhanced absorptive capacity [36]. The trophic effect may well be mediated by gut hormones in response to feeding. It has been documented that there are large postprandial surges in enteroglucagon, gastric inhibitory peptide, gastrin, motilin and neurotensin, mediating gastrointestinal and pancreatic secretion, gastric emptying and intestinal motility [3,25].

Enteral nutrition

Food intolerances are not infrequent in the neonate, especially following bowel resection or ischaemic injury. Intestinal motility is also impaired following bowel resection. Babies who have had bowel resection, necrotizing enterocolitis, Hirschsprung's enterocolitis or meconium ileus are especially prone to intolerances. These are principally manifested as diarrhoea. A recovery from these intolerances is expected (taking from 4 weeks to 3 years depending on severity), and during this period a gradual introduction of sugar and protein can be made, whilst nutrition is maintained by parenteral feeds.

Wherever possible, enteral nutrition by breast, bottle or tube (nasogastric, nasojejunal, gastrostomy, transanastomotic or enterostomy) should be given. Many surgical neonates have no gastrointestinal contraindications to enteral feeding, and this should always be considered and tried first.

The introduction of enteral feeds into a compromised bowel requires planning. Small frequent quantities of full strength feed can be introduced slowly, while hydration (and nutritional support) is provided by parenteral fluids. The overall volume of feed per day must be computed with both oral and intravenous inputs adjusted to meet the total requirements. Feeds are better tolerated if the osmotic load is spread over the whole day, and gastrointestinal secretion is reduced with continuous rather than bolus feeds.

The current choice of formulae for infant feeds is considerable. The surgeon is urged to become

Table 5.5 Comparison of composition of infant milks (in 100 ml normal dilution)

	Breast	Cow & Gate Premium	Gold Cap SMA	Formula S	Pregestimil	Full strength chicken mix
Protein	1.1 g casein/whey 32/68%	1.5 g casein/whey 40/60%	1.5 g casein/whey 40/60%	1.8 g soya	1.9 g hydrolysed casein	1.5 g–3 g comminuted chicken
Carbohydrate	7.4 g lactose	7.2 g lactose	7.2 g lactose	6.7 g glucose maltodextrin	9.1 g glucose maltose oligosaccharide	6 g–9 g glucose polymer
Fat	4.2 g	3.8 g	3.6 g	3.6 g vegetable oils	2.7 g 40% medium chain triglycerides 60% corn oil	2.5 g–3.5 g medium chain triglycerides
(kcal/100 ml)	71	68	65	67	67	variable

familiar with a small number of feeds in terms of their composition, uses and limitations. In all infants the use of breast milk should be considered, but because of its high lactose content, its use in the compromised bowel is limited.

Lactose intolerance can be managed by using a soya milk formula. Table 5.5 reflects the formulations currently in use in our own unit. The cost of a casein hydrolysate (e.g. Pregestimil) is four times that of a soy milk (e.g. Formula S) and clearly an extravagance for treating simple lactose intolerance.

With the more compromised bowel, protein and fat intake should be considered in addition to the carbohydrate. Protein is best administered in a predigested form using a casein or whey hydrolysate. Fat is the least well absorbed nutrient because of a diminished bile salt pool and the action of bile salts on gastrointestinal bacteria. The use of medium chain triglyceride oil (e.g. Liquigen, Scientific Hospital Supplies Ltd) which is absorbed without prior digestion is helpful, but too rapid introduction may provoke vomiting. The effect of unabsorbed bile salts on the colon can be treated with an oral chelating agent such as cholestyramine but is often poorly tolerated.

In cases of severe intolerance the use of a chicken based formula is helpful, in that the individual constituents of protein, carbohydrate and fat can be varied depending upon tolerance, and different combinations can be used.

In many cases of diarrhoea following gastrointestinal tract insult simple measures suffice. Osmotic diarrhoea confirmed by chromatography of liquid stools can be managed by the use of a lactose-free milk (e.g. soy formula) of low osmolality, with the osmolar load spread by giving small frequent feeds. The use of corn syrup sugars (glucose polymers) utilizes the glucosidase system which can digest short glucose polymers, maltose and limit dextrins. This system is present as early as 26–34 weeks' gestation and is distributed throughout the small bowel [13]. The use of such carbohydrate sources has also been shown to have a beneficial effect on gastric emptying [7].

Bacterial overgrowth may produce diarrhoea as a result of hydrolysis of non-absorbed sugars in the gut [37]. The diagnosis can be confirmed by the early rise in breath hydrogen following an oral sugar load or by aerobic and anaerobic culture of jejunal juice. Treatment is with *oral* broad spectrum antibiotics (e.g. gentamicin 25 mg/kg per day in divided doses). If abnormal bowel dynamics continue, overgrowth is likely to persist particularly with anastomoses of bowel of different calibres. The problem may resolve as bowel diameters become equal.

Non-specific measures to reduce gastric secretion with H_2 blockers and intestinal secretions with antiprostaglandins (e.g. loperamide up to 2.0 mg/kg per day) may be helpful with very short bowel problems. The latter agent also has a useful anti-motility action.

Likely deficiencies through abnormal losses can often be forseen. A high zinc and magnesium requirement is likely in any infant with large stool losses for any reason, e.g. enterostomies, rapid gut transit time. Zinc binding ligands in breast milk make absorption from this source more efficient. Sodium losses are usually also increased, with specialized formulae often requiring supplementation. Calcium requirements are also high partly because of the complexing with unabsorbed fatty acids and also partly because of the exclusion of lactose, which enhances absorption, from all specialized feeds [11,35].

Vitamin deficiencies should also be anticipated. Although most milks are nutritionally complete, insidious B_{12} deficiency is often overlooked. B_{12} supplements (200–1000 µg/month) may need to be given indefinitely if terminal ileal resection has been performed. Onset of overt deficiency may be delayed for many years, often only appearing at a time of increased physiological demand such as puberty [34].

Table 5.6 Basic requirements in a parenteral feeding regimen for a neonate

Fluids and electrolytes	See Tables 5.1a and 5.1b	
Calories (kcal)	100–140	per kg per 24 h
Non-protein kcal/g nitrogen	200–250	per kg per 24 h
Protein (g)	2.5–3.0	per kg per 24 h
Nitrogen (g)	0.4–0.5	per kg per 24 h
Carbohydrate (g)	10–20	per kg per 24 h
Fat (g) (<40% total calories)	1–4	per kg per 24 h
Trace element solution (e.g. Ped-El[a])	2–3 ml	per kg per 24 h
Vitamin solution (e.g. MVI-Paed[a])	1–2 ml	per kg per 24 h

[a]Ped-El (KabiVitrum) and MVI-Paediatric (Armour) are commercially available solutions

The more specialized the feed, the more likely are nutritional deficiencies in terms of vitamins and trace elements, and supplements should be started if appropriate. Every attempt should be made to return the patient to a normal feed as soon as possible.

Parenteral nutrition

The nutritional reserves of a neonate at term are poor compared with the adult and are even more limited in the premature infant. The neonatal period is also a time of rapid growth and development. Failure therefore, to establish full enteral nutrition within the first few days of life (and earlier in preterm infants) is an indication for the provision of an adequate caloric intake by the intravenous route. It is indicated in all infants whose surgical conditions preclude oral intake for periods longer than a few days, e.g. gastroschisis, short bowel syndromes, severe necrotizing enterocolitis.

Regimens for intravenous nutrition must provide adequate fluid, electrolytes, calories, protein in the form of amino acids, carbohydrate, essential fatty acids, vitamins and trace elements.

The basic requirements in a parenteral feeding regimen for a neonate are shown in Table 5.6. Fluid and electrolyte requirements follow the same guidelines as described earlier in this chapter.

Energy sources

Many non-protein sources have been tried, but only glucose and fat are now widely used (see Table 5.7).

Using glucose as the only energy source is problematic (Table 5.8). High concentrations of glucose, and hence high osmolality solutions (Table 5.9) are required to provide sufficient calories. Glucose tolerance is limited in the sick neonate and excessive infusion will precipitate an osmotic diuresis. Infusions of glucose in excess of 5 mg/kg per min are unlikely to be used as energy, and conversion to fat leads to a raised respiratory quotient [10] and fatty liver. Hypoglycaemia is likely if the infusion is stopped abruptly.

Glucose tolerance in sick and preterm neonates is often poor. Insulin infusions may therefore be needed to improve carbohydrate tolerance. Infusions of 0.01–0.02 units/kg per h may be needed, but each case needs individual monitoring. Insulin should be mixed in with the glucose infusion in order to avoid hypoglycaemia occurring if the glucose solution is inadvertently discontinued.

Although it has been shown [16] that intravenous alimentation can be given without using fat emulsions, fat reserves in infants are limited, and catabolism of these to provide essential fatty acids rapidly depletes these reserves. In the older child and the adult lipolysis of endogenous fat will stave off the onset of fatty acid deficiency, for long periods, whereas in the small infant biochemical

Table 5.7 Non-protein calorie sources

Solution		Energy density (kcal/ml) (approx. values)
Intralipid	10%	1
Intralipid	20%	2
Glucose	5%	0.2
Glucose	10%	0.4
Glucose	20%	0.8

Table 5.8 Complications associated with glucose as sole energy source

Hyperglycaemia
Osmotic diuresis
Rebound hypoglycaemia
Hyperosmolar non-ketotic dehydration
Hypophosphataemia
Essential fatty acid deficiency

Table 5.9 Osmolality of solutions

	mOsmol/kg water
Plasma	290
0.9% sodium chloride	308
10% intralipid	300
20% intralipid	350
5% glucose	278
10% glucose	523
20% glucose	1250
8.4% sodium bicarbonate	2000

evidence of fatty acid deficiency has been detected as early as 2 days after starting intravenous feeding [17], with clinical signs and symptoms within 28 days.

Fat emulsions provide high calorific input in low volumes, and also prevent essential fatty acid deficiency. It is therefore reasonable to use a combination of fat and glucose to supply energy requirements.

Complications have been described associated with the infusion of fat emulsions, of which fat embolism in the cerebral and pulmonary circulation and cholestatic jaundice are the most relevant. Factors predisposing to cholestasis are prematurity, a high protein intake, abdominal surgery and sepsis. These complications associated with fat are mostly related to an excessive rate of infusion (>0.15 g/kg per h) so it is important to infuse all the solutions concurrently, thereby spreading the fat infusion over the whole day.

The ability of each patient to clear the fat should be monitored individually. In jaundiced neonates, fat infusions should be used sparingly as they may increase the risk of kernicterus [33] but they can be started in the second week of life without increasing the risk of kernicterus, so long as the bilirubin is less than half the exchange transfusion value for that patient [23].

There is little doubt that a mixture of amino acids, sugars and fat emulsion is more physiological and often tolerated better and therefore preferred [24].

Protein

The ideal amino acid profile for infants is not yet available. In addition to the eight essential amino acids required by adults, infants also need histidine, cystine, tyrosine and possibly taurine. The only solutions currently available in the UK which are complete in these (apart from taurine) are Vamin 9 Glucose (KabiVitrum), and Aminoplasmal Ped (Braun).

Vitamins and trace elements

Water- and fat-soluble vitamins and trace elements should be given or deficiency states will occur. Commercially produced solutions are available. Trace element solutions should be avoided in preterm infants for the first week because of reduced renal clearance and also in infants with hepatic or renal failure.

Trace element requirements are shown in Table 5.10. We use Pedel (see Table 5.11) which is sufficient for most elements except iron and selenium. If iron supplements cannot be tolerated orally, top-up transfusions are given when necessary. The use of highly purified protein solutions for intravenous feeding carries a risk of selenium

deficiency in the long term [18]. Supplements will therefore be required if parenteral or modified enteral feeds are used over a long period.

A comparison of multivitamin solutions for parenteral feeding is given in Table 5.12. We use MVI-Paediatric solution (see Table 5.6).

Table 5.10 Daily trace element requirements [21]

Element	Dose/kg neonates	Dose/kg preterm
Iron	20 µmol	12.6 µmol
Zinc	1.5 µmol	7.5 µmol
Copper	0.3 µmol	1.5 µmol
Manganese	0.12 µmol	0.14 µmol
Chromium	3 nmol	105 nmol
Selenium	0.02 µmol	no figure

Table 5.11 Trace element solutions

	Pedel[a] (4 ml)	Addamel[b] (0.5 ml)	
Calcium (mmol)	0.6	0.25	dose/kg per day
Magnesium (mmol)	0.1	0.075	dose/kg per day
Iron (µmol)	2.0	2.5	dose/kg per day
Zinc (µmol)	0.6	1.0	dose/kg per day
Manganese (µmol)	1.0	2.0	dose/kg per day
Copper (µmol)	0.3	0.25	dose/kg per day
Fluoride (µmol)	0.3	2.5	dose/kg per day
Iodine (µmol)	0.04	0.05	dose/kg per day
Phosphate (mmol)	0.3	—	dose/kg per day
Chloride (mmol)	1.4	0.66	dose/kg per day
Sorbitol (mg)	1200	150	dose/kg per day

[a]Pedel (KabiVitrum) 3–4 ml/kg/day to max of 30 ml
[b]Addamel (KabiVitrum) 0.25–0.5 ml/kg/day to max of 10 ml

Table 5.12 Multivitamin preparations for neonatal use

Solution	Solivito[a] (dose/kg)	MVI-Paed[b] (dose/kg)	Vitlipid infant[a] (dose/kg)
Thiamine (B$_1$) (mg)	0.12	0.12	
Riboflavin (B$_2$) (mg)	0.18	0.14	
Nicotinamide (mg)	1.0	1.7	
Pyridoxine (B$_6$) (mg)	0.2	0.1	
Pantothenic acid (mg)	1.0	0.5	
Biotin (mg)	0.03	0.002	
Folic acid (mg)	0.02	0.014	
Cyanocobalamin (µg)	0.2	0.1	
Ascorbic acid (mg)	3.0	8.0	
Retinol (A) (IU)		230	333
Calciferol (D) (IU)		40	100
Phytomenactione (µg)		20	50
Tocopherol (E) (IU)		0.7	

[a]KabiVitrum
[b]Armour

Intravenous feeding at Alder Hey

Long-term intravenous alimentation of infants requires specialized skills from the medical, nursing and pharmacy staff, and therefore is not for the occasional user, but it can be life-saving. Normal growth and development have been seen in infants receiving total parenteral nutrition for several years. However, long-term therapy has many dangers and should not be carried out except in special centres with staff experienced in this type of therapy.

In a 2-year period, 135 children had total parenteral nutrition at Alder Hey Children's Hospital, Liverpool; 58 of these were surgical neonates (of whom 22 were preterm) and they received total parenteral nutrition for a range of 4–101 days (mean 24 days).

These children suffered from a variety of surgical conditions, including all the seven children admitted with gastroschisis during that period, four out of the six cases of meconium ileus, four children with Hirschsprung's colitis (out of 15 neonates presenting with Hirschsprung's disease), and 17 of the 21 patients with necrotizing enterocolitis.

Practical guidelines

The solutions should be mixed using a full aseptic technique, preferably by the pharmacy in a laminar airflow cabinet. Addition of electrolytes or drugs on the ward risks the introduction of bacteria with possible resultant sepsis. The fat solution is not mixed with the glucose, amino acid and electrolyte solution because of instability of the emulsion with the high concentration of divalent cations used in paediatric regimens.

Carbohydrates are introduced in a stepwise fashion, increasing the quantity daily, to allow the appropriate endogenous insulin response to occur, and thus prevent hyperglycaemia and subsequent osmotic diuresis. To achieve efficient protein utilization 200–250 non-protein calories are required per gram of nitrogen infused. Acidosis may occur with excessive amino acid infusions, and hence the protein should also be introduced stepwise along with the carbohydrates.

Monitoring

Monitoring of the various blood parameters needs to be more frequent initially as the parenteral nutrition is being introduced. As fat infusions may interfere with the estimation of urea and electrolytes, the fat should be discontinued 4 h before the blood is sampled. If the plasma is still lipaemic, fat clearance is impaired, and the fat infusion rate should be reduced.

Urea, glucose, sodium, potassium, chloride, protein, albumin, calcium and phosphate should be measured on a daily basis initially. Alterations to the electrolyte content of the feed are then made according to these results. The decision whether to add insulin should be reviewed each day as the glucose concentration in the parenteral feed is increased.

Magnesium, acid-base balance and liver function tests should be measured weekly. Monthly measurements of clotting, iron, copper, zinc, vitamin B_{12} and folate levels, and 3-monthly measurements of thyroxine and selenium levels should also be made in those patients receiving long-term parenteral or specialized enteral nutrition.

Techniques of intravenous therapy

Most neonates requiring surgery need intravenous infusions or blood transfusion during operation. Postoperatively they will require fluids by the intravenous route until enteral feeding can be established. With the recent advances in delivery systems (i.e. fine bore cannulas and central venous catheters, and volumetric infusion pumps) fluids, electrolytes and nutrition can be given to neonates for periods of many weeks, and even months. The non-volumetric pumps (i.e. drip counting devices) are too inaccurate for use in small infants, and should not be used.

Peripheral infusion

The use of peripheral veins is always preferred so as to reduce infective complications. Neonates can be managed for considerable periods in this way as they have many peripheral veins in the scalp and limbs which can be cannulated in rotation with the currently available fine cannulas.

The parenteral nutrition infusion into a peripheral vein should be limited to a glucose solution of about 10% as the more hypertonic solutions may produce local necrosis if extravasation occurs.

Fixation of the cannula is very important, to ensure that it does not move. Various methods are available, which are very much of personal preference, but the site of entry of the cannula into the vein must be visible, so that extravasation can be detected as soon as possible.

Central venous infusion

This becomes necessary when peripheral sites have been exhausted, or may be selected if intravenous nutrition is anticipated to be long term or if solutions of glucose stronger than 10% need to be used.

Percutaneous techniques

Fine silastic catheters can be introduced via a scalp or arm vein, e.g. the brachial vein [29]. Silastic tubing can be threaded into the vein and advanced into the superior vena cava. Percutaneous puncture of the external jugular vein is often easy, as it distends when the baby is lying with a head-down tilt; unfortunately however, the catheter cannot always be advanced into the superior vena cava because of the angle the vein forms behind the clavicle.

It is becoming increasingly common for cannulation of the internal jugular or subclavian veins to be done percutaneously. It is well recognized that thrombosis can occur if the catheter tip is in the axillary, subclavian or jugular veins and is used for hypertonic parenteral nutrition solutions. It is important that the catheter tip lies in the superior vena cava or right atrium, where there is enough flow of blood to facilitate mixing of blood and nutrient fluid, so as to minimize the risk of venous thrombosis. The correct positioning of the catheter tip must be checked with an X-ray before using it for hypertonic solutions.

In adults it has been found that when using the inferior vena cava via the femoral vein (which can be reached by direct puncture of the femoral vein, or by cannulation of the long saphenous vein at the ankle or knee level) there is an increased risk of thrombotic and septic complications. The same holds good for neonates, and femoral veins should never be used unless all other sites are unavailable.

It is usually only possible to cannulate these larger veins when the baby is under general anaesthesia. The procedure should be carried out under strict aseptic conditions, if possible in the operating theatre. The skin where the stab is to be carried out must be disinfected and surrounded by sterile towels. The operator must scrub up and wear gown, mask and gloves.

Various systems are manufactured specifically for the percutaneous cannulation of central veins in babies, either by threading the catheter directly into the needle which enters the vein, or by the Seldinger technique which involves threading a wire down the needle which has entered the vein. The needle is removed, the catheter is threaded over the wire into position in the central vein and then the wire is removed.

Internal jugular vein

The baby is placed in a slight head-down position. This helps to distend the vein, which can then be punctured more easily, and decreases the risk of air embolus. The head of the patient is turned at 45 degrees away from the midline towards the side which is not being cannulated. The neck is extended by placing a rolled up towel between the shoulder blades, and the arms are placed at the sides of the baby.

The entry site for puncture is halfway down the sternomastoid muscle just lateral to the palpable pulsations of the internal carotid artery (Figure

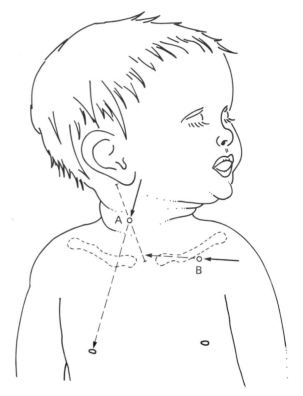

Figure 5.1 A diagrammatic representation of the entry point and needle direction for percutaneous puncture of the right internal jugular vein (A) and left subclavian vein (B)

5.1A). The needle is introduced directly through the muscle and then angled to be parallel to the carotid sheath, aiming towards the nipple on the side of puncture. A 5–10 ml syringe containing a few ml of 0.9% sodium chloride solution is attached to the needle, and the syringe is continuously aspirated during its advancement, so that when the needle enters the internal jugular vein, good backflow of dark venous blood occurs. The sodium chloride solution is then injected and aspirated as the needle is advanced into the vein, to confirm its safe position inside the vein. The syringe is removed, and the catheter (or Seldinger wire and then the catheter) is introduced and advanced into the superior vena cava. The final position is checked with an X-ray, and the catheter is then sutured into position.

Subclavian vein

The technique and position for subclavian puncture is similar to that for the internal jugular. However, the face is turned towards the side of venous puncture to prevent the catheter entering the internal jugular vein instead of the superior vena cava.

The skin is punctured below and just lateral to the midpoint of the clavicle (Figure 5.1B). The needle is then advanced tangentially to the thorax below the clavicle in the direction of the suprasternal notch. Free return of blood into the syringe again confirms its position in the subclavian vein, and when the needle is safely inside the vein, the catheter is introduced as long as there is no resistance. The position of the catheter must again be checked with an X-ray, which will also allow the operator to exclude the complication of pneumothorax.

Operative techniques

Where peripheral infusions or percutaneous central infusion techniques are not possible, we are currently using a Broviac silastic catheter, 4 Fr gauge, inside diameter 0.7 mm. This catheter has a Dacron cuff attached which ensures firm fixation by fibrous tissue. There are various manufacturers of these Broviac catheters, but we are currently using the Evermed (Schuco Ltd).

The size of the catheter is such that in neonates the internal jugular vein has to be used, either directly, as described below, or indirectly via the common facial vein. This is approached via a transverse cervical incision above the clavicle. The

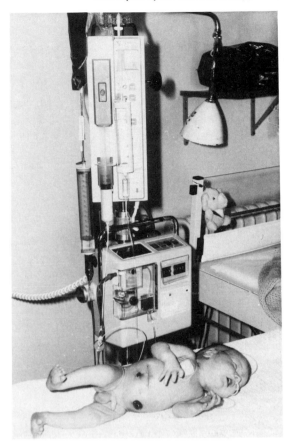

Figure 5.3 A neonate with a central line *in situ*, attached to his IV feeding solutions

sternomastoid muscle is split, and the internal jugular vein is mobilized between two sloops. The catheter is then tunnelled from an entry point on the chest wall (avoiding the future breast area), and the Dacron cuff is positioned subcutaneously, close to the skin entry site.

The catheter entry site into the vein is immobilized and haemostasis achieved by using a purse-string stitch (e.g. 5/0 silk). The use of this technique (rather than ligation of the vein) has enabled us to re-use the same internal jugular vein on subsequent occasions in patients who require very long-term intravenous feeding.

The catheter length required to reach the superior vena cava and right atrium from the entry point in the internal jugular vein is estimated by equating that point with the nipple on that side. The catheter is cut to length and introduced inside the purse-string stitch via a small transverse venotomy. Haemostasis is maintained by the assistant's retraction on the two sloops around the internal jugular vein, apart from the moment of catheter introduction when the assistant relaxes on the lower sloop,

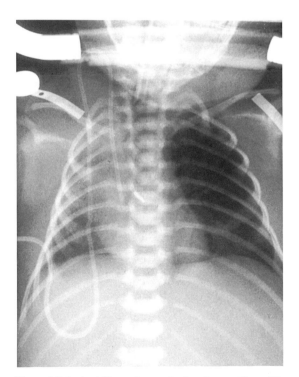

Figure 5.2 A chest X-ray demonstrating the position of the central vein catheter

allowing the catheter to enter the internal jugular vein and then the superior vena cava.

The catheter position is checked with an X-ray (Figure 5.2), and if it is in a satisfactory position, the purse-string is tied gently but firmly around the catheter to produce haemostasis but without occluding the catheter. The wounds are then closed; subcuticular sutures can be used in the neck incision, but we generally use a nylon suture at the skin entry site to hold the catheter steady until the wound heals and the Dacron cuff 'beds' in.

The central vein catheter can then be connected to the total parenteral feeding system (Figure 5.3).

Complications of central venous access

Placement of central venous catheters can cause damage to adjacent structures, including nerves, arteries and pleura, but the danger is minimized if the catheter is introduced under direct vision by an operative technique. This may be preferred in neonates, except when percutaneous puncture can be carried out by experienced staff.

Air embolus could be a hazard, and great care must be taken to ensure that air is never allowed to enter the administration set or line leading to the central venous catheter. The routine use of an air-venting filter is recommended in neonates with a central vein catheter *in situ*.

Infection in a central venous catheter can be a major problem, and a scrupulous aseptic technique must be adhered to for all access procedures.

Septicaemia is not necessarily an indication for removal of the line. Initially central line and peripheral vein blood cultures should be taken, along with a complete septic screen, and intravenous broad spectrum antibiotics (e.g. cefuroxime and gentamicin) should be commenced, given via the central line. The initial antibiotics must be anti-staphylococcal as the commonest pathogen is coagulase negative staphylococcus. The antibiotics are changed if necessary when the cultures are available with the appropriate sensitivity patterns. The fat infusion is discontinued until the septicaemia is under control and when it is recommenced, lipid clearance is monitored and the flow rate of the fat adjusted if necessary.

We have found it possible to sterilize infected catheters in this manner, and have been able to continue using them for parenteral nutrition throughout the episode of infection; this is especially valuable in neonates with their limited venous access.

References

1. Anderson, J.M., Bain, A.D., Brown, J.K., Cockburn, F., Forfar, J.O., Machin, G.A. *et al.*, (1976) Hyaline membrane disease, alkaline buffer treatment and cerebral intraventricular haemorrhage. *Lancet*, **i**, 117–119

2. Atwell, J.D. (1966) Magnesium deficiency following neonatal surgical procedure. *J. Pediat. Surg.*, **1**, 427–440

3. Aynsley-Green, A., Lucas, A. and Bloom, S.R. (1980) The control of the adaptation of the human neonate to postnatal nutrition. *Acta Chir. Scand.*, (Suppl.), **507**, 269–281

4. Banister, A., Matin-Siddiqi, S.A. and Hatcher, G.W. (1975) Treatment of hypernatraemic dehydration in infancy. *Arch. Dis. Child.*, **50**, 179–186

5. Bell, E.F., Warburton, D., Stonestreet, B.S. and Oh, W. (1979) High volume fluid intake predisposes premature infants to necrotizing enterocolitis. *Lancet*, **ii**, 90

6. Bell, E.F., Warburton, D., Stonestreet, B.S. and Oh, W. (1980) Effect of fluid administration on the development of symptomatic patent ductus arteriosus and congestive heart failure in premature infants. *New Engl. J. Med.*, **302**, 598–604

7. Bieberdorf, F.A., Morawski, S. and Fordtran, J.S. (1975) Effect of sodium, mannitol and magnesium on glucose, galactose, 3-*O*-methylglucose and fructose absorption in the human ileum. *Gastroenterology*, **68**, 58–66

8. Brans, Y.W. (1977) Parenteral nutrition of the very low birth weight neonate: a critical view. *Clin. Perinatol.*, **4**, 367–376

9. Brooke, O.G. (1982) Low birth weight babies, nutrition and feeding. *Br. J. Hosp. Med.*, **28**, 462–469

10. Burke, J.F., Wolfe, R.R., Mullany, C.J., Mathews, D.E. and Bier, D.M. (1979) Glucose requirements following burn injury. Parameters of optimal glucose infusion and possible hepatic and respiratory abnormalities following excessive glucose intake. *Ann. Surg.*, **190**, 274–285

11. Charley, P. and Saltman, P. (1963) Chelation of calcium by lactose; its role in transport mechanisms. *Science*, **139**, 1205–1206

12. Coran, A.G., Das, J.B. and Eraklis, A.J. (1971) Use of osmometry in the preoperative and postoperative management of the newborn. *J. Pediat. Surg.*, **6**, 529–534

13. Dahlqist, A. and Lindberg, T. (1966) Development of the intestinal disaccharidase and alkaline phosphatase activities in the human fetus. *Clin. Sci.*, **30**, 517–528

14. Davidson, A.N. and Dobbing, J. (1968) The developing brain. In *Applied Neurochemistry* (ed. A.N. Davidson and J. Dobbing), Blackwell Scientific Publications, Oxford

15. Dobbing, J. and Sands, J. (1973) Quantitative growth and development of human brain. *Arch. Dis. Child.*, **48**, 757–767

16. Dudrick, S.J., Wilmore, D.W., Vars, H.M. and Rhoads, J.E. (1969) Can intravenous feeding as the sole means of nutrition support growth in the child and restore weight loss in the adult?. *Ann. Surg.*, **169**, 974–984

17. Friedman, Z., Danon, A., Stahlman, M.T. and Oates, J.A. (1976) Rapid onset of essential fatty acid deficiency in the newborn. *Pediatrics*, **58**, 640–649

18. Fleming, C.R., Lee, J.T., McCall, J.T. *et al.* (1982) Selenium deficiency and fatal cardiomyopathy in a patient on home parenteral nutrition. *Gastroenterology*, **83**, 689–693

19. Gross, S.J., Oehler, J.M. and Eckerman, C.O. (1983) Head growth and developmental outcome in very low birth weight infants. *Pediatrics*, **71**, 70–75

20. Heird, W.C., Driscoll, J.M., Schullinger, J.N., Grebin, B. and Winters, R.W. (1972) Intravenous alimentation in pediatric patients. *J. Pediat.*, **80**, 351–372

21. James, B.E., Hendry, P.G. and MacMahon, R.A. (1979) Total parenteral nutrition of premature infants. 2. Requirement for micronutrient elements. *Aust. Paediat. J.*, **15**, 67–71

22. Jones, M.D. Jr, Gresham, E.L. and Battaglia, F.C. (1972) Urinary flow rates and urea excretion rates in newborn infants. *Biol. Neonat.*, **21**, 321–329

23. Kerner, J.A. Jr (ed.) *Manual of Pediatric Parenteral Nutrition*, John Wiley & Sons, New York, 1983

24. Kim, S.H. and Rickham, P.P. (1972) Parenteral lipids and amino acids in surgical neonates. *Z. Kinderchir.*, **11**, 277

25. Lucas, A., Aynsley-Green, A. and Bloom, S.R. (1981) Gut hormones and the first meals. *Clin. Sci.*, **60**, 349–353

26. McCance, R.A., Naylor, N.J.B. and Widdowson, E.M. (1954) The response of infants to a large dose of water. *Arch. Dis. Child.*, **29**, 104–109

27. McLean, F. and Hastings, A. (1935) The state of calcium in the fluids of the body. I. The conditions affecting the ionization of calcium. *J. Biol. Chem.*, **108**, 285–322

28. Oh, W. (1982) Fluid and electrolyte therapy and parenteral nutrition in low birth weight infants. *Clin. Perinatol.*, **9**, 637–643

29. Puntis, J.W.L. (1986) Percutaneous insertion of central venous feeding catheters. *Arch. Dis. Child.*, **61**, 1138–1140

30. Roy, R.N. and Sinclair, J.C. (1975) Hydration of the low birth weight infant. *Clin. Perinatol.*, **2**, 393–417

31. Shires, T., Williams, J. and Brown, F. (1961) Acute change in extracellular fluids associated with major surgical procedures. *Ann. Surg.*, **154**, 803–810

32. Stewart, A.L., Reynolds, E.O.R. and Lipscomb, A.P. (1981) Outcome for infants of very low birth weight: survey of world literature. *Lancet*, **i**, 1038–1041

33. Thiessen, H., Jacobsen, J. and Brodersen, R. (1972) Displacement of albumin-bound bilirubin by fatty acids. *Acta Paediat. Scand.*, **61**, 285–288

34. Valman, H.B. and Roberts, P.D. (1974) Vitamin B_{12} absorption after resection of ileum in childhood. *Arch. Dis. Child.*, **49**, 932 935

35. Wasserman, R.H. (1964) Lactose-stimulated intestinal absorption of calcium; a theory. *Nature*, **201**, 997–999

36. Weinstein, L.D., Shoemaker, C.P., Hersh, T. and Wright, H.K. (1969) Enhanced intestinal absorption after small bowel resection in man. *Arch. Surg.*, **99**, 560–562

37. Weser, E. (1979) Nutritional aspects of malabsorption: short gut adaptation. *Am. J. Med.*, **67**, 1014–1020

38. Wilmore, D.W. (1972) Factors correlating with a successful outcome following extensive intestinal resection in newborn infants. *J. Pediat.*, **80**, 88–95

39. Winick, M. and Rosso, P. (1969) Head circumference and cellular growth of the brain in normal and marasmic children. *J. Pediat.*, **74**, 774–778

40. Winick, M. and Rosso, P. (1969) The effect of severe early malnutrition on cellular growth of human brain. *Pediat. Res.*, **3**, 181–184

41. Wu, P.Y.K. and Hodgman, J.E. (1974) Insensible water loss in preterm infants; changes with postnatal development and non-ionizing radiant energy. *Pediatrics*, **54**, 704–712

6

General operative techniques and equipment

R.E. Cudmore

Positioning the infant prior to surgery

The baby is taken to the operating theatre either in an incubator or overhead warmer.

The operating theatre should already have been pre-warmed to a temperature of 28–30°C with a thermostatically controlled water blanket already in place and warmed up pre-operatively. The warm water blanket seems to be the best arrangement for keeping a baby warm during surgery. A disposable aluminium foil diathermy pad is placed on the operating table but will not be connected to the diathermy machine until the baby is on the table. The infant is then transferred directly from the incubator to the operating table and covered with thick gamgee, previously warmed, in order to preserve body heat during induction of anaesthesia. Once anaesthesia has been commenced and the monitoring devices and intravenous catheters securely fixed, the baby is positioned appropriately for the operation. Suitable preparation of the skin is achieved with an antiseptic solution, Hibitane 5% in methylated spirit being our usual skin preparation material. When the alcohol in the skin preparation has evaporated a large adherent plastic drape is laid over the baby so that it is completely covered by the plastic material. Care is taken to ensure that the plastic sheet does not adhere to the anaesthetic tubes or drip sites by covering these areas with gauze. This method is much better than placing gamgee around the baby as has been previously recommended. With the plastic sheeting in place, the usual sterile drapes are placed around the operation site and the operation is commenced.

Incisions

Abdominal

Abdominal incisions for specialized procedures are described in the relevant chapters. The most useful and frequently employed incision is a transverse supraumbilical one (Figure 6.1) which provides easy access to virtually every part of the peritoneal cavity and allows stomata to be placed in the lower abdomen away from the main incision. It also leaves the lower abdomen free of scars for later definitive surgery in colorectal problems. It heals well and even in the presence of infection it rarely disrupts. The incision is best placed more to the right than left of the mid-line although it can be extended in either direction as indicated by the findings at laparotomy. In duodenal obstruction the incision may be made further towards the right flank whilst procedures in the lower abdomen may be best carried out through a more oblique left-sided lower abdominal incision.

After the skin has been incised, fat and muscle can be divided easily and fairly bloodlessly with the cutting diathermy. The rectus muscle is divided, care being taken to coagulate the superior epigastric vessels. It is not always necessary to ligate and divide the umbilical vein, if for instance, the incision is placed towards the right as when approaching the duodenum. The peritoneum is picked up with forceps and opened with scissors. Diathermy should not be used since bowel is at risk, especially if it is dilated. At the end of the operative procedure, the abdominal wall is closed in layers. The peritoneum in a small baby is very fragile and it is therefore

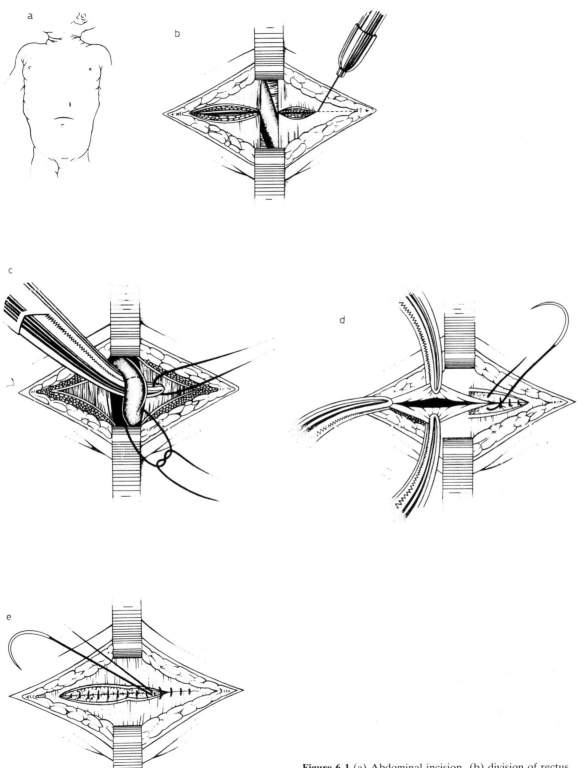

Figure 6.1 (a) Abdominal incision, (b) division of rectus,
(c) ligation of umbilical vein, (d) closure of peritoneum,
(e) closure of anterior rectus sheath

necessary to place the first layer of stitches through the posterior rectus sheath and peritoneum together. The anterior sheath is then apposed in the usual way using a continuous stitch of 3/0 Vicryl (Ethicon Ltd) which we have found much better than chromic catgut. Closure of the fat can be obtained with a few sutures of 4/0 chromic catgut and the skin itself closed using Steristrips or subcuticular Vicryl. There is no need to close the skin wound with sutures. In the infant who has been grossly distended and in whom there is thought to be a definite risk of wound dehiscence, deep tension sutures can be used, being tied over 'dental rolls' as indicated in Figure 6.2.

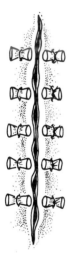

Figure 6.2 Method of tying horizontal mattress, deep tension sutures over 'dental rolls' of compressed cotton wool

More recently, interest has been shown in mass closure of the wound using PDS (polydioxazone sulphate) of 3/0 or 2/0 strength. This mass closure has been shown to be a superior technique in adults [6] and has long been used for the closure of a burst abdomen [8]. Kiely and Spitz [9], in a prospective study of 507 children including 108 neonates, found no significant differences in the incidence of wound dehiscence or incisional hernias related to the use of mass or layered techniques for abdominal closure. The mass technique is simple and quick provided an adequate length of suture (three to four times the length of the wound) is used and is entirely reliable. Long experience with layered closures has led us to use this technique as a routine, but if there is gross abdominal distension there is certainly a place for mass closure.

Occasionally, for pelvic pathology, a subumbilical incision may be indicated. The suprapubic transverse incision is made in an identical manner to the supraumbilical one. Care must be taken to coagulate the inferior epigastric vessels running deeply along the lateral border of the rectus. The two umbilical arteries and the urachus are then isolated and tied. As the neonatal bladder is largely an abdominal organ, the peritoneal incision has to be made at a considerably higher level than the skin incision. The wound is closed in a similar way to the supraumbilical transverse incision.

In infants who are very distended and in infants who have free pus in the abdominal cavity, wound dehiscence is a definite risk. In these children the use of deep tension sutures is recommended. If wound dehiscence does occur the incision must be repaired with the aid of tension sutures. If the breakdown produces a sizeable abdominal wall defect, repair by direct suture may be extremely difficult. In these cases the defect may be covered by sewing a piece of Silastic sheeting over the defect to the margins of the abdominal defect. This sheeting can be removed a week later, leaving an area covered with granulation tissue which may either be allowed to epithelialize or be covered by a skin graft [2].

Thoracotomy

The baby is placed on the operating table in the lateral position with a rolled towel beneath the heating blanket. This allows the chest wall to be bowed convexly so that the ribs separate much more easily once the incision is started. The upper arm is abducted to a suitable position and secured by adhesive strapping. Entry into the chest is usually made through the 4th/5th intercostal space commencing posteriorly just lateral to the spine and extending below the scapula to the anterior axillary line (Figure 6.3).

Having made the skin incision with a scalpel, the muscles are divided with diathermy and the intercostal space exposed. There is no need to remove a rib in small babies and the easiest way of entering the chest at this point is to incise the periosteum with diathermy along the superior border of the rib and elevate it from the bone. This prevents damage to the intercostal vessels and nerve and allows easy division of the intercostal muscles. As most thoracotomies in small babies are used for approaching the oesophagus, where an extrapleural approach is desirable, the intercostal muscle can then be reflected using a Macdonald dissector which allows easy access to the pleura and will not damage it. If a transpleural approach is to be used the pleura is easily opened by scissors, otherwise the pleura is swept away with dabs as described in Chapter 21. Once the initial opening has been made into the intercostal space a Finochietto infant rib spreader (Figure 6.4) is inserted between the ribs and by

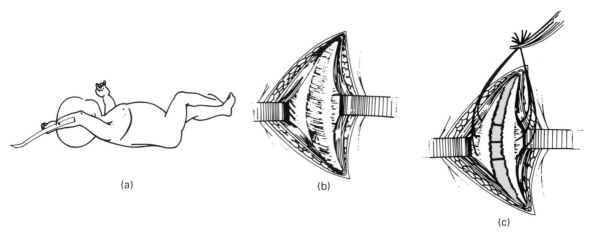

(a) (b) (c)

Figure 6.3 (a) Thoracotomy incision, (b) exposure of ribs and intercostal space, (c) closure of incision

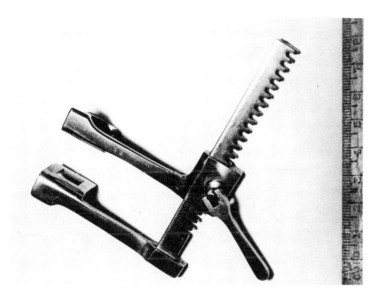

Figure 6.4 Finochietto infant rib spreader

cutting the muscle further forward and backwards, the retractor can be spread more widely.

Closure of the chest wound is very simple; three of four 3/0 vicryl sutures are placed around the ribs to draw them together and then the muscles are closed in layers using the same material with interrupted sutures. The position of the thoracic muscles is not always easy to identify and care is needed to ensure that each layer is closed in the right way. Sometimes it is useful to mark the muscles as the incision is made but most surgeons will learn by experience how the muscles are apposed. The skin and superficial fat are then closed as in closure of an abdominal incision.

Oesophagoscopy

Both rigid and fibre-optic oesophagoscopy can be carried out in small infants. Rigid oesophagoscopy is usually reserved for dilating the oesophagus if necessary after tracheo-oesophageal surgery. The standard Negus oesophagoscope with fibre-optic illumination is perfectly adequate.

Technique

The infant is placed supine on the operating table and after induction of anaesthesia, the endotracheal tube should be moved to one corner of the mouth so that easy access can be obtained to the pharynx and the oesophagus. The operator's left index finger is inserted onto the upper gum margin and acts both to steady the tube and to protect the baby's gum and upper lip. The assistant places a hand into the small of the back between the shoulder blades so that the chest can be elevated as required. The oesophago-scope is passed gently over the tongue into the pharynx and down the oesophagus. There is usually some hold up at the cricopharyngeus but this can be overcome with gentle advancement of the scope. Frequent suction is often necessary. Once the strictured area is seen, dilators can be passed at will. Gum-elastic bougies are preferable and, when well lubricated, are easily passed up to the required diameter. Dilatation should be performed under direct vision and with great gentleness. In experi-enced hands it can often be done, using a gum-elastic bougie, by feel and without direct vision, but it is important to look at the size of the stricture before attempting the dilatation.

Oesophago-gastroscopy

Oesophago-gastroscopy is carried out using a fibre-optic instrument such as the Olympus GIF P020. The diameter of the smallest instrument is about 7 mm and this can easily be passed down a small baby's oesophagus without any damage. Direct vision will give an indication of the size of an oesophageal stricture, reflux if present, the degree of this and erosion of the lower oesophagus. It is rarely necessary to gastroscope small infants though if need be this can easily be achieved. Dilatation with gum-elastic bougies has to some extent been replaced by balloon dilatation in recent years; the

gastroscope can be used to identify the strictured area through which a guide wire is passed prior to passage of the balloon (see Chapter 19).

Laparoscopy

Indications

Laparoscopy has by now been widely practised in adult medicine and surgery. Although there are relatively few indications for its use in neonates it can be of great value, especially in hepatic problems and in intersex conditions [1,3,4,5].

As it allows the taking of much larger specimens than those obtained by needle biopsy, it has been proved to be a very useful procedure in the diagnosis of metabolic diseases of the liver and in the differential diagnosis between neonatal hepatitis and biliary atresia. It has also proved to be useful in the diagnosis of hepatic and other intra-abdominal neoplasms. Finally, it has become the method of choice in the evaluation of the various intersex conditions because the intra-abdominal genitalia can be directly observed and, if necessary, biopsies can be taken.

Instruments

The standard equipment for laparoscopy comprises the following instruments (Figure 6.5). (a) Special pneumoperitoneum needle with spring-controlled blunt stylet stopcock and Luer-Lock connection (Veress needle), trocar and cannula. (b) Hopkins rod lens telescope, 30 degrees with insufflation sheath and stopcock. (c) Smaller cannula and trocar for separate manipulation. (d) Insulated biopsy forceps which can also be used for coagulation.

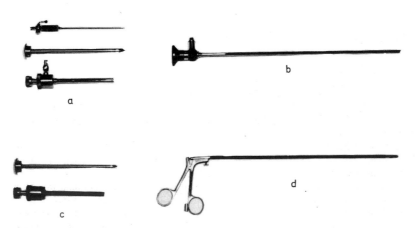

Figure 6.5 For description, see text

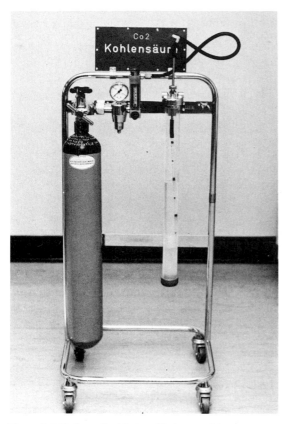

Figure 6.6 Carbon dioxide insufflation machine

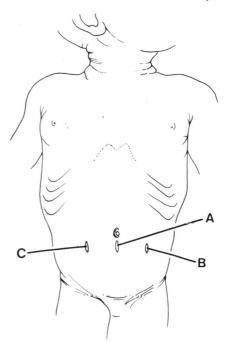

Figure 6.7 Schematic drawing showing punctures for laparoscopy. For description, see text

In addition, a carbon dioxide insufflator has to be used to produce a pneumoperitoneum (Figure 6.6).

Technique [7]

In infants, laparoscopy must always be carried out under general anaesthesia and muscle relaxants as the pneumoperitoneum causes a marked restriction of the diaphragmatic movements.

A small incision is made below the umbilicus (Figure 6.7) (A) and the abdomen is punctured with a Veress needle. The peritoneal cavity is filled with the aid of the carbon dioxide insufflator until the intra-abdominal pressure is raised to about 10 mmHg. Insufflation is carried out slowly to avoid cardiovascular or respiratory difficulties.

The Veress needle is withdrawn and the trocar and cannula are inserted. The trocar is withdrawn and replaced by the telescope. The abdominal cavity can now be inspected. For more complicated manipulation in the region of the liver and right ovary, the smaller cannula for the biopsy forceps can be inserted at point B (Figure 6.7). For inspection of the left ovary, point C (Figure 6.7) may be found to be more advantageous.

References

1. Cognat, M., Papathanassiou, Z. and Gomel, V. (1974) Laparoscopy in infants and adolescents. *J. Reprod. Med.*, **13**, 11–12
2. Cudmore, R.E., Zachary, R.B. and Lister, J. (1970) Silastic sheeting for abdominal wall defects. *Lancet*, **ii**, 666
3. Estrada, R.M. and Cordova, V.L. (1974) Laparoscopia infantil. *Rev. Cuba Pediat.*, **46**, 1283–1286
4. Gans, S.L. and Berci, G. (1971) Advances in endoscopy of infants and children. *J. Pediat. Surg.*, **6**, 199–233
5. Gans, S.L. and Berci, G. (1973) Peritoneoscopy in infants and children. *J. Pediat. Surg.*, **8**, 399–405
6. Goligher, J.C., Irvin, T.T., Johnston, D., De Dombal, F.T., Hill, G.L. and Horrocks, J.C. (1975) A controlled clinical trial of three methods of closure of laparotomy wounds. *Br. J. Surg.*, **62**, 823–829
7. Karamehmedovic, O., Dangel, P., Hirsig, J. and Rickham, P.P. (1977) Laparoscopy in childhood. *J. Pediat. Surg.*, **12**, 75–81
8. Jenkins, T.P.N. (1976) The burst abdominal wound: a mechanical aproach. *Br. J. Surg.*, **63**, 873–876
9. Kiely, E.M. and Spitz, L. (1985) Layered versus mass closure of abdominal wounds in infants and children. *Br. J. Surg.*, **72**, 739–740

7

Antenatal diagnosis and its relevance to paediatric surgeons

D.W. Pilling

The most important method of antenatal diagnosis in the 1980s is the ultrasound examination but this is not the only method of diagnosing or screening for fetal abnormality. This chapter will deal only with the ultrasound aspect of antenatal diagnosis but serum alpha-fetoprotein screening, amniocentesis for alpha-fetoprotein assay and for chromosome culture and, more recently, chorionic biopsy are methods which all have a very important part to play. Magnetic resonance imaging [14] has been used but is unlikely to be widely available nor as valuable as ultrasound because of long exposure times and the problems of fetal movement.

Great changes occurred in paediatric surgery in the 1970s due to prenatal diagnosis, particularly in reducing the number of children born with spina bifida. Since that time improvement in ultrasound equipment and widespread use of real-time equipment in particular has taken antenatal diagnosis even further and increased its relevance to paediatric surgeons. Prior to the widespread availability of real-time ultrasound in the early 1980s it was possible only to undertake comprehensive ultrasound scanning of a small number of fetuses because compound static B scanning, whilst being a high resolution technique, was very time consuming and required a very high degree of operator skill (and patience) and this was only available in a small number of teaching centres.

The technological improvement in ultrasound has meant increasing rapidity of scanning, the training of radiographers and technicians has meant wider availability, and the possibility of 'routine' scanning for fetal abnormalities has become feasible in many district general hospitals. It is, however, very time consuming and there is a relatively small return (2.3/1000 live births even for the commonest abnormality–spina bifida) so that some method of

Table 7.1 Clinical indicators for comprehensive ultrasound scans

Previous fetal abnormality
Raised maternal serum alpha-fetoprotein
Maternal diabetes
Multiple pregnancies
Abnormalities associated with the pregnancy, e.g. oligohydramnios, polyhydramnios or evidence of intrauterine growth retardation

selecting high risk cases has to be considered in most centres. A suggested list of clinical indications justifying comprehensive scanning is given in Table 7.1.

The ultrasound literature in the last few years contains innumerable reports of fetal abnormalities diagnosable by ultrasound and if sufficient time can be given to the examination the conditions which can be recognized include most of those with a macroscopic anomaly. It can, however, be argued that as well as this being an expensive and time-consuming technique, telling the mother that the fetus she is bearing has an abnormality about which nothing can be done will inevitably cause anxiety for some weeks prior to delivery. It is equally difficult, however, for a doctor to know about an abnormality and not to inform the patient. Whilst errors in diagnosis are becoming less common some unnecessary anxiety is caused when an abnormality previously suggested by ultrasound is not confirmed when the infant is delivered. Only increasing experience and training are likely to reduce this problem but it will never be abolished.

Ultrasound diagnosis of fetal abnormality has two aims. The first is to diagnose abnormalities which are so severe that if the baby were to survive it would be either severely handicapped or early death could be predicted. The early diagnosis of these conditions and the offer of termination of pregnancy should be the aim, to save the mother carrying an abnormal fetus to term for which the outlook would be hopeless. Such diagnoses should obviously be made ideally before 20 weeks of pregnancy, so that later termination can be avoided. The second aim of antenatal diagnosis should be, in the case of the less severe abnormalities, to enable counselling of the parents as to the likely outcome of the pregnancy and to aid the obstetrician in determining any modification of the management of the pregnancy and labour which might be necessary in the light of the known fetal abnormality. It is essential in these circumstances to involve the paediatrician and a paediatric surgeon in the counselling as their wide experience of the management of fetal abnormalities is very helpful in giving an accurate prognosis and reassurance to the parents.

One problem that has become evident recently is that it is not always possible to extrapolate prognosis of a surgical condition diagnosed at birth back to the same abnormality diagnosed in the second trimester of pregnancy. Examples of this include diaphragmatic hernia where the prognosis is very poor for those diagnosed early in pregnancy because of the prolonged lung compression and consequent pulmonary hypoplasia. It is clear from the work of Allen *et al.* [3] that the prognosis for cardiac lesions is similarly not as good when diagnosed early in pregnancy as for the same lesion diagnosed postnatally. The outcome for antenatally diagnosed hydronephrosis is similarly less predictable than in the postnatal situation, although sometimes the outcome for renal function and dilatation of collecting systems is better than would be predicted from the prenatal and immediate postnatal appearances.

The literature on antenatal diagnosis by ultrasound is very extensive but much of it is not relevant to paediatric surgery; hence only those conditions directly relevant to paediatric surgery will be discussed here. The reader is referred to Campbell and Pearce [5] for a review of the subject.

The discussion of the individual abnormalities diagnosed by ultrasound in the succeeding paragraphs follows the order in which these conditions appear in the remainder of the book and is not in order of incidence or of ease of diagnosis.

The skull and central nervous system

The most frequently encountered fetal abnormalities which can be diagnosed by ultrasound and towards which most antenatal diagnosis is aimed are abnormalities of the central nervous system. Hydrocephalus is a relatively straightforward diagnosis which can be made in some cases as early as 14

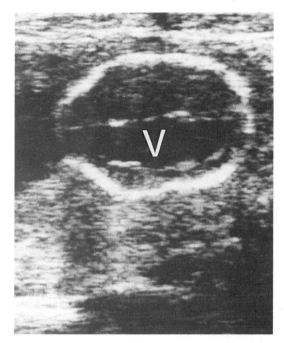

Figure 7.1 Transverse section of brain with hydrocephalus. V = dilated lateral ventricle

weeks' gestation (Figure 7.1). There are, however, some causes of hydrocephalus which may only be manifest much later in pregnancy and there are also described cases where hydrocephalus has been diagnosed in the early weeks of pregnancy and has disappeared by term [10]. This has important practical implications since in the absence of a diagnosable cause for ventricular dilatation, e.g. myelomeningocele, Dandy Walker cyst (Figure 7.2) or other associated abnormalities it is very difficult to advise the parents with regard to prognosis.

Less experienced observers may also have difficulty in the mid trimester with an appearance mimicking hydrocephalus [8]. This is caused by the fact that the normal ventricles are filled with choroid plexus in early pregnancy and that this is more echogenic than the surrounding brain substance. On occasions the normal brain substance will appear almost echo free and could be confused with dilated fluid-filled ventricles but these echo-free areas are more laterally placed within the skull than the ventricles in hydrocephalus, and confusion should not arise if the operator is aware of this.

Encephaloceles can be diagnosed *in utero* (Figure 7.3), the larger ones early in pregnancy but small ones at the base of the skull can easily be missed on an early scan.

Anencephaly can often be suspected as early as 10 weeks' gestation (Figure 7.4) but the normal skull vault is on some occasions not easily visualized until

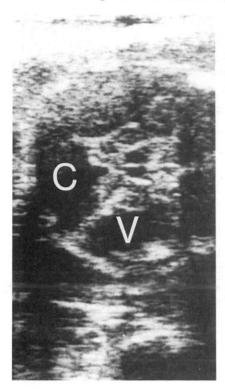

Figure 7.2 Dandy Walker syndrome. Transverse section through base of brain. C = Dandy Walker cyst; V = lateral ventricle

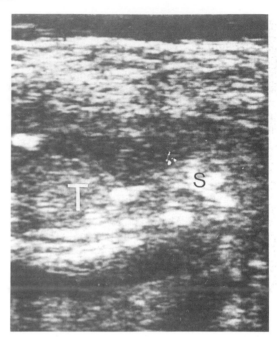

Figure 7.4 Longitudinal section of fetal body showing upper thorax (T) and base of skull (S). Note absence of skull vault structures

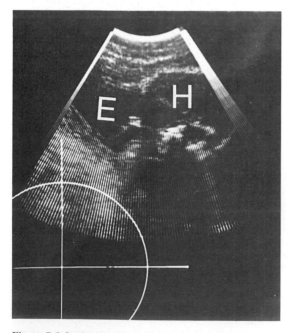

Figure 7.3 Sagittal section of head. H = head; E = encephalocele

after 12 weeks and a confident diagnosis of anencephaly should not be made before this time.

The diagnosis of microcephaly is one of the more difficult diagnoses and unless gross can only be made in the third trimester. In a baby with a normal abdominal circumference for gestational age in whom the head circumference is diminished (the reverse of the situation seen in intrauterine growth retardation), microcephaly is the most likely diagnosis, although the cause of the microcephaly can rarely be determined by ultrasound.

An enormous amount of effort is made to exclude the diagnosis of myelomeningocele by ultrasound (Figures 7.5–7.7) because of the long-term disabilities from which such a baby will suffer. Scanning of the fetal spine should always be undertaken in two views, the coronal longitudinal scan and the transverse scan. In the longitudinal scan the structures forming the spinal canal consisting of the vertebral body centrally and the two laminae laterally should form three parallel lines, although all three elements are not always seen on each section due to the curvature of the spine. The lower lumbar and sacral region is often obscured by the iliac bones and this accounts for the difficulty in diagnosis of small lower lumbar and sacral lesions. The transverse scan is often technically easier but suffers the same disadvantage in the lower lumbar and sacral regions. On this view the elements seen are a vertebral body

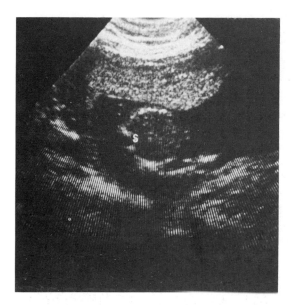

Figure 7.5 Transverse section upper lumbar spine and trunk. S = spine showing divergence of laminae in spina bifida

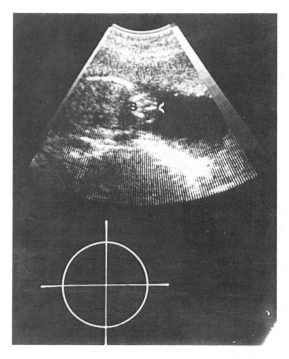

Figure 7.7 Transverse section of fetal trunk and spine. S = spine; < = diastematomyelia

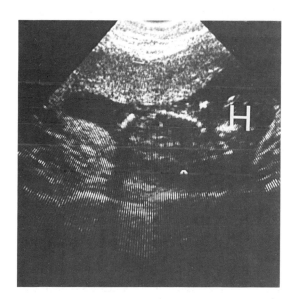

Figure 7.6 Longitudinal section of spine. H = fetal head; ∧ = divergence of laminae at site of spina bifida

anteriorly and two parallel lateral echoes representing the laminae.

Attention should also be paid to the skin surface overlying the spine. When there is surrounding amniotic fluid this is relatively straightforward but if the fetal back is against the uterine wall or placenta, exclusion of a small lesion can be difficult. The presence of a myelomeningocele is indicated by loss

of parallelism of laminae on either or both of the views (longitudinal and transverse) and usually by an overlying soft tissue defect. In the presence of a myelomeningocele this is seen as a shallow plaque but in the presence of a closed meningocele a thin-walled fluid-containing sac which is easy to demonstrate can be seen. The bony lesion is often less marked in these circumstances. The most suitable time to exclude these lesions is between 16 and 20 weeks, as prior to 16 weeks the fetus is frequently too small to exclude the smaller lesions. If the diagnosis is made much after 20 weeks the difficulty of terminating a viable pregnancy becomes a problem.

Neck

This region is often difficult to image satisfactorily due to flexion of the fetus, and the structures of the jaw often overlap. Large tumours can, however, be confidently diagnosed. The commonest of these are cystic hygromas and teratomas. The former often have a multi-loculated cystic appearance and the latter a more mixed appearance although the histology cannot be determined by ultrasound. Cervical meningoceles are unlikely to produce diagnostic difficulties due to their posterior position and usually relatively smaller size. They are rarely multi-loculated. Oedema of the soft tissues of the neck which is a feature of both Turner's syndrome and Down's syndrome enter the differential diagnosis but are rarely a problem as thickening of the soft tissues does not usually have the multi-locular or tumour-like appearance [15].

Abdominal tumours

These are very rare *in utero* and obtaining a definitive diagnosis is not usually possible. The organ of origin can sometimes be determined, particularly if liver [17] or kidney are involved but such diagnoses are rarely feasible in practice.

Pelvic tumours

Sacrococcygeal teratomas [7] (Figure 7.8) have a fairly characteristic appearance with bulging of the soft tissues of the lower back and buttocks and have a mixed echo pattern. They can usually be fairly easily differentiated from meningoceles (Figure 7.9)

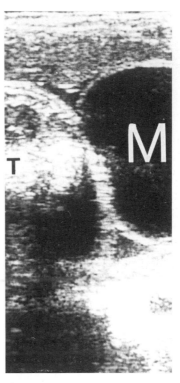

Figure 7.9 Transverse section of fetal trunk and meningocele. T = trunk; M = meningocele

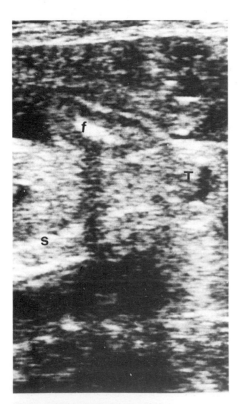

Figure 7.8 Sagittal section of lower abdomen. S = spine; f = femur; T = sacrococcygeal teratoma

which are the only other common 'tumours' in this region in the fetus. As well as assessing the tumour it is advisable to check the kidneys for hydronephrosis secondary to ureteric pressure from the tumour.

Conjoined twins

This abnormality is very rare but several ultrasound diagnoses have been described in the literature [9]. The actual diagnosis is fairly straightforward due to the fixed position of the fetuses with relation to one another on successive examinations. The main purpose of ultrasound is to assess the connection between the twins so as to enable the feasibility of separation to be discussed in the antenatal period.

Diaphragmatic hernia

This condition can be diagnosed as early as 16 weeks by demonstrating the presence of fluid-filled spaces within the chest, usually on the left side, and cardiac displacement (Figure 7.10). It is not possible to assess the size of the defect accurately. It seems that the prognosis is not good in patients with very early prenatal diagnosis, almost certainly related to the

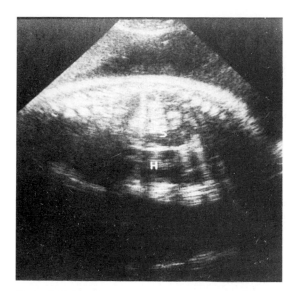

Figure 7.10 Longitudinal section of fetal trunk. H = fetal heart; S = fetal bowel herniating into the chest behind the heart

associated pulmonary hypoplasia resulting from compression of the lung over a prolonged period. The condition should be differentiated from cystic adenomatoid malformation [1] which can also give a multi-loculated appearance within the chest but is often associated with fetal ascites. It is usually possible to identify a normal diaphragm and normally positioned abdominal organs in the latter condition.

Oesophageal atresia

Exclusion of the diagnosis of oesophageal atresia depends on the identification of the normal fluid-filled fetal stomach. It is, however, not unusual to fail to identify the fetal stomach in the first and early second trimester, at least on a single examination. If the stomach is not identified on repeated examination up to 20 weeks' gestation this is significant but not diagnostic. This sign is only reliable in the small group of patients with oesophageal atresia without a fistula as those patients with a fistula will tend to have a demonstrable fluid-filled stomach. Personal experience suggests that a significant number of patients with oesophageal atresia with a fistula do not have a fluid-filled stomach demonstrated by ultrasound in early pregnancy but this is not reliable in a positive diagnostic way.

Cardiac lesions

It is possible to diagnose with considerable confidence some of the more complex cardiac lesions but the expertise required is very great and is only available in a very small number of centres. The interested reader is referred to the work of Allen [2] and her colleagues.

Exomphalos/gastroschisis

The differentiation between these two conditions is important from the point of view of management of the pregnancy [6]. In exomphalos (Figure 7.11) the

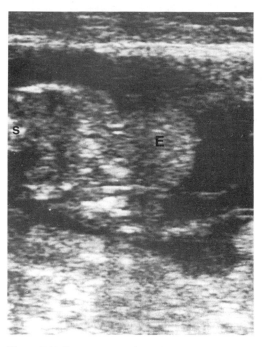

Figure 7.11 Transverse section of abdomen. E = exomphalos; S = spine

herniation of the abdominal contents occurs into the base of the umbilical cord and it is usually possible to identify the cord entering the apex of the sac. In gastroschisis (Figure 7.12) the herniation is to the right of the umbilical cord and the cord can often be traced to the abdominal wall adjacent to the herniated bowel. As well as diagnosing the lesion it is important to realize that gastroschisis is usually an isolated lesion and if small the prognosis for the infant is good. Exomphalos, however, is associated in 67% of cases with other anomalies, 37% of which are life threatening. Therefore, regardless of the size of the exomphalos it is important to exclude other anomalies as the recommendation for continuation or termination of the pregnancy may well revolve

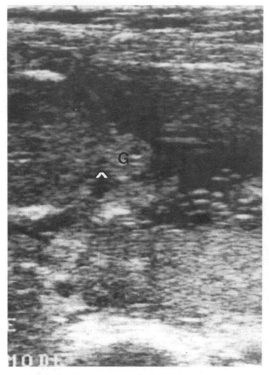

Figure 7.12 Transverse section of abdomen. G = gastroschisis; ∧ = site of cord insertion to left of the hernia

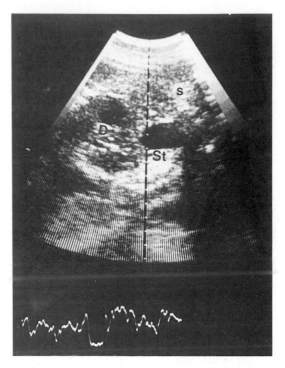

Figure 7.13 Transverse section of abdomen in duodenal. S = spine; St = stomach; D = dilated duodenum

around these anomalies as much as the presence of the exomphalos itself.

Bowel obstruction

Duodenal atresia (Figure 7.13) can be confidently diagnosed by the presence of two fluid-filled structures in the upper abdomen anterior to the kidneys in the late second and third trimesters. The suggestion of such a diagnosis is an indication for amniocentesis in order to exclude Down's syndrome by analysis of the chromosomes. Many attempts have been made to identify ultrasound criteria for the diagnosis of Down's syndrome but these do not appear to be successful.

Lower intestinal atresias

The presence of lower intestinal atresia can be suggested by the detection of many dilated fluid-filled structures in the fetal abdomen in later pregnancy but diagnosis on the basis of a single examination should not be attempted as the normal large bowel has a very variable size in later

pregnancy and can easily be mistaken for dilated loops of small bowel.

Duplication cysts and mesenteric cysts

Duplication cysts (Figure 7.14) and mesenteric cysts have been diagnosed *in utero*, the latter being more commonly multi-locular, but it is not possible to make a confident diagnosis and only a differential diagnosis can be given including these conditions and ovarian cyst if the fetus is female.

Meconium ileus

Meconium ileus can present in the late second and third trimester as an echogenic mass in the abdomen but a confident diagnosis is not usually possible until after delivery. On the other hand if an echogenic mass with calcification is seen within the abdomen (Figure 7.15), whilst calcified abdominal teratoma is possible, the most likely diagnosis is meconium peritonitis, either as a result of meconium ileus or resulting from an intra-uterine perforation the cause of which is not usually diagnosable by ultrasound [13].

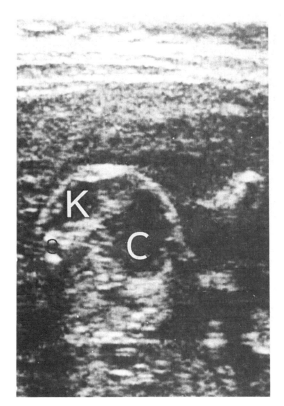

Figure 7.14 Transverse section of fetal trunk. S = spine; K = kidney; C = duplication cust

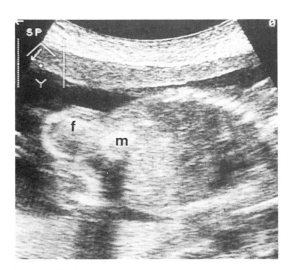

Figure 7.15 Coronal section of fetal trunk. H = heart; f = femur; m = calcified meconium mass resulting from intrauterine bowel perforation

Urinary tract abnormalities

Hydronephrosis

Hydronephrosis can be diagnosed as early as 14 weeks. The normal kidney is not easily defined at this stage but the presence of a fluid-filled lesion in the centre of the area where the kidney would be expected is strongly suggestive of hydronephrosis (Figure 7.16). As pregnancy progresses increasingly

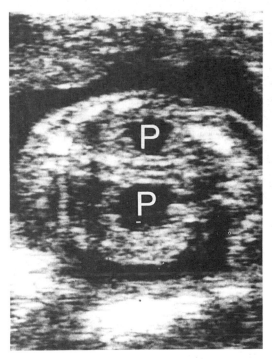

Figure 7.16 Coronal section of abdomen. P = dilated renal pelves in bilateral pelvic-ureteric junction obstruction

lesser degrees of dilatation of the renal pelvis can be determined. The effect of hydronephrosis is usually such that it severely damages the developing kidney so that postnatal function is almost always severely impaired. The separation of cases of extrarenal pelvis which are of no significance from mild hydronephrosis is very difficult by ultrasound. Recently it has been suggested [4] that if the renal pelvis at any stage in pregnancy is more than 10 mm in diameter this is abnormal; between 5 and 10 mm is probably normal and less than 5 mm is undoubtedly normal. The group between 5 and 10 mm can sometimes be further subdivided by determining if the pelvic diameter is greater or less than one-third of the renal diameter at that point. Where the pelvic diameter is greater than one-third this is almost certainly indicative of hydronephrosis.

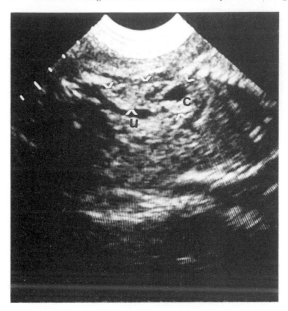

Figure 7.17 Longitudinal section of fetal duplex kidney. C = upper pole calyx; U = ureter from upper pole. Arrowheads indicate renal outline

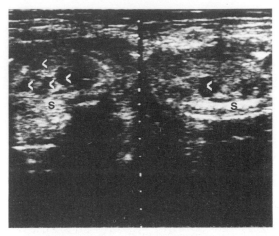

Figure 7.18 Sagittal sections of both kidneys with bilateral multicystic kidneys. < = cyst; S = spine

Only further experience will show whether these figures are reliable or not. As well as looking for renal pelvic and calyceal dilatation the diagnosis of hydronephrosis is incomplete without examination for the presence of dilated ureters (Figure 7.17). These are sometimes confused with loops of bowel and minor degrees of dilatation cannot be diagnosed by ultrasound *in utero*. The size of the fetal bladder is also important as bladder outlet obstruction is usually manifested by a persistently dilated fetal bladder. This can only be adequately assessed by serial examinations. It is also important to determine the sex of the child in order to give a more accurate diagnosis in the presence of bladder outlet obstruction, the commonest cause of which in the male is posterior urethral valves. Hydronephrosis of part of a kidney can sometimes be seen in late pregnancy and a complicated duplex kidney thus suggested. Accurate diagnosis of the complex situations can usually only be achieved after delivery [18].

Multicystic kidney

This condition is thought by many to be the end stage of early *in utero* obstruction. The ultrasound appearances are those of transonic areas (of different size) within the region of the kidney (Figure 7.18), completely replacing the kidney. It is not possible to differentiate this with certainty from a severe hydronephrosis although, if the most medial lying loculus is not the largest, if the loculi are of differing size and if the normal renal shape is lost a multicystic kidney is more likely to be the diagnosis than severe hydronephrosis.

Infantile polycystic disease

The kidneys in infantile polycystic disease are more echogenic than normal and considerably enlarged. These can usually be detected *in utero* prior to 20 weeks' gestation and the ultrasound appearances are virtually diagnostic.

Most urinary tract abnormalities do not affect the conduct of the pregnancy in any way and there is no indication for intervention in the presence of unilateral hydronephrosis [12]. In the presence of infantile polycystic disease or where a renal abnormality or bladder abnormality are demonstrated with the presence of severe oligohydramnios then termination of pregnancy should probably be recommended as not only will the renal function be severely impaired but the infant is unlikely to survive because of the concomitant pulmonary hypoplasia.

The presence of bilateral hydronephrosis raises certain problems. If it is detected early in pregnancy then the question arises as to whether the kidney should be drained into the amniotic cavity to relieve obstruction and preserve renal function or whether such intervention is more hazardous than is justified. It seems that there are very few patients in whom intervention of this sort in pregnancy is justified, particularly as there is no proof that renal function is preserved by these procedures. Many authors suggest that by the time the diagnosis is made irrecoverable renal damage has occurred. It is not possible to show whether pelvi-calyceal dilatation is due to obstruction, which may possibly benefit from drainage, or due to vesico-ureteric reflux, for which treatment would be of no value, and this further limits the value of the procedure.

Potter's syndrome

Every pregnancy in which oligohydramnios is suggested clinically should have an ultrasound examination (Figure 7.19). The two major causes of oligohydramnios are intrauterine growth retardation and

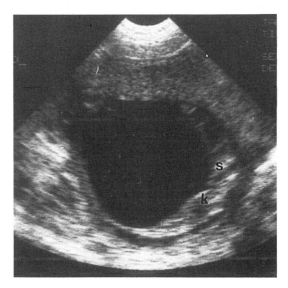

Figure 7.19 Transverse section of fetal trunk. Hugely distended bladder due to posterior urethral valves. S = spine; K = cystic dysplastic kidney. Note almost complete absence of amniotic fluid around the baby

fetal renal disease. It is difficult in the absence of amniotic fluid to obtain good scans of the kidneys but it is usually possible to identify normal kidneys. Hydronephrotic kidneys or cystic dysplastic kidneys can also usually be demonstrated but very small kidneys without presence of cysts or hydronephrosis can be very difficult to demonstrate. A search is also made for the urinary bladder and if this is demonstrated and of normal size, whilst not excluding Potter's syndrome, it makes that diagnosis less likely. In the absence of demonstrable kidneys and particularly if no urine is seen in the fetal bladder after repeated scanning, including stimulation by administration of Lasix to the mother then termination is advised.

The presence of a renal abnormality diagnosed by ultrasound may also be a pointer to other abnormalities and the presence, particularly, of oligohydramnios with renal anomaly or bilateral hydronephrosis

should lead to a search for other anomalies as 50% of this group will have them [11,16].

Further improvement in image quality will continue to improve ultrasound diagnosis antenatally. Only by expansion of routine comprehensive scanning will the number of fetuses reaching viability with abnormalities be further reduced and this is a very costly exercise. The use of karyotyping using fetal blood samples obtained by fetoscopy to exclude chromosome abnormalities in fetuses with other abnormalities will help in counselling parents with regard to termination or continuing the pregnancy.

A multidisciplinary team consisting of a radiologist, obstetrician, paediatrician and paediatric surgeon is absolutely essential for the efficient management of the fetal abnormalities for which termination is not appropriate as the parents and baby need much expert help and no single person can give this adequately.

References

1. Adzick, N.S., Harrison, M.R., Glick, P.L., Colbus, M.S., Anderson, R.L., Mahony, B.S., *et al.* (1985) Fetal cystic adenomatoid malformation: prenatal diagnosis and natural history. *J. Pediat. Surg.*, **20**, 483–488
2. Allen, L.D. (1983) Early detection of congenital heart disease in pre-natal life. *Clin. Obstet. Gynaec.*, **10**, 507–514
3. Allen, L.D., Crawford, D.C., Anderson, R.H. and Tynan, M. (1985) Spectrum of congenital heart disease detected echocardiographically in prenatal life. *Br. Heart J.*, **54**, 523–526
4. Arger, P.H., Coleman, B.G., Mintz, M.C., Snyder, H.P., Camardese, T., Arenson, R.L., *et al.* (1985) Routine fetal genitourinary tract screening. *Radiology*, **156**, 584–489
5. Campbell, S. and Pearce, J.M. (1983) Pre-natal diagnosis of foetal structural anomalies by ultrasound. *Clin. Obstet. Gynaecol.*, **10**, 475–506
6. Campbell, S., Rodeck, C., Thorn, A., Little, D. and Roberts, A. (1978) Early diagnosis of exomphalos. *Lancet*, **i**, 1098
7. Chervenak, F.A., Isaacson, G., Rouloukion, R., Tortora, M., Berkowitz, R. and Hobbins, J.C. (1985) Diagnosis and management of fetal teratomas. *Obstet. Gynaec.*, **66**, 666–671
8. Fisher, C.E. and Filly, R.A. (1982) Ultrasound evaluation of the normal and abnormal foetal neural axis. *Radiol. Clin. N. Am.*, **20**, 285–296
9. Fitzgerald, E.J., Toi, A. and Cochlin, D.L. (1985) Conjoined twins. Antenatal ultrasound diagnosis and a review of the literature. *Br. J. Radiol.*, **58**, 1053–1056
10. Glick, P.L., Harrison, M.R., Nakayara, D.K., Edwards, M.S.B., Filly, R.A., Chinn, D.H. *et al.*

(1984) Management of ventriculomegaly in the foetus. *J. Pediat.*, **105**, 97–105

11. Gruenewald, S.M., Crocker, E.F., Walker, A.G. and Trudinger, B.J. (1984) Antenatal diagnosis of urinary tract abnormalities: correlation of ultrasound appearance with postnatal diagnosis. *Am. J. Obstet. Gynaecol.*, **148**, 278–283

12. Harrison, M.R., Golbus, M.S., Filly, R.A., Nakayama, D.K., Callen, P.W., de Lorimier, A.A. *et al.* (1982) Management of the foetus with congenital hydronephrosis. *J. Pediat. Surg.*, **17**, 728–742

13. Lince, D.M., Pretorius, D.H., Marco-Johnson, M.L., Manchester, D. and Clewell, W.H. (1985) The clinical significance of increased echogenicity in the fetal abdomen. *Am. J. Roent.*, **145**, 683–686

14. McCarthy, S.M., Filly, R.A., Stark, D.D., Callen, P.W., Golbus, M.S. and Hricak, H. (1985) Magnetic resonance imaging of fetal anomalies: early experience. *Am. J. Roent.*, **145**, 677–682

15. Nakazato, Y., Gilsarz, V. and Falk, R.E. (1985) Fetal cystic hygroma, web neck and trisomy 13 syndrome. *Br. J. Radiol.*, **58**, 1011–1013

16. Nicolaides, K.H., Rodeck, C.H. and Gorden, C.M. (1986) Rapid karyotyping in non-lethal fetal malformations. *Lancet*, **i**, 283–287

17. Platt, L.D., Devore, G.R., Benner, P., Siassi, B., Ralls, P.W. and Mikity, V.G. (1983) Antenatal diagnosis of a fetal liver mass. *Ultrasound Med.*, **2(11)**, 521–522

18. Thomas, D.F.M. (1984) Urological diagnosis *in utero*. *Arch. Dis. Child.*, **59**, 913–915

8

Radiology of the newborn

Helen M.L. Carty

The full range of imaging procedures that are now encompassed in the term diagnostic radiology all have a role to play in the diagnosis of diseases of the newborn. The clinician and radiologist must work closely together in deciding the most appropriate investigations so that maximum diagnostic information can be gained with efficient use of resources.

The information gained from the different techniques is complementary but often overlaps. Briefly, conventional X-rays provide anatomical information in two dimensions, some structural information as to the composition of a substance, i.e. gas, fat calcium and bone, but no information as to the functional state of the organ. Information is gained from ultrasound about cross-sectional anatomy and structure of a substance, i.e. solid or cystic, but as bone and air are impervious to ultrasound, visualization of some parts of the body is impossible. In addition, there is little information about the functional state of the organ under investigation. Ultrasound has the great advantage of being without radiation hazard and can, therefore, be repeated frequently. It can be performed successfully in an incubator in the intensive care unit. It is also cheap in material cost though expensive in medical time.

Nuclear medicine studies provide excellent pathophysiological information about the organ under investigation but give relatively crude anatomical detail. Most studies require injection of the pharmaceutical. Functional studies of kidneys and heart can be obtained by a mobile camera in the intensive care unit, but for good quality images of bones, etc., the infant will nearly always have to be moved to the nuclear medicine department. Nuclear medicine services are frequently not available on site in paediatric hospitals, thus limiting their usefulness.

Computed tomography (CT) imaging provides a superb demonstration of cross-sectional anatomy in the axial plane and by using reconstructed images sagittal and coronal information can be obtained. It is now possible to obtain direct coronal and sometimes direct sagittal imaging of the neonate in modern scanners. The images obtained by direct imaging are much sharper than reconstructed ones. The quality of image in the neonatal body is not as good as in the older patient due to the relative lack of body fat and oral or intravenous contrast medium may have to be administered to provide the necessary contrast. The lack of fat does not interfere with brain imaging. Use of CT in neonates is again often limited by the practical problem of the scanner not being available on site.

Magnetic resonance imaging (MRI) is the newest of the imaging parameters, and its use in neonates is still largely for research purposes. It shares with ultrasound the benefits of achieving images without the use of ionizing radiation. It provides cross-sectional anatomical information in any desired plane without the necessity for reconstruction of the image. There are, however, logistical problems of monitoring of the baby in the imaging tunnel, the necessity of ensuring that all monitoring equipment is not ferromagnetic and of ensuring that the infant remains still for the relatively long acquisition times of the images. MR spectroscopy of the infant brain is being successfully achieved but it will be some time before MRI becomes available as a routine clinical tool, suitable for use in neonates.

General problems of X-raying babies

Routine radiography of the neonate should be carried out by experienced staff and not delegated to the most junior member of the department. Due to the potential hazards of ionizing radiation, films should be centred on that area of the body which one wishes to see, i.e. if a chest X-ray is required the beam should be restricted to this area and not include the abdomen. Badly centred and rotated films cause problems of interpretation. It is easier to ensure good positioning with the infant supine. Most neonatal films should be performed with the infant supine and the erect position reserved for those infants in whom one wishes to see fluid levels and free air. Even in these infants a decubitus film within the incubator will provide the required information, and is much easier to carry out. Protection of the staff, which would be necessary if they had to hold the infant for erect filming, is not required as no holding is necessary. If an infant has to be taken out of an incubator or positioned within it for an X-ray, care must be taken not to disturb drips, tubes, etc. and close cooperation between radiographic and nursing staff is therefore essential. Immobilization of arms and legs within an incubator is achieved by the use of lead gloves and sandbags.

The contrast quality of the radiograph is a decision for the radiologist. The author's preference is for a low contrast film with good soft-tissue detail. Initial abdominal films are taken without gonadal protection, and include hernial orifices. Gonadal protection is used on repeat films in boys where it is practicable but we do not attempt to use it in infant girls. Radiographers must be warned about the dangers of heat loss in the infant and care must be taken to keep this to a minimum.

X-ray and imaging equipment

Much of the radiography of the sick infant is done with portable equipment in the special care baby unit and not within the main X-ray department. The equipment does not need to be sophisticated but it has to have accurate short exposure capability. This is best achieved with modern mobile X-ray units. These also have accurate beam collimation, important in reducing unnecessary irradiation.

Environment

Environmental temperature in X-ray rooms used for X-raying neonates should be at least 70°F. Oxygen and resuscitation equipment must be available always in the room for the benefit of sick infants. If adequate environmental temperatures cannot be sustained then the infant must be kept wrapped in protective clothing and only the minimum area of the body exposed. Simple plastic-backed incontinence pads provide very good insulation.

Screening equipment

There are now some specialized screening units available for paediatrics. The tables are suitably small and have a series of cradles into which an infant can be securely and safely strapped. The intensifier is under the table. Access to the infant is easier than it is with the over-couch intensifier systems. Decubitus films such as are required in oesophageal studies when seeking an H-type fistula are easy to achieve as are double-contrast erect views of the stomach. While these units are ideal for procedures on small babies, they are not essential and the more conventional equipment, though a little more awkward, is satisfactory. Full remote-control units are not suitable for neonatal work. To reduce radiation dose, screening films should be taken with a camera attached to the image intensifier via an optical system. The radiation dose is reduced by a factor of approximately 90% by this. Further dose reduction is achieved by screening without a grid.

Ultrasound

Most paediatric radiologists find sector scanning more appropriate for neonatal ultrasound work than scanning with linear array systems. Real-time scanning is now universally used. A small probe is essential for good contact with the body. Frequencies in the 5–7.5 MHz range are necessary for neonatal work. A video attachment is useful and hard copy image recording essential. While contact scanning is generally satisfactory a system that provides some stand off of the probe from the skin will allow visualization of the first 2 cm which is often not visible due to the focal length of the probe. There are a variety of 'water bag' systems available commercially.

Nuclear medicine

High resolution gamma cameras with fast acquisition times are necessary to ensure optimum quality for static images and dynamic studies. Analogue images or very fine matrix digital images are essential for interpretation. Coarse matrix digital images are useless for infants and studies should not be done if this is the only equipment available. A clean injection is essential, especially for quantitative studies. Loss of part of the dose into the tissues will destroy quantitation.

Computed tomography

All modern CT scanners are suitable for imaging neonates. Care must be taken to ensure that the baby does not get chilled during the examination. Most scanners are in air-conditioned rooms and the ambient temperature is usually too cool for a sick infant. The infant must not be left unattended. Sedation and general anaesthesia are not required for infants. They will remain still enough for most examinations if they are kept warm, securely wrapped and, if possible, recently fed. One of the indications for imaging neonates is to identify the extent of masses such as cystic hygromas. These can cause airway obstruction and it may be necessary to image the infant in the prone position to maintain a free airway. Full resuscitation facilities must be available on site in the CT suite. The choice of scan parameters, the thickness of the slice and the administration of oral or intravenous contrast media are dependent on the nature of the expected pathology and should be decided locally. In general, fast scan times are not needed in examining the infant brain but are necessary in the infant thorax and abdomen.

Contrast media

There have been two major developments in the use of contrast media in recent years which have increased the safety of contrast examinations. The major advance has been the development of low osmolar non-ionic contrast media (for both intravenous and intra-arterial injection), as a replacement for the older high osmolar ionic media. Endothelial damage and the risk of a hypersensitivity reaction are greatly reduced. The main danger in neonates with the older contrast media was the development of pulmonary oedema if too high a dose was given – which was partly due to the volume of the contrast medium and partly due to the sodium load. Modern non-ionic media are not in sodium-rich solutions and it is possible to give higher volumes safely. Whilst intravenous urography is now rarely done in the neonate, following the advent of ultrasound and radionuclides, the increased safety margin is of great importance in paediatric cardiology. These non-ionic contrast media are also safe for intrathecal injection. Oral use of the older contrast medium carried the same hazards as Gastrografin; the danger of pulmonary oedema if there was pulmonary aspiration, and circulatory collapse which could occur due to depletion of the extracellular volume by the hyperosmolar intraluminal contrast medium. The non-ionic contrast media are not irritant to the bronchial mucosa. The low osmolarity obviates shift of fluid into the bowel lumen. This has the advantage that there is no dilution of the contrast medium and as it is also not absorbed from the bowel excellent images can be obtained even 4–5 days after oral administration. There is no danger of impaction such as can occur with barium. They are now the contrast media of choice in neonates suspected of a leak from an anastomosis or a

perforation, in the identification of strictures following necrotizing entercolitis or in localizing the site of intestinal obstruction, particularly postoperatively. Their relative inertness means that they are not suitable for use in relieving meconium ileus in the newborn. The hyperosmolarity of Gastrografin and its wetting agent (Tween 80) are required for this.

Clinical applications

Technically the relief of intestinal obstruction by contrast enemas could be classed as interventional radiology. The term is, however, more usually reserved for the insertion of percutaneous drains, and fine needle aspiration biopsy procedures under fluoroscopic ultrasound or CT control. These techniques are now well established radiological procedures, and where indicated are also applicable in the neonate. The indications in the neonate are fewer than in the older child but when used in an appropriate clinical situation are extremely helpful. Examples of their use in our hospital over the last 5 years include antegrade pyelography and nephrostomy to diagnose the site of and to relieve obstruction in sick infants with obstructive uropathy, diagnostic aspiration and the drainage of encysted fluid collections in the chest, tumour and liver biopsies, and percutaneous cholangiography and cholecystocholangiography under ultrasound control. More recently balloon dilatation of oesophageal strictures following repair of oesophageal atresia has been successfully undertaken.

Ultrasound in the neonate

Details of the precise role of ultrasound in specific pathological situations will be found in the appropriate chapters elsewhere in this book. A brief outline of the main indications follows. There are several excellent textbooks of paediatric ultrasound and more detailed information can be obtained from these.

The head

The patent anterior fontanelle provides an acoustic window on the infant brain. It is now part of routine assessment in the premature infant to identify and monitor intraventricular and intracranial haemorrhage. A major complication of such haemorrhage is the development of hydrocephalus. It is possible with ultrasound to identify this, to localize residual intracerebral and porencephalic cysts, to identify the position of intraventricular shunts and to localize areas which may require additional shunts. In the more complex cases CT will be required to demonstrate the full extent of the problem.

Ultrasound is indicated in any infant with a full or bulging fontanelle, apnoea attacks and fits. Underlying lesions found in these situations will include hydrocephalus, intraventricular and intracranial haemorrhage, subdural haematoma and, more rarely, tumour. It is usually possible to identify congenital malformations that cause the hydrocephalus. Ultrasound is also indicated in infants at risk of congenital malformation of the brain, even though there is no obvious clinical problem. Such situations include children with odd facies, chromosomal abnormalities and failure of normal development. Whilst the ultrasound examination will be normal in most of these children, it is reassuring to the parent and clinician to know that there is no structural anomaly.

Cranial ultrasound is indicated in children who are the victims of child abuse, especially if there is clinical evidence of intracranial pathology. Subdural collections will be the most frequent finding. Small collections may be missed. CT is more sensitive in their detection. Cerebral oedema in such cases and also in meningitis can be shown by ultrasound; the ventricles become narrowed and slit shaped, and gyral detail may be obscured.

Ultrasound is a useful and simple means of excluding underlying hydrocephalus in children with big heads which are growing rapidly but who are otherwise behaving normally. It is also worth doing cranial ultrasound in children with cranial bruits – underlying arteriovenous malformations may be detected and subsequent CT and angiography tailored to further resolve a known problem.

Cranial ultrasound can be very helpful in localizing the cause of CSF shunt malfunction. It is usually possible to locate the tip of the ventricular catheter, and to see that it is not actually on the ventricular wall, surrounded and obstructed by the choroid plexus and to ensure that it is intraventricular and not located within the cerebral substance. Cerebrospinal fluid collections around the tip of the intraperitoneal shunt tubing, which also cause valve malfunction, are easily identified by ultrasound.

Abdominal ultrasound

The two main roles of ultrasound in the neonatal abdomen are the follow-up and further elucidation of masses detected antenatally where these are clinically silent, and as an initial diagnostic procedure in infants with clinically palpable masses so as to determine the organ of origin. Two other major indications are the routine assessment of the kidneys in children at risk for renal anomalies, e.g. those with oesophageal or anorectal atresia, and in the assessment of the jaundiced infant thought to have biliary atresia or neonatal hepatitis. Ultrasound examination will determine whether a mass is solid or cystic, identify secondary obstructive uropathy and detect ascites.

In children who present with a palpable mass, it is the author's practice to first request anterior and lateral radiographs of the abdomen to determine the distribution of bowel gas relative to the mass and to proceed immediately to ultrasound. If the mass is not clinically detectable then X-rays are unlikely to contribute further information and I proceed immediately to ultrasound.

Renal ultrasound

Details of the specific ultrasonic appearances of the varied renal lesions will be found in the appropriate chapters in this book. The main roles of renal ultrasound in the neonate are:

1. To establish the presence of kidneys in children at risk of partial or complete renal agenesis.
2. To confirm that a mass detected antenatally is renal in origin.
3. To confirm that a palpable mass thought to be a kidney is in fact renal in origin; e.g. a mass due to neonatal adrenal haemorrhage can mimic a palpable kidney.
4. To determine whether the mass is solid or cystic and thus get a likely indication of the pathology.
5. If cystic, to distinguish between a multicystic kidney and an obstructed kidney.
6. To determine the likely level of obstruction by identifying dilated ureters, and/or a dilated posterior urethra.
7. To detect ureteroceles as a cause of obstruction.
8. To detect other pelvic masses causing obstructive uropathy, e.g. sacrococcygeal teratomas, hydrocolpos and anterior sacral meningoceles.
9. To diagnose renal vein thrombosis.
10. To assess the kidneys in congenital nephrosis.
11. To identify the classic changes of infantile polycystic kidneys or other variants of cystic dysplasia.
12. To diagnose pyonephrosis, and identify candida fungus balls in a kidney.

While the list is long, the actual examination time is short and most of these conditions are readily identified by an experienced paediatric radiologist.

Liver ultrasound

Congenital liver masses are rare but if present ultrasound will rapidly confirm that a mass is of hepatic origin and indicate if it is solid or cystic. The more usual indications for liver ultrasound in the neonate are:

1. To assess an enlarged liver and to exclude an intrinsic mass lesion as a cause of this.
2. To identify intrahepatic, subhepatic and subphrenic abscesses in septicaemic ill infants, and if

necessary to perform diagnostic aspirations for bacteriology and subsequent percutaneous drainage.

3. To assess the presence of a gall bladder in a jaundiced infant. The finding of a normal gall bladder in a fasting infant virtually excludes the diagnosis of biliary atresia.

4. To diagnose choledochal cysts, either following antenatal detection or in the course of investigation of jaundice.

5. To assess the presence of a patent portal vein in infants with portal hypertension. A specific ultrasonic sign of portal hypertension is visualization of a patent ductus venosus.

Ascites

Ascites is a rare cause of abdominal distension in the neonate and nowadays is most commonly due to cardiac failure or to renal or biliary pathology. Although perforation of the bowel and peritonitis can also cause ascites this is usually clinically obvious and ultrasound is directed to the assessment of loculated collections. Urinary ascites tends to be completely free of echoes unless infected. Most other causes of ascites will cause debris to be seen as echogenic material within the ascitic fluid. Rhesus incompatibility is now a rare cause of neonatal ascites.

Antenatal abdominal 'cysts'

Masses discovered incidentally antenatally will include duplication cysts of the bowel, omental and retroperitoneal lymphangiomas and ovarian cysts. Ovarian cysts in the neonatal abdomen can be very variable in position and can wander, to appear even in the epigastrium. Lymphangiomas invariably have septae which serves to distinguish them from duplication and ovarian cysts which are more commonly unilocular. Normal female infants may have multiple small ovarian cysts in normally placed ovaries. These will disappear as the influence of maternal hormones fades.

Sacrococcygeal teratoma

Ultrasound examination will determine if the tumour is dominantly solid or cystic and will identify intra-abdominal extension and secondary obstructive uropathy. A sacral X-ray must be done to identify the extent of bony involvement. CT may be required to assess more fully any extension through the obturator foramina.

Chest ultrasound

The likely nature of a chest mass is usually obvious from the chest X-ray and ultrasound has little part

to play. If the nature of the mass is obscure then ultrasound may give useful information. We have found it of most benefit in diagnosing encysted effusions and in distinguishing these from true masses in the neonatal chest. In the older child chest ultrasound is more useful.

Neck ultrasound

The nature and consistency of a neck mass is usually obvious clinically. Ultrasound will confirm clinical impressions but seldom contributes any significant additional information. It is possible to see mediastinal extension of a cystic hygroma with ultrasound, but the full extent is better seen with contrast-enhanced CT, as is the relationship of the lesion to the neck vessels.

Spinal ultrasound

It is possible to see the spinal cord and identify its lower level ultrasonically in the neonatal back. This is useful in assessing children with a hairy patch or sacral dimple who are at risk of a tethered cord.

Hip ultrasound

It is now possible to confirm the diagnosis of congenital dislocation of the hip (CDH) and to identify acetabular dysplasia in children with subluxing hips, thus identifying the ones which are likely to proceed to dislocation. It is likely that hip ultrasound will become a screening procedure for CDH but the exact cost of this and, therefore, its practicality has yet to be established.

Cardiac ultrasound

Echocardiography has revolutionized the investigation of cardiac problems in the neonate. Cardiac ultrasound is mainly done by paediatric cardiologists and is discussed in the section on heart disease. The paediatric radiologist can easily determine the presence of a pericardial effusion if this is thought to be the clinical problem.

Radionuclide studies in the neonate

Radionuclide studies make an important contribution in the diagnosis of some cardiac, gastrointestinal, kidney, bone, hepatic, pulmonary and thyroid diseases of the neonate. The details of the abnormalities will be found in the respective chapters. Only an outline of the indications will be given here.

GI bleeding

Bleeding from a Meckel's diverticulum rarely occurs in the neonatal period but if suspected a technetium pertechnetate scan to detect ectopic gastric mucosa is indicated. A positive scan confirms the diagnosis. A negative scan does not exclude a Meckel's as the cause of the bleed but makes it less likely. A positive scan is dependent on sufficient gastric mucosa being present within the Meckel's to take up enough pertechnetate for it to be imaged. Scanning of the neonatal abdomen with technetium-99m methylene diphosphonate (MDP) has been described as a means of diagnosis of bowel necrosis in necrotizing enterocolitis but we have not found it particularly helpful.

Cardiac scanning

Even in small neonates it is possible to identify the level and size of an intracardiac shunt by nuclear first pass angiography. It can be done in the intensive care unit with a mobile camera. There are very few centres in the UK performing neonatal cardiac surgery which have access to nuclear cardiological services, so enthusiasm is limited. Much of the information can be gained from echocardiography. Advantages of nuclear angiography include lower radiation dose than from contrast angiography, non-invasiveness other than an intravenous injection, good quantitative functional information, reproducibility, no contrast hazard and the facility to do it in the intensive care unit. It cannot provide pressure measurements. Advance knowledge of the likely pathology can help to tailor a subsequent angiogram, so that it is swifter and requires a lower contrast volume.

Renal studies

There are two radionuclide techniques of value in assessing neonatal kidneys:

1. Renal cortical imaging usually using technetium-99m dimercaptosuccinic acid (DMSA) which also provides functional information.
2. Diuresis renography using either technetium-99m, diethylene triamine penta-acetic acid (DTPA) or iodine-123 hippuran, mainly to detect obstruction in hydronephrosis.

Renal cortical imaging provides an excellent image of functioning renal cortex even when kidneys are ectopically placed or renal function is poor. It is possible to get a reliable, reproducible assessment of divided renal function by calculating the relative uptakes of the two kidneys. One can also see the relative function of the two poles of a duplex kidney which aids surgical decisions about preservation of tissue versus nephrectomy or heminephrectomy.

Indications for DMSA scanning in the neonate include:

1. Assessment of kidney size, the detection of scars and assessment of baseline divided renal function in infants with reflux.
2. Visualization of ectopic, e.g. pelvic, kidneys which are not properly seen on ultrasound and intravenous urogram (IVU).
3. Assessment of baseline cortical function in urethral valves.

Diuresis renography also provides valuable information about renal function in the neonatal kidney. Indications for its use include:

1. The detection or exclusion of obstruction in the presence of hydronephrosis.
2. Provision of baseline assessment of function and of the degree of obstruction in infants with mild hydronephrosis, which is mainly detected antenatally. It is now becoming apparent that many of these infants improve spontaneously.

Isotope cystography

Radionuclide cystography can be carried out in infants via a catheter technique similar to that used in conventional contrast micturating cystourethrography (MCU). Its advantage is a very significant reduction in radiation dose, but this is gained at the expense of detailed anatomical information. Most clinicians prefer the contrast MCU as a first examination in the neonate but if future examinations are required for the monitoring of reflux, then these should be by a radionuclide method.

Bone scanning

The main indication for radionuclide bone scanning in the neonate is the detection of a focus of osteomyelitis. Technetium-99m MDP is the radiopharmaceutical used. Whilst bone scanning is a fairly reliable method of detecting osteomyelitis in the older child, it has a high false negative rate in the neonatal period. A negative scan does not exclude a focus of infection, and clinical sense must prevail. If the scan is positive then it facilitates management decisions and for this reason it is worth doing. It is important that the scan is done with meticulous care, and that great attention is paid to imaging the limbs symmetrically. A bladder catheter may need to be passed to avoid obscuring detail of the infant's pelvis and hips. The scan must be interpreted by a radiologist who is familiar with the infant's nuclear scans so as to avoid errors of interpretation.

Fractures of child abuse in the neonatal period are less common than in the slightly older child. If suspected, bone scintigraphy can be very helpful in confirming the presence of suspected fractures particularly in the metaphyses and in the ribs.

Liver and biliary scanning

There are two radionuclide methods of imaging the liver and biliary tree. Technetium-99m sulphur colloid is taken up by the reticulo-endothelial systems in the liver and spleen, thus producing a functional image of these systems. This is rarely indicated in neonates but can be useful in assessing functional disturbance in metabolic liver disease, such as is found in galactosaemia.

The main role of radionuclide liver studies in the infant is the demonstration of a patent biliary tree by imaging the excretion of a radionuclide into the bowel following intravenous injection. The most widely used radiopharmaceutical is one of the technetium-labelled iminodiacetic acid complexes. The demonstration of gastrointestinal radioactivity following injection is good evidence of a patent biliary system and excludes a diagnosis of biliary atresia. However, these agents can be excreted via alternative pathways in the presence of severe jaundice, producing false negative studies. More recently Rose Bengal and bromosulphthalein labelled with iodine-123 have been used and are proving more reliable in distinguishing neonatal hepatitis from biliary atresia.

Lung scanning

Both ventilation and perfusion lung scanning are easily performed in the neonate but there are very limited applications for primary diagnosis. Most of the lesions can be easily diagnosed on the plain chest radiographs. Technetium-99m-labelled macroaggregate is the radiopharmaceutical most favoured for perfusion scanning. Krypton-81m which has a half-life of only 13 s is ideal for showing regional ventilation. It cannot positively demonstrate air trapping because of its short half-life. The indications are postoperative assessment of the lungs following repair of a diaphragmatic hernia, confirmation of pulmonary aplasia, confirmation of pulmonary hypoplasia and detection of any V/Q mismatch and occasionally in the assessment of the lung in congenital lesions, such as scimitar syndrome and pulmonary sequestration if these are detected in the neonate.

Thyroid scanning

Congenital thyroid anomalies are more a problem of neonatal medicine than surgery and thyroid scanning is mainly concerned with the detection and localization of thyroid tissue in congenital hypothyroidism. If there is any doubt about the nature of a small neck nodule, before excision, a radionuclide thyroid scan will confirm that it is not functioning thyroid tissue.

Computed tomography

As with ultrasound and nuclear medicine, the role of CT in the investigation of specific problems in the neonate will be discussed in the individual chapters. An outline of the main indications follows.

Cranial CT

The main indication for CT in the neonate is the confirmation of suspected intracranial pathology. Before CT is undertaken the infant should have an ultrasound examination. In many infants this will provide the necessary information. CT is, however, indicated in infants in whom a tumour or a complex malformation is suspected on ultrasound. It is also indicated in those infants in whom a congenital brain infection is suspected. Calcification of this type will not be seen on cranial ultrasound. CT is also indicated for further assessment of subdural collections discovered on ultrasound or for their detection when ultrasound is negative. Contrast-enhanced CT will frequently confirm the presence of suspected arteriovenous malformations, enabling one to select those cases which require angiography. CT is not routinely indicated in the pre-operative assessment of hydrocephalus but it is very helpful in some cases of post-haemorrhagic hydrocephalus, e.g. those which are multiloculated and may need the insertion of more than one shunt system for successful drainage. A baseline scan done postoperatively when the child is well is extremely helpful in the subsequent assessment of suspected shunt malfunction.

CT is also of immense value in defining the bony malformations of the face and orbits that accompany many of the craniostenosis malformations. This is especially true of the asymmetrical lesions. Further information may be gained from three-dimensional reconstruction of the images in these infants.

CT is indicated in the pre-operative assessment of infants born with occipital and cervical encephaloceles and meningoceles. It is not routinely indicated in infants with spina bifida and dorsal or lumbar meningoceles. It is, however, indicated in the full assessment of infants with sacral lipomas, closed meningoceles and lipomeningoceles so that the full intrathecal extent of the lesion is displayed. Where facilities are available MR imaging is a better method of assessing these infants but such facilities are so limited that for practical purposes CT is the only investigation available.

Chest and abdomen

As previously stated the lack of body fat in the neonate reduces the inherent contrast and limits the resolution and quality of images that can be obtained. Much of the information required in the assessment of infant tumours and other abdominal masses can be obtained by a combination of conventional radiographs, contrast radiography and ultrasound. In this hospital we find CT valuable in demonstrating the full extent of sacrococcygeal teratomas and in gaining information about the relationship of the tumour to main vessels and the extension through the obturator foramen that cannot be obtained by other means. Direct sagittal imaging which has become possible with the advent of larger gantry apertures gives additional information in these infants. CT is also helpful in the further assessment of masses the nature of which is not clear from ultrasound.

CT with and without contrast is often diagnostic in identifying the type of tumour in the infant liver; for example a haemangioma has a characteristic enhancing pattern. As with abdominal masses, the nature and extent of most chest masses can be diagnosed by conventional radiology and ultrasound. We have found CT is of most use in displaying the chest extension of cystic hygromas and the relationship of the mass to the major vessels. Direct sagittal CT can be used to identify the extent of the atretic segment in infants with oesophageal atresia and a fistula but is not routinely indicated. We reserve this for difficult cases.

Further reading

General radiography of neonates

Cohen, G., Wagner, L., McDaniel, D. and Robinson, L. (1984) Dose efficiency of screen film systems used in paediatric radiography. *Radiology*, **152**, 187–193

Drury, P. and Robinson, A. (1980) Fluoroscopy without the grid: a method of reducing the radiation dose. *Br. J. Radiol.*, **53**, 93–100

Gyll, C. and Blake, N. (1986) *Paediatric Diagnostic Imaging*. W.M. Heinemann Medical Books, London

Murdoch, D. and Darlon, B. (1984) Handling during neonatal intensive care. *Arch. Dis. Child.*, **59**, 957–962

Singleton, E. (1981) Radiologic considerations of intensive care in the premature infant: annual oration in honour of Wm Henry Neil. *Radiology*, **140**, 291–300

Werner, A. and Isdale, J. (1986) Radiation hazards in a paediatric intensive care unit. *Paed. Radiol.*, **16**, 275–277

Wesenberg, R. and Amundson, G. (1984) Fluoroscopy in children: low exposure technology. *Radiology*, **153**, 243–249

Nuclear medicine

Ash, J. and Gilday, D. (1980) The futility of bone scanning in neonatal osteomyelitis. *J. Nucl. Med.*, **21**, 417–420

Barnes, N. (1985) Screening for congenital hypothyroidism: the first decade. *Arch. Dis. Child.*, **60**, 587–593

Bressler, E., Conway, J. and Weiss, S. (1984) Neonatal osteomyelitis examined by bone scintigraphy. *Radiology*, **152**, 685–689

Carty, H., Pilling, D. and Majury, C. (1986) 123I BSP scanning in neonatal jaundice. *Ann. Radiol.*, **29**(8), 647–650

Howie, D., Savage, J., Wilson, T. and Paterson, D. (1983) Technetium phosphate bone scanning in the diagnosis of osteomyelitis in childhood. *J. Bone Jt Surg.*, **65A**, 431–437

Kirks, D., Coleman, R. and Filston, H. (1984) Imaging approach to persistent neonatal jaundice. *Am. J. Roent.*, **142**, 461–465

Minford, J., Hardy, J., Johnston, D. and Wastie, M. (1984) The investigation of neonatal obstructive jaundice using 123I Rose Bengal. *Br. J. Radiol.*, **57**, 213–217

Piepsz, A., Georges, B., Perlmutter, N., Rodesch, P. and Cadranel, S. (1981) Gastrooesophageal scintiscan in children. *Paed. Radiol.*, **11**, 71–74

Saul, P., Lloyd, D. and Smith, F. (1983) The role of bone scanning in neonatal rickets. *Paed. Radiol.*, **13**, 89–91

Siegel, J., Wu, R., Knight, L., Zelac, R., Stern, H. and Malmund, L. (1983) Radiation dose estimates for oral agents used in upper GI disease. *J. Nucl. Med.*, **24**, 835–837

Smith, F., Gilday, D., Ash, J. and Green, M. (1980) Non accidental injury: costovertebral injuries shown with bone scanning. *Paed. Radiol.*, **10**, 103–106

Sty, J. and Starshak, R. (1983) The role of bone scintigraphy in the evaluation of the suspected abused child. *Radiology*, **146**, 369–377

Sty, J., Starshak, R. and Miller, J. (1983) *Pediatric Nuclear Medicine*. Appleton-Century-Crofts,

Willi, U. and Treves, S. (1983) Radionuclide voiding cystography. *Urol. Radiol.*, **5**, 161–173

Computed tomography

Altman, N., Altman, D. and Wolfe, S. (1986) Three dimensional CT reformation in children. *Am. J. Roent.*, **146**, 1261–1267

Altman, N., Harwood-Nash, D. and Fitz, C. (1985) Evaluation of the infant spine by direct saggital computed tomography. *Am. J. Neuroradiol.*, **6**, 65–69

Bergen, P., Kuhn, J. and Brusehaber, J. (1981) Techniques for computed tomography in infants and children. *Radiol. Clin. N. Am.*, **19**, 399–408

Daneman, A. (1987) *Pediatric Body CT*. Springer Verlag, Berlin, New York

Day, D. (1985) Aortic arch in neonates with oesophageal atresia: preoperative assessment using CT. *Radiology*, **155**, 99–100

Kalifa, G. and Meunier, S. (1984) Indications for body CT in children (abs). *Radiology*, **152**, 853

Kirks, D. and Korobkin, M. (1981) Computed tomography of the chest in infants and children: techniques and mediastinal evaluation. *Rad. Clin. N. Am.*, **19**, 409–413

Kirks, D. (ed.) (1983) Practical techniques for paediatric CT. *Paed. Radiol.*, **13**, 148–155

Lassen, M. (1986) Dedicated CT for scanning neonates. *Radiology*, **161**, 363–366

Lee, S. and Rao, K. (1987) *Cranial CT and MRI*. McGraw Hill

Lipinski, J. and Cremin, B. (1986) Ultrasound and computed tomography of the infant brain. *Clin. Radiol.*, **37**, 365–369

Siegel, M., Nadel, S., Glazer, H. and Sagel, S. (1986) Mediastinal lesions in children: a comparison of CT and MR. *Radiology*, **160**, 241–244

Siegel, M., Patel, J., Gado, M. and Schackleford, G. (1983) Cranial computed tomography and real time sonography in full term neonates and infants. *Radiology*, **149**, 111–116

Tschappler, H. (1984) CT evaluation of the paediatric mediastinum. *Ann. Radiol.*, **27**, 160–165

Magnetic resonance imaging

Dubowitz, L. and Pennock, J. (1986) High resolution magnetic resonance imaging of the brain in children. *Clin. Radiol.*, **37**, 113–117

Fletcher, B., Dearborn, D. and Mulopulos, G. (1986) MR imaging in infants with airway obstruction: preliminary observations. *Radiology*, **160**, 245–249

Laurin, S., Williams, J. and Fitzsimmons, J. (1986) Magnetic resonance imaging of the paediatric thorax: initial experience. *Eur. J. Radiol.*, **6**, 36–41

McArdle, C., Nicholas, D., Richardson, C. and Amporo, E. (1986) Monitoring of the neonate undergoing MR imaging: technical considerations: work in progress. *Radiology*, **159**, 223–226

Siegel, M., Nadel, S., Glazer, H. and Sagel, S. (1986) Mediastinal lesions in children: comparison of CT and MR. *Radiology*, **160**, 241–244

Smith, F. (1983) Value of NMR in paediatric practice. *Paed. Radiol.*, **13**, 141–147

Wilson, D. and Steiner, R. (1986) Periventricular leukomalacia: evaluation with MR imaging. *Radiology*, **160**, 507–511

Zimmerman, R. and Bilaniuk, L. (1986) Application of magnetic resonance imaging in disease of the paediatric central nervous system. *Magn. Res. Imag.*, **4**, 11–24

Contrast media

Ansell, G. (1970) Fatal overdose of contrast media in infants. *Br. J. Radiol.*, **43**, 395–396

Cohen, M. (1982) Prolonged visualization of the GI tract with metrizamide. *Radiology*, **144**, 327–329

Cohen, M. (1987) Choosing contrast media for the evaluation of the GI tract of neonates and infants. *Radiology*, **162**, 447–457

McAllister, W., Siegel, M. and Schackleford, G. (1979) Pulmonary oedema following IV urography in a neonate. *Br. J. Radiol.*, **52**, 410–411

Ratcliffe, J. (1986) The use of low osmolality water soluble contrast media in the paediatric GI tract. *Paed. Radiol.*, **16**, 47–53

Wood, B. and Smith, W. (1981) Pulmonary oedema in infants following injection of contrast media for urography. *Radiology*, **139**, 377–379

Interventional radiology

Baran, G., Haagan, J., Shurin, S. and Alfidi, R (1984) CT guided percutaneous biopsies in the paediatric patient. *Paed. Radiol.*, **14**, 161–165

Couanet, D., Caillaud, J., Geoffrey, A., Montague, J. and Aubier, F. (1986) Percutaneous thin needle biopsy of paediatric tumours. *Ann. Radiol.*, **29**, 293–300

Diament, M., Stanley, P. and Taylor, S. (1985) Percutaneous fine needle biopsy in paediatrics. *Paed. Radiol.*, **15**, 409–411

Dux, A., Hall, C. and Spitz, L. (1984) Balloon catheter dilatation of oesophageal stricture in children. *Br. J. Radiol.*, **57**, 251–254

Hoffer, F., Winter, H., Fellows, K. and Folkman, J. (1987) The treatment of postoperative and peptic oesophageal strictures after oesophageal atresia repair: a program including dilatation with a balloon catheter. *Paed. Radiol.*, **17**, 454–459

Towbin, R. and Strife, J. (1985) Percutaneous aspiration, drainage and biopsies in children. *Radiology*, **157**, 81–85

Winfield, A., Kirchner, S., Brun, M., Mazer, M., Braren, H. and Kirchner, F. (1984) Percutaneous nephrostomy in neonates, infants and children. *Radiology*, **151**, 617–621

General ultrasound

Amodio, J., Abramson, S., Berdon, W., Bell, J., Winchester, P., Stolar, C. and Liebert, P. (1987) Postnatal resolution of large ovarian cysts detected in utero: report of two cases. *Paed. Radiol.*, **17**, 467–470

Avni, E., Godart, S., Israel, C. and Schmitz, C. (1983) Ovarian torsion cyst presenting as a wandering tumour in a newborn. *Paed. Radiol.*, **13**, 169–171

Avni, E., Rodesch, F. and Schillmer, C. (1985) Foetal uropathies: diagnostic pitfalls and management. *J. Urol.*, **134**, 921–925

Blane, C., Jongeward, R. and Silver, T. (1983) Sonographic features of hepatocellular disease in neonates and infants. *Am. J. Roent.*, **141**, 1313–1316

Blumhager, J. (1986) Role of ultrasound in evaluating vomiting in infants. *Paed. Radiol.*, **16**, 267–271

Brum, P., Gauthier, F., Boucher, D. and Brunelle, F. (1985) Ultrasound findings in biliary atresia in children. *Ann. Radiol.*, **28**, 259–263

Cochlin, D. (1982) Ultrasound of the foetal spine. *Clin. Radiol.*, **33**, 641–651

Geer, L., Mitterstaedt, G., Staabe, E. and Gaisie, G. (1984) Mesenteric cyst: sonographic appearance with CT correlation. *Paed. Radiol.*, **14**, 102–104

Graif, M., Itxchak, Y., Avigad, I., Strauss, S. and Ben-Ami, T. (1984) The pylorus in infancy: overall sonographic assessment. *Paed. Radiol.*, **14**, 14–17

Graif, M., Lison, M., Strauss, S., Manon, A., Itzchak, Y. and Sack, J. (1982) Congenital nephrosis: ultrasound features. *Paed. Radiol.*, **12**, 154–155

Grignon, A., Filatrault, D., Homsy, Y., Robitaille, P., Filon, R., Boutin, H. and Leblond, R. (1986) Antenatal ultrasonographic diagnosis: postnatal investigation and follow-up. *Radiology*, **160**, 649–653

Haller, J., Berdon, W. and Friedman, A. (1982) Increased renal cortical echogenicity: a normal finding in neonates and infants. *Radiology*, **142**, 173–175

Hayden, C. and Swischuk, L. (1987) *Paediatric Ultrasonography*. Williams and Wilkins, Baltimore

Jequier, S., Cramer, B. and O'Gorman, A. (1985) Ultrasound of the spinal cord in neonates and infants. *Ann. Radiol.*, **28**, 225–231

Kalifa, G. (ed.) (1986) *Paediatric Ultrasonography*. Springer-Verlag, Berlin, New York, London

Miller, J. and Kembering, C. (1984) Ultrasound scanning of the GIT in children: subject review. *Radiology*, **152**, 671–679

Ros, P., Olmsted, W., Moser, R., Dachman, A., Hjermstad, B. and Sobin, L. (1987) Mesenteric and omental cysts: histological classification with imaging correlation. *Radiology*, **164**, 327–333

Stunder, R., LeQuesne, G. and Little, K. (1986) The improved ultrasound diagnosis of pyloric stenosis. *Paed. Radiol.*, **16**, 200–206

Head ultrasound

Babcock, D. and Bokyung, K. (1981) The accuracy of high resolution real time ultrasound of the head in infants. *Radiology*, **139**, 665–676

Babcock, D. (1984) The normal, absent and abnormal corpus callosum sonographic findings. *Radiology*, **151**, 449–455

Chambers, S., Hendry, G. and Wild, R. (1985) Real time ultrasound scanning of the head in neonates and infants including a correlation between ultrasound and CT. *Paed. Radiol.*, **15**, 4–8

Cremin, B., Lipinski, K., Sharp, J. and Peacock, W. (1984) Ultrasound detection of subdural collections. *Paed. Radiol.*, **14**, 191–195

Flodmark, O., Roland, F., Hill, A. and Whitfield, M. (1987) Periventricular leukomalacia: radiologic diagnosis. *Radiology*, **162**, 119–124

Grant, E., Williams, A., Schellinger, D. and Slovis, T. (1985) Intracranial calcification in the infant and neonate: evaluation by sonography and CT. *Radiology*, **157**, 63–68

Han, B., Babcock, D. and McAdams, L. (1985) Bacterial meningitis in infants: sonographic finding. *Radiology*, **154**, 645–651

Hecht, S., Filly, R., Callen, B. and Wilson Davis, S. (1983) Intracranial haemorrhage: late onset in the preterm neonate. *Radiology*, **149**, 697–699

Kirks, D. and Bowie, J. (1986) Cranial ultrasound of the neonatal periventricular and intraventricular haemorrhage: who, how, why and when? *Paed. Radiol.*, **16**, 114–120

Strassburg, H., Sauer, M., Weber, S. and Gilsbach, J. (1984) Ultrasonographic diagnosis of brain tumours in infancy. *Paed. Radiol.*, **14**, 284–288

Veyrac, C. and Couture, A. (1985) Normal and pathologic choroid plexus ultrasound. *Ann. Radiol.*, **28**, 215–223

Hip ultrasound

Berman, L. and Hollingdale, J. (1987) The ultrasound appearances of positive hip instability tests. *Clin. Radiol.*, **38**, 117–119

Faure, C., Schmidt, P. and Salvat, D. (1984) Cost benefit evaluation of systematic radiological diagnosis of CDH. *Paed. Radiol.*, **14**, 407–413

Graf, R. (1981) The ultrasound image of the acetabular rim in infants. *Arch. Orthop. Trauma Surg.*, **99**, 35–44

Graf, R. (1984) Fundamentals of the sonographic diagnosis of infant hip dysplasia. *J. Paed. Orthopaed.*, **4**, 735–740

Special report (1986) Screening for the detection of congenital dislocation of the hip. *Arch. Dis. Child.*, **61**, 921–927

9

The low birth weight baby

R.W.I. Cooke

Introduction

Infants born with a birth weight of less than 2500 g are defined as being of low birth weight (LBW). The rate of low birth weight varies greatly from one part of the world to another being between 4 and 7% in Europe and North America, but as high as 40% in some developing nations. Babies may be of LBW because they have been born too early (preterm), or because they have had their growth retarded *in utero* by genetic or adverse environmental causes. Growth retarded infants whose birth weight is lower than the 10th percentile for that expected at the gestational age at birth are called 'small for dates' (SFD). Some authors define growth retardation in terms of the 5th percentile or as 2 standard deviations (SD) below the mean (approximately the 3rd percentile). Many infants may, of course, be both growth retarded and born preterm as the terms are not mutually exclusive. Overall, LBW infants have a mortality ten times that of full-sized infants,

and problems related to LBW are associated with more than three-quarters of perinatal mortality.

There are several reasons why the problems of LBW are of importance to the paediatric surgeon. The rate of anatomical malformations in LBW infants is higher than at term, the physiological problems of LBW may interfere with the surgical management of these malformations, and also the medical management of diseases of LBW in intensive care units produces a number of important complications which may be amenable to surgical treatment.

Intrauterine growth retardation (IUGR)

Poor growth *in utero* resulting in a SFD infant may be due to fetal or maternal factors. Major chromosomal defects such as the trisomies, all tend to produce a fetus that is smaller than average (Figure 9.1). The presence of many malformations is also

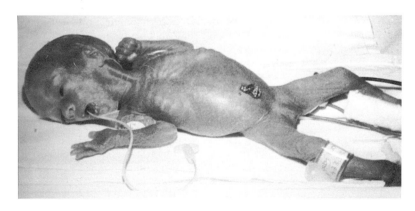

Figure 9.1 Extreme growth retardation. A 27-week gestation baby weighing 500 g

associated with smaller babies, although it is not known if the malformation is responsible for this or if the same adverse factor which caused the IUGR also led to the production of the malformation. Parental size, particularly that of the mother, has a marked effect on fetal size. On a worldwide basis problems such as chronic maternal undernutrition and endemic diseases such as malaria are responsible for most IUGR. In developed countries the major cause is maternal hypertension either associated with pregnancy or as an exacerbation of pre-existing essential hypertension. Probably as great an influence is cigarette smoking, and to a lesser extent alcohol consumption during pregnancy. Intrauterine infections with viruses such as rubella and cytomegalovirus, whilst widely recognized as producing IUGR and malformations, probably are only responsible for about 5% of SFD infants. High altitude may cause IUGR because of hypoxia in some parts of the world such as the Andes and the Himalayas.

Effects of IUGR

Where poor growth in the fetus has been due to genetic factors, the effects on the newborn infant may not be a problem. In most cases, however, chronic undernutrition and/or hypoxia in the fetus lead to a recognizable SFD syndrome of asymmetrical growth retardation, poor fat and glycogen stores, polycythaemia, and a degree of acceleration of maturation of systems such as the lung phospholipids. A major part of antenatal care is concentrated on the identification of the IUGR fetus. Methods vary from the simple use of a tape measure to record fundal height above the symphysis pubis, to ultrasound scan measurements of the fetal head and abdominal circumferences. When identified, the fetal condition can be further estimated by using fetal heart rate monitoring, and most recently, by blood flow velocity measurements in the placenta, umbilical artery or in fetal vessels using Doppler ultrasound. Ultrasound may also be used to identify the cause of IUGR if this is associated with malformation, and amniocentesis or chorionic villus biopsy may be used to diagnose chromosomal defects.

The most serious problems of SFD infants are at around the time of birth, when low fetal reserves may result in asphyxia, aspiration syndromes and persistent fetal circulation. After birth, hypothermia, hypoglycaemia, hyperviscosity, and hyperbilirubinaemia may all occur.

Preterm infants

In Europe and North America the preterm birth rate varies between 5 and 8%. Such infants are more likely to develop disorders associated with organ or system immaturity, and their mortality rises with decreasing gestational age. Survival rates of under 10% are seen for infants of 24 weeks' gestation, rising to 75% or higher at 28 weeks, and over 95% at 32 weeks' gestation [24]. About 2% of the UK population born are 32 weeks of gestation or less [2].

Many preterm deliveries are unexplained. Maternal illness is an important cause and preterm delivery occurs more often in mothers with cardiac and renal disease, as well as with acute infections where the mother is febrile, such as urinary infection or influenza. Abnormal fetuses are more often born early, although the mechanism for this is unclear.

Hypertension in the mother, usually due to pre-eclampsia, may force the obstetrician to intervene at an early stage, resulting in a premature delivery. Uterine abnormalities such as bicornuate uterus and 'cervical incompetence' may be the cause for a smaller number of early births, and recent work has also shown the importance of local endocervical infection and cigarette smoking in preterm labour [7].

Asphyxia, aspiration and persistent pulmonary hypertension

Because many IUGR fetuses have experienced chronic hypoxia and poor placental perfusion during gestation, they have low reserves of glycogen in liver and muscle, and are less able to withstand further intrapartum hypoxia by means of anaerobic respiration. The low fetal arterial oxygen tension leads to hypertrophy of the pulmonary arteriolar musculature with the result that pulmonary vasodilatation following birth and the commencement of air breathing is incomplete leading to pulmonary hypertension and low lung blood flow. Pulmonary hypertension may complicate other lung disorders in the newborn and be part of the pathology of cardiac malformations and diaphragmatic hernia. Aspiration, usually of meconium, frequently occurs in IUGR infants with birth asphyxia. If the trachea is adequately suctioned at birth the resulting respiratory distress is fairly short-lived, although it may be complicated by pneumothorax or a secondary pneumonia. Severe pulmonary hypertension is present in some infants with meconium aspiration, and is responsible for the mortality seen [5]. Management is largely supportive. Hyperventilation may reduce the pulmonary hypertension, and pulmonary vasodilators such as tolazoline or prostacyclin are often used in more severe cases.

The degree of birth asphyxia experienced by

IUGR infants is important in determining their ultimate developmental outcome, and its frequent occurrence may explain the poorer long-term developmental progress often seen in these babies. Preterm babies also frequently suffer birth asphyxia, usually in association with early placental separation, cord compression or antepartum haemorrhage. Asphyxiated preterm infants develop more periventricular cerebral haemorrhage and have worse respiratory distress. Prevention of perinatal asphyxia is therefore essential if a good outcome is to be achieved with low birthweight infants.

Water and heat loss

All low birthweight infants lose heat very readily. This is a particular problem at birth when resuscitation is to be carried out, and later if a small infant comes to surgery. Part of the problem stems from the relatively large surface area of small infants (which determines their rate of heat loss) and their small body mass (which determines their rate of heat production). In addition both IUGR and preterm infants have minimal 'brown-fat' stores for thermogenesis, and no subcutaneous fat for insulation [12]. Preterm infants have an immature skin that allows rapid transudation of water which evaporates, taking heat from the infant. This effect becomes less after the first week of life as the epidermis becomes thicker [21]. Other heat loss is caused by radiation, convection and conduction, but is not usually as great as that caused by evaporation. Hypothermia is associated with a poorer outcome in most studies. With the smallest infants use of an incubator is often not enough and covering the infant with plastic film or the use of a high humidity environment may avoid cold. The use of overhead radiant heaters or 'open' cribs makes the avoidance of hypothermia easier, but care must be taken to avoid dehydration from excessive evaporation. Damage to the skin by adhesive electrode rings and tape allows increased evaporation and heat loss and care should be taken in very preterm babies to avoid this. Large wet wound dressings or packs also have the same cooling effect. If exposed gut or spinal tissue needs to be kept moist prior to surgery, it is better to cover it with a non-stick impermeable dressing than a wet pack.

Nutrition and hypoglycaemia

Well infants of 34 weeks' gestation or more will usually feed normally from birth. Smaller infants may feed less well and require some or all their feeds to be given by gastric tube. Signs of gastrointestinal stasis, recurrent apnoea, or tachypnoea are reasons to withhold oral feeds, and to maintain calories, electrolytes and fluids are given by intravenous infusion. Some neonatal units will also feed infants of less than 1500 g intravenously for at least the first few days of life until it is clear that they are well. Ill infants are best fed intravenously, although it is possible to feed infants on mechanical ventilation by gastric tube when the acute phase of their illness is over. Feeding by jejunal tube was popular for a while but has no clear advantages over gastric feeding. Gastric tubes are best placed through the mouth in small infants rather than the nose in order to avoid increasing the work of breathing by nasal obstruction. Human milk is tolerated better than artificial milks, but may not always be available. Special preterm formulas will often promote faster growth and avoid problems such as rickets later. However, some are hypertonic and others may cause milk curd obstruction. The rate of increase of feeding should be gradual, making up any deficit with parenteral fluids. A total energy intake of over 100 kcal/kg per day is usually recommended, although growth may occur on less than this if the infant is otherwise well.

Hypoglycaemia most commonly occurs in the neonatal period in SFD infants and may be seen symptomatically in 10% of infants of birth weights more than 2 SD below the mean for age [1]. Symptoms are not usually seen until the blood glucose falls below 2 mmol/l. Jitteriness, apnoea, and eventually convulsions occur. SFD infants should be fed early or given a dextrose infusion to avoid this. Infants should in addition be screened prior to each feed using a bedside 'stick' test for blood sugar, during the first 48 h of life. Hypoglycaemia with symptoms, or not responding to a feed, should be treated with a dextrose infusion. This may need to be maintained for 2–3 days in some cases until some glycogen storage is built up. The long-term outcome for infants with symptomatic hypoglycaemia is poor, although whether this is a direct result of the low blood sugar or results from the period of growth retardation is not clear.

Respiratory problems

Respiratory disorders are common in the low birthweight infant, and especially in preterm babies. They present as respiratory distress, which is seen as cyanosis, tachypnoea, sternal and intercostal recession, and grunting respiration. The commonest cause of respiratory distress is transient tachypnoea of the newborn (TTN), which is seen in infants of any gestational age up to term. Its aetiology is thought to be delayed clearance of lung fluid from the lungs after birth. Lung fluid is produced in large amounts before birth, but its rate of secretion falls rapidly on commencement of air breathing. This change is mediated by catecholamine release during the stress of birth, and this may account for the high incidence of TTN in babies born by elective caesarean section [21]. The baby is rarely very ill and mechanical ventilation is not required. Most infants are improving on the second day of life, and need only some supplemental oxygen for a few days. The chest X-ray shows a streaky appearance from fluid-filled lymphatics, and sometimes fluid in the interlobar fissure can be seen.

Respiratory distress syndrome (RDS), also called hyaline membrane disease or surfactant deficiency syndrome, is a disease of preterm infants, and a major cause of morbidity and mortality in this age group. It is almost universal in infants of 28 weeks or less, and occurs with decreasing frequency up until term. Lung maturity is determined by the release of phospholipids (surfactant) from type 2 pneumatocytes in the lung which are responsible for the reduction of surface tension in lung fluid, allowing the lung to be easily expanded and for it to maintain a residual capacity in expiration.

Surfactant synthesis begins in the lung before the end of the last trimester, but release does not usually occur until around 34 weeks of gestation. The stress of early delivery or even of growth retardation is often enough to stimulate release before this time, allowing many small infants to avoid RDS [13]. This stress can be mimicked by giving the mother corticosteroids prior to preterm birth, and thus avoiding or reducing the severity of RDS. The signs of RDS are those of respiratory distress, usually very marked, and appearing within 4 h of birth (Figure 9.2). The less mature the infant, the earlier the signs appear, and very preterm infants are often unable to initiate adequate respiration at birth. The chest X-ray shows a fine granular appearance in the peripheral lung fields with the bronchi outlined ('air-bronchogram') (Figure 9.3).

The management of RDS is essentially supportive. Mechanical ventilation is required in all but the mildest cases, but attention to other aspects of supportive care such as fluid and electrolyte balance and adequate nutritional support is essential if treatment is to be successful. The recent introduction of surfactant therapy is the first major improvement in the treatment of RDS in 20 years. Both artificial and animal and human derived surfactant mixtures have been used, for both the treatment of established RDS and prophylaxis in high risk newborns [6,23]. Commercial surfactant mixtures will shortly be available.

Larger infants with RDS are breathing air alone by 7–10 days after birth and in general the prognosis is very good. For smaller infants (under 1250 g) the period of treatment may last weeks or even months in some cases. In the short term, complications such as pneumothorax (Figure 9.4), persistent ductus arteriosus, and intraventricular cerebral haemorrhage are common. Later the problems of chronic lung disease (bronchopulmonary dysplasia) and ischaemic brain injury become more important.

In very preterm infants, recurrent apnoea is common. This is in part due to the rather immature respiratory patterns of the preterm, and partly to the ease with which they become exhausted with the effort of the work of breathing. The chest wall is very compliant in the preterm infant and this results in a waste of respiratory effort as the sternum indraws with each contraction of the diaphragm. In most preterm infants, recurrent apnoea may be managed by repeated stimulation. It is essential that all such infants are adequately monitored using an

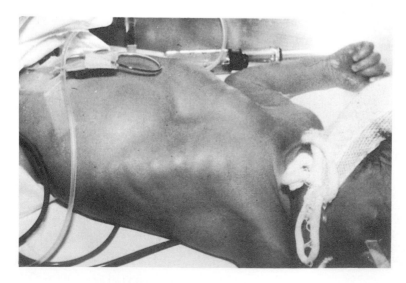

Figure 9.2 Sternal recession in an infant with respiratory distress syndrome

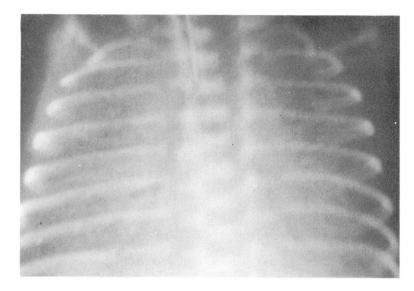

Figure 9.3 Chest X-ray of infant with respiratory distress syndrome showing 'air-bronchogram'

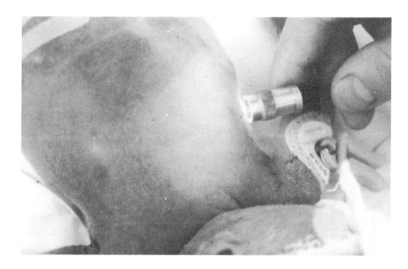

Figure 9.4 Pneumothorax in ventilated infant demonstrated by transillumination

apnoea mattress or ECG monitor. Where apnoea is persistent, and other neonatal illnesses such as sugar or electrolyte disorder and infections have been excluded, treatment with methylxanthines such as theophylline or aminophylline are often effective. In resistant cases intubation and positive airways pressure or mechanical ventilation may become necessary.

Respiratory problems from lung infection are common in the neonatal period. Early infections (within the first 2 days) are usually due to infections acquired before or during birth. The risk of such infection is increased if the amniotic membranes ruptured more than 24 h before delivery. The usual organisms responsible are group B beta-haemolytic streptococci, and various Gram-negative organisms from the maternal urogenital tract or rectum. The diagnosis of pneumonia in the newborn is not always easy, and depends on a high index of suspicion. Ruptured membranes, or an atypical respiratory illness in a mature infant are pointers. Many infants with pneumonia, however, are clinically and radiologically indistinguishable from infants with hyaline membrane disease. Antibiotic therapy with a penicillin and an aminoglycoside is begun after a full septic screen in all infants suspected of pneumonia. If cultures are negative after 2 days the antibiotics may be discontinued if the baby appears to be improving. Later lung infections usually occur in infants who are being ventilated, and may be caused by staphylococci or enterobacilli usually from the infant's own gastrointestinal tract.

Hyperbilirubinaemia

Visible jaundice occurs in as many as 50% of newborn infants, but in the majority it is of little consequence. Serum levels of bilirubin do not usually exceed 250 μmol/l, and no treatment is needed, the jaundice resolving within 10 days or so. This is commonly called 'physiological' jaundice, and is related to the relatively high rate of turnover of haemoglobin at this time. The importance of pathological neonatal jaundice is as a sign of underlying illness, or in some cases as a cause of central nervous system damage. High levels of bilirubin may result from increased haemolysis of red cells, reduced conjugation and excretion at the hepatic level, obstruction of the biliary system or an increase in the enterohepatic circulation because of increased transit time in the gut. Severe hyperbilirubinaemia may also be seen in infants who have suffered intrapartum infections such as cytomegalovirus, with bacterial infections such as septicaemia or urinary tract infections, and with metabolic disorders such as hypothyroidism and galactosaemia. Preterm infants are more likely to develop 'pathological' levels of jaundice, although often a specific cause cannot be found. In the past, infants with isoimmunization from the Rhesus (D) factor were the main source of infants with very high levels of bilirubin. With the introduction of anti-D prophylaxis, this is much less commonly seen, although isoimmunization with the formation of anti-C and anti-E is still seen.

Bilirubin is neurotoxic if it enters the central nervous system. It normally does not cross the cerebral capillary endothelium easily (blood-brain barrier), and the small amounts entering the brain are rapidly hydrolysed by a specific enzyme. This protective mechanism is fragile, and in a number of states such as severe asphyxia, acidosis or sepsis, the endothelium leaks allowing excessive amounts of bilirubin in. It is the state of the blood-brain barrier rather than the absolute plasma level of bilirubin that determines entry of bilirubin [12]. However, in conditions with a high level of bilirubin, acidosis or sepsis frequently co-exists. There is no clinical test for the integrity of the blood-brain barrier, and neonatal management of hyperbilirubinaemia is largely based on keeping the plasma bilirubin at a low level where possible. The classic picture of bilirubin neurotoxicity is rarely seen today. Fits and hypertonicity in the neonatal period are followed by death, or in survivors by hypotonicity and later deafness, mental retardation and athetoid cerebral

palsy. Autopsy shows yellow staining of the basal ganglia of the brain (kernicterus) and neuronal death and gliosis are seen microscopically. Although there is no direct evidence, it is commonly supposed that the high level of nerve deafness seen in very low birthweight infants is due to bilirubin induced auditory nerve damage. Management of neonatal jaundice is primarily aimed at the diagnosis and treatment of underlying causative illnesses such as infection. Treatment of hyperbilirubinaemia is by exchange transfusion of about 180 ml/kg blood via an umbilical artery or vein catheter. In preterm infants the need for exchange transfusion can be reduced by the early use of phototherapy. The infant is exposed to blue or green light which causes photoisomerization of bilirubin in the skin. Certain photoisomers of bilirubin produced by bright light are more readily excreted by the liver. Phototherapy results in more rapid excretion of bilirubin into the gut. It may produce loose stools and skin erythema in treated infants. The eyes of the infant are usually covered, but the risk of retinal damage in those not covered is not known.

Infection

Infection in the neonatal period is much more common in the low birthweight than the full-term infant and in infants in intensive care units an infection rate of 10% is not uncommon [8]. Although reduced cellular and humoral immunity exists in low birthweight infants, the main factors predisposing to their high infection rates are other illnesses and the high rate of skin damage from surgery, catheterization and other injuries. Infections may be localized such as omphalitis or wound infections, but may rapidly disseminate as a septicaemia. Failure to localize infection is common, making the signs of infection in the newborn non-specific and difficult to identify. A low threshold of suspicion is needed, and it is usually necessary to treat infants with antibiotics before any confirmation of infection is available from laboratory tests. No one test is specific for neonatal infection and several authors have tried to use batteries of tests to increase diagnostic sensitivity and specificity [19]. Absolute neutrophil counts and percentage of 'band forms' present are quick and widely available. Acute phase proteins such as C reactive protein are now easier to measure using kits, but are more useful for following the course of an infection than in making the original diagnosis.

Although a wide range of differing antibiotic regimens have been suggested, the combination of a penicillin with an aminoglycoside until culture results are known is the most usually used, treatment being changed to a more specific drug later if necessary. It is important to appreciate that treatment of neonatal infection often involves support of respiration, blood pressure, fluid balance and nutrition, etc, and is not confined to antibiotic therapy alone. Antibiotic therapy is continued for 5 days, or longer if recovery is delayed. If culture results are negative it is prudent to stop antibiotic therapy, thus reducing the chances of encouraging drug resistance.

Early neonatal infection is mainly related to organisms derived from the mother's birth canal including Gram-positive organisms such as group B beta-haemolytic streptococci and a wide range of gut-derived Gram-negative organisms such as *Escherichia coli*, *Proteus*, *Enterobacter*, etc. Later infections which tend to be nosocomial, include *Staphylococcus aureus* and epidermidis, and often multiply drug resistant Gram-negative organisms such as *Pseudomonas*, *Proteus*, *Klebsiella* and *Serratia*. Extensive handling of infants by personnel and lowered resistance in sick infants make the latter group a particular threat in intensive care units.

Neurological disorders

The ultimate quality of survival of a sick newborn infant is largely determined by the absence of neurological sequelae. The brain of the preterm or growth retarded infant is very vulnerable to injury due to its relatively large size, and to its immature and developing state.

Apart from direct physical trauma, the brain may be injured by intrauterine viral infection, growth retardation, toxins such as alcohol or bilirubin, or by drugs or radiation. The majority of cerebral injury in low birthweight infants is attributable to haemorrhagic and ischaemic lesions, and our understanding of these has greatly increased since the introduction of portable real-time ultrasound scanners to neonatal practice [16]. The cerebral circulation in the preterm newborn with hyaline membrane disease or following birth asphyxia is unstable, and liable to fluctuate with changes in cardiac output and variations in blood pressure. Most cerebral haemorrhage in the preterm infant occurs around the cerebral ventricles and is referred to as periventricular haemorrhage. The site of origin of the bleeding is the germinal matrix, which lies on the lateral border of the lateral ventricles overlying the caudate nucleus [17]. About 50% of all very low birthweight infants have some degree of periventricular haemorrhage detectable on cerebral ultrasound scanning in the first week of life [18]. Most of these haemorrhages are small and confined to the germinal matrix. They are not associated with adverse outcome. These small haemorrhages may extend into the cerebral ventricles by rupture, or into the brain parenchyma by a process of venous infarction. Extensive ventricular haemorrhage is associated

with a high risk of post-haemorrhagic hydrocephalus. Parenchymal extension of haemorrhage is followed by the formation of porencephalic cysts at the site of the extension, and often subsequent hemiplegia [4].

Ischaemic injury to the preterm brain may be in the form of extensive infarction, or as periventricular leucomalacia. Major infarction may occur as the consequence of antepartum haemorrhage, or later following septicaemia. Periventricular leucomalacia is seen on cerebral ultrasound scan at 2–3 weeks of age or later, although some signs may be present before this. Leucomalacia is usually clinically silent, although late onset convulsions are often seen. Extensive leucomalacia is strongly associated with later cerebral palsy and cortical blindness [4]. The aetiology of leucomalacia is unclear, although local reduction in cerebral blood flow, possibly following haemorrhage, would seem likely.

Haemorrhagic disorders

Haemorrhagic disease in the newborn due to lack of vitamin K dependent clotting factors is now rarely seen because of routine administration of vitamin K to newborn infants immediately after birth. Bleeding in sick low birthweight infants is most likely to be due to a consumption coagulopathy or to thrombocytopenia. Consumption coagulopathy is seen after birth asphyxia, severe maternal pre-eclampsia, septicaemia or extensive haemorrhage such as intraventricular haemorrhage. It is best managed by transfusion of fresh frozen plasma or by exchange transfusion with fresh whole blood. The prognosis depends on the removal or treatment of the causative factor, rather than on direct treatment of the coagulopathy.

Thrombocytopenia is most often seen in this age group in association with sepsis. Platelet consumption such as in necrotizing enterocolitis is also seen. If bleeding is a major problem, platelet transfusions may be given, although their effect is short-lived and correction of the causative factor is essential. Thrombocytopenia due to isoimmunization or to maternal idiopathic thrombocytopenic purpura is not often seen in low birthweight infants. Exchange transfusion may be used to treat it but this is not usually needed. A short course of corticosteroids or intravenous immunoglobulin is usually effective.

Surgical disorders arising from the care of low birthweight infants

Patent ductus arteriosus

Closure of the ductus normally occurs within hours of birth, but in the preterm infant, particularly when respiratory distress is present, this may be delayed for days or even weeks. In the first few days after birth the patent ductus causes little problem as the pulmonary artery pressure remains high. As the infant's pulmonary resistance falls, a left-to-right shunt develops from aorta to pulmonary artery. This may result eventually in a pulmonary blood flow which exceeds the systemic flow by two to three times, causing pulmonary plethora and a low blood flow to the lower body, in particular to the kidneys and gut. A systolic murmur and full pulses are usually present. Other clinical signs are weight gain, apnoeic attacks or an inability to 'wean' ventilated infants. Complications include necrotizing enterocolitis and possibly cerebral haemorrhage, and the incidence of chronic lung disease is increased. By restricting fluid intake to below 130 ml/kg/day, in the early stages, the incidence of symptomatic ductus can be minimized. Ductal signs may often be reduced to acceptable levels by correction of anaemia or by giving a small dose of frusemide. If problems persist, closure of the duct is indicated. In the past this was done surgically, but now is mainly effected by treatment with indomethacin, a cyclo-oxygenase inhibitor which reduces the production of prostaglandins [9]. A dose of 0.2 mg/kg is used and given 8-hourly for three doses. Recent work suggests that a smaller daily dose for 6 days is just as effective and produces fewer side effects. The only serious problem with indomethacin is gastrointestinal bleeding, although temporary oliguria is common. Treatment is more often successful with intravenous rather than oral therapy. Surgical ligation is effective and may be carried out by a skilled surgeon without removing the infant from the intensive care unit. The mortality and the reported complication rate is low, although recurrent laryngeal nerve palsy and accidental ligation of a pulmonary artery have been described.

Bronchopulmonary dysplasia

Following prolonged ventilator therapy, particularly in very preterm infants, chronic lung disease develops. This is called bronchopulmonary dysplasia by pathologists, but 'ventilator lung' or chronic lung disease by clinicians. The chest X-ray shows a patchy and varying consolidation interspersed with areas of hyperinflation or frank cystic development. Prolonged oxygen dependence occurs, and weaning from the ventilator may be difficult. In the worst cases, cor pulmonale develops and the infant dies. However, with care the majority will survive. The use of a regular dose of a diuretic often improves the respiratory state, as does a short course of a corticosteroid [14]. The latter carries the risk of sepsis, and the long-term benefits of such therapy are questioned. Occasionally, a portion of the lung

with cystic damage will become hyperinflated and compromise the function of the remaining lung. This is distinct from congenital malformations of the lung, although it has often been confused with them. Surgical intervention is rarely indicated, and a satisfactory short-term solution is usually to aspirate the cysts with a needle and syringe, and this may need to be repeated once or twice a day until they finally resolve.

Upper airway damage

Because of prolonged intubation of the airway in intensive care, a number of injuries are seen which may require surgical attention. Tracheal stenosis was most common when red rubber endotracheal tubes were used. The advent of modern inert and siliconized tubes has greatly reduced the problem. A few very small infants do still develop tracheal obstruction on extubation. Some of this is due to oedema, and may be helped with a dose of corticosteroid a few hours before extubation. In the minority tracheostomy is indicated. In the very small infant this is not easy, and damage to the trachea may result in difficulty in closing the tracheostomy later.

Damage to the nasal septum or to the palate may also result from prolonged intubation. Septal damage is due to pressure necrosis, and may be avoided by not using too large a nasal tube, and by alternating the side of intubation regularly. Palatal deformity occurs with prolonged orotracheal intubation, a deep groove forming in the midline. It slowly improves with growth in survivors.

Necrotizing enterocolitis

Necrotizing enterocolitis is a common complication occurring in low birthweight infants in intensive care. Although a large number of clinical associations are described, they are mainly descriptive of infants with a low gut blood flow; high haematocrit, patent ductus arteriosus, umbilical vessel catheterization, recurrent apnoea and birth asphyxia [11]. The fully developed picture of abdominal distension, bloody diarrhoea, bile-stained vomiting, and pneumatosis is not always seen in the very low birthweight infant (Figure 9.5). This is because oral feeds are often withheld for several weeks in sick ventilated babies. The lack of bacterial substrate in the gut does not permit gas formation and the rapid bacterial invasion of the ischaemic gut that usually occurs. The clinical picture may simply be of abdominal distension with ascites, abdominal wall discoloration, and X-ray appearances of a gas-free bowel or a fixed solitary loop of gas-filled gut in the region of the terminal ileum.

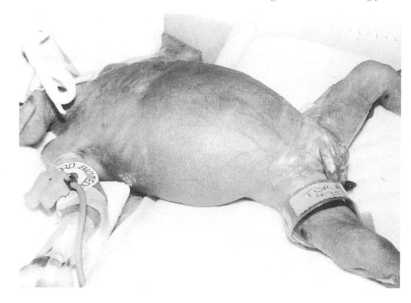

Figure 9.5 Very low birthweight infant with necrotizing enterocolitis. Note distended and discoloured abdomen and bloody stools

The treatment of choice is initially conservative with general supportive measures and antibiotics. If improvement is not obvious within 24–48 h, laparotomy is indicated, and extensive disease is to be expected. In conservatively managed cases, later deterioration may be due to perforation, which is also usually considered an indication for laparotomy, although conservative measures with insertion of an abdominal drain have been reported. Even in infants responding well to conservative measures, later stricture information is common, and 'cold' resection may be required. In the long term, most survivors do well, and the incidence of 'short-gut syndrome' is very low with initial conservative management. Closure of the ileostomy formed after resection may need to be carried out earlier than anticipated in some tiny infants in order to minimize fluid losses.

Hernias

Umbilical and inguinal hernias are both common in very low birthweight survivors [20]. The former, although often very large, invariably resolve during the first year of life. Inguinal hernias occur in both male and female low birthweight infants, and are usually repaired as soon as is practicable, often as a day case on the day of discharge from the baby unit. Unfortunately the thin abdominal wall and poor musculature in these infants means that they may recur after repair.

Skin loss

Frequent placement of peripheral intravenous infusions in tiny infants inevitably means a number of infusions which run into the tissues around the vein, with resultant necrosis (Figure 9.6). The hypertonic composition of intravenous feeding solutions make this more likely. Although most of the necrotic lesions produced will heal with straightforward nursing care, some of the larger ones will require skin grafting in order to avoid very extensive scar formation or damage to underlying muscles or tendons. Such lesions may to some degree be avoided by the use of central venous access, surgically implanted, though this may increase the risk of septicaemia.

Retinopathy of prematurity

About 5% of infants of less than 1000 g birth weight will develop retinopathy of prematurity of such a degree as to have no useful vision. A much larger number will have lesser damage or lesions which will resolve with time. The exact aetiology is unknown, and although there is strong circumstantial evidence that in larger infants uncontrolled administration of oxygen was responsible in the 1940s and 1950s, the situation is more complex in very low birthweight infants. Prevention by vitamin E prophylaxis has

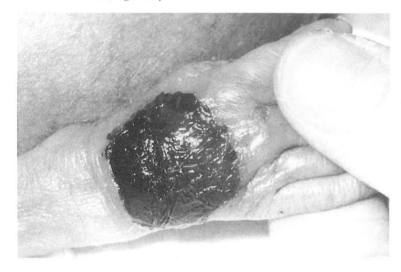

Figure 9.6 Superficial skin necrosis produced by extravasation of parenteral nutrition infusion

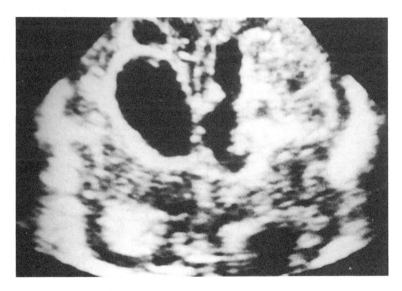

Figure 9.7 Coronal ultrasound scan of infant brain showing intraventricular haemorrhage and early ventricular dilatation

been tried in several controlled trials, but the evidence of long-term benefit is unconvincing. Surgical management using laser treatment to control the proliferation of new retinal vessels formed has not been evaluated in a controlled manner and must be seen as experimental [15]. A recent collaborative controlled trial of early cryotherapy in infants with stage 3+ or worse retinopathy of prematurity has shown a significant improvement in outcome in treated infants [25].

Post-haemorrhagic hydrocephalus

In a busy intensive care unit with a referral service, as many as 1–2% of low birthweight survivors will develop post-haemorrhagic hydrocephalus after extensive intraventricular haemorrhage [3]. A few of these infants will have clear evidence of gross neurological deficit, and a decision not to treat further may be made. For the majority however some form of treatment will become necessary.

Following the haemorrhage, the cerebral ventricles will begin to enlarge almost immediately, and this can be seen on ultrasound scanning (Figure 9.7). In many infants this initial ventriculomegaly is a temporary phenomenon, and spontaneous arrest occurs followed by slow resolution. Where the enlargement continues to progress, the head circumference only begins to enlarge 2–3 weeks later, the brain filling the large subarachnoid space before this time. At about the same time, symptoms of recurrent apnoea, vomiting or convulsions may be observed. Many infants are asymptomatic, however. Attempts to slow down the rate of enlargement with drugs such as isosorbide, glycerine, frusemide and acetazolamide have been made, and are partly successful. There is no evidence that such treatment has any long-term advantage. Alternatively, removal of cerebrospinal fluid (CSF) using spinal or ventricular punctures will slow the progress of enlargement and relieve symptoms. Equally, however, no long-term benefit has yet been demonstrated. Most centres use some form of temporizing measure where infants are considered to be too small for insertion of a ventriculoperitoneal shunt. The repeated removal of CSF also serves to lower the protein and blood content of the CSF which some surgeons believe is responsible for early blockage of the shunt system. Ventriculo-atrial shunts are difficult to insert in very small infants, have a higher risk of infection, and will need earlier replacement. During the first years of life complications of shunt block are common, and are frequently associated with low-grade infections with *Staph. epidermidis*. The long-term prognosis for infants treated for post-haemorrhagic hydrocephalus is very variable, but largely depends on the extent of parenchymal brain damage present following the initial bleed [3].

References

1. Aynsley-Green, A. and Soltesz, G. (1986) Metabolic and endocrine disorders. In *Textbook of Neonatology*, (ed. N.R.C. Roberton) Churchill Livingstone, Edinburgh

2. Chamberlain, R. (1975) Birthweight and length of gestation. In *British Births 1970*. Heinemann, London

3. Cooke, R.W.I. (1987) Determinants of major handicap in post-haemorrhagic hydrocephalus. *Arch. Dis. Child.*, **62**, 504–506

4. Cooke, R.W.I. (1987) Early and late cranial ultrasonographic appearances and outcome in very low birthweight infants. *Arch. Dis. Child.*, **62**, 931–937

5. Fox, W.W., Gewitz, M.H. and Dinwiddie, R. (1977) Pulmonary hypertension in the perinatal aspiration syndrome. *Pediatrics*, **59**, 205

6. Hallman, M., Merritt, T.A. and Jarvenpas, A.L. (1985) Exogenous human surfactant for treatment of severe respiratory distress syndrome: a randomised prospective clinical trial. *J. Pediat.*, **106**, 963–969

7. Harvey, J., Agustsson, P., Patel, N. and Anderson, J. (1985) The role of infection in the aetiology of preterm labour. In *Preterm Labour and its Consequences* (ed. R.W. Beard and F. Sharp) Royal College of Obstetricians and Gynaecologists, London

8. Hensey, O.J., Hart, C.A. and Cooke, R.W.I. (1985) Serious infection in a neonatal intensive care unit: a 2 year survey. *J. Hyg. Camb.*, **95**, 289–297

9. Heymann, M.A., Rudolph, A.M. and Silverman, N.H. (1976) Closure of the ductus arteriosus in premature infants by inhibition of prostaglandin synthesis. *New Engl. J. Med.*, **295**, 530–533

10. Hull, D. (1975) The storage and supply of fatty acids before and after birth. *Br. Med. Bull.*, **31**, 32–36

11. Kleigman, R.M. and Fanaroff, A.A. (1984) Necrotizing enterocolitis. *New Engl. J. Med.*, **310**, 1093–1103

12. Levine, R.L., Fredericks, W.R., Rapoport, A.B. and Rapoport, S.I. (1982) Entry of bilirubin into the brain due to opening of the blood-brain barrier. *Pediatrics*, **69**, 255–258

13. Liggins, G.C. and Howie, R.N. (1972) A controlled trial of antepartum glucocorticoid treatment for prevention of the respiratory distress syndrome in premature infants. *Pediatrics*, **50**, 515–525

14. Mammel, M.C., Green, T.P. and Johnson, D.E. (1983) Controlled trial of dexamethasone therapy in infants with bronchopulmonary dysplasia. *Lancet*, **i**, 1356–1357

15. Palmer, E.A., Biglan, A.W. and Hardy, R.J. (1986) Retinal ablative therapy for active proliferative retinopathy of prematurity: history, current status and prospects. In *Retinopathy of Prematurity* (ed. W.A. Silverman and J.T. Flynn) Blackwell Scientific Publications, Oxford

16. Pape, K.E., Cusick, G., Houang, M.T.W. *et al.* (1979) Ultrasound detection of brain damage in preterm infants. *Lancet*, **i**, 1261–1263

17. Pape, K.E. and Wigglesworth, J.S. (1979) *Haemorrhage, Ischaemia and the Perinatal Brain*. Heinemann, London

18. Papile, L.-A., Burstein, J., Burstein, R. and Koffler, H. (1978) Incidence and evolution of subependymal and intraventricular haemorrhage: a study of infants with birthweights less than 1500 g. *J. Pediat.*, **92**, 529

19. Philip, A.G.S. and Hewitt, J.R. (1980) Early diagnosis of neonatal sepsis. *Pediatrics*, **65**, 1036–1041

20. Powell, T.G., Hallows, J.A., Cooke, R.W.I. and Pharoah, P.O.D. (1986) Why do so many infants develop an inguinal hernia? *Arch. Dis. Child.*, **61**, 991–995

21. Rutter, N. and Hull, D. (1979) Water loss from the skin of term and preterm babies. *Arch. Dis. Child.*, **54**, 858–868

22. Strang, L.B. (1977) Fetal lung liquid. In *Neonatal Respiration* (ed. L.C. Strang) Blackwell Scientific Publications, Oxford
23. Ten Centre Study Group (1987) Ten Centre trial of artificial surfactant (artificial lung expanding compound) in very premature babies. *Br. Med. J.*, **294**, 991–996
24. Yu, V.Y.H. (1987) Survival and neurodevelopmental outcome of preterm infants. In *Prematurity* (ed. V.Y.H. Yu and C.E. Wood) Churchill Livingstone, Edinburgh
25. Cryotherapy for Retinopathy of Prematurity Cooperative Group (1988) *Arch. Ophthalmol.* **106**, 471–479

10

Neonatal infections and antibiotics

C.A. Hart

Introduction

The neonate, and in particular the premature neonate, is at increased risk of infection compared with older children or adults. Rates of infection vary with the prematurity of the baby. For example, the prevalence of bacterial septicaemia and meningitis for infants born weighing more than 2500 g is respectively 1.1 cases and 0.04 cases per 1000 live births but for those weighing less than 2500 g is 13.3 cases of septicaemia and 2.3 cases of meningitis per 1000 live births [48]. A more recent survey in Germany has indicated that the overall prevalence has increased from 0.88 cases of septicaemia per 1000 live births over the period 1962–74 to 2.0 cases per 1000 births from 1975–82 [73]. This presumably represents improved intensive care facilities that allow babies of increasing prematurity to survive. In general it is estimated that between 10 and 22% of neonates admitted to neonatal intensive care units (NICU) develop septicaemia [7,40,44]. These figures of course vary with the intensity of management. Unfortunately there is very little information on infection in neonatal surgical units. Not only are neonates at increased risk of serious infection but they are at increased risk of dying from their infections. For example, mortality rates in septicaemia of 40% rising to 62% in infants born weighing less than 1000 g have been recorded [45]. However mortality rates do seem to be improving with earlier diagnosis, rapid institution of antimicrobial chemotherapy and better management [42,63,73]. Nevertheless the frequency and gravity of severe neonatal infection is high and, in part, is a reflection of the impairment of the host's defence mechanisms [18].

The neonate as an immune-compromised host

The immune system is divided into the non-specific and specific arms and the neonate has defects in both.

Non-specific immune system

The non-specific immune system acts as both a barrier to or to remove invading microorganisms but is not directed against any specific invader. It may be sub-divided conveniently into that present at body surfaces (skin and mucous membranes) and that within the tissues. The neonate is deficient in each of these areas (Table 10.1).

Table 10.1 Defects in neonatal non-specific immunity

At skin surfaces
    Umbilical stump
    Intravenous or intra-arterial lines
    Lack of normal flora
At mucous membranes
    Ventilation
    Gastric acidity
    Intestinal permeability
    Lack of normal flora
In the tissues
    Decreased complement levels
    Poor temperature control
    Diminished inflammatory response
    Diminished phagocytic activity

At body surfaces

The umbilical stump represents both a breach in the skin surface and a reservoir for microorganisms. If cord care is not optimal, it can act as a rich culture medium for both aerobic and anaerobic bacteria particularly if it is moist. This may merely represent abnormal colonization but may progress to produce bacterial omphalitis [12] which can prove fatal. Figure 10.1 shows a Gram film of peritoneal pus obtained at autopsy from a neonate who died with omphalitis due to *Clostridium perfringens*. A Gram-positive bacterium can be seen in close association with a neutrophil that has been lysed by the clostridial lecithinase. In addition because catheters are often inserted into the umbilical artery, bacteria

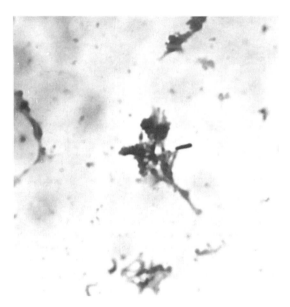

Figure 10.1 Gram-stained film of peritoneal pus in a neonate with omphalitis due to *Clostridium perfringens*, showing a bacillus with disrupted pus cells

may gain access from the umbilicus into the blood. It is noteworthy that of 139 neonates in Liverpool with septicaemia, 79 (52%) had umbilical artery catheters *in situ* and 71 (90%) of these showed umbilical colonization with their infecting bacteria [42]. Other intravenous and arterial lines may also provide a means by which microorganisms gain direct access to the blood stream, bypassing the skin's natural defences. Such microorganisms are derived either from the skin itself or from the infused fluid [31].

Non-specific defences at mucosal surfaces include factors such as the mucociliary escalator in the bronchi, lysozyme and lactoferrin on most mucosae, and intestinal secretions, peristalsis and normal flora.

It appears that for both lysozyme (which cleaves bacterial peptidoglycan) and lactoferrin (which starves bacteria of the iron necessary for replication) synthesis begins early in fetal life (from 10–12 weeks) [1] and deficiency is rare. In addition, both lactoferrin and lysozyme are present in breast milk and colostrum.

The use of endotracheal tubes in mechanical ventilation will in part bypass one of the lung's most important defences, the mucociliary escalator. If improperly managed, endotracheal tubes will deliver microorganisms either from the oropharynx or via the lumen of the tube directly into the bronchi. The trauma associated with the introduction of an endotracheal tube may also lead to bacteraemia [23]. In the gastrointestinal tract, secretion of gastric acid, secretion of mucin, and the mechanical cleansing activity of peristalsis are important and there is evidence that these activities are impaired [79] especially if the neonate is being fed parenterally.

It has been estimated that the adult human comprises 10^{14} cells but that only 10% of these are human. The remainder are microorganisms, principally bacteria, that form the 'normal flora'. *In utero*, the developing fetus is uncontaminated by microorganisms, indeed amniotic fluid contains peptides that prevent bacterial growth [76]. However if there is premature rupture of membranes, and when the neonate is being born, microorganisms derived from the maternal vagina are acquired. The 'normal flora' of the oropharynx and intestine are of great importance both as a defence mechanism and because, if abnormal colonization occurs, it can provide a reservoir from which bacteria may be translocated to cause bacteraemia. The latter is particularly important since it appears that the neonatal intestine is more permeable than that of adults to large molecules and perhaps therefore to bacteria [79].

In adults, 'normal flora' consist of large numbers of anaerobes (about 10^{12}/ml of colonic contents) in particular *Bifidobacterium*, *Veillonella* and *Eubacteria* with much smaller numbers of aerobes such as *Escherichia coli* (about 10^{7}/ml). Other enterobacteria such as *Klebsiella*, *Enterobacter*, *Citrobacter* and *Serratia* are not usually part of the normal flora. The majority of the intestinal 'normal flora' are found in the lower ileum, caecum, colon and rectum where intestinal movement is slowest.

The neonate begins to be colonized within 24 h of birth but the types of microorganisms and speed of colonization are dependent on many factors (Table 10.2).

In general, breast-fed, term babies show early colonization with facultative anaerobes such as *E.coli* and *Lactobacillus*, followed by large numbers of *Bifidobacterium* as the redox potential in the

Table 10.2 Factors important in the development of normal flora

Premature rupture of membranes
Prematurity
Enteral feeding
Breast feeding
Maternal contact
Administration of antibiotics
Admission to intensive care units

intestine falls [11,15,75]. This tends to prevent colonization by enterobacteria such as *Klebsiella* and pathogenic anaerobes such as *Bacteroides fragilis*. Bottle-fed term neonates and preterm neonates tend to be less readily colonized by *Bifidobacterium* and more frequently with *Klebsiella, Enterobacter, Serratia, Pseudomonas aeruginosa* and *Clostridium* [15,30,35,36,69]. In general, administration of broad-spectrum antibiotics, being admitted to NICU and supplementary formula feeding will predispose to the development of abnormal flora.

In the tissues

Since the barrier defence of body surfaces is impaired, non-specific defences in the tissues assume greater importance. However, these too are less than optimal.

Adult serum has a natural bactericidal activity which is mediated primarily by the complement cascade. This activity is deficient in the neonate. For example, *E.coli* K1 is able to multiply in neonatal serum whereas adult serum inhibits its growth [4]. The haemolytic activity of complement (CH_{50}) in neonates is about half that of adults with levels of individual components being 50–70% of adult levels [1].

Microorganisms grow optimally within a fairly narrow temperature range and the growth of many human pathogens is slowed at temperatures above 37°C. Thus a febrile response may help to limit infection. Unfortunately, the premature neonate has poor temperature control and cannot mount a febrile response. Indeed in a survey of serious infection that occurred in neonates in Liverpool, only seven (5%) of 151 episodes were accompanied by pyrexia [42].

The inflammatory response is of importance in bringing defence components such as antibody, complement and phagocytes from the bloodstream to the sites in the tissues of microbial invasion. Secondly, the inflammatory response is highly effective in localizing infections and preventing dissemination. There is evidence that the inflammatory response is less than fully efficient in the premature neonate. This can be illustrated by our experience

with neonates in Liverpool. Of 160 episodes of serious infection 135 (84%) presented as bacteraemia alone and 16 (10%) as focal infection that became disseminated [42].

The inflammatory response brings professional phagocytes from the bloodstream to the site of attack and is maintained in part by the continuing presence of the phagocytes.

Professional phagocytes are divided into those that are in the circulation such as the neutrophilic polymorphonuclear leucocytes (neutrophils) and monocytes and those that are fixed in tissues, namely macrophages. Monocytes are only weakly phagocytic and their main function is to be turned into macrophages by interferon at the site of microbial invasion. The neutrophils are very potent microbial killers and actively migrate towards invading microorganisms. The macrophages form the reticulo-endothelial system and act to remove particles such as bacteria from the bloodstream. Phagocytosis occurs naturally as part of the non-specific immune system but can also be the final stage following activation of the specific immune system. For example, neutrophils and macrophages have specific receptors for the Fc portion of antibodies and for the C_{3b} component of the complement cascade. The importance of the phagocyte in defence against infection is well demonstrated by the numerous congenital and acquired defects in phagocytosis that have been described [68].

The stages in phagocytosis are chemotaxis, adherence/opsonization, endocytosis, oxygen-dependent killing and finally phagolysosome fusion. Although there are conflicting data, most authors consider that the later stages of phagocytosis are fully active in neonatal blood [56]. However, neonatal neutrophils are deficient in the crucial initial stage of chemotaxis. It has been found that the chemotactic response of neonatal neutrophils *in vitro* is impaired both in healthy term and preterm babies and that this activity is even more impaired in stressed neonates [50,51]. Thus, although neonatal neutrophils have the capacity to kill microorganisms they have difficulty in actually getting to the site of infection.

Specific immune system

The specific immune system is divided into that mediated by antibody – the humoral immune system, and that mediated by activated T-lymphocytes – the cell-mediated immune system.

Humoral immunity

Although the neonate has B-lymphocytes capable of producing antibody, they show little activity and the vast majority of circulating immunoglobulin is derived from the maternal blood.

B-cells with the capacity to produce antibody appear in the fetal circulation by about 11–12 weeks post conception and have reached adult levels by 16 weeks. These B-cells have the ability to produce IgM, IgG or IgA but are inactive perhaps due to T-suppressor cell activity [56]. Fetal IgM production does not begin until 16 weeks and at term is only 18% of adult levels. IgG production begins at 28 weeks and at term is 5% of adult levels. IgA production does not begin until birth.

It is however possible for the fetus to respond to specific antigens as has been observed following intrauterine infection with rubella virus [19] and hepatitis B virus [64]. In addition administration of tetanus toxoid to pregnant women at as early as 5 months of gestation can result in production of fetal IgM anti-tetanus toxoid [34]. However the placenta does act as a barrier and only certain antigens can gain access to fetal lymphocytes. It is clear that the neonate is grossly deficient in producing its own antibody.

The antibody that it does possess comes mainly from the maternal blood. Only IgG (each of the subclasses) can cross the placenta. Transplacental transmission is an active process which involves specific Fc to receptors on the trophoblast membrane [47]. Transmission begins at about the 10th week of gestation and is maximal by the 33rd week. The activity of such antibodies has not yet been fully determined although there is some evidence that antiviral antibodies are concentrated on the fetal side of the placenta [37]. Of course premature neonates born before 30 weeks will not have optimal amounts of antibody necessary for protection.

Cell mediated immunity

T-lymphocytes can be detected as early as 6 weeks of gestation and cells showing T-cell function (mixed lymphocyte reaction and response to mitogens) are seen by week 10. At birth the neonate's T-lymphocyte system is fully developed and so at least in this aspect of immunity it is not at a disadvantage [56].

Neonatal infections

Neonates can be infected by the transplacental route, during delivery or postnatally. In general, transplacental infections are acquired from the maternal blood, those in delivery from the birth canal and those post-delivery from the ward environment either animate or inanimate, directly or indirectly.

Transplacental infections

Although many infective agents are reported to infect the fetus *in utero* only a few are well-

Table 10.3 Transplacental infection

I. *Well established agents*

Agent	Incidence of infection (% of live births)	Incidence of damage (% of those infected)
Cytomegalovirus	0.24%–2.2%	about 10%
Herpes simplex	unknown	rare
Varicella-zoster	unknown	rare
Rubella virus	0.1%	40–50%
Human parvovirus	unknown	unknown
Treponema pallidum	rare	50–70%
Listeria monocytogenes	unknown	high
Toxoplasma gondii	0.05%	10%

II. *Less well established agents*

Viruses	Bacteria	Protozoa
Epstein–Barr	*Mycobacterium tuberculosis*	Plasmodium
Hepatitis B		Trypanosomes
Human immune deficiency virus		
Influenza virus		
Enterovirus		
Measles virus		
Japanese encephalitis virus		

established as agents that can cross the placenta (Table 10.3).

The clinical spectrum of congenital rubella is well-known and it is not appropriate to discuss it here. Fortunately with the advent of effective vaccination campaigns the incidence of congenital infection has fallen. Nevertheless, cases still occur both due to poor uptake of the vaccine and because the live rubella vaccine itself can also cause transplacental infection, although the risk is less than for wild-type rubella virus [58].

The majority of infections due to herpes simplex virus (and the most serious) are acquired during delivery. However, transplacental spread has been described and there are about 50 recorded cases of congenital malformations due to this virus.

Varicella zoster virus can also cross the placenta to cause congenital malformation [14] but this is rare. If the mother develops chickenpox up to 5 days before delivery, the neonate is at grave risk of developing fatal varicella [25]. If maternal infection occurs earlier, it is possible that the neonate will develop shingles at 4–6 months of age.

The recently described DNA virus, human parvovirus can cross the placenta to infect the fetus. Such infections may lead to fetal loss, hydrops foetalis or may be inapparent [5].

Cytomegalovirus (CMV) is undoubtedly the commonest viral infection of the human fetus, and it is estimated that between 0.24 and 2.2% of pregnancies are complicated by congenital CMV infection [66] depending upon geographical and social factors.

Of course not all of these infections result in malformation and it is estimated that up to 10% of such infections cause congenital malformation. The congenital defects range through a spectrum from mild deafness, failure to perform as well as expected at school, hepatosplenomegaly with a rash to severe brain damage with hydranencephaly. There is no safe and effective vaccine available and though it was previously thought that only primary maternal infections could result in fetal infection, it is now clear that secondary infection or reactivations may produce disease in the fetus [74].

It should also be remembered that with congenital virus infections the infected neonate will excrete large numbers of virus particles for some considerable time. Thus, congenitally infected neonates may act as a source for infection in neonatal units which can be spread via hands or even by the airborne route.

Congenital syphilis is an avoidable disease and should not occur in developed countries with screening programmes for antibodies against *Treponema pallidum*. The spirochaete is still highly susceptible to penicillin, an antibiotic which is not harmful to the developing fetus, yet congenital syphilis still occurs.

The protozoon parasite *Toxoplasma gondii* may cause symptomatic or asymptomatic infection in humans but does have the ability to cross the placenta. Infection is most often acquired from the domestic cat. In Britain congenital infection is rare (0.05% of births) but it is commoner in other European countries, such as France. Congenital infection occurs most readily following maternal infection in the last months of pregnancy but is less likely to result in severe disease [67]. Approximately 10% of infected fetuses are clinically affected. This can range from stillbirth to the classic triad of hydrocephalus, chorioretinitis and intracranial calcification, but other clinical manifestations have been recorded [67]. If *in utero* infection is diagnosed early enough, treatment with pyrimethamine and sulfadoxine is of value [21].

Infections acquired during delivery

These infections are acquired from the birth canal either during delivery or by microorganisms ascending into the uterus following premature rupture of membranes. In general, infections presenting within 48 h of delivery are acquired in this fashion. Many different microorganisms can be acquired during delivery and some are listed in Table 10.4. Infecting agents may be pathogens or commensals of the vagina or may be enteric pathogens that contaminate the vagina due to the close proximity of the anus.

Enteroviruses such as ECHO 11 [62], and Coxsackie B5 [49] may be acquired during delivery and subsequently lead to unit outbreaks. Such infections

Table 10.4 Infections acquired during delivery

Viruses	Bacteria	Protozoa
Enteroviruses	Group B streptococci	*Plasmodium*
Rotavirus	*Listeria monocytogenes*	
Human immune deficiency virus	*Neisseria gonorrhoea*	
Hepatitis B virus	*Neisseria meningitidis*	
Herpes simplex virus	*Pasteurella multocida*	
	Salmonella spp.	
	Shigella spp.	
	Chlamydia trachomatis	

are often serious with high mortality. In contrast, neonatal rotavirus infections are frequently asymptomatic and all babies on a unit could be infected, with only sporadic cases being clinically apparent [60]. Such outbreaks can be extremely difficult to control, often necessitating closure of the unit. *Salmonella* infections are also much less likely to cause enteritis and more likely to cause bacteraemia and meningitis.

Listeria monocytogenes may be acquired transplacentally or during delivery probably following vaginal contamination from the anus [52]. Treatment is with penicillin or ampicillin; the bacterium is resistant to the cephalosporins.

Premature rupture of membranes also predisposes the neonate to infection with vaginal commensals. The risk of infection is increased in premature neonates, in males and if there is amnionitis [77]. Among vaginal commensals Group B streptococci are particularly likely to cause serious infection [65]. Neonatal Group B streptococci infections are apparently more common in the USA than the UK. Prompt treatment with penicillin G can be life saving.

Of the genital tract pathogens *Neisseria gonorrhoeae* and *Chlamydia trachomatis* both cause neonatal conjunctivitis. In general that due to the gonococcus is apparent by day 3 post delivery or earlier whereas *C.trachomatis* conjunctivitis does not appear until days 5 to 7 [43]. It should be remembered in the case of each pathogen that the mother is also infected and will need treatment. Optimal treatment for *C.trachomatis* conjunctivitis is tetracycline ointment to the eye and erythromycin orally. If incompletely treated there is a risk of *C.trachomatis* causing pneumonia.

Herpes simplex virus remains latent in the sacral ganglia and re-emerges either asymptomatically or with the production of cervicitis, vaginitis or localized lesions on the vulva. If a neonate is born through the sea of virus particles then it runs the risk of developing infection. Neonatal herpes simplex infections have high mortality (60–65%) and high morbidity. The incidence of infection in the USA is estimated at between 1 in 300 and 1 in 1000 births but is apparently much lower in Britain [54].

Strategies for preventing such infection include caesarean section for at-risk neonates or pre-emptive treatment with acycloguanosine, but there are no trials establishing efficacy or need. Acycloguanosine is an effective and relatively non-toxic treatment for neonatal herpes.

Finally, since delivery is a fairly bloody business, there is a risk that blood-borne viral infections such as hepatitis B and human immune deficiency (HIV) viruses could be acquired at this time. World-wide this is probably the major way in which hepatitis B virus (HBV) is transmitted. With the advent of safe and effective vaccines transmission of the HBV from mother to neonate can be prevented [80].

Unfortunately this option is not available for HIV; it is estimated that approximately 70% of neonates born to infected mothers will themselves become infected.

Infections acquired post partum

In terms of both numbers of cases and morbidity and mortality, infections acquired by neonates after delivery are undoubtedly the most important. A recent survey of the prevalence of hospital-acquired infections revealed that 16.8% of babies in neonatal intensive care units (NICU) were infected [55]. This was a survey of bacterial infection only and there is little systematic information available on virus infections in NICU. Certainly viruses such as CMV, varicella zoster virus (VZV), rotavirus and entero-viruses can spread with ease amongst neonates in NICU, but the frequency with which this occurs is unknown. Some viruses such as CMV can also be acquired from blood transfusions or breast milk and can produce considerable morbidity [2].

The types of bacteria causing neonatal infection are constantly changing. In the second quarter of the century *Staphylococcus aureus* and Group A beta-haemolytic streptococci were the predominant pathogens. In the third quarter, Gram-negative bacteria such as *E.coli* assumed greater importance [32]. Latterly an increase in infections due to Group B streptococci [65], coagulase negative staphylo-cocci [23,31,42] and multidrug resistant *Klebsiella* and *Enterobacter* [57,59] have been described. In addition, because premature neonates are so immune deficient, infection with unusual pathogens such as *Hansenula anomala*, a yeast contaminant in the brewing industry, can occur [61].

The implication of the above is that there must be continuous surveillance of infecting microorganisms and their susceptibility to antibiotics in order to provide the optimal combination for both surgical prophylaxis and for treatment of infection.

General surgical infections

Although there is a wealth of information on surgical infection and its prevention in adults [26],

there is little available in paediatric surgery and virtually none in neonatal surgery. This is particularly unfortunate since, as indicated previously, the neonate is in effect an immune compromised host. In general the infecting microorganisms will be endogenous, i.e. derived from the neonate's own microflora. Operations in which mucosal surfaces are transected will of course increase the risk of infection since such surfaces will have a rich normal flora. This is less predictable for neonates since their normal flora are not properly developed and if they have been in hospital since birth, have received broad-spectrum antibiotics or have been formula fed they may be colonized by potential pathogens such as klebsiellae and pseudomonads.

Surveys of infection in paediatric surgery have reported rates of between 3.1% [24] and 8.0% [27] for clean operations, higher than that (2.0%) reported for such operations in adults [20]. In the former survey [24] infection rates of 7.8% for clean/contaminated, 17% for contaminated and 10% for dirty operations were observed. However, it is difficult to extrapolate these results to neonatal surgery since the mean age of those studied was around 6 months.

Preliminary results from a survey of infections in neonates in the neonatal surgical unit at Alder Hey indicate that up to 32% of patients are affected [53]. However the infections were not necessarily directly related to surgery. They ranged from stomatitis, urinary tract infection, pneumonia, intravenous line related infection to wound infection which occurred in half of those infected. Nevertheless two neonates died from overwhelming *Pseudomonas* infection. The infecting microorganisms were principally Gram-negative bacteria (*E.coli*, *Enterobacter cloacae*, *Klebsiella aerogenes* and *Pseudomonas aeruginosa*) and yeasts such as *Candida albicans*. Interestingly, anaerobes were not a problem in the 40 neonates studied. In each case the neonates were colonized by their infecting microorganism prior to the development of infection. The prevalence of colonization with the above Gram-negative bacteria increased with duration of stay in the unit with 90% of neonates being colonized within 40 days of admission. This would suggest that techniques developed to prevent infection by selective decon-tamination of severely traumatized adults in intensive care units might be of value [78].

Shunt infections

Ventriculo-peritoneal (VP) and ventriculo-atrial (VA) shunts have been developed to control hydro-cephalus. Infection is one of the major causes of shunt failure. Infections may occur either as a wound infection around the exterior surface of the catheter or in the lumen of the system. In the former, *Staph.aureus* is the major pathogen. Such infections can be managed by local wound toilet and systemic antibiotics such as flucloxacillin. Unfortunately intraluminal infections occur more frequently and are much more difficult to manage. Reported shunt infection rates vary from 1 to 39% [8]. Approximately 10% of the shunts inserted at Alder Hey become infected and Table 10.5 shows the pathogens most frequently isolated. Coagulase negative staphylococci (CONS) account for the vast majority (90%) of infections and of these *Staph. epidermidis* [70] is most frequently isolated followed by *Staph.capitis*.

Table 10.5 Pathogens associated with shunt infection

Organism	% of cases
Coagulase negative staphylococci	90
Staphylococcus aureus	2–3
Corynebacteria	1–2
Propionibacterium acnes	1–2
Streptococci	1
Coliforms	2–3

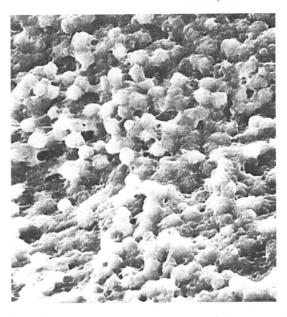

Figure 10.2 A scanning electron micrograph of the luminal surface of a ventriculo-peritoneal catheter showing a microcolony of *Staphylococcus epidermidis* with extracellular slime

Shunt infection may develop at any time after insertion and it is thought that the microorganisms gain access to the system at the time of operation [10]. Exceptions to this will of course include VA shunts that become colonized at the atrial end by blood-borne bacteria, VP shunts that erode into the intestines thus acquiring Gram-negative bacteria, and external ventricular drains. However, in the majority of cases infecting microorganisms gain access at the time of operation. As can be seen from Table 10.5 the pathogens responsible are largely derived from the normal skin flora of the patient or operating theatre staff.

The development of symptoms and signs of shunt infection can take many years especially with CONS. Often with CONS infection there is little evidence of inflammation either as meningitis or ventriculitis, and the infection presents as a blockage of the system with raised intracranial pressure. In contrast shunt infection with more aggressive bacteria such as *S.aureus* and *E.coli* often produces fulminant infection. For example, of 35 cases of shunt infection with CONS only three patients had CSF leucocyte counts of more than 400/mm^3 and none were more than 2000/mm^3, whereas in all four cases of infection with *Staph.aureus* leucocyte counts of more than 4000/mm^3 were seen [8].

The strains of CONS which produce shunt infections all have in common the ability to produce an extracellular slime [9]. Following introduction of CONS into the system, they first adhere to the plastic, perhaps by electrostatic forces, and bacteria adhere to different plastics with different degrees of

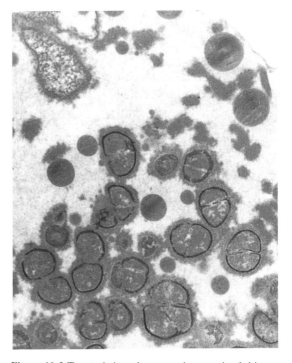

Figure 10.3 Transmission electron micrograph of thin sections of a ventriculo-peritoneal catheter showing dividing cocci with extracellular slime

efficiency [6]. The CONS then grow to produce microcolonies that are firmly attached to the surface of the catheter. The slime that is produced by the bacteria is apparently hydrophobic [13] which tends to cement the bacteria to the catheter wall.

Figure 10.2 is a scanning electron micrograph looking down on the luminal surface of a VP catheter. It shows numerous cocci anchored by strands of slime. Figure 10.3 is a transmission electron micrograph of the same catheter showing dividing cocci surrounded by electron-dense slime. CONS were isolated from this shunt and from the patient's CSF. Much more slime is present *in vivo* but it has been lost during the processing of these specimens for electron microscopy. This is of some significance when considering the management of shunt infections. In general, although it is possible to sterilize CSF in infected shunts with antibiotics, once therapy ceases then the infection recrudesces. This is because the antibiotic is unable to penetrate completely through the slimy adherent colonies. Therefore it is generally agreed that effective treatment of CONS shunt infections involves both the use of appropriate antimicrobial chemotherapy and subsequent removal of the shunt [46]. It is unclear whether this follows for shunt infections with bacteria that do not adhere as firmly as CONS. However, since there is no evidence either way it is probably safer to manage all shunt infections as if due to CONS.

CONS are becoming increasingly resistant to antibiotics. Initially CONS shunt infections were treated successfully with penicillin [16] but now up to 90% of such isolates are resistant to penicillin and ampicillin [39]. In addition, a third of these isolates were resistant to cloxacillin, 45% to cefuroxime, 55% to trimethoprim and 55% to gentamicin. In contrast all Gram-positive shunt pathogens (CONS, propionibacteria, corynebacteria and *Staph.aureus*) tested were inhibited by vancomycin at a concentration of 4 mg/l or less, and almost all (98%) by rifampicin at the same concentration.

Because there is little inflammatory response with the majority of shunt infections antibiotics administered orally, intravenously or intramuscularly will rarely achieve therapeutic levels in the CSF. Thus antibiotics must be given directly into the ventricles via the shunt. Naturally if a VA shunt is infected it will also be necessary to give intravenous antibiotics. Intraventricular vancomycin has proved effective in treating shunt infections [8], with little of the toxicity associated with intravenous administration. CSF vancomycin levels should be monitored and should not exceed 30 mg/l, but even with levels up to 1000 mg/l toxicity was not observed. However the system should be first exteriorized and once the CSF is sterile (which usually takes 3–5 days) the system replaced under vancomycin cover.

Prevention is obviously better than the cure and meticulous attention to detail, the use of prophylactic antibiotics, skin antisepsis and the use of laminar air flow might be of benefit.

Prevention of neonatal infections

Neonates are at great risk of developing infection and in the majority of cases the infecting microorganism is endogenous (i.e. derived from the patient's own microflora). However the neonate does not have a normal flora at birth and can easily become colonized by potentially pathogenic bacteria. The reservoirs of these potential pathogens are other neonates, attendant staff, visitors and occasionally the inanimate environment. Although transmission by the airborne route has been documented for CMV, VZV and some respiratory pathogens, hand carriage remains the most important mode of transmission of most pathogens [17,38,71]. The transmission of infection can be decreased by frequent hand-washing with appropriate soaps and disinfectants [17,38]. However, even with the most cooperative staff only 75% compliance can be expected [3].

The efficacy of gowning in preventing cross-infection is often questioned and there seems little evidence to support its use [28]. Similarly the use of masks and overshoes may be of little value. Certainly unless hands are washed, putting on overshoes seems to be a very good way of transferring bacteria from shoes to patients via hands.

Once infection becomes apparent cohorting infants together is a method for controlling further spread. If possible a group of staff should be assigned to care only for the infected infants. The concept of replacing virulent colonizing bacteria with less virulent ones is worthy of consideration. However its value remains unproven.

Antibiotics and neonatal surgery

There is a bewildering array of antimicrobials available for the treatment of infection and it is often difficult to choose the most appropriate agent. Before discussing individual antibiotics it is worthwhile considering strategies for their use. In general, antimicrobials will be given for treatment or for prevention of infection. Signs of neonatal infection are non-specific but the results of such infection can be catastrophic. Therefore antimicrobial chemotherapy is initiated pre-emptively, in the knowledge that in 80–89% of cases the neonate will not be infected. The neonate can be regarded as an immune compromised host and it is preferable to use bactericidal (e.g. aminoglycosides, beta-lactams) rather than bacteriostatic (e.g. erythromycin) antibiotics. The antibiotics should be given intravenously rather than orally or intramuscularly to achieve high levels rapidly. The least toxic agents should be used and if aminoglycosides or vancomycin are used their levels should be monitored.

Because in the majority of cases of pre-emptive therapy there is no infection there should be a firm policy on when to stop treatment (generally after 48 h if there is no objective evidence of infection). In choosing the antimicrobials to be used the site of infection should be considered. For example, gentamicin does not cross the blood-brain barrier well, only 25% of the serum level being achieved in the CSF. It is therefore unlikely to be effective in treating meningitis. The choice of antibiotic is also governed by a knowledge of the pathogens prevalent in the unit and their antimicrobial susceptibility. Constant surveillance of the prevalent pathogens is of importance since different pathogens emerge over a period [42,57,59]. Currently a combination of ampicillin and gentamicin is used to give broad-spectrum pre-emptive cover. If there is a suspicion that a mucous surface has been breached, e.g. in severe necrotizing enterocolitis or following colonic surgery then anaerobic cover (e.g. metronidazole) should be added. If meningitis is suspected it would be advisable to substitute cefotaxime or ceftazidime for ampicillin since most coliforms are resistant to the latter (there is a risk that *Listeria monocytogenes* would not be covered with this regimen but such infections are rare). If an intravenous or intra-arterial line infection is suspected, it might be necessary to use cefuroxime or vancomycin. Finally disseminated fungal (especially candidal) infections can occur [41,61], they can be difficult to treat but our experience, using a combination of amphotericin B and 5-flucytosine, has been good.

In order to use chemoprophylaxis in surgery effectively several factors should be considered. It is useful to have an idea of the incidence and consequences of infection in the absence of chemoprophylaxis. For example, it is unlikely that the benefits will outweigh the disadvantages of antimicrobial chemoprophylaxis if the incidence of infection is 2% or less, unless the results of infection are dire. There is little information about chemoprophylaxis in neonatal surgery. It is necessary to know when the microorganisms are likely to gain access to the tissues, what are the likely pathogens and to which antibiotics they are sensitive. Again there is little information in neonatal surgery. It would, however, seem appropriate to extrapolate from the data available for adult surgical practice [26]. For example, if mucous surfaces are transected then the normal flora resident are likely to be inoculated into the surrounding tissues. If the operation involves the colon then it would seem appropriate to use chemoprophylaxis covering both anaerobes and aerobes (e.g. metronidazole and gentamicin).

It would be inappropriate to discuss individual antibiotics here and there are several reviews available of antibiotics and their use in neonates [22,29,33].

Finally it is worthwhile considering other forms of treatment and prophylaxis, for example, the use of hyperimmune serum or plasma, granulocyte transfusions or selective decontamination.

References

1. Adinolfi, M. (1981) Complement, lysozyme and lactoferrin in man. In *Immunological Aspects of Infection in the Fetus and New-born* (ed. H.P. Lambert and C.B.S. Wood) Academic Press, London, pp. 19–47

2. Adler, S.P., Chandrika, T., Lawrence, L. and Baggett, J. (1983) Cytomegalovirus infections in neonates acquired by blood transfusions. *Pediat. Infect. Dis.*, **2**, 114–118

3. Albert, R.K. and Condie, F. (1981) Hand-washing patterns in medical intensive care units. *New Engl. J. Med.*, **304**, 1465–1466

4. Allen, P.M., Roberts, I., Boulnois, G., Saunders, J.R. and Hart, C.A. (1987) Contribution of capsular polysaccharides and surface properties to virulence of *Escherichia coli* Kl. *Infect. Immun.*, **55**, 2662–2668

5. Anand, A., Gray, E.S., Brown, T., Clowley, J.P. and Cohen, B.J. (1987) Human parvovirus infection in pregnancy and hydrops fetalis. *New Engl. J. Med.*, **316**, 183–186

6. Ashkenazi, S. (1984) Bacterial adherence to plastics. *Lancet*, **i**, 1075–1976

7. Battisti, O., Mitchison, R. and Davies, P.A. (1981) Changing blood culture isolates in a referral neonatal intensive care unit. *Arch. Dis. Child.*, **56**, 775–778

8. Bayston, R., Hart, C.A. and Barnicoat, M. (1987) Intraventricular vancomycin in the treatment of ventriculitis associated with cerebrospinal fluid shunting and drainage. *J. Neurol., Neurosurg. Psychiat.*, **50**, 1419–1423

9. Bayston, R. and Penny, S.R. (1972) Excessive production of mucoid substance in staphylococcus S IIA. *Dev. Med. Childh. Neurol.*, (Suppl.) **27**, 25–28

10. Bayston, R. and Lari, J. (1974) A study of the sources of infection in colonised shunts. *Dev. Med. Childh. Neurol.*, (Suppl.) **32**, 16–22

11. Blakey, J.L., Lubitz, L., Barnes, G.L., Bishop, R.F., Campbell, N.T. and Gillam, G.L. (1982) Development of gut colonisation in pre-term neonates. *J. Med. Microbiol.*, **15**, 519–529

12. Brook, I. (1982) Bacteriology of neonatal omphalitis. *J. Infect.*, **5**, 127–131

13. Bruce, D.L., Fisher, D. and Hart, C.A. (1987) The partitioning of *Staphylococcus epidermidis* in aqueous two-phase system. *J. Med. Microbiol.*, **24**, 181–184

14. Brunell, P.A. (1981) Epidemiology of varicella-zoster virus infections. In *The Human Herpesviruses* (ed. A.J. Nahmias, W.R. Dowdle and R.F. Schinazi) Elsevier, New York, pp. 153–158

15. Bullen, J.J. (1981) The role of milk and gut flora in

protection of the newborn against infection. In *Immunological Aspects of Infection in the Fetus and New-born* (ed. H.P. Lambert and C.B.S. Wood), Academic Press, London, pp. 123–129

16. Callaghan, R.P., Cohen, S.J. and Stewart, G.T. (1961) Septicaemia due to colonisation of Spitz-Holter valves by staphylococci: five cases treated with penicillin. *Br. Med. J.*, **1**, 860–863

17. Casewell, M.W. (1980) The role of hand disinfection in specific problems today. *Roy. Soc. Med. Congr. Symp.*, **23**, 21–27

18. Chiswick, M. (1983) Infection and defenses in neonates. *Br. Med. J.*, **286**, 1377–1378

19. Craddock-Watson, J.E., Ridehalgh, M.K.S., Anderson, M.J., Pattison, J.R. and Kangro, H.O. (1980) Foetal infection resulting from maternal rubella after the first trimester of pregnancy. *J. Hyg. (Camb.)*, **85**, 381–391

20. Cruse, P.J.E. and Foord, R. (1980) The epidemiology of wound infection: a 10 year prospective study of 62,939 wounds. *Surg. Clin. N. Am.*, **60**, 27–40

21. Daffos, F., Forestier, F., Capella-Pavlovsky, M., Thulliez, P., Aufrant, C., Valenti, D. and Cox, W.L. (1988) Prenatal management of 746 pregnancies at risk for congenital toxoplasmosis. *New Engl. J. Med.*, **318**, 271–275

22. Davies, P.A. (1978) Treatment of neonatal bacterial infection. *Br. Med. J.*, **ii**, 676–679

23. Davies, A.J., Ward-Platt, M., Kirk, R., Marshall, R., Speidel, B.D. and Reeves, D.S. (1984) Is coagulase-negative staphylococcal bacteraemia in neonates a consequence of mechanical ventilation? *J. Hosp. Infect.*, **5**, 260–269

24. Davis, S.D., Sobocinski, K., Hoffmann, R.G., Mohr, B. and Nelson, D.B. (1984) Postoperative wound infections in a children's hospital. *Pediat. Infect. Dis.*, **3**, 114–116

25. De Nicola, L.K. and Hanshaw, J.D. (1979) Congenital and neonatal varicella. *J. Pediat.*, **94**, 175–176

26. DiPiro, J.T., Bivins, B.A., Record, K.E., Bell, R.M. and Griffen, W.O. (1983) The prophylactic use of antimicrobials in surgery. *Curr. Prob. Surg.*, **20**, 75–132

27. Doig, C.M. and Wilkinson, A.W. (1976) Wound infections in a children's hospital. *Br. J. Surg.*, **63**, 647–650

28. Donowitz, L.G. (1986) Failure of the overgown to prevent nosocomial infection in a Pediatric Intensive Care Unit. *Pediatrics*, **77**, 35–38

29. Eichenwald, H.F. and McCracken, G.H. (1978) Antimicrobial therapy in infants and children. *J. Pediat.*, **93**, 337–377

30. Feeney, A.R., Cooke, A.M. and Shinebaum, R. (1980) A comparative study of gram-negative aerobic bacilli in the faeces of babies born in hospital and at home. *J. Hyg. (Camb.)*, **84**, 91–96

31. Fleer, A., Senders, R.C., Visser, M.R., Bijlmer, R.P., Gerards, L.J., Kraaijeveld, C.A. *et al.* (1983) Septicaemia due to coagulase-negative staphylococci

in a neonatal intensive care unit: clinical and bacteriological features and contaminated parenteral fluids as a source of sepsis. *Pediat. Infect. Dis.*, **2**, 426–428

32. Freedman, R.M., Ingram, D.L., Gross, I., Ehrenkranz, R.A., Warkshaw, J.B. and Baltimore, R.S. (1981) A half century of neonatal sepsis at Yale: 1928 to 1978. *Am. J. Dis. Childh.*, **135**, 140–144

33. Geddes, A.M. (1988) Antibiotic therapy–a resume. *Lancet*, **i**, 286–289

34. Gill, T.J., Repetti, C.F., Metlay, L.A., Rabin, B.S., Taylor, F.H., Thompson, D.S. *et al.* (1983) Transplacental immunization of the human fetus to tetanus by immunization of the mother. *J. Clin. Invest.*, **72**, 987–996

35. Goldman, D.A. (1981) Bacterial colonization and infection in the neonate. *Am. J. Med.*, **70**, 417–422

35A. Goldman, D.A., Durbin, W.A. and Freeman, J. (1981) Nosocomial infections in a neonatal intensive care unit. *J. Infect. Dis.*, **144**, 449–459

36. Goldman, D.A., Leclair, J. and Macone, A. (1978) Bacterial colonization of neonates admitted to an intensive care environment. *J. Pediat.*, **93**, 288–293

37. Griffiths, P.D., Berney, S.I., Argent, S. and Heath, R.B. (1982) Antibody against viruses in maternal and cord sera: specific antibody is concentrated on the fetal side of the circulation. *J. Hyg. (Camb.)*, **89**, 303–310

38. Hart, C.A. (1986) Nosocomial *Klebsiella pneumoniae* in a neonatal special care unit. *Ann. Trop. Paediat.*, **6**, 127–128

39. Hart, C.A., Bayston, R. and Barnicoat, M., unpublished

40. Hemming, V.G., Overall, J.C. and Britt, M.R. (1976) Nosocomial infections in a newborn intensive care unit. *New Engl. J. Med.*, **294**, 1310–1316

41. Hensey, O.J., Hart, C.A. and Cooke, R.W.I. (1984) *Candida albicans* skin abscesses. *Arch. Dis. Child.*, **59**, 479–480

42. Hensey, O.J., Hart, C.A. and Cooke, R.W.I. (1985) Serious infection in a neonatal intensive care unit: A two year survey. *J. Hyg. (Camb.)*, **95**, 289–297

43. Hobson, D., Rees, E. and Viswalinham, N.D. (1983) Chlamydial infections in children. *Br. Med. Bull.*, **39**, 128–132

44. Hoogkamp-Korstanje, J.A.A., Cats, B., Senders, R.C. and van Ertbruggen, I. (1982) Analysis of bacterial infections in a neonatal intensive care unit. *J. Hosp. Infect.*, **3**, 275–284

45. Hurley, R. (1982) Neonatal septicaemia and meningitis. *J. Hosp. Infect.*, **3**, 323–328

46. James, H.E., Walsh, J.W., Wilson, H.D., Connor, J.D., Bean, J.R. and Tibbs, P.A. (1980) Prospective randomised study of therapy in cerebrospinal fluid shunt infection. *Neurosurgery*, **7**, 459–463

47. Johnson, P.M. and Brown, P.J. (1981) Fc-γ receptors in the placenta. *Placenta*, **2**, 355–370

48. Klein, J.O. and Marcy, S.M. (1976) Bacterial infections. In *Infectious Diseases of the Fetus and Newborn* (ed. J.S. Remington and J.O. Klein), W.B. Saunders Co., Philadelphia, pp. 747–796

49. Krajden, S. and Middleton, P.J. (1983) Enterovirus infections in the neonate. *Clin. Pediat.*, **22**, 87–92

50. Krause, P., Herson, V.C., Boutin-Liebowitz, J., Eisenfeld, L., Block, C., Lobelle, T. *et al.* (1986) Polymorphonuclear leucocyte adherence and chemotaxis in stressed and healthy neonates. *Pediat. Res.*, **20**, 296–300

51. Laurenti, F., Ferro, R., Marzetti, G., Rossini, M. and Bucci, G. (1980) Neutrophil chemotaxis in preterm infants with infections. *J. Pediat.*, **96**, 468–470

52. Lennon, D., Lewis, B., Mantell, C., Becroft, D., Dove, B., Farmer, K. *et al.* (1984) Epidemic perinatal listeriosis. *Pediat. Infect. Dis.*, **3**, 30–34

53. Leonard, E.M., Van Saene, H.K.F., Walker, J., Tam, P. and Lloyd, D., unpublished

54. Marshall, W.C. and Peckham, C.S. (1983) The management of herpes simplex in pregnant women and neonates. *J. Infect.*, **6** (Suppl. 1), 23–29

55. Mccrs, P.D., Ayliffe, G.A.J., Emmerson, A.M., Leigh, D.A., Mayon-White, R.T., Mackintosh, C.A. *et al.* (1981) Report on the National Survey of Infection in Hospitals. *J. Hosp. Infect.*, **2**, 13–18

56. Miler, I. (1983) *The Immunity of the Human Fetus and Newborn Infant.* Martinus Nijhoff, London

57. Modi, N., Damjanovic, V. and Cooke, R.W.I. (1987) Outbreak of cephalosporin resistant *Enterobacter cloacae* infection in a neonatal intensive care unit. *Arch. Dis. Child.*, **62**, 148–151

58. Modlin, J.F., Herrman, K., Brandling-Bennett, A.D., Eddins, D.L. and Hayden, G. (1976) Risk of congenital abnormality after inadvertent rubella vaccination of pregnant women. *New Engl. J. Med.*, **294**, 272–274

59. Morgan, M.E.I., Hart, C.A. and Cooke, R.W.I. (1984) Klebsiella infection in a neonatal intensive care unit: Role of bacteriological surveillance. *J. Hosp. Infect.*, **5**, 377–385

60. Murphy, A.M., Albrey, M.B. and Crewe, E.B. (1977) Rotavirus infections of neonates. *Lancet*, **ii**, 1149

61. Murphy, N., Buchanan, C.R., Damjanovic, V., Whitaker, R., Hart, C.A. and Cooke, R.W.I. (1986) Infection and colonization of neonates by *Hansenula anomala*. *Lancet*, **i**, 291–293

62. Nagington, J., Gandy, G., Walker, J. and Gray, J.J. (1983) Use of normal immunoglobulin in an Echovirus 11 outbreak in a special care baby unit. *Lancet*, **ii**, 443–446

63. Oto, A. (1982) Major bacterial infection in a referral intensive care unit. *J. Infect:*, **5**, 117–126

64. Papaevangelou, G., Hoofnagle, J. and Kremastinou, J. (1974) Transplacental transmission of hepatitis B virus by symptom-free chronic carrier mothers. *Lancet*, **ii**, 746–748

65. Parker, M.T. (1979) Infections with group-B streptococci. *J. Antimicrob. Chemother.*, **5**, (Suppl. 5) 27–37

66. Peckham, C.S., Chin, K.S., Coleman, J.C., Henderson, C., Hurley, R. and Preece, P.M. (1983) Cytomegalovirus infection in pregnancy: preliminary findings from a prospective study. *Lancet*, **i**, 1352–1355

67. Remington, J.S. and Desmonts, G. (1976) Toxoplasmosis. In *Infectious Diseases of the Fetus and Newborn Infant* (ed. J.S. Remington and J.O. Klein) W.B. Saunders Co., Philadelphia, pp. 191–332

68. Rotrosen, D. and Gallin, J.I. (1987) Disorders of phagocyte function. *Ann. Rev. Immunol.*, **5**, 127–159

69. Shinebaum, R., Cooke, E.M. and Brayson, J.C. (1979) Acquisition of *Klebsiella aerogenes* by neonates. *J. Med. Microbiol.*, **12**, 201–205

70. Shurtleff, D.B., Foltz, E.L., Weeks, R.D. and Losser, J. (1974) Therapy of *Staphylococcus epidermidis* infections associated with cerebrospinal fluid shunts. *Pediatrics*, **53**, 55–62

71. Siegel, J. (1985) Controlling infection in the nursery. *Pediat. Infect. Dis.*, **4**, S36–S41

72. Siegel, J.D. and McCracken, G.H. (1981) Sepsis neonatorum. *New Engl. J. Med.*, **304**, 642–647

73. Speer, C.P., Hauptmann, D., Stubbe, P. and Gahr, M. (1985) Neonatal septicaemia and meningitis in Gottingen, West Germany. *Pediat. Infect. Dis.*, **4**, 36–41

74. Stagno, S., Pass, R.F., Dworsky, M.E. (1982) Congenital cytomegalovirus: The relative importance of primary and recurrent maternal infection. *New Engl. J. Med.*, **306**, 945–949

75. Stark, P.L. and Lee, A. (1982) The bacterial colonization of the large bowel of pre-term low birth weight neonates. *J. Hyg. (Camb.)*, **89**, 59–67

76. Stern, C.M.M. (1981) Bactericidal glycopeptide in human amniotic fluid. *J. Antimicrob. Chemother.*, **8**, 3–4

77. St Geme, J.W., Murray, D.L., Carter, J., Hobel, C., Leake, R.D., Anthony, B.F. *et al.* (1984) Perinatal bacterial infection after prolonged rupture of amniotic membranes: An analysis of risk and management. *J. Pediat.*, **104**, 608–613

78. van Saene, H.K.F. and Stoutenbeek, C.P. (1987) Selective decontamination. *J. Antimicrob. Chemother.*, **20**, 462–465

79. Walker, W.A. (1981) Intestinal immunity in the newborn. In *Immunological Aspects of Infection in the Fetus and New-born* (ed. H.P. Lambert and C.B.S. Woods), Academic Press, London, pp. 83–99

80. Wong, V.C.W., Ip, H.M.H., Reesink, H.W., Lelie, P.N., Reerink-Brongers, E.E., Yeung, C.Y. *et al.* (1984) Prevention of the HBsAg carrier state in newborn infants of mothers who are chronic carriers of HBsAg and HBeAg by administration of hepatitis B vaccine and hepatitis B immunoglobulin. *Lancet*, **i**, 921–926

Part II

Trauma, tumours and twins

11

Birth injuries

Margaretha Lehner

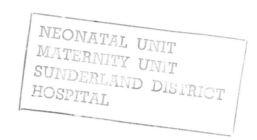

Introduction

The majority of traumatic birth injuries are mild and have a favourable outcome. Severe injuries can cause infant death or permanent handicaps. Prompt evaluation and rapid appropriate therapy will minimize the morbidity and mortality caused by birth trauma.

In this chapter only the more important birth injuries which necessitate treatment during the neonatal period are described. Specialist literature should be referred to for injuries to the spinal cord, brain, special sensory organs and certain orthopaedic problems.

Incidence

Although the more liberal use of caesarean section and the regionalization of high-risk obstetric services contributes to a declining frequency, in the USA birth trauma was still the sixth leading cause of neonatal mortality in 1981 [32].

It is extremely difficult to be certain about the incidence of birth injuries, partly because minor injuries are often neither diagnosed nor require any treatment, and partly because severe injuries often cause death directly after birth and are only diagnosed at autopsy [31].

The varying frequencies of certain injuries depend on the living standard of the population being studied. The higher the standard the rarer are birth injuries. For instance, in 1962 Adler [1] reported a frequency of brachial plexus paralysis of 0.38 per 1000 live births found in the New York Hospital Center; Gordon [12] reported a frequency of 1.89 per 1000 live births, studying a population of families with low income.

Cephalhaematoma has been reported to occur in 0.4–2.5% of liveborn infants. Reports about the frequency of underlying skull fractures range from 5.4–25% [20]. Estimates of the frequency of injuries to the bones lie between 0.2 and 2% and are most probably below 1% [33]. Apart from clavicular injuries which are commonly missed the most common bony injuries are epiphyseal separation of femur and humerus followed by midshaft fracture of the same bones. Distal epiphyseal separations are less common, fracture of the forearm or lower leg are exceedingly rare, as is congenital dislocation of the glenohumeral joint [10].

Improvement in obstetrical care has reduced the incidence of plexus paralysis in this century [16]. Reports range now from 0.38 to 0.87 per 1000 live births [4,9,14,29]. Erb's palsy is seen in approximately 58–72% of all brachial plexus injuries [16].

Ruptures of the parenchymatous abdominal organs following birth trauma have been reported by Cywes to cause 3% of the deaths found at autopsy on newborn African infants; rupture of the liver was the most common cause of death [7]. The rapid advances in neonatology have allowed more and more newborn infants to be treated successfully for rupture of liver, spleen, kidney and adrenal gland due to birth injury [5,7,13,19,21,28]. Presence of a neuroblastoma is a predisposing factor for rupture of adrenal gland [2,23]. Severe genital trauma is a rare occurrence [5,11].

Aetiology

Birth injuries are caused by mechanical influence on the fetus during birth due either to pressure in the birth canal or to traction and pressure produced by manipulations during delivery. A narrow pelvis, rigidity of the mother's soft tissues as well as prematurity or a high birth weight of the infant predispose to birth injury. Many of these risk factors are also associated with hypoxic ischaemic injury so that it must be remembered that mechanical and hypoxic injury may coexist and it may be difficult to separate the effects [10].

Cephalhaematoma occurs as result of shearing forces causing a disruption of the vessels passing from skull to periosteum, produced by forceps or prolonged labour. Pressure of the mother's symphysis pubis, sacral promontory or perineum can cause dislocation of the triangular cartilage of the nasal septum of the infant. Fracture of the clavicle is more common in cephalic deliveries: the fracture is usually in the clavicle that is in contact with the maternal symphysis. Injuries to bone and joint occur more often with complicated obstetrical procedures or breech deliveries than with spontaneous labour.

Facial nerve palsy is often associated with forceps deliveries and facial presentation. Central palsy may be due to brain injury, the peripheral one to direct compression; brachial plexus paralysis is mainly seen in breech presentations. They are caused by the pressure of the obstetrician's second and third fingers upon the plexus in the supraclavicular fossa or by the expansion by arm release respectively. During spontaneous births the plexus can be overstretched when the head has a sideways slant against rigid shoulders.

Ruptures of parenchymatous abdominal organs are usually seen following spontaneous births and the children thus affected commonly have a high birth weight. Genital trauma occurs with breech delivery.

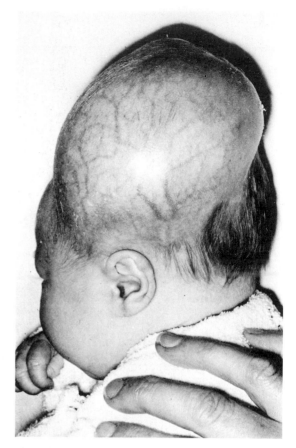

Figure 11.1 Enormous parietal cephalhaematoma in a 14-day old infant. Delivery had been normal. The swelling had become tense and erythematous 1 day before admission. Incision and vacuum drainage required; 180 ml dark blood evacuated; *E. coli* grown on culture

Clinical picture and treatment of the various injuries

Cephalhaematoma and skull fracture

Since cephalhaematoma represents subperiosteal blood accumulation the fluctuant swelling does not cross suture lines. Treatment is not necessary because spontaneous resorption occurs within 6 weeks and aspiration can introduce infection. Superinfection is rare (Figure 11.1) and aspiration and drainage and antibiotic therapy is indicated; we treated five such cases during a period of 10 years in our neonatal service at the Olgahospital, Stuttgart (FRG), where we see about 8000 newborns a year.

Linear skull fractures – fracture of the parietal bone is the most common – need no treatment. Growing fracture is very rare.

Depressed skull fracture may require elevation. Closed elevation of ping-pong ball fracture by breast pump vacuum extractor or thump compression

[25,31] has been described. Open elevation is indicated if there is increased intracranial pressure or neurological defect, or bony fragments project into cerebral tissue, or if the depression is more than three times the thickness of the skull.

Intracranial haemorrhage

Epidural, subdural and primary subarachnoidal haemorrhages can be caused by birth trauma and must be treated by neurosurgical procedures.

Dislocation of the triangular cartilage of the nasal septum

This injury is quite common and can be easily diagnosed when examining the septum of the nose (Figure 11.2a). Compression of the tip of the nose increases the dislocation (Figure 11.2b). After the

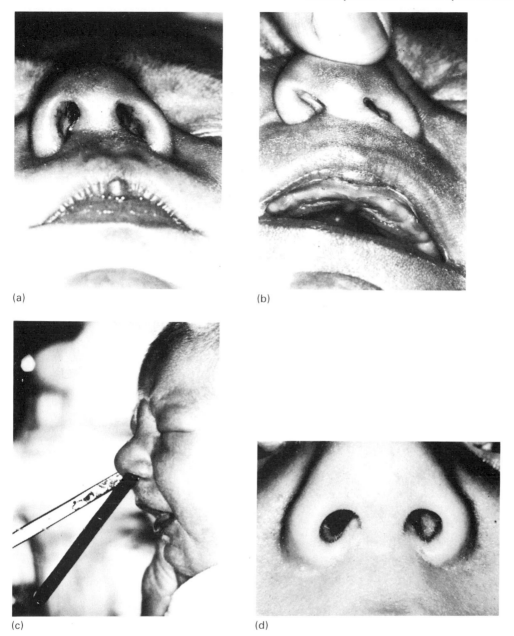

Figure 11.2 (a) Dislocation of the nasal septum in a 1-day-old child. (b) The displacement is increased by pressing on the tip of the nose. (c) Reposition. (d) One week after reposition

pressure has been discontinued the septum slips to its original position.

Replacement can usually be carried out without anaesthetic on the second or third day of life (Figure 11.2c,d). Fixation is unnecessary. If the septum is not replaced the child will suffer from obstruction of the air passages later [27,30].

Fractures of the clavicle

Greenstick fractures are rarely associated with clinical symptoms and become apparent only during the second week of life because of excessive callus formation. If a complete fracture has occurred, the newborn infant will not actively move the affected

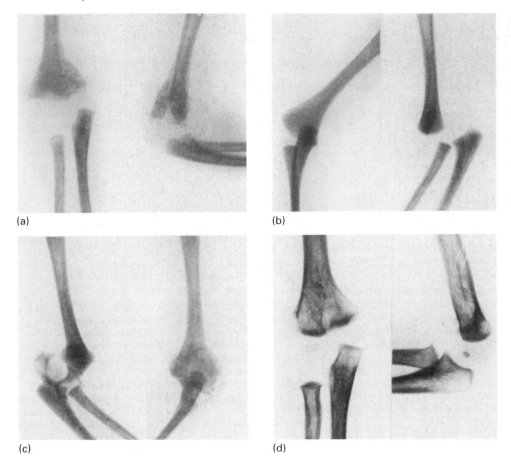

(a)

(b)

(c)

(d)

Figure 11.3 Epiphysiolysis of the epiphysis of the distal end of the humerus. (a) Formation of callus 1 month after birth. (b) Radiograph 2 days after birth, resembling dislocation of the elbow. (c) Arthrography shows epiphysis in the correct position. (d) Radiograph at the age of 8 months

arm and will cry when the arm is passively moved. The Moro reflex is missing on the affected side, and swelling and deformity are noticed in the area of the clavicle. Treatment is not necessary.

Epiphysiolysis

Clinically epiphysiolysis presents as a swelling of the affected joint and possibly a slight shortening of the extremity. Active movements will be absent and passive movement is painful. Often the diagnosis of osteomyelitis is made. Radiologically the diagnosis is easy if the ossification centre can already be recognized after birth. Since the ossification centre of both ends of humerus and the proximal femur are not visible in epiphyseal separation no radiological signs are primarily shown if there is no displacement. One or 2 weeks after the trauma the development of a callus will reveal that an epiphysiolysis has occurred (Figure 11.3a). If displacement is present

a simple dislocation will be diagnosed radiologically (Figure 11.3b). In arthrography (Figure 11.3c) the presence of a normally placed epiphysis can be confirmed. Recent reports [34] that epiphysiolysis can be studied by sonography suggest that the diagnosis can be made with arthrography (Figure 11.4).

Epiphyseal separation of the proximal humerus is often associated with brachial plexus palsy. The arm is held extended and outwardly rotated. Treatment in cases with marked displacement consists in closed reduction and immobilization of the arm by bandaging to the chest.

In distal humerus epiphysiolysis the bones of the forearm are usually displaced in a posterior and lateral direction. Treatment consists in reduction and immobilization in a splint for about 3 weeks.

Epiphysiolysis of the proximal femur is sometimes confused with a congenital dislocation of the hip and septic arthritis. The normally developed acetabulum

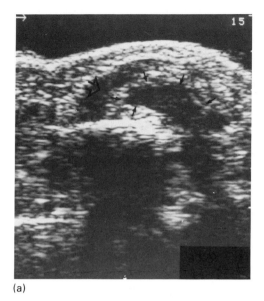

(a)

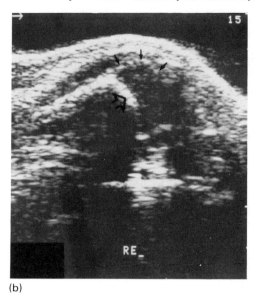

(b)

Figure 11.4 (a) Coronal sonographic section through a normal shoulder of a newborn. Epiphysis (arrows), growth plate (open arrow). (b) Coronal sonographic section of the left shoulder in a 1-day-old newborn, showing a dislocated epiphysis with thickening of the joint capsule and atypical shaped deltoid muscle (open arrow) (Courtesy of Dr Schulz, Head of the Department of Ultrasound, Olgahospital, Stuttgart, FRG)

will make the diagnosis of congenital dislocated hip unlikely. A traumatic hip dislocation by birth trauma has not been described yet. Similar to slipped capital epiphysis the femoral neck is displaced anteriorly with outward rotation. Treatment consists in closed reduction and immobilization in a spica cast. Internal fixation is required if instability is present. Necrosis of the head of the femur has not been described yet. Coxa vara frequently results, which will only rarely require a correction osteotomy.

Fractures of the shaft of the long bones

These are rare and the diagnosis is not difficult. Treatment consists in restriction of movement by traction, splinting or suitable bandaging for a period of 3 weeks. Care must be taken to avoid vascular complications.

Injuries of the peripheral nerves

Paralysis of the phrenic nerve

These are described in Chapter 19.

Injuries of the brachial plexus

Birth trauma can result in mild to severe partial and even complete tears of the roots of the brachial plexus. The first clinical sign is usually the absent Moro reflex on the affected side; occasionally a swelling is noted above the clavicle. There are no active movements of the muscles supplied by the affected nerves but passive movements are full. In the common Erb's palsy C5 and C6 are injured and the upper arm is extended, medially rotated and adducted; the forearm is pronated. The flexors of the hand and the fingers and the small muscles of the hand have normal functions. In Klumpke's paralysis (which is much rarer) there has been damage to the C8 and T1 roots and the flexors of the hand and fingers do not function. A Horner's syndrome is frequently observed because of damage to the communicating ramus from the first thoracic root. Total paralysis of the plexus is rare and will result in complete flaccidity of the whole arm. Isolated radial paralysis is also very uncommon.

In the differential diagnosis, fracture of the clavicle and traumatic epiphysiolysis of the proximal epiphysis of the humerus must be considered. These injuries can of course occur in addition to the plexus paralysis. A radiograph of the shoulder and of the upper arm should be taken. It must be remembered that in a percentage of brachial plexus lesions a paralysis of the phrenic nerve and even an eventration of the diaphragm may occur.

In adults, severe damage of the brachial plexus is only caused by very severe trauma. Trauma of such severity is rarely seen at birth. Most of the brachial plexus paralyses caused at birth will therefore heal spontaneously either completely or partially. The treatment of brachial plexus paralysis in the new-born is therefore primarily conservative. The aim is, on the one hand, the immobilization of the stretched nerve fibres for a period of 3–4 weeks following the trauma, which will allow a spontaneous cure; on the other hand, muscle and joint contractures must be prevented. It must be stressed that the immobilization position of abduction and external rotation of the shoulder is dangerous, as in this position the brachial plexus is under considerable tension [24]. If the brachial plexus is exposed at operation, one can easily recognize that tension is minimal if the arm is adducted to the thorax, whilst external rotation and abduction of the upper arm will cause marked tension of the nerve roots. Further contraindications to the abduction-external rotation position are abduction contracture as described by Adler [1] and secondary dislocation of the shoulder as described by Babbit [3].

During the first 4 weeks, abduction and external rotation of the shoulder are prevented by fixing the upper arm to the thorax. In the other joints careful passive physiotherapy should be carried out. After 4 weeks, passive abduction and external rotation of the shoulder are carefully carried out until, at the age of about 2 months, an abduction of 90 degrees has been achieved. Electrical stimulation is not used.

The prognosis of brachial plexus paralysis is better in the Erb's than in the Klumpke's variety or in cases of total paralysis. In the majority of cases of Erb's palsy, a partial or complete recovery can be achieved [9]. If recovery does not occur within the first 6 months, an electromyographic examination [17] should be performed and myelography should eliminate the possibility of an intraspinal lesion. Operative revision neurolysis and, in cases of complete severance of the nerves, bridging the gap with a nerve transplant taken from the suralis nerve should then be performed [24].

Facial paralysis

The nerves can be injured by lesions in the internal auditory meatus, in the mastoid or more distally in the region of the parotid or masseter muscle. Injuries in the last-mentioned region are caused by pressure of prominences in a narrow birth canal or by pressure of the delivery forceps. These injuries are usually incomplete and have a good prognosis. If however, electromyographic and electroneurographic tests reveal a worsening of the degeneration, neurolysis and a nerve cable transplant are advised if the facial nerve has degenerated [18,22].

Rupture of the solid organs

Rupture of the liver, suprarenal gland, spleen and kidney occur in that order of frequency. The symptoms become apparent after a symptom-free interval of a few hours or even a few days after birth. Clinically, two groups of patients can be recognized: (1) ruptures causing haemorrhage into the perito-neal cavity and (2) subcapsular or retroperitoneal rupture with delayed haemorrhage. The former group includes ruptures of liver and spleen with a tear of the capsule as well as ruptures of the suprarenal gland with a tear of the peritoneum. The presenting symptoms are severe shock and abdominal distension. If the processus vaginalis is still open a scrotal swelling may be observed. Severe anaemia is nearly always present and if the state of shock persists, a gradual decrease of the platelets and consequent coagulopathy will develop.

Ultrasonic and radiological investigations

Plain radiography of the abdomen is usually not very helpful. Ultrasonography shows free fluid in the abdomen in cases with intraperitoneal bleeding. Acute subcapsular haematoma of the liver (Figure 11.5) spleen and kidney are usually transonic while

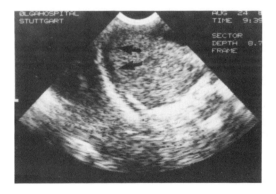

Figure 11.5 Longitudinal section of the right upper abdomen in a newborn. Between the diaphragm and the liver surface, sickle-like anechoic formation (arrows): haematoma of the liver capsule. (Courtesy of Dr Schulz. Head of the Department of Ultrasound, Olgahospital, Stuttgart, FRG)

chronic haematomas may have high intensity echoes [15]. In cases of injury of the kidney an excretory urogram is primarily indicated. Arteriography is indicated if there is neither excretion nor any spill of radio-opaque dye through the renal parenchyma into the perirenal space. In adrenal haemorrhage serial ultrasound (Figure 11.6) and computer tomographic examinations as well as quantitative urine and serum catecholamine assays are necessary to rule out neuroblastoma.

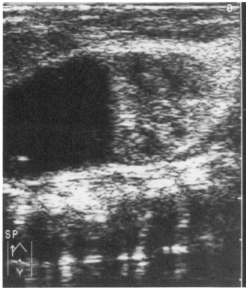

(a)

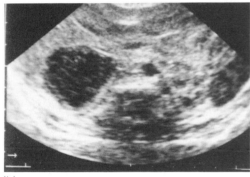

(b)

Figure 11.6 (a) Longitudinal section of the right upper abdomen. Trapezoid anechoic formation directly upon the upper part of the kidney: bleeding of the right adrenal gland. (b) Transverse section of the upper abdomen. On the right paravertebral side and subhepatical well distinctable round anechoic formation: bleeding of the right adrenal gland. (Courtesy of Dr Schulz. Head of the Department of Ultrasound, Olgahospital, Stuttgart, FRG)

Treatment

A haemoperitoneum caused by traumatic rupture of the liver or spleen or intraperitoneal rupture of a bleeding suprarenal gland should be submitted to immediate laparotomy after the shock has been treated. Ruptures of the liver are sutured or repaired with fibrin glue [33]. Because of the danger of severe infections following splenectomy it is of great importance to preserve as much as possible of the organ with fibrin glue, sutures or partial

splenectomy [6,21]. Small subcapsular haematomas and small ruptures can be treated conservatively [13]. If big haematomas or rupture of capsule with bleeding into the abdomen should occur immediate intervention is necessary. In unilateral rupture of the suprarenal gland adrenalectomy can be performed and there will be no danger of later adrenal insufficiency but it may be possible to arrest the haemorrhage by suturing the rent in the capsule. Suprarenal haemorrhages inside the perinephric fascia usually arrest spontaneously. It must be remembered that the underlying pathology may be a neuroblastoma [2,23,28] and a biopsy should always be taken. Renal injury must be treated conservatively if possible. Only severe bleeding and total rupture of parenchyma such as rupture of pelvis or ureter must be repaired [28]. As with the spleen preservation of all functioning renal tissue is indicated.

Genital trauma

Following breech delivery oedema and haematoma of the scrotum may occur. The differential diagnosis should include neonatal torsion and bleeding into a patent processus vaginalis [11]. No treatment is necessary. A single case of gangrene has been reported as a complication.

References

1. Adler, J.B. and Patterson, R.L. (1967) Erb's palsy: long-term results of treatment in eighty-eight cases *J. Bone Jt Surg.*, **49A**, 1052–1064
2. Angerpointner, T.A. (1985) Ein Fall von Geburtstraumatisch rupturiertem kongenitalem Neuroblastom. *Monatsschr, Kinderheilk.*, **133**, 241–242
3. Babbit, D.P. and Cassidy, R.H. (1968) Obstetrical paralysis and dislocation of the shoulder in infancy. *J. Bone Jt Surg.*, **50A**, 1447–1452
4. Bennet, G.C. and Harold, A.J. (1976) Prognosis and early management of birth injuries to the brachial plexus. *Br. Med. J.*, **1**, 1520–1521
5. Blocker, S.H. and Ternberg, J.L. (1986) Traumatic liver laceration in the newborn: repair with Fibringlue. *J. Pediat. Surg.*, **21**, 369–371
6. Chryss, C. and Aaron, W.S. (1980) Successful treatment of rupture of normal spleen in a newborn. *Am. J. Dis. Child.*, **134**, 418–419
7. Cywes, S. (1967) Haemoperitoneum in the newborn. *S. Afr. Med. J.*, **41**, 1050–1057
8. Denes, J., Lukacs, F.V. and Leb, J. (1972) Spontaneous idiopathic rupture of the stomach in the neonatal period. *Acta Paediat. Acad. Sci. Hung.*, **13**, 253–258
9. Donn, S.M. and Faix, R.G. (1983) Long-term prognosis for the infant with severe birth trauma. *Clin. Perinatol.*, **10**, 507–520

10. Faix, R.G. and Donn, S.M. (1983) Immediate management of the traumatized infant. *Clin. Perinatol.*, **10**, 487–505
11. Finan, B.F. and Redman, J.F. (1985) Neonatal genital trauma. *Urology*, **25**, 532–533
12. Gordon, M., Rich, H., Deutschberger, J. *et al.* (1973) The immediate and longterm outcome of obstetric birth trauma. 1. Brachial plexus paralysis. *Am. J. Obstet. Gynecol.*, **117**, 51–56
13. Hadley, G.P. and Mickel, R.E. (1984) Splenic artery ligation – an adjunct to splenorraph in children. Case reports. *S. Afr. J. Surg.*, **22**, 97–101
14. Hardy, A.E. (1981) Birth injuries of the brachial plexus: incidence and prognosis. *J. Bone Jt Surg.*, **63B**, 98–101
15. Hendry, G.M. (1981) The ultrasonic appearances of intra-abdominal haematomas. *Ann. Radiol.*, **24**, 91–98
16. Hensinger, R.N. and Jones, E.T. (1981) *Neonatal Orthopedics*. Grune & Stratton, New York
17. Hoffmann, W., Bickel, A. and Ullrich, K.P. (1985) Die Prognose von geburtstraumatisch bedingten Paresen des Plexus brachialis. *Pediat. Grenzeb.*, **24**, 259–264
18. Kornblut, A.D. (1977) Facial nerve injuries in children. *Ear, Nose Throat J.*, **56**, 369–376
19. Lehner, M. (1974) Geburtstraumatische Rupturen parenchymatöser Abdominalorgane. *Z. Kinderchir.*, **14**, 265–273
20. Mangurten, H.H. (1983) Birth injuries. In *Neonatal Perinatal Medicine: Diseases of the Fetus and Infant*, 3rd edn. (eds) Fanaroff, A.A. and Martin, R.J. C.V. Mosby, St. Louis
21. Matsuyama, S. and Suzuki, N. (1976) Rupture of the spleen in the newborn: treatment without splenectomy. *J. Pediat. Surg.*, **11**, 115–116
22. Miehlke, A. (1973) *Surgery of the Facial Nerve*. 2nd edn, Urban and Schwarzenberg, Munich
23. Murthy, T.V.M., Irving, I.M. and Lister, J. (1978) Massive adrenal hemorrhage in neonatal neuroblastoma. *J. Pediat. Surg.*, **13**, 31–34
24. Narakas, A. (1976) Clinique chirurgicale et permanence de longeraie. Personal communication
25. Raynor, R. and Parsa, M. (1968) Non-surgical elevation of depressed skull fracture in an infant. *J. Pediat.*, **72**, 262–264
26. Schrager, G.O. (1970) Elevation of depressed skull fracture with a breast pump. *J. Pediat.*, **77**, 300–301
27. Silverman, S.H. and Leibow, S.G. (1975) Dislocation of the triangular cartilage of the nasal septum. *J. Pediat.*, **87**, 456–458
28. Sober, I. and Hirsch, M. (1965) Unilateral massive adrenal hemorrhage in newborn infant. *J. Urol.*, **93**, 430–434
29. Specht, E.E. (1975) Brachial plexus palsy in the newborn: incidence and prognosis. *Clin. Orthop.*, **110**, 32–34
30. Stocksted, P. and Schønsted-Madsen, U. (1979) Traumatology of the newborn's nose. *Rhinology*, **17**, 77–82
31. Tan, K.L. (1974) Elevation of congenital depressed features of the skull by the vacuum extractor. *Acta Paediat. Scand.*, **63**, 562–564
32. Valdes-Dapena, M.A. and Arey, J.B. (1970) The causes of neonatal mortality: an analysis of 501 autopsies on newborn infants. *J. Pediat.*, **77**, 366–375
33. Wegmann, M.E. (1982) Annual summary of vital statistics – 1980. *Pediatrics*, **68**, 755–762
34. Zieger, M., Dorr, U. and Schulz, R.D. (1987) Sonography of slipped humeral epiphysis due to birth injury. *Pediat. Radiol.*, **17**, 425–426

12

Tumours of the head and neck

Irene M. Irving

Nasal glioma

Historical notes and incidence

The term nasal glioma was introduced by Schmidt [61] in 1900 and his was the first well documented case. By 1977, 138 cases had been reported in the literature [37]. During the period 1953–85 only four newborns with the condition were admitted to the Liverpool Regional Neonatal Surgical Centre. All of these were cases of the extranasal form of glioma, but during the period 1960–80 a further five cases were treated by our ENT colleagues, three of these being intranasal and two combined extranasal and intranasal tumours [11].

Pathology and embryology

The tumour consists of astrocytic neuroglial tissue separated into islets by dense fibrous tissue trabeculae. There is no capsule and no covering of meninges. Overlying skin is usually normal but may be atrophic [24]. Mitotic activity is not seen and neuronal differentiation is a very rare feature [48]. About 60% of cases are entirely extranasal, 30% are intranasal whilst the remainder are combined defects. In 20% of the reported cases an intracranial connection, usually fibrous, has been demonstrated, the bony defect being usually in the cribriform plate [37]. Such connections are very rare in the case of extranasal tumours.

Many theories have been advanced about the origin of the nasal glioma [37,72] but most authors subscribe to the view that the lesion is a sequestrated encephalocele completely or, less commonly, partially separated from the frontal lobes by closure of the cranial sutures. Strictly speaking, it is a choristoma, i.e. a tumour-like malformation composed of tissue not normally present in the affected part.

Clinical picture

Extranasal gliomas present at birth as a firm subcutaneous lump with red or bluish discoloration, lying on one side of the nasal bridge (Figure 12.1). Widening of the nasal bridge and hypertelorism may be observed. The mass is firmly attached to the skin, does not pulsate and does not increase in size on crying or straining. The tumours are usually not large, reaching a diameter of 2–3 cm. Intranasal lesions present at or shortly after birth as a polyp-like mass causing unilateral nasal airway obstruction. In the presence of an extranasal glioma the

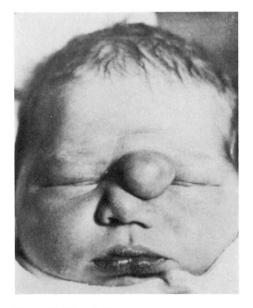

Figure 12.1 Nasal glioma

possibility of an intranasal component must be borne in mind and the nasal passages must be examined. In the case of extranasal tumours radiography of the skull will not show any abnormality, but in the case of intranasal or combined tumours full evaluation of the skull by tomography and CT scanning is necessary [11].

Treatment

The surgery of intranasal gliomas does not come within the scope of this chapter and the reader is referred to the literature [11,66,72].

Gliomas which are entirely extranasal can be removed safely by simple excision. Small skin flaps are fashioned at the base of the tumour but the remainder of the closely adherent skin is removed with the tumour. A thin fibrous stalk attached to the deep aspect of the tumour usually passes upwards for a short distance under the nasal bone. If the child is otherwise fit, excision should be performed during the neonatal period as the tumour is unsightly and will interfere with vision.

Results

These are benign tumours which only recur if the initial excision has been incomplete [37]. Our three infants are alive and without recurrence.

Congenital epulis

'Epulis' is a term which includes all soft tissue tumours arising from the alveolus, but the meaning of 'congenital epulis' has become restricted to a distinct entity known also as congenital granular cell epulis, congenital granular cell myoblastoma and gingival granular cell tumour.

Historical notes and incidence

Neumann [49], in 1871, gave the first description of a soft tissue tumour which may be found on the maxillary alveolus of newborn infants. In a centennial review, Fuhr and Krogh [22] reviewed 113 reported cases, to which an additional 51 cases had been added by 1984 [71]. Girls are affected much more commonly than boys, in a ratio of 8:1 [22]. Since 1953 we have treated four cases in the Liverpool Neonatal Surgical Centre.

Pathology

The tumour, which is covered by stratified squamous epithelium and is non-encapsulated, has a homogeneous structure consisting of large cells with pale eosinophilic granular cytoplasm. There have been numerous theories concerning the tissue

of origin of these cells [22]; Abrikossoff's myoblastoma theory [1] has been the most widely held although many workers have disputed it [8,19]. Recent ultrastructural and immunohistochemical studies indicate a different histogenesis to the granular cell myoblastoma [41], and support a mesenchymal origin [40,42]. In view of the marked predilection for females, a hormonal factor or factors may be important in the development of these lesions [18,40].

Clinical picture

The child is born with a pea- to walnut-sized brown or bluish-red lobulated mass attached to the incisor or canine region of the maxillary or mandibular alveolus (Figure 12.2), the former being the more

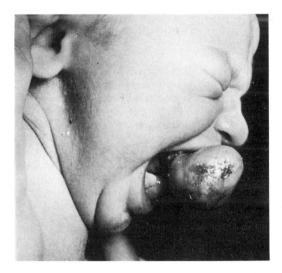

Figure 12.2 Congenital epulis (by courtesy of Mr K. Richards)

common. The attachment to the alveolus is usually broad-based but may be pedunculated. Overlying mucosa may be ulcerated in the case of larger lesions. Rarely, multiple tumours may be present [16,53]. If the swelling is large, the infant is unable to close his mouth and may have difficulty in feeding or even have respiratory obstruction [14].

Treatment

A congenital epulis should be removed during early infancy because of the disabilities which it causes and for cosmetic reasons. If left alone, however, it will not grow in size and may regress [18].

The lesion is entirely benign, and the surgeon must not be misled by the term myoblastoma (which should be abandoned in this context) into thinking that wide excision is required. The operation, which is best performed under endotracheal anaesthesia, is not difficult. The excision can be performed close to the tumour but the periosteum can be removed. The wound does not need to be sutured and will heal rapidly.

Results

Even if the excision of these tumours is incomplete recurrence does not occur; metastases have never been described. Minor dental anomalies, probably resulting from intraoperative damage to the tooth-buds, have been documented [14,65]. Our own four cases recovered without complications.

Teratomas of the head and neck

Teratomas of the head and neck constitute only a small fraction of childhood teratomas. Those occurring in the neck or in the oronasopharynx are usually present at birth and although rare are of importance because they can cause life-threatening respiratory obstruction.

Cervical teratoma

Historical notes and incidence

The first authentic case of cervical teratoma was that reported by Hess in 1856 [29]. These tumours are rare; in a recent review Jordan and Gauderer could trace only 212 cases in the literature, to which they added a further five. Our own experience is of five cases since 1953. These comprised only 11% of the total number of neonatal teratomas treated over the same period (Table 12.1). The corresponding figure in four reviews of teratomas in infancy and childhood ranged from 2.3 to 9.3% [5,7,26,67]. The sexes are affected equally. One instance of cervical teratoma in two siblings is on record [32].

Table 12.1 Anatomical location of neonatal teratomas treated in the Liverpool Neonatal Surgical Unit 1953–85

Sacrococcygeal	35
Presacral	2
Rectal	1
Retroperitoneal	2
Mediastinal	1
Cervical	5
Total	46

Pathology and histogenesis

Cervical teratomas are usually large tumours, partly cystic and partly solid and well encapsulated. They are true neoplasms, being composed of tissues foreign to the site of origin, with derivatives of all three germ layers, often with a preponderance of central nervous tissue. The great majority of childhood cervical teratomas are benign but there are a few well-documented instances of malignant metastatic tumours in newborns and young infants [52] as well as some cases with histological evidence of local lymph node involvement but with a non-aggressive clinical course [35]. One of our five cases was malignant; a large tumour in a premature baby, removed on the day of birth, consisted mainly of malignant embryonic mesenchyme differentiating in parts into nephroblastoma, retinoblastoma and neuroblastoma.

Most cervical teratomas are associated with the thyroid gland, either by being in direct continuity with it or by replacing part of the gland [38,58]. Roediger and Spitz propose a common origin for all cervical teratomas, from totipotential cells of each germ cell layer, found in the thyroid gland [58].

Clinical picture

Maternal hydramnios, present in three of our five cases, is a common feature [38] and is thought to be due to the tumour preventing fetal swallowing of the amniotic fluid [64]. Large tumours may cause dystocia. Seventy-five percent of cervical teratomas present at birth and although some may be relatively small, the majority are large and are associated with respiratory distress [27,35], sometimes amounting to total respiratory obstruction.

The tumour is a firm well-defined mass with multiple bosses which can be seen as well as felt (Figure 12.3). Some areas may feel more solid than others and, as in one of our cases, spurs of solid tissue may be palpable within cysts. The mass, which is mobile from side to side, is situated anteriorly or to one side of the neck and extends from mandible to clavicle, with very occasional extension into the superior mediastinum or into the floor of the mouth [35]. The mass does not transilluminate.

Imaging studies

Prenatal ultrasound diagnosis of these tumours, first described by Schoenfeld in 1978 [62], is now well established [59] and is based on the presence of a fetal cervical mass which is part cystic and part solid. Postnatal ultrasound evaluation is useful only as a means of demonstrating the mixture of cystic and solid components in the mass as an aid to differential diagnosis from cystic hygroma if doubt exists on clinical grounds.

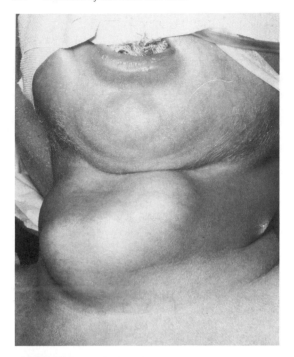

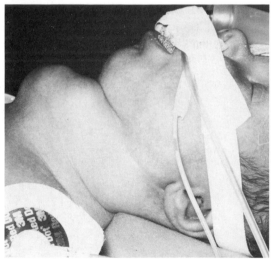

Figure 12.3 Large cervical teratoma which caused tracheal obstruction at birth

Plain radiography (anteroposterior and lateral views) is indicated in all cases, as it may demonstrate the diagnostic feature of calcification within the tumour and will also reveal the presence of tracheal compression and deviation.

Pre-operative radioisotope thyroid scanning should not be undertaken routinely; it is unlikely to yield helpful information and may actually be misleading [70]. Likewise, CT scanning is rarely, if ever, indicated.

Laboratory studies

There are insufficient data in the literature to indicate whether the serum alpha-fetoprotein level is useful as a tumour 'marker' in cervical teratomas and our own cases predated the use of this investigation. It is possible, however, that rapidly growing embryonal tissue within these tumours could increase serum AFP levels [35] and blood should be taken pre- or intraoperatively to establish a baseline level.

Treatment

Newborns with respiratory obstruction due to a cervical teratoma require immediate intubation and resuscitation. This may be a life-saving procedure as in one of our patients who could achieve no air entry despite vigorous respiratory effort. It is in such cases that prenatal diagnosis is of great value as it affords the opportunity for arranging the timing, location and mode of delivery for optimal management of the airway and subsequent surgery [30]. In such cases operation should obviously be carried out without delay, but this applies also to tumours not causing respiratory embarrassment as cysts may enlarge rapidly and cause tracheal compression.

Operation

This is carried out through a long transverse incision along a cervical skin crease. The nodular tumour is exposed (Figure 12.4). This will usually necessitate division of the strap muscles although sometimes the tumour is found to be lying superficial to the musculature. The tumour may have no attachment to vital structures, may be connected by just a flimsy

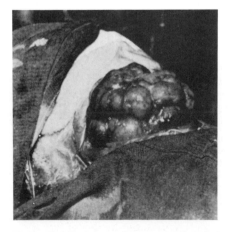

Figure 12.4 Exposure of teratoma of neck through a transverse cervical incision

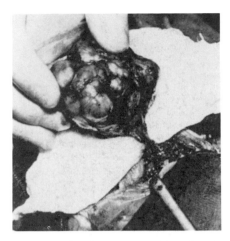

Figure 12.5 Cervical teratoma. There is only a flimsy pedicle attached to the thyroid gland

pedicle to the thyroid gland (Figure 12.5) or may be more intimately connected to the thyroid, necessitating partial thyroidectomy [27,51]. Enucleation is usually not difficult, although in one of our cases a retropharyngeal extension caused problems. The wound should be drained with suction for 48 h. Ventilation may be required for 2 or 3 days.

In cases where no normal residual thyroid gland can be identified, thyroid function studies should be done postoperatively, but there are no cases on record of postoperative thyroid (or parathyroid) deficiency.

Results

Jordan and Gauderer [35] propose a helpful prognostic classification based on clinical presentation and age. Of their five groups, three are applicable to neonates: Group I, stillborn and moribund live born (100% mortality); group II, newborn with respiratory distress (43% mortality) and group III, newborn without respiratory distress (2.7% mortality). Group II, which includes 61% of reported neonatal cases is clearly the group in which the survival rate could be improved by accurate diagnosis, both prenatal and postnatal, prompt attention to the airway and early surgery.

Of our own four cases of benign cervical teratoma, two had respiratory distress and two did not. All survived early surgery but one has a residual unilateral Horner's syndrome.

Our single case of malignant cervical teratoma, a huge, solid tumour which had caused respiratory obstruction, was removed on the day of birth. The child, who was premature, with respiratory distress syndrome, did not survive.

Teratoid tumours of the oronasopharynx

Teratomas arising within the nasopharynx or oropharynx are rare; they accounted for only two of 91 cases of teratomas treated at the Hospital for Sick Children, Great Ormond Street between 1925 and 1969 [68] and two of 245 cases treated at the Children's Hospital, Boston [30] between 1928 and 1982.

Pathology

Ewing [21] classified oronasopharyngeal teratoid tumours into three types:

Type I: dermoids, composed of ecto- and mesodermal derivatives. These tumours are often pedunculated and are covered by skin and hair.
Type II: teratomas, composed of tissues derived from all three germ layers. They differ from type I by their more marked structural differentiation and larger size. Skull deformities are often associated.
Type III: epignathus. These are highly organized teratomas containing recognizable organs.

Type I is the most common and tends to affect adults, although this type of lesion has been described in the newborn [10,44]. In types II and III associated malformations are very common. Females are much more commonly affected than males [10].

The tumours may arise from a variety of sites, typically from the wall of the nasopharynx above the level of the soft palate, but also from the soft or hard palate, the uvula or the tonsillar area [69]. There may be a cleft palate because the mass of the tumour has prevented fusion of the two halves of the palate [56]. In the majority of cases the tumour is a pedunculated, rounded nodular whitish mass which is only a few centimetres in diameter. The most gross variant of the condition is the so-called giant epignathus which fills the mouth and protrudes from it [6,28]. On rare occasions a teratoma of the nasopharynx may extend into the neck [2] or into the cranium [28,56].

Clinical picture

In many cases large teratomas and epignathi have been found in deformed stillborn infants [10] or have resulted in death on delivery [56]. In the case of tumours which are not visible externally, respiratory symptoms are the usual presenting problem; dyspnoea may be noted from the time of birth or may occur later, typically after a change in posture which can cause a pedunculated mass to shift and block the nasopharyngeal airway. The sudden onset of, and also the relief of, obstruction related to changes in posture should suggest the diagnosis [34].

Excessive nasal mucus and feeding problems may also occur. Routine examination may reveal the tumour but a small mass confined to the nasopharynx can be missed on visual inspection and may only be diagnosed by palpation or by radiography [10]. Other features are forward displacement or absence of the soft palate or replacement of the hard palate by tumour [2].

Radiography

If the tumour is calcified it can easily be seen in a lateral radiograph; non-calcified masses can also be delineated as filling defects in the nasopharyngeal air shadow [10]. Tomography and CT scanning can be useful in defining bony defects [2,69].

Treatment

The airway must be secured either by endotracheal intubation or, if necessary, by tracheostomy. The tumour should be removed promptly once the diagnosis is established. Removal of pedunculated tumours is relatively easy; a snare can be used for a narrow pedicle [44], but usually excision with diathermy is necessary so as to minimize blood loss. Giant tumours necessitate extensive dissection of tumour from soft tissues, jaws and base of skull. Total excision may prove impossible in such cases, and incomplete removal is preferable to grossly mutilating surgery since these tumours have a low potential for malignant change [69].

Results

The prognosis after operation for dermoid cysts is good. Survival has been unusual in cases of teratoma and epignathus but at least ten such cases are now on record [69]. These patients need prolonged follow-up for detection of local recurrence and for correction of residual deformities [6,56,69]. A solitary case of malignant dissemination is recorded [67].

Cystic hygroma of the neck

Terminology

A cystic hygroma is a benign hamartomatous lesion of lymphatic origin. Strictly speaking, the term should be reserved for the variety of lymphangioma which is composed of cysts rather than of dilated lymphatic channels. In practice, there is a tendency to use the terms cystic hygroma and lymphangioma synonymously and this is reasonable as there is no sharp dividing line between the two. However, as lymphangiomas of the neck are typically of the cystic

type [9], we have elected to use the term cystic hygroma in this chapter.

Historical notes

The condition was first described by Redenbacker [55] in 1828. Although it had previously been suspected that cystic hygroma was of lymphatic origin, it was not until the beginning of this century, when Sabin [60] studied the embryology of the lymphatic system in detail, that the lymphatic nature of these tumours was fully recognized.

Aetiology

Sabin [60] postulated that human lymphatics originate by centrifugal growth from veins and lymphatic cavities. This theory was subsequently disproved by Huntington [31] in studies on cats and by Kampmeier [36] who showed that at the 9–12 mm stage of human fetal development mesenchymal slits appear in the reticulum of the large venous plexuses of the cervical region. These slits coalesce to form lymphatic cavities, which open secondarily into the venous system. If these primary lymphatic spaces fail to join up with the central system, cyst formation results; the more peripheral the sequestration the smaller the cysts [25]. The cystic mass enlarges because lymph formed in the cystic spaces cannot drain away from the sequestrated areas.

Pathology

Cystic hygroma is a multilocular mass composed of a large number of individual cysts lined with endothelium and containing clear, slightly yellowish fluid which is identical with lymph [3]. Following even minor trauma the fluid may become blood-stained. This is not surprising as capillaries and even cavernous venous spaces are often intimately associated with cystic hygromas. The majority of cystic hygromas do not constitute a neonatal emergency, but giant hygromas of the neck can cause grave emergencies in the newborn period. These swellings may fill the whole of one side of the neck, may cross the midline and may invade the muscles of the neck and also the pharynx and larynx [17] which are frequently studded with numerous small submucosal cysts. Invasion of the tongue may also occur, causing macroglossia (Figure 12.6). They may extend behind the clavicle into the axilla (Figure 12.7) or through the thoracic inlet into the mediastinum. These tumours are benign but they grow locally and infiltrate by insinuation along blood vessels and nerve trunks [9]. Sudden and rapid enlargement of the mass may occur as a result of haemorrhage, or because of adjacent inflammation as in upper respiratory tract infection, and in infection of the cystic hygroma itself.

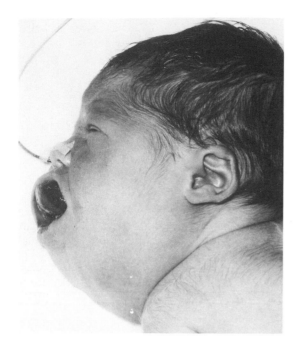

Figure 12.6 Large cystic hygroma of neck with infiltration of the tongue

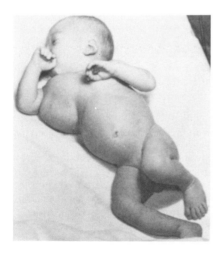

Figure 12.7 Large cystic hygroma of neck extending into the axilla

Incidence

Cystic hygroma is a comparatively uncommon condition. The sexes are affected equally. Approximately 75% of these lesions are situated in the neck [54] and between 50 and 65% are present at birth [9]. Tumours giving rise to acute symptoms in the neonatal period are very uncommon. Between 1953

and 1985 12 neonates with large cystic hygromas were treated in the Liverpool Neonatal Surgical Centre; ten of these were situated in the neck, five being confined to the neck whilst in the other five cases there were varying degrees of involvement of face, tongue, floor of mouth, larynx and pharynx. Mediastinal involvement was found in only one case. Nine of our ten patients had no other congenital anomalies but one child had Turner's syndrome. Recent reports [12,15,23,45] of fetal cystic hygroma of the neck diagnosed by ultrasound emphasize the high proportion of Turner's syndrome amongst these cases; Ba'geel and Kidess [4] found an incidence of 60% Turner's syndrome amongst 83 such cases collected from the literature and a high association with hydrops fetalis and intrauterine death. There is evidence to suggest that intrauterine resolution of cystic hygroma can occur and that this may be the forerunner of the webbed neck of Turner's syndrome [15,63].

Clinical picture

The infant is born with a large soft cystic mass, usually in the posterior triangle of the neck but sometimes in the anterior triangle. The mass fluctuates, and transilluminates brilliantly unless there has been haemorrhage into it. The tumour is not attached to skin unless infection has occurred previously, but it is not movable on its deep aspect. The boundaries of the lesion are typically ill-defined and the one case in our series which was a well-defined mass proved to be an unusual unilocular lymphatic cyst (Figure 12.8). The skin overlying large lesions is thin and bluish. Infection causes erythema of the overlying skin whilst haemorrhage causes bluish-red discoloration [13]. The lesion may cause respiratory distress immediately after birth

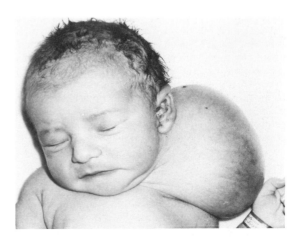

Figure 12.8 Unilocular cystic hygroma of neck

because of laryngeal and tracheal compression and
also because of direct extension into the pharynx,
larynx, floor of mouth and tongue (Figure 12.6).
The tongue, when involved, is enlarged and beefy,
often with superficial vesicles which exude blood-
stained fluid. Oral feeding may be difficult or
impossible. In some cases there may be no symptoms at birth but acute respiratory embarrassment
may occur later because of sudden enlargement of
the lesion due to haemorrhage, upper respiratory
tract infection or bacterial infection of the lesion
itself. In the event of such complications, the lesion
may become tender. Hygromas with extension into
the mediastinum are especially prone to these
complications. Axillary involvement may produce
brachial plexus compression with pain and hyperaes-
thesia [13]. Laboratory investigations are almost
always normal but in patients with infected cystic
hygromas leucocytosis and granulocytosis are
observed, and we have seen a newborn with
septicaemia associated with an infected cystic hygroma. Haemorrhage into the tumour may be sufficiently severe to cause anaemia.

Imaging

Radiography of the neck will reveal any displacement or compression of the trachea, and in cases
with mediastinal extension the chest radiogram will
show a mediastinal mass (Figure 12.9). Sonography
shows a primarily cystic mass with septa of varying
thickness and is useful in determining the full extent
of the lesion before surgery and in assessing
postoperative complications and recurrences [63].

Differential diagnosis

This should present little difficulty in the neonate.
Cervical teratoma is much more solid than a cystic
hygroma, is neither fluctuant nor translucent and
has a different sonographic appearance. A lesion
which can present in the neonate as a soft lateral
cervical swelling is the rare third branchial pouch
remnant [46,57], which is invariably left-sided and is
prone to early infection because of its fistulous
connection with the pyriform fossa. In the unusual
event of the cystic hygroma being confined to the
tongue or floor of the mouth, thyroglossal cyst,
gastroenteric duplication cyst [43], dermoid cyst and
retention cyst of the sublingual gland must be
considered in the differential diagnosis.

Treatment

Surgical excision is the only effective treatment.
Radiotherapy has been tried but is ineffective [50]
and should never be used because of the risk of
severe complications. The injection of sclerosing
agents was often advocated in times past but has

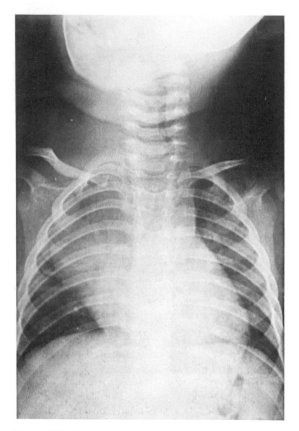

Figure 12.9 Cystic hygroma of neck with mediastinal
extension

never been satisfactory, with the possible exception
of bleomycin injections which have been reported as
beneficial in residual tumour after incomplete
surgery for massive infiltrating lesions [33]. The
presence of infection is a contraindication to
surgery, which must be delayed until antibiotics
have been given and the infection has resolved.

Although spontaneous resolution of these lesions
has been documented it is a rare event [50] and
postponement of surgery in the hope of improvement is not rewarding; it is, in fact, hazardous in
extensive lesions, particularly those involving the
tongue and the floor of the mouth and those with a
mediastinal extension, as the cystic mass may
enlarge rapidly and cause respiratory obstruction. In
some cases emergency tracheostomy (and gastrostomy) may be required in the first few days of life.
Early surgery may obviate the necessity for these
procedures and should be performed without delay
if the infant is otherwise fit.

Operation

The operation is carried out under routine endotracheal anaesthesia. The patient's head and neck should be covered by transparent adhesive drape to enable the surgeon to see any twitching of the muscles of the face and neck. A faradic nerve stimulator should be at hand. The patient is placed flat on his back with a small rolled-up towel behind his shoulders. The cystic hygroma is best removed through a long transverse cervical incision over the most prominent part of the tumour. Ideally the whole mass of cysts should be completely removed but this may be very difficult as the deep aspect of the tumour is often found to be infiltrating the cervical muscles and the pharynx as well as surrounding the nerves. The nerves should be identified by use of the nerve stimulator and dissected free of the tumour as far as possible; the most vulnerable are the cervical branch of the facial nerve, the superior laryngeal nerve and the spinal accessory nerve. Submucous cysts of the pharynx and larynx should be removed if possible but it is often wise to leave some of the endothelial lining *in situ* as it is closely attached to the mucosa. Similarly, the large vessels are often completely surrounded by cysts and it is often impossible to peel off all the endothelial lining from the vessels. In two of our cases one internal jugular vein was sacrificed. It has been our experience that provided irremovable cysts are opened and as much as possible of their lining is removed, the remaining endothelium usually stops secreting lymph, although there may be some extravasation of lymph during the immediate postoperative period.

It must be remembered that cystic hygromas are not malignant tumours, that total excision of the massive infiltrating lesions is impossible and that grossly mutilating surgery is not justifiable. Staged surgery will almost certainly be necessary in those cases involving mouth, tongue, pharynx, larynx, etc. If the tumour extends into the axilla, the cervical part of the tumour is first dissected down to clavicular level, following which the dissection is continued from below, through a separate transverse axillary incision. Extreme care has to be taken to avoid damage to the brachial plexus and subclavian vessels; if necessary the clavicle can be divided so as to improve access. Some axillary hygromas infiltrate the skin, which has the appearance of peau d'orange. It is most unwise to leave this skin as it will be a constant source of trouble (oedema, lymphangitis, etc.); it should therefore be excised together with the hygroma.

A mediastinal extension of a cervical cystic hygroma can usually be removed together with the main tumour. If the mediastinal component is not extensive and not firmly adherent to the pleura it may be possible to deal with it from the neck.

Otherwise it must be exposed through a median sternotomy and dissected free. A single stage procedure [39,47] is preferable to two-stage procedures because of the particular danger of respiratory obstruction in these cases.

The neck wound should be drained in all cases using a vacuum drain, and antibiotics should be given as there is a considerable danger of infection. Collections of lymph or blood may accumulate despite wound drainage and can be treated by needle aspiration. After extensive dissection involving the pharynx, larynx and trachea, intubation, or occasionally tracheostomy, may be required,

In the massive infiltrating lesions further surgery will be required, often extending over many years, for the treatment in particular of lingual and laryngeal disease. Laser surgery is proving to be particularly useful in the treatment of these extremely difficult cases [17,20].

References

1. Abrikossoff, A. (1926) Ueber Myone, ausgehend von der quergestrieften, willkurlichen Muskulatur. *Virchow's Archiv path. Anat. Physiol. Klin. Med.*, **260**, 215–233

2. Alter, A.D. and Cove, J.K. (1987) Congenital nasopharyngeal teratoma: report of a case and review of the literature. *J. Pediat. Surg.*, **22**, 179–181

3. von Ammon, A. Cited by Wernher, A. (1843) *Die angeborenen Kysten Hygrome und die ihnen verwandten Geschwülste in anatomischer, diagnosticher und therapeutischer Beziehung.* G.F. Heyer, Giessen

4. Ba'aqueel, H.S. and Kidess, E.A. (1988) Fetal cystic hygroma – its significance and clinical behaviour. *Saudi Med. J.*, **9**, 194–204

5. Bale, P.M., Painter, D.M. and Cohen, D. (1975) Teratomas in childhood. *Pathology*, **7**, 209–218

6. Bennett, J.P. (1970) A case of epignathus with long term survival. *Br. J. Plastic Surg.*, **23**, 360–364

7. Berry, C.L., Keeling, J. and Hilton, C. (1969) Teratoma in infancy and childhood: a review of 91 cases. *J. Path.*, **98**, 241–252

8. Bhaskar, S.N. (1963) Oral tumours of infancy and childhood. *J. Pediat.*, **63**, 195–210

9. Bill, A.H. and Sumner, D.S. (1965) A unified concept of lymphangioma and cystic hygroma. *Surg. Gynecol. Obstet.*, **120**, 79–86

10. Boeckman, C.R. (1968) Teratoid tumours of the nasopharynx in children. *J. Pediat. Surg.*, **3**, 735–739

11. Bradley, P.J. and Singh, S.D. (1982) Congenital nasal masses: diagnosis and management. *Clin. Otolaryngol.*, **7**, 87–97

12. Carr, R.F., Ochs, R.H., Ritter, D.A., Kenny, J.D., Fridey, J.L. and Ming, P.L. (1986) Fetal cystic hygroma and Turner's syndrome. *Am. J. Dis. Child.*, **140**, 580–583

13. Chait, D., Yonkers, A.J., Beddoe, G.M. and Yarington, C.T. (1974) Management of cystic hygromas. *Surg. Gynec. Obstet.*, **139**, 55–57

14. Chamberlain, J.W. (1967) Congenital epulis. *J. Pediat. Surg.*, **2**, 158–163

15. Chervenak, F.A., Isaacson, G., Blakemore, K.J., Breg, W.R., Hobbins, J.C., Berkowitz, R.L. *et al.* (1983) Fetal cystic hygroma. Cause and natural history. *New Engl. J. Med.*, **309**, 822–825

16. Cigliano, B., De Fazio, P., Esposito, P. and Insabato, L. (1985) Neonatal congenital epulis. *Int. J. Oral Surg.*, **14**, 456–457

17. Cohen, S.R. and Thompson, J.W. (1986) Lymphangiomas of the larynx in infants and children. A survey of pediatric lymphagioma. *Ann. Otol. Rhinol. Laryngol.* (Suppl.), **127**, 1–20

18. Cussen, L.J. and MacMahon, R.A. (1975) Congenital granular-cell myoblastoma. *J. Pediat. Surg.*, **10**, 249–253

19. Custer, R.P. and Fust, J.A. (1952) Congenital epulis. *Am. J. Clin. Path.*, **2**, 1044–1053

20. Dixon, J.A., Davis, R.K. and Gilbertson, J.J. (1986) Laser photocoagulation of vascular malformations of the tongue. *Laryngoscope*, **96**, 537–541

21. Ewing, J. (1940) *Neoplastic Diseases*, 4th edn. W.B. Saunders, Philadelphia

22. Fuhr, A.H. and Krogh, P.H.J. (1972) Congenital epulis of the newborn. *J. Oral Surg.*, **30**, 30–35

23. Garden, A.S., Benzie, R.J., Miskin, M. and Gardner, H.A. (1986) Fetal cystic hygroma colli: Antenatal diagnosis, significance and management. *Am. J. Obstet. Gynec.*, **154**, 221–225

24. Gebhart, W., Hohlbrugger, H., Lassmann, H. and Ramadan, W. (1982) Nasal glioma. *Int. J. Dermat.*, **21**, 212–215

25. Godart, S. (1966) Embryological significance of lymphangioma. *Arch. Dis. Child.*, **41**, 204–206

26. Grosfeld, J.L., Ballantine, T.V.N., Lowe, D. and Baehner, R.L. (1976) Benign and malignant teratomas in children: Analysis of 85 patients. *Surgery*, **80**, 297–305

27. Gundry, S.R., Wesley, J.R., Klein, M.D., Barr, M. and Coran, A.G. (1983) Cervical teratomas in the newborn. *J. Pediat. Surg.*, **18**, 382–386

28. Hatzihaberis, F., Stamatis, D. and Staurinos, D. (1978) Giant epignathus. *J. Pediat. Surg.*, **13**, 517–518

29. Hess, W. (1854) Beitrag zur Casuistik der Geschwülste mit zeugungsähnlichem Inhalte, p. 24. Inaug.-Diss., Giessen. Cited by Keynes, W.M. (1959) Teratoma of the neck in relation to the thyroid gland. *Br. J. Surg.*, **46**, 466–472

30. Holinger, L.D. and Birnholz, J.C. (1987) Management of infants with prenatal ultrasound diagnosis of airway obstruction by teratoma. *Ann. Otol. Rhinol. Laryngol.*, **96**, 61–64

31. Huntington, G.S. (1911) *The Anatomy and Development of Systemic Lymphatic Vessels in the Domestic Cat*. Wistar Institute, Philadelphia

32. Hurlbut, H.J., Webb, H.W. and Mosely, T. (1967) Cervical teratoma in infant siblings. *J. Pediat. Surg.*, **2**, 424–426

33. Ikeda, K., Suita, S., Hayashida, Y. and Yakabe, S. (1977) Massive infiltrating cystic hygroma of the neck in infancy with special reference to Bleomycin therapy. *Z. Kinderchir.*, **20**, 227–236

34. Jones, P.G. and Campbell, P.E. (1976) *Tumours of Infancy and Childhood*, Blackwell Scientific Publications, Oxford, pp. 348–350

35. Jordan, R.B. and Gauderer, M.W.L. (1988) Cervical teratomas: an analysis. Literature review and proposed classification. *J. Pediat. Surg.*, **23**, 583–591

36. Kampmeier, O.F. (1931) Ursprung und Entwicklungsgeschichte des Ductus thoracicus nebst Saccus Lymphaticus jugularis und Cysternachyli beim Menschen. *Morphologisches Jahrbuch*, **67**, 157

37. Karma, P., Rasanen, O. and Karja, J. (1977) Nasal gliomas. A review and report of two cases. *Laryngoscope*, **73**, 93–107

38. Keynes, W.M. (1959) Teratoma of the neck in relation to the thyroid gland. *Br. J. Surg.*, **46**, 466–472

39. Kirschner, P.A. (1966) Cervicomediastinal cystic hygroma. *Surgery*, **60**, 1104–1107

40. Lack, E.E., Perez-Atadye, A.R., McGill, T.J. and Vawter, G.F. (1982) Gingival granular cell tumour of the newborn (congenital 'epulis'): ultrastructural observations relating to histogenesis. *Human Path.*, **13**, 686–688

41. Lauriola, L., Musiani, P., Bracaglia, R., Maggiano, N. and Dina, M.A. (1984) Congenital epulis: an ultrastructural and immunohistochemical study. *Appl. Path.*, **2**, 153–159

42. Lifshitz, M.S., Flotte, T.J. and Alba Greco, M. (1984) Congenital granular cell epulis. Immunohistochemical and ultrastructural observations. *Cancer*, **53**, 1845–1848

43. Lister, J. and Zachary, R.B. (1968) Cystic duplications in the tongue. *J. Pediat. Surg.*, **3**, 491–493

44. Loeb, W.J. and Smith, E.E. (1967) Airway obstruction in the newborn by pedunculated pharyngeal dermoid. *Pediatrics*, **40**, 20–23

45. Lyngbye, T., Haugaard, L. and Klebe, J.G. (1986) Antenatal sonographic diagnosis of giant cystic hygroma of the neck. A problem for the clinician. *Acta Obstet. Gynecol. Scand.*, **65**, 873–875

46. Miller, D., Hill, J.L., Sun, C-C., O'Brien, D.S. and Haller, J.A. (1983) The diagnosis and management of pyriform sinus fistulae in infants and young children. *J. Pediat. Surg.*, **18**, 377–381

47. Mills, N.L. and Grosfeld, J.L. (1973) One-stage operation for cervicomediastinal cystic hygroma in infancy. *J. Thorac. Cardiovasc. Surg.*, **65**, 608–609

48. Mirra, S.S., Pearl, G.S., Hoffman, J.C. and Campbell, W.G. (1981) Nasal 'glioma' with prominent neuronal component. *Arch. Path. Lab. Med.*, **105**, 540–541

49. Neumann, E. (1871) Ein Fall von kongenitaler Epulis. *Arch. Heilk.*, **12**, 180. Cited by Fuhr, A.H. and Krogh, P.H.J. (1972). Congenital epulis of the newborn. *J.*

Oral Surg., **30**, 30–35

50. Ninh, T.N. and Ninh, T.X. (1974) Cystic hygroma in children: A report of 126 cases. *J. Pediat. Surg.*, **9**, 191–195

51. Numanoglu, I., Asku, Y. and Mutaf, O. (1970) Teratoma of thyroid gland in newborn infant. *J. Pediat. Surg.*, **5**, 381–382

52. Pearl, R.M., Wisnicki, J. and Sinclair, G. (1986) Metastatic cervical teratoma of infancy. *Plastic Reconstr. Surg.*, **77**, 469–473

53. Rainey, J.B. and Smith, I.J. (1984) Congenital epulis of the newborn. *J. Pediat. Surg.*, **19**, 305–306

54. Ravitch, M.M. and Rush, B.F. (1986) Cystic Hygroma. In *Paediatric Surgery* (ed. K.J. Welch, J.G. Randolph, M.M. Ravitch, J.A. O'Neill and M.I. Rowe), 4th Edn. Year Book Medical Publishers, Inc., Chicago pp. 533–539

55. Redenbacker. Cited by Wenher, A. (1843) *Die angeborenen Kysten Hygrome und die ihnen verwandten Geschwülste in anatomischer, diagnosticher und therapeutischer Beziehung.* G.F. Heger, Giessen

56. Rintala, A. and Ranta, R. (1974) Separate epignathi of the mandible and the nasopharynx with cleft palate: case report. *Br. J. Plast. Surg.*, **27**, 103–106

57. Roediger, W.E.W., Kalk, F., Spitz, L. and Schmaman, A. (1977) Congenital thyroid cyst of ultimobranchial gland origin. *J. Pediat. Surg.*, **12**, 575–576

58. Roediger, W.E., Spitz, L. and Schmaman, A. (1974) Histogenesis of benign cervical teratomas. *Teratology*, **10**, 111–118

59. Roodhooft, A.M., Delbeke, L. and Vaneerdeweg, W. (1987) Cervical teratoma: Prenatal detection and management in the neonate. *Pediat. Surg. Int.*, **21**, 181–184

60. Sabin, F.R. (1912) The development of the lymphatic system. In *Manual of Human Embryology* (ed. F. Kiebel and F.P. Mall), Lippincott, Philadelphia

61. Schmidt, M.B. (1900) Ueber seltene Spaltbildungen im Bereich des mittleren Stirnfortsatzes. *Arch. Pathol. Anat. Physiol. klin. Med.*, **162**, 340–370

62. Schoenfield, A., Edelstein, T. and Joel-Cohen, S.J. (1978) Prenatal ultrasonic diagnosis of fetal teratoma of the neck. *Br. J. Radiol.*, **51**, 742–744

63. Sheth, S., Nussbaum, A.R., Hutchins, G.M. and Sanders, R.C. (1987) Cystic hygromas in children: sonographic-pathologic correlation. *Radiology*, **162**, 821–824

64. Silberman, R. and Mendelson, I.R. (1960) Teratoma of the neck. Report of two cases and review of the literature. *Arch. Dis. Child.*, **35**, 159–170

65. Sunderland, R., Sunderland, E.P. and Smith, C.J. (1984) Hypoplasia following congenital epulis. *Br. Dental J.*, **157**, 353

66. Swift, A.C. and Singh, S.D. (1985) The presentation and management of the nasal glioma. *Int. J. Pediat. Otorhinolaryng.*, **10**, 253–261

67. Tapper, D. and Lack, E.E. (1983) Teratomas in infancy and childhood. A 54 year experience at the Children's Hospital Medical Center. *Ann. Surg.*, **198**, 398–410

68. Tsingoglou, S.T. (1970) Unusual tumours of the oral cavity in the newborn. *Ann. Clin. Paed. Univ. Atheniensis*, **17**, 210

69. Valente, A., Grant, C., Orr, J.D. and Brereton, R.J. (1988) Neonatal tonsillar teratoma. *J. Pediat. Surg.*, **23**, 364–366

70. Walker, J. and Johnston, D.I. (1985) Two cases of cervical teratoma. *Br. J. Clin. Pract.*, **39**, 446–448

71. Webb, D.J., Wescott, W.B. and Correll, R.W. (1984) Firm swelling on the anterior maxillary gingiva of an infant. *J. Am. Dental Ass.*, **109**, 307–308

72. Whitaker, S.R., Sprinkle, P.M. and Chou, S.M. (1981) Nasal glioma. *Arch. Otolaryngol.*, **107**, 550–554

13

Abdominal tumours

Irene M. Irving

Abdominal tumours are rarely found at birth or during the first month of life; only 27 such cases were treated in the Regional Neonatal Surgical Centre in Alder Hey Children's Hospital over a period of 33 years (1953–85) and of these only 17 were neoplastic, the remainder being classifiable as hamartomas (haemangioma or lymphangioma) or as being 'physiological' (ovarian cysts) (Table 13.1).

Table 13.1 Abdominal tumours admitted to Liverpool Neonatal Surgical Centre 1953 to 1985

	Cases	Deaths
Neuroblastoma	10	3
Ovarian cysts	5	—
Haemangioma of liver	3	2
Mesoblastic nephroma	2	—
Retroperitoneal teratoma	2	—
Lymphangioma	2	1
Hepatoblastoma	1	1
Islet cell adenoma	1	—
Leiomyosarcoma	1	—
Total	27	7

The presenting features were varied: four were admitted with complications, including severe intra-peritoneal haemorrhage from an adrenal neuroblastoma, perforation of the ileum at the site of a leiomyosarcoma, intestinal obstruction due to a lymphangioma and hypoglycaemia due to an islet cell adenoma; three tumours were incidental findings at autopsies on babies dying from other causes; four (three ovarian cysts and one mesoblastic nephroma) were diagnosed prenatally by ultrasound; the remaining 16 babies had asymptomatic abdominal masses.

Twelve of the 17 neoplasms were frankly malignant; two (the mesoblastic nephromas) could be regarded as being 'borderline' in this respect whilst the retroperitoneal teratomas and the islet-cell adenoma were benign lesions. Four of the 12 infants with malignant tumours died but only two died as a direct result of cancer. This low mortality largely reflects the long-recognized fact that the prognosis in neuroblastoma is better during the first year of life than thereafter [80].

Surgery plays a major role in the treatment of solid tumours in the neonate; few neonates have metastatic disease at the time of diagnosis, so that total excision alone is often curative. The routine use of adjuvant chemotherapy and radiation therapy is therefore not indicated in the neonate; not only because it is usually unnecessary, but because the rapidly-growing and immature tissues of the new-born child are uniquely vulnerable to the damaging effects of cytotoxic drugs and radiotherapy, with resultant deaths and long-term morbidity. On the rare occasions when chemotherapy is indicated, for a non-resectable lesion or for metastatic disease, it must be borne in mind that the pharmacokinetic behaviour of these drugs in the neonate is different from that in the older child or adult [47] and that careful choice of agents and of dosage are essential.

Renal tumours

Although in the past neonatal renal tumours were generally classified as 'congenital Wilms' tumour' it is now a well-accepted fact that the typical renal tumour in patients under the age of 6 months is the relatively benign mesoblastic nephroma.

History

Nephroblastoma has carried the eponymous name of Wilms' tumour since that author's thesis in 1899 [154]. Rance [116], however, is credited with the first description of a malignant renal tumour in childhood some 60 years earlier. Paul [107], reporting in 1886 a case of 'congenital adenosarcoma of the kidney' in a 2½-year-old child, made reference to a 7-month fetus presented at a meeting 3 years previously in Liverpool in which both kidneys were enlarged and on section showed considerable amounts of trabeculated connective tissue surrounding small masses of normal renal tissue; this description closely resembles the congenital mesoblastic nephroma of infancy described below.

Bolande and colleagues [12,13,14] are credited [10] with having been the first to delineate clearly the fibromatosis-like renal tumour of infancy as a distinct clinicopathological entity associated with a favourable outcome following nephrectomy alone. They chose to refer to this tumour as congenital mesoblastic nephroma and this is now the accepted name although many alternative names have been suggested (sarcoma [71,101]; leiomyoma [89,118,158]; leiomyosarcoma [6]; fibrosarcoma [98]; hamartoma [78,153]; embryoma [136]). Along with the recognition of the essentially benign nature of this tumour came the establishment of the fact that classic Wilms' tumour is very rare in the neonate [153], although it has been recorded [68,152]. Subsequently it became apparent that the situation with regard to congenital mesoblastic nephroma was not so simple as originally thought as as a few infants had suffered recurrences of these tumours; this fact led Beckwith [8] to propose that congenital mesoblastic nephroma comprised a spectrum of malignant potential, with most lesions falling towards the more benign end of the spectrum. Recently, Joshi and colleagues [74] suggested the use of the term atypical mesoblastic nephroma for lesions having gross and microscopical features which they view as ominous. Beckwith and Weeks [10], however, in reviewing this concept express concern that this approach could lead to overtreatment of some patients and they emphasize the fact that of 11 cases involving relapse, only one patient was under 3 months of age at the time of the original nephrectomy. There is, therefore, good reason to regard renal neoplasms which present in the neonatal period as being different, not only in structure but also in behaviour, to those found in later infancy and childhood.

Pathology

The classic Wilms' tumour arises from the metanephric mesoderm; it is encapsulated until the disease is advanced; the cut surface is lobulated and

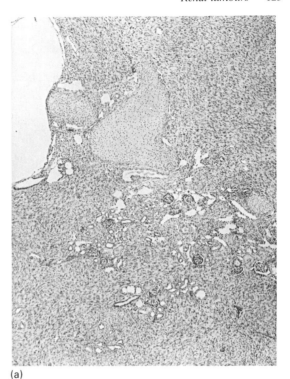

(a)

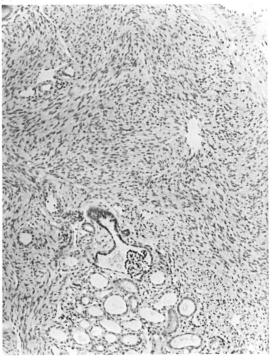

(b)

Figure 13.1 Congenital mesoblastic nephroma. (a) Cellular fibromatous stroma with areas of imperfect primitive glomeruli and tubules, cartilage and cyst formation (× 32). (b) Higher-power view showing spindle-celled stromal pattern with tubular and glomerular differentiation (× 80)

white or yellowish with areas of necrosis and haemorrhage and possibly cysts. Histologically, the tumour is composed of undifferentiated cellular tissue, possibly with occasional attempts at formation of tubules and glomeruli and a varying background of myxomatous material, smooth and striped muscle, cartilage and bone. Local spread is into adjacent tissues or into the pelvis and ureter. There is a marked tendency to invasion of the renal vein with consequent blood-borne tumour embolization of the lungs. Metastases also occur in the regional lymph glands and the liver.

The congenital mesoblastic nephroma, in contrast, has no capsule and infiltrates the greater part of the renal parenchyma; it is rubbery in consistency and the cut surface is pale and whorled, resembling a uterine fibroid, and does not show areas of haemorrhage or necrosis although very occasionally cysts are seen. Histologically, the tumour consists largely of sheets of interlacing spindle-shaped immature connective-tissue cells (Figure 13.1) which extend into the perirenal soft tissues; especially at the periphery there are inclusions of normal mature nephrons, but there are also areas of dysplastic glomeruli and tubules and occasional hypercellular areas resembling a Wilms' tumour. The ground meshwork of spindle-shaped cells may show mature fibrous, leiomyomatous or rhabdomyomatous cells, and amongst it are vascular spaces; occasional areas of cartilage are seen and, especially in the very young child, areas of haemopoiesis.

The term atypical mesoblastic nephroma has been suggested [74] for lesions having at least one atypical gross feature, such as fleshy areas, haemorrhage, necrosis, involvement of surrounding structures other than perirenal or hilar connective tissue, as well as one or both of two atypical microscopic features – hypercellularity and high mitotic index.

Aniridia, hemihypertrophy, hypospadias, undescended testis and Beckwith's syndrome have all been found more frequently than expected in association with Wilms' tumour [7,96,109], which may also arise in an abnormal kidney or in an extrarenal site. None of these features has been recorded in association with congenital mesoblastic nephroma, although it is interesting to note that one of our two cases of neonatal mesoblastic nephroma is the first cousin of one of our Beckwith's syndrome patients. Bilateral congenital mesoblastic nephroma has not been reported.

Clinical features

Boys are affected more commonly than girls. Maternal polyhydramnios has been reported in a number of cases without any explanation of its cause [91,120]. The tumour may be detected by antenatal ultrasound, as in one of our cases.

A palpable loin mass is the most common presenting feature; gross or microscopic haematuria may also be found. Hypertension is rare but is on record [22,64], as is hypercalcaemia [130] and consumption coagulopathy [112]. A plain radiograph of the abdomen will show a soft tissue mass displacing bowel and intravenous urography will usually show distortion of the collecting system with compression or elongation of the pelvis and calyces. The urogram, combined with ultrasonography, will serve to differentiate the tumour from a multicystic kidney and from a tense hydronephrosis. Ultrasonography will confirm the diagnosis of renal tumour, and Chan and colleagues [22] describe a distinctive 'ring sign' (concentric alternating echogenic and poorly echoic rings) in cases of typical congenital mesoblastic nephroma. A chest X-ray is done as a routine to exclude metastases.

Treatment and prognosis

Prompt surgical excision of the tumour is indicated. A transperitoneal approach through a transverse upper abdominal incision gives the best access. After dividing the posterior peritoneum laterally, the colon is reflected medially. It is usually recommended that the vascular pedicle should be ligated and divided very early in the procedure so as to reduce the risk of displacement of tumour emboli from the renal vein. However, when the tumour is very large, and especially in right-sided lesions, the venous anatomy may be distorted and mobilization of the kidney with full exposure of the vascular anatomy is preferable to inadvertent ligation of or damage to the inferior vena cava or opposite renal vein. In patients who are hypertensive preoperatively, careful monitoring is essential at the time of renal vein ligation as there is a risk of cardiac arrest due to hypotension [64]. The kidney and tumour should be mobilized together with the fatty capsule and the adrenal removed with the mass unless it is clearly separate from the tumour. The ureter should be divided as low as possible. Visible para-aortic lymph glands should be removed.

The use of postoperative radiotherapy and cytotoxic drugs is not indicated; firstly because the great majority of neonatal renal tumours will be found on histological examination to be the relatively benign mesoblastic nephroma, and secondly because both radiotherapy and chemotherapy carry considerable risks in the very young patient. Richmond and Dougall in a review of 28 cases in 1970 [120] found that of the four deaths three were attributable to complications of radiotherapy or chemotherapy. Seven of their patients had radiotherapy; one died of radiation necrosis of the bowel and four developed some degree of kyphoscoliosis. Three patients had actinomycin D; one died of bleeding during treatment and another of sepsis. Of the 19 patients who had no record of treatment by radiotherapy or chemotherapy only one died and he was a crib death aged 7 weeks on whom no autopsy was performed. Howell and colleagues [64] in a report of 51 patients in the National Wilms' Tumour Study with mesoblastic nephroma found that the only death was in newborn who was given postoperative chemotherapy in full dosage, which led to neutropenia and lethal sepsis; they also report several non-fatal severe complications of chemotherapy. Furthermore, although atypical features [74] may be found in the histology of mesoblastic nephromas in neonates, these do not appear to have the same sinister significance as in patients over the age of 3 months. Beckwith and Weeks [10], having reviewed the microscopic sections from 11 collected cases of locally recurrent or metastatic mesoblastic nephromas stress the point that only one of these patients was under 3 months of age at the time of the original nephrectomy. In this case, originally reported by two separate authors [46,75], a tumour resected from a 1-day-old infant showed some microscopic evidence of increased cellularity and mitotic activity as well as infiltration of the ureteral margin of the specimen. The tumour recurred massively and was unresectable 4 months after nephrectomy. The infant responded initially to radiation and chemotherapy but died at 18 months after a second recurrence. It can be argued [10] that recurrence occurred in this case because of incomplete resection but on the other hand many cases can be cited [22] of survival without recurrence after nephrectomy alone despite demonstrable involvement of the surgical margins and the perinephric connective tissues by tumour. This situation should not, therefore, be regarded as an indication for chemotherapy or radiotherapy, but rather for careful follow-up with serial imaging studies or possibly a second-look procedure [64] in the very rare situation in the newborn of a tumour that is very invasive.

A frank Wilms' tumour is extremely rare in the newborn [147,153], so much so that it has been suggested that operative treatment of a neonatal renal tumour can safely be postponed until the child has been allowed to regain his birth weight [97]. We cannot accept this recommendation; in a properly equipped unit the operative risk of nephrectomy in a neonate is minimal, and there are, albeit extremely rarely, instances of frankly malignant mesenchymal tumours in the neonate [147]. Furthermore, the natural history of congenital mesoblastic nephroma suggests that delay in treatment may worsen the prognosis.

Neuroblastoma

Pathology

Neuroblastoma is the most primitive of the tumours which arise from the embryonic neural crest. It may occur in the adrenal medulla or in any of the sympathetic ganglia in the abdomen, thorax or neck. Macroscopically, the tumour forms a large very vascular, nodular mass which grows rapidly and tends to infiltrate adjacent structures; areas of haemorrhage, necrosis and cystic degeneration may be present. Histologically, the tumour may be composed entirely of undifferentiated small round cells or there may be rosette-like clusters of cells enclosing a tangle of nerve fibres; some examples, so-called ganglioneuroblastoma, contain in addition mature nerve cells. Electron microscopy reveals neurofibrils and neurosecretory granules; these ultrastructural findings will usually allow the undifferentiated tumours to be distinguished from other small-cell tumours.

Congenital neuroblastoma is the most common form of intra-abdominal malignancy in the newborn. Neuroblastomas (all sites) constituted 25% of 250 cases of congenital malignant tumours reviewed by Wells [151] in 1940 and 47% of 102 neonatal malignant tumours reported from Toronto by Campbell and colleagues in 1987 [20]; whereas these 102 cases represented only 2% of the total number of paediatric malignancies treated over a period of 60 years, neonatal cases accounted for 12% of the total number of neuroblastomas. Of their 48 neonatal cases, 16 were instances of unsuspected adrenal neuroblastoma *in situ* discovered at autopsy after death from other causes; 14 had adrenal tumours of which five were bilateral, eight had thoracoabdominal paraspinal tumours, seven had cervical tumours and three had pelvic neuroblastomas. In Schneider, Becker and Krasna's [126] collected series of 60 neonatal neuroblastomas, metastases were present in 52% at the time of initial examination. The location of metastases in the young infant differs from that in the older child; osseous deposits (other than those confined to marrow) are much less common, whereas liver involvement and cutaneous metastases are commoner in the neonate.

Staging

Several different staging methods have been proposed but the one most commonly used is that drawn up by Evans and colleagues in 1971 [38], as follows:

Stage I is a tumour confined to a single organ or structure and completely resectable.

Stage II is a tumour extending in continuity beyond the organ or structure of origin but not crossing the midline. Regional lymph nodes on the ipsilateral side may be involved.

Stage III denotes a tumour extending in continuity beyond the midline, often unresectable. Regional lymph nodes may be involved bilaterally.

Stage IV denotes cases with remote disease involving skeleton, parenchymatous organs, soft tissues or distant lymph node groups.

Stage IV-S (S for special) includes patients who would be classed as stage I or II but who have remote disease, confined to one or more of the following sites: liver, skin or bone marrow (without radiographic evidence of bone metastases on complete skeletal survey).

The special feature of stage IV-S is the remarkably good prognosis, even when little or no treatment is given [35,36]. The great majority of patients who fulfil the IV-S criteria are young infants; four out of 17 cases reviewed by Evans and colleagues were newborn, 11 were 3 months old or younger and none was older than 11 months [36]. Typically the primary tumour is infradiaphragmatic, the large majority being of adrenal origin [35,52]. Hepatic disease is a major component of the IV-S complex being present in all 17 of the above-mentioned series and in 30 of 31 patients included in a multicentre study, also reported by Evans [35]. It is not known why the IV-S subgroup behave differently to stage IV patients. It has been suggested that IV-S patients do not have true metastatic deposits, but rather that they have widely disseminated multiple primary tumours in the liver, skin or both [30], arising from cells of neural crest origin in those sites. Regression of IV-S tumours appears to result from necrobiosis [36] with only rare maturation to ganglioneuroma, although this has been described, both in IV-S patients [50,117] and others [27,81]. Everson and Cole [39] reviewed 29 recorded examples of spontaneous regression, all being in patients under 2 years of age and most under 6 months. Spontaneous regression has also been regarded as providing the explanation for the disparity between the reported incidence of neuroblastoma *in situ* and that of the clinical incidence of tumour; Beckwith and Perrin [9], studying the adrenal glands obtained at autopsies of stillborn infants and infants up to 3 months of age, found minute neuroblastomas at 40 times the expected incidence and similar findings were reported by Shanklin [131] and by Guin [55]. In studies done in Liverpool of fetal adrenals for tumour precursors, neuroblast clusters closely resembling neuroblastoma *in situ* were found in all fetal adrenals at 14–18 weeks [67]. Previous workers [146] had suggested that persistence of aggregates of such clusters into neonatal life could explain the neuroblastoma *in situ*. Our studies pointed to the importance of measurement of nuclear size in the distinction between a true malignant focus and a normal benign residual neuroblast nodule. The debate will doubtless continue.

A great deal of both laboratory and clinical research has been devoted to the immunological aspects of neuroblastoma since such a mechanism could explain the phenomenon of spontaneous regression and, if exploitable, could provide a valuable method of treatment. The resemblance of the placenta to that found in erythroblastosis foetalis has been noted in some cases of fetal neuroblastoma [72]; one of our neonatal cases had a very large placenta, possibly resembling that found in isoimmune disease but not invaded by tumour cells; this may be a reaction to circulating tumour cells. Hellstrom *et al.* found that lymphocytes from neuroblastoma patients are lethal against neuroblastoma cells in tissue culture [61], and it has been found [11] that there is a correlation between high peripheral blood lymphocyte counts at diagnosis and survival in children under 1 year. The finding of lymphocytic infiltration of the tumour itself is also an indication of good prognosis [61,117]. The sera from some patients with progressive disease contain a humoral 'blocking antibody' which nullifies the otherwise lethal effect of the lymphocytes [60]; these often disappear after the primary tumour is removed [52]. Ziegler and Koop [157] found that, in mouse neuroblastoma, electrocoagulation of the tumour (as opposed to clean surgical excision) potentiates the host's anti-tumour immune response, and they recommend the use of electrocoagulation in debulking procedures. To date no effective immunotherapy has been developed.

Our ten cases of abdominal neuroblastoma in neonates included six cases of adrenal tumour, bilateral in one case and arising in an accessory gland in a further case. The remainder were of sympathetic origin. Two were found only at autopsy. Seven cases were stage I (including the two found at autopsy), one was stage III and two were IV-S cases (one of these being the child with bilateral adrenal tumours).

Clinical features

As in the case of neonatal renal tumours, the commonest presentation of neuroblastoma in the newborn is as a mass, which may have been picked up prenatally on ultrasound scanning. The mass is typically fixed and nodular and may extend across the midline; in seven of our ten cases an abdominal mass was palpable and in the other three abdominal distension was recorded. Haemorrhage into the tumour may occur and be sufficient to necessitate urgent transfusion; in one of our cases abdominal distension and shock were attributed (correctly) to intraperitoneal haemorrhage thought (incorrectly) to be the result of damage to the liver during birth; laparotomy revealed a retroperitoneal haematoma which had ruptured into the peritoneal cavity, the source of the bleeding being a haemorrhagic right adrenal gland. No obvious tumour was seen and the diagnosis was made only on microscopy of a biopsy taken from the edge of the ruptured capsule of the adrenal [100]. A similar case has been reported by Brock and Ricketts [16]. A further two of our six neonatal adrenal tumours were haemorrhagic and we consider neuroblastoma to be an important cause of neonatal adrenal haemorrhage [100]. Occasionally the newborn may present with subcutaneous metastases which are widespread and numerous and often blue in colour so that the condition has been termed 'blueberry muffin baby', a term sometimes used to describe the purpuric patches seen in the rubella syndrome [133]. The neonate may also present with obvious liver enlargement which may be massive enough to cause respiratory embarrassment as well as vena caval or renal vascular occlusion [36]. In older infants and children with neural crest tumours severe excretory diarrhoea, hypokalaemia, dehydration and weight loss can occur as a result of production of VIP (vasoactive intestinal polypeptide) by the tumour. We are not aware of this having been reported under the age of 6 months [25], but one of our neonates had intestinal hurry and what appeared to be considerable abdominal colic during the period when her catecholamines were high; at the time these symptoms were attributed to catecholamines. Excessive production of catecholamines can cause hypertension, flushing, sweating and irritability, symptoms which have been experienced during late pregnancy by mothers of babies with congenital neuroblastoma [73].

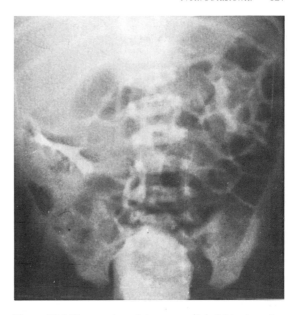

Figure 13.2 Haemorrhage into congenital right adrenal neuroblastoma. Intravenous urogram, showing downwards and lateral displacement of the kidney. A loin swelling and general signs of haemorrhage appeared on the third day of life. The urinary catecholamine levels were within the range of normality

Diagnosis

Radiography

Radiography may show the tumour as a soft-tissue shadow, sometimes displacing bowel gas and often with finely stippled calcification. On intravenous urography, the kidney is seen to be displaced downwards and laterally in the case of an adrenal tumour (Figure 13.2) whilst a neuroblastoma arising from the lumbar sympathetic chain may cause lateral displacement and distortion of the kidney or ureter (Figure 13.3). Although cortical bony metastases are rare in congenital cases, radiography of the long bones, skull, pelvis, vertebrae and ribs is indicated. In the long bones, the metaphyses are affected first; localized areas of rarefaction are seen and there may be new bone formation under the periosteum in the form either of radiating spicules or of onion-layer laminae.

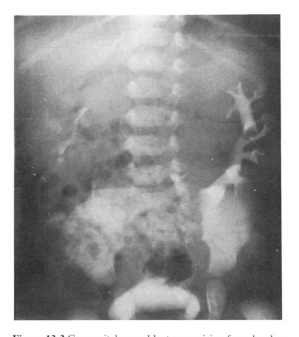

Figure 13.3 Congenital neuroblastoma arising from lumbar sympathetic ganglion. Intravenous urogram, showing displacement and distortion of left kidney. Cure followed excision of the tumour and of the intimately involved left kidney. The cystogram demonstrates well the inguinal protrusions commonly seen in the neonate

Other imaging studies

Ultrasonography is extremely useful in distinguishing between solid and cystic lesions and in distinguishing between extrarenal and renal pathology and is best done in conjunction with the straight X-ray, before the intravenous urogram. Sonography also reveals any distortion of the inferior vena cava, and if the liver is enlarged this can also be evaluated. Radionuclide bone scans can be useful in patients found to have marrow infiltration as they may reveal bony metastases that have not been revealed by radiology. A recently described technique, I-MIBG (meta-iodobenzylguanidine) scanning relies on the affinity of MIBG for adrenergic nervous tissue. It competes with, and displaces, catecholamines and is useful in location of a primary tumour as well as in the detection of residual, recurrent or metastatic disease [62]. CT scanning is not necessary as a routine investigation but could be valuable in determining the exact extent of advanced tumours.

Bone marrow

Bone marrow aspirates should be obtained from several sites in every patient in whom neuroblastoma is diagnosed or suspected; clusters of tumour cells will frequently be found even in the absence of radiological changes.

Urinary catecholamines

The secretion and increased urinary excretion of catecholamines and their derivatives by neuroblastomas was first demonstrated by Mason and his colleagues [95]. Estimation of the amounts of these substances in the urine is of value in diagnosis and also in assessing the effects of treatment. The pathway of synthesis and breakdown of the adrenal hormones is shown in Figure 13.4. The pattern of catecholamines and of their metabolites in the urine varies from case to case and can be correlated with prognosis; Laug and colleagues [86] found that in stage IV patients the VMA/HVA (vanilmandelic acid/homovanillic acid) ratio had a predictive value; the higher the value the better the prognosis. The presence of VLA (vanillactic acid), a metabolite of DOPA (dihydroxyphenyl alanine), was found to be an indicator of poor prognosis. It is therefore necessary to use a scheme of investigation which covers all the potential excretion products. Different laboratories may employ different combinations of analyses and different techniques; these considerations are relevant in the clinical interpretation of the biochemical results. Although a VMA 'spot test' is useful as a screening technique [124], a full analysis necessitates collection of a 24-h specimen of urine for examination. Because of difficulties in obtaining complete collections, the excretion of catecholamines may alternatively be related to creatinine output but it should be noted that in the newborn in particular, creatinine excretion may be variable.

Very rarely the excretion of catecholamines may be normal. This may indicate a very poorly differentiated tumour [149], a parasympathetic neuroblastoma which secretes acetylcholine but does not metabolize tyrosine to DOPA [110], or haemorrhage into the tumour which can produce a temporary drop in the excretion rates of catecholamines and their metabolites; in such cases the clinical, radiological and biochemical features can simulate those of simple adrenal haematoma of the newborn (see Figure 13.2).

Neuron-specific enolase

Raised serum levels of neuron-specific enolase have been found at diagnosis in all stages of neuroblastoma, including a case with negative urinary VMA

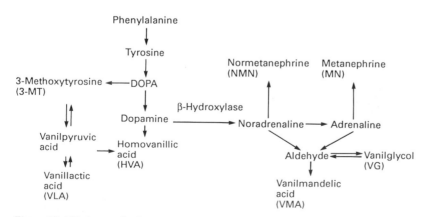

Figure 13.4 Pathway of adrenal hormone synthesis and breakdown

and HVA [145]. Serum levels are related to the stage of the disease at diagnosis and can be used as a marker to monitor progress, having been shown to decline to normal or near-normal values during remission and to become elevated upon clinical relapse.

Treatment

Total excision of the primary tumour must remain the treatment of choice; it is usually possible in stage I, stage II and stage IV-S cases, as was so in six of the eight cases in our series who had laparotomies. No further treatment is required in stages I and II and the same usually applies to IV-S cases. The question of whether it is strictly necessary to remove the primary tumour in IV-S cases is debatable; many cases are on record of survival without removal of the primary [36], but it is recommended that it should be resected some time during the course of the disease [36] since there are rare patients who develop a late recurrence at the site of the primary even though the remainder of the disease has regressed [117]. Gross abdominal distension in a IV-S case would be an indication for delay in resection and maybe for abdominal decompression by creation of a temporary ventral hernia, using silastic sheeting as recommended by Schnaufer and Koop [125].

Tumour excision is performed transperitoneally through a transverse supra-umbilical excision; the tumour is exposed by medial reflection of the colon. The tumour may be very friable and must be handled gently to avoid spillage. Not uncommonly, as in two of our cases, it is necessary to remove the ipsilateral kidney along with an adrenal or paraspinal tumour, but excessively aggressive surgery is not warranted; if a tumour is judged to be unresectable the options are firstly, a debulking procedure [81,82] with or without subsequent chemotherapy or, secondly, shrinkage of the tumour by chemotherapy followed by secondary resection [83]. A liver biopsy should always be taken, regardless of the gross appearance of the liver.

In the neonate radiotherapy should be avoided; it carries very high risks of skeletal deformities as indicated previously and is unlikely to affect the outcome. Chemotherapy, if given at all, should be reserved for stage III and stage IV patients and should be given in dosage suitable for the neonate, namely: vincristine $1.5 \, mg/m^2$ weekly for 6 weeks, cyclophosphamide $300 \, mg/m^2$, also weekly for 6 weeks but with omission of doses if the total neutrophil count falls below $1 \times 10^9/l$.

Prognosis

The overall survival rate in neuroblastoma has scarcely altered over the last two to three decades,

a fact which reflects the lack of influence of chemotherapy and irradiation on survival [37]. It has long been recognized that in infants diagnosed before the age of 1 year the prognosis is better than in older age groups [80]; this may be due in part to easier and hence earlier recognition but also appears to depend on a greater tendency to spontaneous regression [29,35]. Evans, D'Angio and Koop [37], reporting on 49 patients with stage I-III disease recorded 91% 2-year relapse-free survival in stage I, 75% in stage II and 50% in stage III; there was not a single death amongst 13 patients diagnosed in the first year of life, but details of the staging in these 13 infants is not given. In the group of 31 IV-S patients referred to earlier, Evans and colleagues [35] found a projected 2-year survival rate of 87%. The four deaths in this series were all in the first 2 months of life and all resulted from complications of gross hepatomegaly. These authors contrast the favourable IV-S prognosis with a survival of 42% in reported stage IV patients under the age of 1 year. Bleak though the latter figure may seem, it compares very favourably with the disease-free survival rate of 7% for stage IV patients of all ages [51].

Of our own ten neonatal cases, one stage IV-S child died (33 years ago) after liver biopsy alone; another IV-S case is disease-free at age 12 years. A boy, aged 1 week, with stage III disease was treated 21 years ago by partial excision of the tumour, irradiation and chemotherapy and survived; nowadays this would be regarded as overtreatment in a neonate. Of seven stage I tumours, two were discovered at autopsy following death from unrelated causes; the remaining five patients are all alive and disease-free following surgery.

Pelvic rhabdomyosarcoma

Rhabdomyosarcoma (sarcoma botryoides) is a highly malignant, embryonic mesenchymal tumour. In the male, it may arise in the bladder or the prostate; in the female the vagina is the commonest site. As a rule, the tumour is multicentric in its viscus of origin. In gross structure, the neoplasm consists of polypoid masses which project into the lumen of the affected viscus. Histologically, it is composed of a loose or myxomatous matrix containing fusiform or stellate cells; striated muscle fibres or multinucleated rhabdomyoblasts may be recognizable. The tumour infiltrates through the wall of the vagina or bladder to invade the pelvic cellular tissues, but as a rule distant metastases are late in appearing.

Fortunately, these tumours are very rare in the newborn [33], but occasional cases are encountered. Khoury and Speer [79] in 1944 described in detail a congenital rhabdomyosarcoma of the bladder in a boy. The condition presents with dysuria and palpable vesical enlargement; infection and haematuria follow and an umbilical urinary fistula may form spontaneously. Intravenous urography reveals upper urinary tract dilatation and cystography demonstrates the typical lobulated filling defects in the bladder.

Ober, Smith and Rouillard [106] described two newborn infants whom they considered to have sarcoma botryoides of the vagina. Unlike the older child, who usually presents with a bleeding polypoid mass at the vulva, these babies each had a solitary polyp; the diagnosis of malignancy was made on histological examination. Benign hymenal polyp is, however, not uncommon in the newborn and is regarded as being the result of maternal oestrogenic stimulation. Borglin and Selander [15] found such lesions in 6% of the 1000 infants examined by them. Norris and Taylor [104] described benign polyps originating both from the hymen and from within the vaginal introitus and drew attention to the difficulties which exist in their histological assessment. These benign polyps regress spontaneously.

More recently Campbell and colleagues listed two congenital rhabdomyosarcomas of the vagina amongst 102 cases of neonatal cancer seen in Toronto over a 60-year period [20]. Ragab and colleagues reported 14 neonates in a total of 1561 children with rhabdomyosarcoma in all sites registered in the Intergroup Rhabdomyosarcoma Study [115]. Infants younger than 1 year of age had a higher rate of bladder-prostate-vagina primary tumour sites than older children (26% versus 10%). In contrast with neuroblastoma cases, an age of less than 1 year was not a favourable prognostic factor.

Treatment and prognosis

Since the 1960s it has been recognized that excellent survival rates (90%) can be achieved in cases of localized pelvic rhabdomyosarcoma by a combination of radical surgical extirpation coupled with radiotherapy and multiple-agent chemotherapy [53,139]. Subsequently, efforts have been directed towards trying to avoid mutilating surgery, as exemplified by the Intergroup Rhabdomyosarcoma Study protocol in which primary treatment was by chemotherapy (monthly vincristine, actinomycin D and cyclophosphamide) followed by irradiation if chemotherapy failed to eradicate the tumour completely, with surgery reserved for patients in whom chemotherapy and radiotherapy failed to eliminate palpable or visible tumour. Excellent results were obtained with vaginal tumours [59], which are very responsive to chemotherapy. Primary bladder-prostate tumours responded less favourably [58], with a poorer survival rate than was achieved by anterior pelvic exenteration. It is apparent that primary chemotherapy is not the treatment of choice for this group.

Ovarian tumours and cysts

History and incidence

True neoplasms of the ovary are extremely rare in the newborn infant. Ziegler [157] described bilateral granulosa cell carcinoma in a 30-week-old fetus and Bulfamonte [18] reported a case of neonatal ovarian cystadenoma but all other recorded congenital ovarian tumours have been retention cysts, which are believed to be the result of an exaggerated response to maternal gonadotrophin stimulation. Karrer and Swenson [76] in 1961 found reports of 15 such cases and added a further one. Marshall [92] found a total of 26 cases and added one of his own; Ahmed [1], in 1971 found 47 cases in the literature and added six of his own. Ovarian cyst in the newborn has not, therefore, been regarded as being a common condition. This was borne out by our own experience; a review of 106 patients with ovarian cysts and tumours treated at the two Liverpool children's hospitals from 1950 to 1982 included only two neonates, both of whom had ovarian cysts (the youngest of the 47 patients with ovarian neoplasms being an 11-month-old baby with a granulosa-cell tumour) [132]. During the present decade, however, there has been a marked increase in the detection rate of large ovarian cysts in the newborn as a result of the widespread use of antenatal ultrasound examination. In Bristol, for example, five cases (four diagnosed antenatally) were treated in 4 years, none having been encountered in the previous 20 years [90]. Ikeda and colleagues have encountered nine cases diagnosed antenatally over 11 years [65]; in the Liverpool Neonatal Surgical Centre we have treated three such cases since the above-mentioned review. The upsurge in numbers suggests that in past years a considerable proportion of neonatal ovarian cysts have resolved without being detected clinically, a concept which raises questions about how asymptomatic cases should be managed.

Pathology

The cyst may be follicular or, less commonly, luteal in type, the former arising from a graafian follicle and the latter from a corpus luteum; in some instances the cyst lining is atrophic or infarcted and the precise origin is uncertain. Most commonly, the cyst is unilateral and unilocular, although in one of our neonatal cases bilateral large cysts were present. Multilocular cysts represent multiple unilocular cysts [2]. Rupture [91,141] or torsion [65,76] (Figure 13.5) may occur. The former complication may cause considerable haemorrhage from the cyst wall

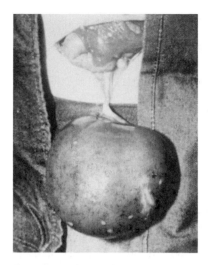

Figure 13.5 Torsion of congenital ovarian cyst in a newborn infant

resulting in haemoperitoneum [91], whereas torsion may result in intestinal obstruction as a result of the bowel becoming adherent to the infarcted cyst [76], or in peritonitis [1]. Occasional cases have been reported of oestradiol-producing ovarian cysts in premature babies [127].

Resolution of cysts has been studied by serial ultrasonography; Nussbaum and colleagues studied three infants with medium-sized (3–5 cm diameter) lower abdominal cysts, presumed to be ovarian in origin, and found that all three had disappeared within 4 months of discovery [105]. Ikeda and colleagues decided on conservative management of four neonates with cysts of less than 4 cm diameter at birth and observed gradual shrinkage of the cysts, with disappearance of three, by the ages of 14 days, 1 month and 12 months; the fourth was still under observation but had shrunk during the first 2 weeks of life [65].

Clinical picture

As already indicated, the presence of an abdominal cyst is likely to have been detected antenatally and confirmed after birth in centres where routine antenatal ultrasound scanning is practised (Figure 13.6). In the majority of cases the abdomen is distended. The cyst can usually be palpated easily as a mobile lower abdominal mass but it may be displaceable into the mid-abdomen or even the epigastrium. A very large cyst will fill the abdomen and can be mistaken for ascites; in such cases there may be respiratory embarrassment. The radiological appearances of such a case are shown in Figure 13.7. Complications such as torsion or rupture will usually

(but not always) be evidenced by increasing abdominal girth and tenderness, vomiting, fever and leucocytosis. A change in the sonographic appearance, notably the appearance of debris in the cyst, may also indicate torsion [65,105].

Treatment

Early surgery is indicated in the case of very large cysts and in those showing evidence of complications. Cystectomy with preservation of the ovary is the treatment of choice; this may be difficult in the neonate, especially as normal ovarian tissue may be splayed out over the cyst, but an effort should be made to create a plane between cyst and ovary and to preserve the latter, which can be oversewn with catgut after removal of the cyst. If normal ovarian tissue cannot be identified at the base of the cyst, then the alternative approach is to aspirate the cyst and resect its wall. Salpingo-oophorectomy may be unavoidable in cases of torsion. Small cysts in the contralateral ovary should be left alone to resolve.

The possibility of significant loss of ovarian tissue as a consequence of surgery (especially in bilateral cases) as well as the danger of postoperative pelvic adhesions affecting future fertility are reasons for considering conservative management of asymptomatic cases. This must be weighed against the potential risks of expectant treatment, notably those of torsion and of incorrect diagnosis; it may be impossible to distinguish on sonography, with absolute certainty, between ovarian cysts and duplication cysts of the bowel.

In the light of the encouraging reports, already referred to, of spontaneous resolution of neonatal ovarian cysts it seems reasonable to opt for conservative management of the smaller (<4 or 5 cm) cysts in the asymptomatic infant provided that (a) regular ultrasound monitoring is feasible, and (b) there is ready access to a paediatric surgical service in the event of an abdominal emergency. In conservatively-managed cases the parents will need to be well informed.

Our own five cases were all treated surgically, two before the advent of ultrasound. Two cysts had undergone torsion and were necrotic, necessitating oophorectomy. The remainder (one luteal cyst and two cases of follicular cyst, one bilateral) were treated by ovarian cystectomy.

Testicular tumours

Congenital testicular tumours are rare but the occurrence of several pathological types has been recorded. Sertoli cell tumour was reported by Culp, Frazier and Butler [26] and later by Mostofi, Theiss

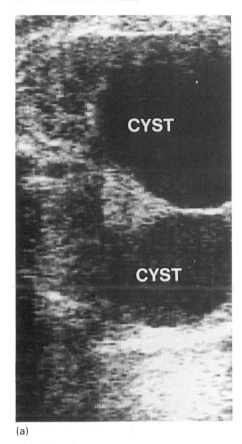

(a)

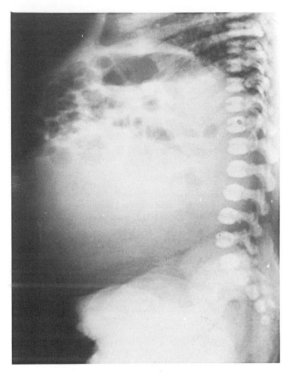

Figure 13.7 Congenital ovarian cyst causing abdominal distension and dystocia. Lateral X-ray of abdomen showing large lower abdominal tumour displacing the intestinal tract

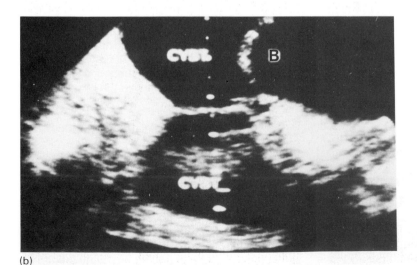

(b)

Figure 13.6 (a) Antenatal transverse lower abdominal ultrasound scan (spine to left) showing large bilateral cysts, presumed to be ovarian. (b) Postnatal scan (oblique sagittal; B = bladder) confirmed the diagnosis. Echoes in the lower cyst indicate haemorrhage. At operation bilateral follicular cysts were found

and Ashley [99]; in each case the tumour was benign and in none did it produce the endocrine effects which may be encountered in older age groups. 'Adult' teratoma containing mature tissues was described by Rusche [123] and by Phelan, Woolner and Hayles [108]; unlike the teratoma of the adult testis, the tumour is benign. The important testicular tumour of infancy is the malignant yolk sac tumour (endodermal sinus tumour). The majority of these occur between 6 months and 3 years of age but some neonatal cases have been reported [94,123,140]. Approximately 90% of these tumours produce alpha-fetoprotein (AFP) [43]. Spread to retroperitoneal lymph nodes occurs in less than 10% of cases [42] but pulmonary metastases can occur in the absence of lymph node involvement, suggesting that haematogenous spread is the commonest route of dissemination [113]. No metastasizing cases have been reported in neonates.

Congenital testicular tumour usually presents as a painless, firm enlargement of the testis, detected on routine examination. In Hansen's patient [56], a 2-month-old infant, there was an abdominal mass which proved to be a teratoma of an intra-abdominal testis which had undergone torsion.

Treatment

Treatment consists of orchidectomy through an inguinal incision, with high ligation of the cord. The spermatic cord should be exposed and occluded with a vascular clamp before any manipulation of the testis is performed. Blood should be taken for AFP assay at the time of surgery. If the tumour proves to be a yolk sac tumour careful follow-up is required, with monthly checking of serum AFP, which should decline steadily and reach normal levels within 3 months [43]. Routine retroperitoneal lymph node dissection is not required, but if serum AFP levels indicate the presence of metastatic tumour a search for retroperitoneal nodes must be made by sonography and CT scan and for lung metastases by chest X-ray and CT scan, with subsequent lymph node dissection and chemotherapy as indicated by the findings [43].

Retroperitoneal teratoma

Retroperitoneal teratoma presents as a large, partly solid and partly cystic mass which may originate in the abdomen or pelvis; the latter type may be regarded as a variant of the sacrococcygeal teratoma in which the growth of the tumour is predominantly internal rather than external, and will be dealt with in the next chapter. The teratoma contains derivatives of all three embryonic layers; mature tissues such as brain, bone and skin are commonly present. In the collected series of Arnheim [4], three (6.8%)

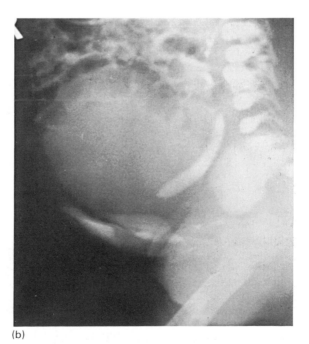

(a)

(b)

Figure 13.8 Intravenous urogram in a case of retroperitoneal teratoma in a newborn girl. (a) Anteroposterior: marked lateral displacement of ureters and hydronephrosis of right kidney. (b) Lateral: ureter stretched over tumour; compression of bladder by tumour

of 44 tumours contained malignant tissue on histological examination. Distribution between the sexes is approximately equal. Most cases present at birth or in early infancy, with abdominal enlargement or discovery of a mass, which is usually sizeable. In our series of neonates there were two cases in which a teratoma was confined to the retroperitoneal region and did not reach the presacral area. Plain radiography demonstrates a soft tissue shadow, often with calcification or ossification. Ultrasonography shows a complex mass with solid and cystic components and will also reveal any associated urinary tract displacement and dilatation, as will intravenous urography (Figure 13.8).

Treatment

Treatment consists of excision of the tumour. Surgery may be difficult because of adherence to the great vessels but the possibility of later malignant change as in sacrococcygeal lesions is always present and complete removal should be attempted. Chemotherapy would be indicated in the unlikely event of there being histological evidence of malignancy.

Hepatic haemangioma

Hepatic haemangioma was first described in 1893 by von Eiselberg [34] and the first successful resection of a hepatic haemangioma in a newborn child was reported in 1949 by Shuller and colleagues [134]. The condition as seen in the newborn child is potentially lethal because of the serious complications associated with it. The majority of cases present during the early weeks of life; of a total of 67 cases detailed in four recent reports [24,28,63,102] 42 were 6 weeks old or less when first seen. In the Toronto series, eight of 14 patients were seen at birth [102]. We have encountered only three cases in neonates since 1953; one found incidentally at autopsy in a child with myelomeningocele, one dying of cardiac failure on the fourth day of life and one treated successfully by resection of the left lobe of the liver.

Pathology

Hepatic vascular hamartomas may occur as localized single cavernous haemangiomas but the more usual pathology is the multiple haemangioendothelioma, which appears grossly as multiple circumscribed lesions, involving the whole liver in the most florid cases; microscopically the nodules are cellular capillary haemangiomas. Hepatic haemangiomas may cause death by necrosis with rupture and fatal haemorrhage [128], by platelet trapping and thrombocytopenia [77] or, more commonly, by high-output cardiac failure due to the large arteriovenous

shunt [31]. Spontaneous regression of the lesions has been reported; Nguyen, Shandling and colleagues reported regression before the age of 1 year in a group of five conservatively managed patients [102]. Such regression is probably rarer in the large cavernous lesions but one such case, deemed inoperable in the neonatal period, was seen in Alder Hey before the current series; 5 years later, having had no treatment, he was well and had a normal liver [122].

Clinical features

Presentation in the neonate is usually with hepatomegaly, less commonly with a localized upper abdominal mass but, if there has been rupture of the lesion, the child may be in oligaemic shock possibly, but not certainly, with haemoperitoneum [49]. Some cases of hepatic haemangioendothelioma present with high-output congestive heart failure, in the absence of any evidence of congenital heart disease but with a systolic bruit over the enlarged liver. In approximately one-quarter of these cases multiple cutaneous haemangiomas are present [28] and these are a valuable diagnostic clue.

Investigation

Straight abdominal X-ray is unlikely to be helpful apart from showing liver enlargement. Ultrasound will locate the lesion and indicate its extent but the echogenic pattern is variable. Technetium-99m scanning will show at least one area, and probably multiple areas, of decreased radioactivity; these areas will appear to be fluid-filled on the ultrasound scan [85].

Selective angiography is the most valuable examination; it shows the vascular character of the lesion, its early venous drainage and the tortuosity of the vessels and gives an indication of whether the lesion is resectable. It is, however, an invasive investigation with a risk of long-term sequelae, and should be reserved for cases in which surgery or hepatic artery embolization is planned. CT scanning with contrast enhancement has been found by Holcomb and colleagues [63] to be as specific as angiography in the diagnosis of haemangioendothelioma.

Treatment

In the absence of symptoms or complications no treatment is required, but the patient has to be observed very closely for evidence of increasing hepatic enlargement, cardiac failure, respiratory distress, thrombocytopenia and anaemia. The first line of treatment in such cases – additional to digitalis, diuretics, etc. – is steroid therapy in the form of prednisone in doses up to 5 mg/kg per day. Since the first reports of their use, in 1969–70

[17,142], many workers have reported a good response to steroids [63], with diminution of hepatomegaly and control of congestive failure; others, however [102], doubt whether steroids provide any benefit, and argue that the administration of steroids may simply have coincided with the period of natural regression of the condition.

Failure to respond to medical management necessitates intervention, in the form of hepatic resection or interruption of the hepatic arterial blood supply by ligation or embolization. Angiography is an essential preliminary to any of these procedures. Resection is only rarely feasible and is recommended only for localized 'tumours', especially if they are complicated by intraperitoneal haemorrhage; excision of the more common widespread lesions is impossible. In such cases ligation of the common hepatic artery, as originally described by DeLorimier [31], usually has a dramatic effect; alternatively embolization of the artery can be undertaken if the technique is available and if the angiographic findings indicate that it is worthwhile [19,63].

Prognosis

Although haemangioma of the liver remains a potentially lethal condition, the last two decades have seen a vast improvement in reported results. Burrows and colleagues [19] reported on 16 patients from the literature and two of their own who had been treated by hepatic devascularization for congestive heart failure secondary to hepatic haemangioma; 15 had survived with 14 (78%) regarded as being cured. Prior to 1967 the survival rate for the same category of severely ill patients was 12% [31]. The experience of Nguyen, Shandling and colleagues suggests, however, that recent improvements in survival are not entirely due to a more aggressive approach; they report excellent results in a conservatively-managed series of patients which included neonates in cardiac failure [102].

Mesenchymal hamartoma of liver

This rare tumour-like malformation almost always presents during the first year of life and may be encountered in the neonate [143] and in the fetus [44]. The tumour, which is often very large, is composed of multiple cysts filled with clear fluid or mucoid material; microscopically, loose myxoid tissue contains branching bile ducts, hepatocytes and often angiomatous elements. The tumour may be pedunculated or may be deeply embedded in the liver substance. Typically it produces rapid abdominal enlargement and a palpable mass in an otherwise asymptomatic child. The serum AFP may be elevated [70]. It should be possible to distinguish this tumour from other liver tumours by clinical evaluation and non-invasive imaging techniques; radionuclide scan and ultrasonography will usually provide an accurate diagnosis. The predominance of cysts on sonography is a good indication that the lesion is benign [114]. Treatment is by resection; this is not difficult in pedunculated lesions but in the case of deeply-situated masses lobectomy or enucleation of the mass is necessary. This is a benign condition, with no reports of malignant change; mortality is associated with operative complications [138].

Malignant tumours of the liver

Malignant primary tumours of the liver account for 0.2–2.8% of all primary malignancies in children from European or North American series [148]. The great majority of these tumours arise from hepatocytes and are divided into two main groups; the hepatoblastomas [23], which occur mostly in infancy and early childhood, being rare over the age of 5 years, and the hepatocarcinomas of adult type which tend to occur in an already diseased liver, usually in children in their teens but occasionally in children under the age of 4 years [69].

Congenital and neonatal cases are very rare but some large series of liver tumours in children include one or two neonates; for example, Gauthier and colleagues had two cases in which the tumour was discovered at birth in a series of 29 cases [48]. Isaacs reported one neonatal hepatoblastoma over a 28-year period in Los Angeles, during which time a total of 42 hepatoblastomas were treated and a total of 51 neonatal malignant tumours were treated [68]. In a similar survey conducted in Toronto, Campbell and colleagues found one neonatal hepatoblastoma amongst 56 cases of liver tumours in children and amongst 102 cases of neonatal cancers [20].

Hepatocarcinoma has been reported in the newborn [45] and a liver tumour was recorded as a cause of dystocia in 1879 [103]. In Liverpool we have encountered only one neonatal hepatoblastoma over a period of 33 years; this was an enormous tumour surrounding the inferior vena cava and invading the posterior abdominal wall; the child died without operation, shortly after admission.

As with other abdominal tumours, presentation in the neonatal period is with an abdominal mass. Plain X-ray of the abdomen shows hepatomegaly but calcification is rarely seen; displacement of the colonic gas shadow will be seen in the case of right lobe lesions and of the stomach gas in the case of left lobe lesions. Ultrasonography is extremely useful as a first-line investigation to rule out such diagnoses as hydronephrosis, choledochal cyst and mesenchymal hamartoma of the liver and to demonstrate the presence of an intrahepatic solid mass. Technetium-99m scanning gives a good indication of exact location and size of the tumour. CT scanning is particularly useful in the identification of multifocal tumour formation within the liver parenchyma [135].

Angiography, preferably performed via an umbilical artery, is essential if resection is being considered, but should be done only if the other imaging studies have not excluded the possibility of resection. Liver function tests are usually normal. Serum AFP levels are raised in approximately 90% of cases of liver cell carcinoma and serve as a very useful tumour 'marker' [111], although in the neonate evaluation of levels is complicated by the high levels which are a normal feature of the early months of life [144].

The only curative treatment is operative removal of the lesion by lobectomy, hemihepatectomy or extended right hepatectomy. In the 1975 survey of the American Academy of Pediatrics [40] 375 hepatic tumours were analysed: 252 were malignant (129 hepatoblastoma, 98 hepatocarcinoma); no patient survived after incomplete excision or biopsy only, but of the hepatoblastomas completely excised 58% survived and of the hepatocarcinomas 36%. In three patients an inoperable tumour was converted to an operable one by combined radiotherapy and multiple cytotoxic drugs. Since that time there have been several reports of successful responses of initially unresectable hepatoblastomas to chemotherapy [3,66,129] with or without irradiation, allowing delayed complete resection. The benefit of irradiation of liver tumours is, however, questionable and such treatment would be inappropriate for the newborn. Chemotherapy, likewise, although of considerable value in both primary and metastatic hepatoblastoma [3,111] carries the risk of severe side effects in the neonate. Surgery should therefore be the primary treatment of choice in the neonate with use of chemotherapy only in the event of the tumour proving to be unresectable.

Pancreas: nesidioblastosis and islet-cell adenoma

Persistent neonatal hypoglycaemia is a potentially serious condition which can lead to seizures, permanent brain damage and even death. Severe symptomatic hypoglycaemia in the newborn is most commonly seen in small-for-gestational-age babies and is attributable to intrauterine starvation; vigorous treatment usually results in the child being able to sustain normal blood glucose levels by the age of 2 weeks. Glycogen storage disease, extrapancreatic endocrine disorders, the Beckwith–Wiedemann syndrome and maternal diabetes are less common causes. Persistence of hypoglycaemia beyond the age of 2 weeks is an indication for thorough investigation. Amongst the cases previously labelled 'idiopathic', hyperinsulinism is the commonest cause of hypoglycaemia and in the majority of these cases the underlying pathology is beta-cell nesidioblastosis or, less commonly, islet cell adenoma [21].

Pathology

Yakovac, in 1971, defined beta-cell nesidioblastosis as 'continuous or continual differentiation of insulin-producing beta cells from any or all divisions of the ductular system of the exocrine pancreas'. In nine out of 12 surgically resected pancreases of infants with 'idiopathic' hypoglycaemia, histochemical staining revealed many beta cells in addition to the normal complement within the islets; the additional beta cells were scattered throughout the pancreas, singly or in small clusters, and were regarded as representing neoformation of islet cells from ductular elements [155]. Islet cell adenoma has been found in one-third of the reported cases of organic hyperinsulinism with onset of symptoms before the age of 2 months [21]. These lesions tend to be small (1 mm–1 cm diameter); when visible they have a reddish-tan appearance but some are identifiable only on microscopy [119,121]. Diffuse and localized lesions may co-exist [21]. In our one case of islet-cell adenoma a 2.5-mm diameter lesion was located in the head of the pancreas and was identified only on microscopy.

Diagnosis and management

The diagnosis of hyperinsulinism depends on the demonstration of inappropriately raised levels of serum insulin in the presence of hypoglycaemia in paired blood samples [5]. Attempts to localize a lesion in the pancreas by any imaging technique is most unlikely to be helpful in a small infant. Surgery is indicated when persistent hyperinsulinism fails to respond to medical treatment with diazoxide [32].

The abdomen is opened through a transverse upper abdominal incision and the pancreas is fully exposed by division of the gastrocolic omentum and Kocher's manoevre. The pancreas is inspected and palpated for adenoma, but identification of a tumour is very unusual in the neonate, even after complete mobilization of the pancreas [119,121]. If a tumour is found, partial pancreatectomy is performed. Otherwise, the procedure of choice is a near-total (95%) pancreatectomy [57,84,93,137] with preservation only of a small portion of the head of the gland between the right side of the common bile duct and the duodenum [21,137,150]. The short gastric vessels are preserved, to protect the spleen in the event of damage to the splenic vessels; it should, however be possible to preserve the splenic vessels if the small branches running from them to the pancreas are dealt with meticulously [93,137].

Carcasonne [21] has suggested a refinement of this technique which involves intraoperative measurement of portal vein blood insulin levels, and for further operative details the reader is referred to his paper and those of Martin [93], Spitz [137] and Warden [150].

Prognosis

The trend towards increasingly radical surgery has occurred because of unacceptably high recurrence rates after sub-total (70–80%) resections; 54 of 85 infants reported in the literature had had recurrent hypoglycaemia, necessitating 36 re-operations [21]. Of 22 infants who had had 95% pancreatectomies eight had had recurrences of hypoglycaemia, but seven of these responded to medical treatment with only one requiring a repeat (total) pancreatectomy [21]. Dunger and colleagues [32] have recently assessed exocrine and endocrine function in seven of their patients 1 to 2 years after 95% pancreatectomy for nesidioblastosis. None had had recurrent hypoglycaemia [37], four had had transient hyperglycaemia after surgery but only one had a frankly diabetic glucose tolerance curve 1 year later. Exocrine function was seriously impaired in one of the seven.

Fetus-in-fetu

In this rare condition, a malformed monozygotic twin lies within the body of its fellow. The enclosed parasite is distinguished from a teratoma by its possession of a spinal column and of limbs and organs arranged appropriately to the spinal axis. Most commonly, the fetus-in-fetu is single and occupies a sac in the retroperitoneum of the upper abdomen of the host [88], but Gross and Clatworthy [54] recorded an example in which the sac contained two fetuses, and in Lee's [87] case three fetuses lay in the pelvis of their 2-month-old brother. Fetus-in-fetu presents clinically as an abdominal mass; the diagnosis may be made radiologically by the demonstration of fetal skeletal parts. Surgical excision of the lesion is indicated.

References

1. Ahmed, S. (1971) Neonatal and childhood ovarian cysts. *J. Pediat. Surg.*, **6**, 702–708
2. Alvear, D.T. and Rayfield, M.M. (1976) Bilateral ovarian cysts in early infancy. *J. Pediat. Surg.*, **11**, 993–995
3. Andrassy, R.J., Brennan, L.P., Siegel, M.M., Weitzman, J.J., Siegel, S.E., Stanley, P. *et al.* (1980) Preoperative chemotherapy for hepatoblastomas in children: report of six cases. *J. Pediat. Surg.*, **15**, 517–522
4. Arnheim, E.E. (1951) Retro-peritoneal teratoma in infancy and childhood. *Pediatrics*, **8**, 309–327
5. Aynsley-Green, A., Polack, J.M., Bloom, S.R., Gough, M.H., Keeling, J., Ashcroft, S.J.H. *et al.* (1981) Nesidioblastosis of the pancreas: definition of the syndrome and the management of the severe neonatal hyperinsulinaemic hypoglycaemia. *Arch. Dis. Child.*, **56**, 496–508
6. Bagolan, P. (1950) Su un caso raro di leiomyosarcoma bilaterale dei reini. *Tumori*, **24**, 75
7. Beckwith, J.B. (1969) Macroglossia, omphalocele, adrenal cytomegaly, gigantism and hyperplastic visceromegaly. *Birth Defects*, **5** (2), 188–196
8. Beckwith, J.B. (1974) Mesenchymal renal neoplasms in infancy revisited. *J. Pediat. Surg.*, **9**, 803–805 (Editorial)
9. Beckwith, J.B. and Perrin, E.V. (1963) In situ neuroblastomas: contribution to the natural history of neural crest tumours. *Am. J. Path.*, **43**, 1089–1104
10. Beckwith, J.B. and Weeks, D.A. (1986) Congenital mesoblastic nephroma. When should we worry? *Arch. Path. Lab. Med.*, **110**, 98–99 (Editorial)
11. Bill, A.H. and Morgan, A. (1970) Evidence for immune reactions to neuroblastoma and future possibilities for investigation. *J. Pediat. Surg.*, **5**, 111–116
12. Bolande, R.P. (1973) Congenital mesoblastic nephroma of infancy. *Perspect. Pediat. Path.*, **1**, 227–250
13. Bolande, R.P. (1974) Congenital and infantile neoplasia of the kidney. *Lancet*, **ii**, 1497–1499
14. Bolande, R.P., Brough, A.J. and Izant, R.J. (1967) Congenital mesoblastic nephroma of infancy. *Pediatrics*, **40**, 272–278
15. Borglin, N.E. and Selander, P. (1962) Hymenal polyps in newborn infants. *Acta Paediat. (Uppsala)*, **51** (Suppl. 135), 28–31
16. Brock, C.E. and Ricketts, R.R. (1982) Haemoperitoneum from spontaneous rupture of neonatal neuroblastoma. *Am. J. Dis. Child.*, **136**, 370–371
17. Brown, S.H. and Fonkalsrud, E. (1969) Successful treatment of hepatic hemangioma with corticosteroids. *J. Am. Med. Ass.*, **208**, 2473–2474
18. Bulfamonte, J.C. (1942) Large ovarian cyst in newborn child. *Am. J. Surg.*, **55**, 175–176
19. Burrows, P.E., Rosenberg, H.C. and Chuang, H.S. (1985) Diffuse hepatic hemangiomas: percutaneous transcatheter embolization with detachable silicone balloons. *Radiology*, **156**, 85–88
20. Campbell, A.N., Chan, H.S.L., O'Brien, A., Smith, C.R. and Becker, L.E. (1987) Malignant tumours in the neonate. *Arch. Dis. Child.*, **62**, 19–23
21. Carcassonne, M., DeLarue, A. and LeTourneau, J.M. (1983) Surgical treatment of organic pancreatic hypoglycaemia in the pediatric age. *J. Pediat. Surg.*, **18**, 75–79
22. Chan, H.S.L., Mancer, K., Weitzman, S.S.,

Kotecha, P. and Daneman, A. (1987) Congenital mesoblastic nephroma: a clinicoradiologic study of 17 cases representing the pathologic spectrum of the disease. *J. Pediat.*, **111**, 64–70

23. Clatworthy, H.W., Boles, E.T. and Newton, W.A. (1960) Primary tumours of the liver in infants and children. *Arch. Dis. Child.*, **35**, 22–28
24. Cohen, R.C. and Myers, N.A. (1986) Diagnosis and management of massive hepatic hemangiomas in childhood. *J. Pediat. Surg.*, **21**, 6–9
25. Cooney, D.R., Voorhess, M.L., Fisher, J.E., Brecher, M., Karp, M.P. and Jewett, T.C. (1982) Vasoactive intestinal peptide producing neuroblastoma. *J. Pediat. Surg.*, **17**, 821–825
26. Culp, D.A., Frazier, R.G. and Butler, J.J. (1965) Sertoli cell tumour in an infant. *J. Urol.*, **76**, 162–167
27. Cushing, H. and Wolbach, S.B. (1927) The transformation of malignant paravertebral sympathicoblastoma into a benign ganglioneuroma. *Am. J. Path.*, **3**, 203–216
28. Dachman, A.H., Lichtenstein, J.E., Friedman, A.C. and Hartman, D.S. (1983) Infantile hemangioendothelioma of the liver. *Am. J. Roent.*, **140**, 1091–1096
29. D'Angio, G.J., Evans, A.E. and Koop, C.E. (1971) Special pattern of widespread neuroblastoma with a favourable prognosis. *Lancet*, **i**, 1046–1049
30. D'Angio, G.J., Lyser, K.M. and Urunay, G. (1971) Neuroblastoma, Stage IV-S: a special entity? *Memorial Sloan-Kettering Cancer Center Bull.*, **2**(2), 61–65
31. DeLorimer, A.A., Simpson, E.B., Baum, R.S. and Carlson, E. (1967) Hepatic artery ligation for hepatic hemangiomatosis. *New Engl. J. Med.*, **227**, 333–336
32. Dunger, D.B., Burns, C., Ghale, G.K., Muller, D.P.R., Spitz, L. and Grant, D.B. (1988) Pancreatic exocrine and endocrine function after subtotal pancreatectomy for nesidioblastosis. *J. Pediat. Surg.*, **23**, 112–115
33. Ehrlich, F.E., Haas, J.E. and Kiesewetter, W.B. (1971) Rhabdomyosarcoma in infants and children: factors affecting long term survival. *J. Pediat. Surg.*, **6**, 572–577
34. von Eiselberg, A.F. (1893) Abtrangung eines cavernous der leber. *Wien. Klin. Wochenschr.*, **6**, 1
35. Evans, A.E., Baum, E. and Chard, R. (1981) Do infants with Stage IV-S neuroblastoma need treatment? *Arch. Dis. Child.*, **56**, 271–274
36. Evans, A.E., Chatten, J., D'Angio, G.J., Gerson, J.M., Robinson, J. and Schnaufer, L. (1980) A review of 17 IV-S neuroblastoma patients at the Children's Hospital of Philadelphia. *Cancer*, **45**, 833–839
37. Evans, A.E., D'Angio, G.J. and Koop, C.E. (1984) The role of multimodal therapy in patients with local and regional neuroblastoma. *J. Pediat. Surg.*, **19**, 77–80
38. Evans, A.E., D'Angio, G.J. and Randolph, J.G. (1971) A proposed staging for children with neuroblastoma. *Cancer*, **27**, 374–378

39. Everson, T.C. and Cole, W.H. (1966) *Spontaneous Regression of Cancer*, Saunders, Philadelphia and London
40. Exelby, P.R., Filler, R.M. and Grosfeld, J.L. (1975) Liver tumours in children in the particular reference to hepatoblastoma and hepatocellular carcinoma. American Academy of Pediatrics Surgical Section Survey. *J. Pediat. Surg.*, **10**, 329–337
41. Favara, B.E., Johnson, W. and Ito, J. (1968) Renal tumours in the neonatal period. *Cancer*, **22**, 845–855
42. Filler, R.M. (1986) Testicular tumours. In *Pediatric Surgery* (ed. K.J. Welch, J.G. Randolph, M.M. Ravitch, J.A. O'Neill, Jr. and M.I. Rowe), 4th Edition, Year Book Medical Publishers, Inc., Chicago, pp. 1326–1330
43. Flamant, F., Nihoul-Fékété, C., Patte, C. and Lemerle, J. (1968) Optimal treatment of Stage I yolk sac tumour of the testis in children. *J. Pediat. Surg.*, **21**, 108–111
44. Foucar, E., Williamson, R.A. and Yiu-Chiu, V. (1982) Mesenchymal hamartoma of the liver identified by fetal sonography. *Am. J. Roent.*, **140**, 970–972
45. Fraumeni, J.F., Miller, R.W. and Hill, J.A. (1968) Primary carcinoma of the liver in children: an epidemiologic study. *J. Nat. Cancer Inst.*, **40**, 1087–1099
46. Fu, Y.S. and Kay, S. (1973) Congenital mesoblastic nephroma and its recurrence. *Arch. Path.*, **96**, 66–70
47. Gale, G.B., D'Angio, G.J., Uri, A., Chatten, J. and Koop, C.E. (1982) Cancer in neonates: the experience at the Children's Hospital of Philadelphia. *Pediatrics*, **70**, 409–413
48. Gauthier, F., Valayer, J., Le Thai, B., Sinico, M. and Kalifa, C. (1986) Hepatoblastoma and hepatocarcinoma in children: analysis of a series of 29 cases. *J. Pediat. Surg.*, **21**, 424–429
49. Graivier, L., Votteler, T.P. and Dorman, G.W. (1967) Hepatic haemangioma in newborn infants. *J. Pediat. Surg.*, **2**, 299–307
50. Griffin, M.E. and Bolande, R.P. (1969) Familial neuroblastoma with regression and maturation to ganglioneurofibroma. *Pediatrics*, **43**, 377–382
51. Grosfeld, J.L. (1986) Neuroblastoma. In *Pediatric Surgery* (ed. K.J. Welch, J.G. Randolph, M.M. Ravitch, J.A. O'Neill, Jr. and M.I. Rowe), 4th Edition. Year Book Medical Publishers, Chicago, pp. 283–293
52. Grosfeld, J.L. and Baehner, R.L. (1980) Neuroblastoma: an analysis of 160 cases. *World J. Surg.*, **4**, 29–38
53. Grosfeld, J.L., Smith, J.P. and Clatworthy, H.W. (1972) Pelvic rhabdomyosarcoma in infants and children. *J. Urol.*, **107**, 673–675
54. Gross, R.E. and Clatworthy, H.W. (1951) Twin fetuses in fetu. *J. Pediat.*, **38**, 502–508
55. Guin, G.H., Gilbert, E.F. and Jones, B. (1969) Incidental neuroblastoma in infants. *Am. J. Clin. Path.*, **51**, 126–136

56. Hansen, J.L. (1967) Tumour of undescended testicle in an infant. *J. Am. Med. Ass.*, **199**, 944–945

57. Harken, A.H., Filler, R.M., AvRuskin, T.W. and Crigler, J.F. Jr (1971) The role of 'total' pancreatectomy in the treatment of unremitting hypoglycemia of infancy. *J. Pediat. Surg.*, **6**, 284–289

58. Hays, D.M., Raney, R.B. Jr, Lawrence, W. Jr, Tefft, M., Soule, E.H., Crist, W.M. *et al.* (1982) Primary chemotherapy in the treatment of children with bladder-prostate tumours in the Intergroup Rhabdomyosarcoma Study (IRS II) *J. Pediat. Surg.*, **17**, 812–820

59. Hays, D.M., Shimada, H., Raney, R.B. Jr., Tefft, M., Newton, W., Crist, W.M. *et al.* (1985) Sarcoma of the vagina and uterus: The Intergroup Rhabdomyosarcoma Study. *J. Pediat. Surg.*, **20**, 718–724

60. Hellström, I.E., Hellström, K.E., Evans, C.A., Heppner, G.H., Pierce, G.E. and Yang, J.P.S. (1969) Serum-mediated protection of neoplastic cells from inhibition by lymphocytes immune to their tumour-specific antigens. *Proc. Nat. Acad. Sci. USA*, **62**, 362–368

61. Hellström, I.E., Hellström, K.E., Pierce, G.E. and Bill, A.H. (1968) Demonstration of a cell bound and humoral immunity against neuroblastoma cells. *Proc. Nat. Acad. Sci USA*, **60**, 1231–1238

62. Hoefnagel, C.A., Voûte, P.A., DeKraker, J. and Marcuse, H.R. (1985) Total-body scintigraphy with I-meta-iodobenzylguanidine for detection of neuroblastoma. *Diag. Imag. Clin. Med.*, **54**, 21–27

63. Holcomb, G.W. III, O'Neill, J.A. Jr, Mahboubi, S. and Bishop, H.C. (1988) Experience with hepatic haemangioendothelioma in infancy and childhood. *J. Pediat. Surg.*, **23**, 661–666

64. Howell, C.G., Othersen, H.B., Kiviat, N.E., Norkool, P., Beckwith, J.B. and D'Angio, G.J. (1982) Therapy and outcome in 51 children with mesoblastic nephroma: A report of the National Wilms' Tumour Study. *J. Pediat. Surg.*, **17**, 826–831

65. Ikeda, K., Suita, S. and Nakano, H. (1988) Management of ovarian cyst detected antenatally. *J. Pediat. Surg.*, **23**, 432–435

66. Ikeda, L., Suita, S. and Nakagawara, A. (1979) Preoperative chemotherapy for initially unresectable hepatoblastoma in children. *Arch. Surg.*, **114**, 203–207

67. Ikeda, Y., Lister, J., Bouton, J.M. and Buyukpamukcu, M. (1981) Congenital neuroblastoma, neuroblastoma in situ, and the normal fetal development of the adrenal. *J. Pediat. Surg.*, **16**, 636–644

68. Issacs, H. Jr (1987) Congenital and neonatal malignant tumours. A 28-year experience at Children's Hospital of Los Angeles. *Am. J. Pediat. Hematol./Oncol.*, **9**, 121–129

69. Ishak, K. and Glunz, P.R. (1967) Hepatoblastoma and hepatocarcinoma in infancy and childhood: report of 47 cases. *Cancer*, **20**, 396–422

70. Ito, H., Kishikawa, T., Toda, T., Arai, M. and Muro, H. (1984) Hepatic mesenchymal hamartoma of an infant. *J. Pediat. Surg.*, **19**, 315–317

71. Jacobi, A. (1886) Primares Sarcom der Niere bei den fotus und den neugeboren kinde. *Jahrbuch für Kinderheilkunde*, **25**, 112

72. Johnson, A.T. and Halbert, D. (1974) Congenital neuroblastoma presenting as hydrops foetalis. *North Carolina Med. J.*, **35**, 289–291

73. Jonte, P.A., Wadman, S.K. and Van Putten, W.J. (1970) Congenital neuroblastoma; symptoms in the mother during pregnancy. *Clin. Pediat.*, **9**, 206

74. Joshi, V.V., Kasznica, J. and Walters, T.R. (1986) Atypical mesoblastic nephroma. Pathologic characterization of a potentially aggressive variant of conventional congenital mesoblastic nephroma. *Arch. Path. Lab. Med.*, **110**, 100–106

75. Joshi, V.V., Kay, S., Milstein Koontz, W. and McWilliams, N.B. (1973) Congenital mesoblastic nephroma of infancy: Report of a case with unusual clinical behaviour. *Am. J. Clin. Path.*, **60**, 811–816

76. Karrer, F.W. and Swenson, S.A. (1961) Twisted ovarian cyst in a newborn infant. *Arch. Surg.*, **83**, 921–924

77. Katz, H.P. and Askin, J. (1968) Multiple haemangiomata with thrombopenia; an unusual case with comments on steroid therapy. *Am. J. Dis. Child.*, **115**, 351–357

78. Kay, S., Pratt, C.B. and Salzberg, A.M. (1966) Hamartoma (leiomyomatous type) of the kidney. *Cancer*, **19**, 1825–1832

79. Khoury, E.N. and Speer, F.D. (1944) Rhabdomyosarcoma of the urinary bladder. *J. Urol.*, **51**, 505–516

80. Koop, C.E. (1968) Factors affecting survival in neuroblastoma. *J. Pediat. Surg.*, **3**, 113–114

81. Koop, C.E. (1972) The neuroblastoma. *Prog. Pediat. Surg.*, **4**, 1–28

82. Koop, C.E. and Hernandez, J.R. (1964) Neuroblastoma: Experience with 100 cases in children. *Surgery*, **56**, 726–733

83. Kumar, A.P.M., Wrenn, E.L., Fleming, I.D., Hustu, H.O., Pratt, C.B. and Pinkel, D. (1975) Preoperative therapy for unresectable malignant tumours in children. *J. Pediat. Surg.*, **10**, 657–670

84. Langer, J.C., Filler, R.M., Wesson, D.E., Sherwood, G. and Cutz, E. (1984) Surgical management of persistent neonatal hypoglycemia due to islet cell dysplasia. *J. Pediat. Surg.*, **19**, 786–792

85. Larcher, V.F., Howard, E.R. and Mowat, A.P. (1981) Hepatic haemangiomata: diagnosis and management. *Arch. Dis. Child.*, **56**, 7–14

86. Laug, W.E., Siegel, S.E., Shaw, K.N.F., Landing, B., Baptista, J. and Gutenstein, M. (1978) Initial urinary catecholamine metabolite concentrations and prognosis in neuroblastoma. *Pediatrics*, **62**, 77–83

87. Lee, E.Y.C. (1965) Foetus in foetu. *Arch. Dis. Child.*, **40**, 689–693

88. Lord, J.M. (1956) Intra-abdominal foetus in foetu. *J. Path. Bact.*, **72**, 627

89. McCune, W.R., Galleher, E.P. and Wood, C. (1964)

Leiomyoma of the kidney in a newborn infant. *J. Urol.*, **91**, 646–648

90. McKeever, P.A. and Andrews, H. (1988) Fetal ovarian cysts: A report of five cases. *J. Pediat. Surg.*, **23**, 354–355

91. Mainolfi, F.G., Standiford, W.E. and Hubbard, T.B. (1968) Ruptured ovarian cyst in newborn. *J. Pediat. Surg.*, **3**, 612–616

92. Marshall, J.R. (1965) Ovarian enlargements in the first year of life. *Ann. Surg.*, **161**, 372–377

93. Martin, L.W., Ryckman, F.C. and Sheldon, C.A. (1984) Experience with 95% pancreatectomy and splenic salvage for neonatal nesidioblastosis. *Ann. Surg.*, **200**, 355–362

94. Martinez-Mora, J., Cerquella, S., Padulles, J., Prats, J., Boix-Ochoa, J., Moragas, A. *et al.* (1980) Management of primary testicular tumours in children. *J. Pediat. Surg.*, **15**, 283–286

95. Mason, G.A., Hart-Mercer, J., Millar, E.J., Strang, L.B. and Wynne, N.A. (1957) Adrenaline-secreting neuroblastoma in an infant. *Lancet*, **ii**, 322–325

96. Miller, R.W., Fraumeni, J.F. and Manning, M.D. (1964) Association of Wilms' tumour with aniridia, hemihypertrophy and other congenital malformations. *New Engl. J. Med.*, **270**, 922–927

97. Minielly, J.A., Tuttle, R.J. and Thompson, G.D. (1974) Fetal hamartoma of the kidney – a benign tumour to be distinguished from Wilms' tumour. *Can. J. Surg.*, **17**, 235–238

98. Mogg, R.A. (1957) Rare renal tumours: with special reference to those occurring in children. *Br. J. Urol.*, **29**, 287–292

99. Mostofi, F.K., Theiss, E.A. and Ashley, D.J.B. (1959) Tumours of specialised gonadal stroma in human male patients. *Cancer*, **12**, 944–957

100. Murthy, T.V.M., Irving, I.M. and Lister, J. (1978) Massive adrenal haemorrhage in neonatal neuroblastoma. *J. Pediat. Surg.*, **13**, 31–34

101. Muto, K. (1941) Renal sarcoma in a seven month fetus. *J. Am. Med. Ass.*, **116**, 786

102. Nguyen, B., Shandling, B., Ein, S. and Stephens, C. (1982) Hepatic hemangioma in childhood: medical management or surgical management? *J. Pediat. Surg.*, **17**, 576–579

103. Noeggerath, E. (1879) Case of carcinoma of liver as a cause of dystocia. *Am. J. Obstet.*, **12**, 692

104. Norris, H.J. and Taylor, H.B. (1966) Polyps of the vagina. *Cancer*, **19**, 227–232

105. Nussbaum, A.R., Sanders, R.C., Benator, R.M., Haller, J.A. and Dudgeon, D.L. (1987) Spontaneous resolution of neonatal ovarian cysts. *Am. J. Roent.*, **148**, 175–176

106. Ober, W.B., Smith, J.A. and Rouillard, F.C. (1958) Congenital sarcoma botryoides of vagina; report of two cases. *Cancer*, **11**, 620–623

107. Paul, F.T. (1886) Congenital adenosarcoma of the kidney. *Proc. Path. Soc. Lond.*, **37**, 292

108. Phelan, J.T., Wollner, L.B. and Hayles, A.B. (1957) Testicular tumours in infants and children. *Surg. Gynec. Obstet.*, **105**, 569–576

109. Pilling, G.P. (1975) Wilms' tumour in seven children with aniridia. *J. Pediat. Surg.*, **10**, 87–96

110. Prasad, K.N., Mandal, B. and Kumar, S. (1973) Demonstration of cholinergic cells in human neuroblastoma and ganglioneuroma. *J. Pediat.*, **82**, 677–679

111. Pritchard, J., da Cunha, A., Cornbleet, M.A. and Carter, C.J. (1982) Alpha fetoprotein monitoring of response to adriamycin therapy in hepatoblastoma. *J. Pediat. Surg.*, **17**, 429–430

112. Procianoy, R.S., Giacomini, C.B., Mattos, T.C. and Roesch, L.H. (1986) Congenital Wilms' tumour associated with consumption coagulopathy and hyperbilirubinemia. *J. Pediat. Surg.*, **21**, 993–994

113. Quintana, J., Beresi, V., Latorre, J.J., Izzo, C., Sanhueza, S. and Del Pozo, H. (1982) Infantile embryonal carcinoma of testis. *J. Urol.*, **128**, 785–787

114. Raffensperger, J.G., Gonzalez-Cruss, F. and Skeehan, T. (1983) Mesenchymal hamartoma of the liver. *J. Pediat. Surg.*, **18**, 585–587

115. Ragab, A.H., Heyn, R., Tefft, M., Hays, D.N., Newton, W.A. and Beltangady, M. (1986) Infants younger than 1 year of age with rhabdomyosarcoma. *Cancer*, **58**, 2606–2610

116. Rance, T.F. (1814) A case of fungus haematoides in the kidney. *Med. Physic. J.*, **32**, 19

117. Rangecroft, L., Lauder, I. and Wagget, J. (1978) Spontaneous maturation of stage IV-S neuroblastoma. *Arch. Dis. Child.*, **53**, 815–817

118. Reeder, F.K. and Morse, T.S. (1962) Renal leiomyoma in a newborn infant. *Am. J. Surg.*, **104**, 788–790

119. Rich, R.H., Dehner, L.P., Okinaga, K., Deeb, L.C., Ulstrom, R.A. and Leonard, A.S. (1978) Surgical management of islet-cell adenoma in infancy. *Surgery*, **84**, 519–526

120. Richmond, H. and Dougal, A.J. (1970) Neonatal renal tumours. *J. Pediat. Surg.*, **5**, 513–417

121. Rickham, P.P. (1975) Islet cell tumours in childhood. *J. Pediat. Surg.*, **10**, 83–86

122. Rickham, P.P. Artigas, J.L.R. (1969) Tumours of the liver in childhood. *Z. Kinderchir.*, **7**, 447

123. Rusche, C. (1952) Twelve cases of testicular tumours occurring during infancy and childhood. *J. Pediat.*, **40**, 192–199

124. Sawada, T., Todo, S., Fujita, K., Iino, F., Imashuku, S. and Kusunoki, T. (1982) Mass screening of neuroblastoma in infancy. *Am. J. Dis. Child.*, **136**, 710–712

125. Schnaufer, L. and Koop, C.E. (1975) Silastic pouch for temporary hepatomegaly in Stage IVs neuroblastoma. *J. Pediat. Surg.*, **10**, 73–75

126. Schneider, K.M., Becker, J.M. and Krasna, I.H. (1965) Neonatal neuroblastoma. *Pediatrics*, **36**, 359–366

127. Sedin, G., Bergquist, C. and Lindgren, P.G. (1985) Ovarian hyperstimulation syndrome in preterm infants. *Pediat. Res.*, **19**, 548–552

128. Sewell, J.H. and Weiss, K. (1961) Spontaneous rupture of haemangioma of the liver; a review of the literature and presentation of illustrative case. *Arch. Surg.*, **83**, 729–733

129. Shafer, A.D. and Selinkoff, P.M. (1977) Preoperative irradiation and chemotherapy for initially unresectable hepatoblastoma. *J. Pediat. Surg.*, **12**, 1001–1007

130. Shanbhogue, L.K.R., Gray, E. and Miller, S.S. (1986) Congenital mesoblastic nephroma of infancy associated with hypercalcemia. *J. Urol.*, **135**, 771–772

131. Shanklin, D.R. and Sotelo-Avila, C. (1969) *In situ* tumours in fetuses, newborns, and young infants. *Biol. Neonat.*, **14**, 283–316

132. Shawis, R.N., El Gohary, A. and Cook, R.C.M. (1985) Ovarian cysts and tumours in infancy and childhood. *Ann. Roy. Coll. Surg. Engl.*, **67**, 17–19

133. Shown, T.E. and Durfee, M.F. (1970) Blueberry muffin baby: neonatal neuroblastoma with subcutaneous metastases. *J. Urol.*, **104**, 193–195

134. Shuller, T., Rosenweig, J.L. and Areg, J.B. (1949) Successful removal of haemangioma of the liver in an infant. *Pediatrics*, **3**, 328–342

135. Snow, J.H., Goldstein, H.M. and Wallace, S. (1979) Comparison of scintigraphy, sonography and computed tomography in the evaluation of hepatic neoplasms. *Am. J. Roent.*, **132**, 915–918

136. Sober, I. and Hirsch, M. (1965) Embryoma of kidney in newborn infant. Case report. *J. Urol.*, **93**, 449–451

137. Spitz, L., Buick, R.G., Grant, D.B., Leonard, J.V. and Pincott, J.R. (1986) Surgical treatment of nesidioblastosis *Paediat. Surg. Int.*, **1**, 26–29

138. Stocker, J.T. and Ishak, K.G. (1983) Mesenchymal hamartoma of the liver: report of 30 cases and review of the literature. *Pediat. Path.*, **1**, 245–267

139. Tefft, M. and Jaffe, N. (1973) Sarcoma of the bladder and prostate in children. Rationale for the role of radiation therapy based on a review of the literature and a report of 14 additional patients. *Cancer*, **12**, 1161–1177

140. Teoh, T.B., Steward, J.K. and Willis, R.A. (1960) The distinctive adenocarcinoma of the infant's testis: an account of 15 cases. *J. Path. Bact.*, **80**, 147–156

141. Tietz, K.G. and Davis, J.B. (1957) Ruptured ovarian cyst in a newborn infant. *J. Pediat.*, **51**, 564–565

142. Touloukian, R.J. (1970) Hepatic hemangioendothelioma during infancy: Pathology, diagnosis and treatment with prednisone. *Pediatrics*, **45**, 71–76

143. Touloukian, R.J. (1986) Non-malignant liver tumours and hepatic infections. In *Pediatric Surgery* (ed. K.J. Welch, J.G. Randolph, M.M. Ravitch, J.A. O'Neill Jr. and M.I. Rowe), 4th Edn, Year Book Medical Publisher, Inc., Chicago, pp. 1067–1974

144. Tsuchida, Y., Endo, Y., Saito, S., Kaneko, M., Shiraki, K. and Ohmi, K. (1978) Evaluation of alpha-fetoprotein in early infancy. *J. Pediat. Surg.*, **13**, 155–156

145. Tsuchida, Y., Honna, T., Iwanaka, T., Saeki, M., Taguchi, N., Kaneko, T. *et al.* (1987) Serial determination of serum neuron-specific enolase in patients with neuroblastoma and other pediatric tumours. *J. Pediat. Surg.*, **22**, 419–424

146. Turkel, S.B. and Itabashi, H.H. (1974) The natural history of neuroblastic cells in fetal adrenal gland. *Am. J. Path.*, **76**, 225–236

147. Ugarte, N., Gonzalez-Crussi, F. and Hsueh, W. (1981) Wilms' tumour: Its morphology in patients under one year of age. *Cancer*, **48**, 346–353

148. Valayer, J. and Lemerle, J. (1978) Tumeurs du foie. In *Maladies du Foie et des Voies Biliares Chez l'Enfant* (ed. D. Alagille and M. Odievre), Flammarion, Paris, pp. 239–259. Cited by Gautier, F., Valayer, J., Le Thai, B., Sinico, M. and Chantal, K. (1986) Hepatoblastoma and hepatocarcinoma in children: Analysis of a series of 29 cases. *J. Pediat. Surg.*, **21**, 424–429

149. Voûte, P.A., de Kraker, J. and Burgers, J.M.V. (1986) Tumours of the Sympathetic Nervous System, In Cancer in Children (ed. P.A. Voûte, A. Barret, H.J.G. Bloom, J. Lemerle and M.K. Neidhardt) 2nd Edn. Springer-Verlag, Berlin, pp. 238–251

150. Warden, M.J., German, J.C. and Buckingham, B.A. (1988) Surgical management of hyperinsulinism in infancy due to nesidioblastosis. *J. Pediat. Surg.*, **23**, 162–165

151. Wells, H.G. (1940) Occurrence and significance of congenital malignant neoplasms. *Arch. Path.*, **30**, 535–601

152. Wexler, H.A., Poole, C.A. and Fojaco, R.M. (1975) Metastatic neonatal Wilms' tumour. *Paediat. Radiol.*, **3**, 179–181

153. Wigger, H.J. (1969) Fetal hamartoma of kidney. *Am. J. Clin. Path.*, **51**, 323–337

154. Wilms, M. (1899) *Die Mischgeschwülste der Niere*. A. Georgi, Leipzig

155. Yakovac, W.C., Baker, L. and Hummeler, K. (1971) Beta cell nesidioblastosis in idiopathic hypoglycemia of infancy. *J. Pediat.*, **79**, 226–231

156. Ziegler, E.E. (1945) Bilateral ovarian carcinoma in a 30 week foetus. *Arch. Path.*, **40**, 279–282

157. Ziegler, M.M. and Koop, C.E. (1980) Electrocoagulation induced immunity–an explanation for regression of neuroblastoma. *J. Pediat. Surg.*, **15**, 34–37

158. Zuckerman, I.C., Kershner, D., Laytner, B.D. and Hirschl, D. (1947) Leiomyoma of the kidney. *Ann. Surg.*, **126**, 220–228

14

Sacrococcygeal teratoma

Irene M. Irving

Congenital tumours are uncommon but amongst them the sacrococcygeal teratoma ranks as not only the most common congenital teratoma but also as the commonest neoplasm of the newborn [31].

Historical notes

The cuneiform tablets of the Chaldeans of about 2000 BC describe what appears to have been a sacrococcygeal teratoma; at least they refer to a baby born with three legs; two normal ones and one between the two normal extremities [4]. This may have been an example of an incomplete twin, of which there are numerous descriptions in the antique and medieval literature.

The first exact description of a sacrococcygeal teratoma in an infant was given by Saxtoph and Duvigneau in 1970 [30]. There is some disagreement as to who was the first surgeon to remove a sacrococcygeal tumour successfully but credit should go to Stanley [28] who reported the first successful operation in 1841. The first to postulate the modern view on the aetiology of this tumour was Steinmann [29] in his doctorate thesis of 1905.

Aetiology

For a long time the difference between a teratoma and an incomplete twin was not appreciated and teratomas were regarded as a sort of fetus-in-fetu, partly because organs or parts of organs may be found in a tumour and partly because in the families of patients with teratoma twins have occurred more commonly than normal [22]. Steinmann [29] was the first to doubt this theory and he suggested that teratomas developed from embryonic cells derived from the primitive knot of Hensen, the caudal part

of the primitive streak. Amongst embryologists, Bremer [7] and amongst pathologists, Willis [35] strongly supported the theory that teratomas arise from totipotent or pluripotent cells separated off from the primitive streak. The more modern view, which has evolved from the work of Teilum [32] is that the totipotential stem cells from which sacrococcygeal (and other non-gonadal) teratomas arise are primitive germ cells which have gone astray during their migration from the endoderm of the yolk sac to the genital ridge in the retroperitoneum. The teratoma is therefore classified as a germ cell tumour [5]. The aberrant germ cell can differentiate either into embryonal structures (giving rise to teratoma) or into extraembryonic structures, namely trophoblast (giving rise to choriocarcinoma) or yolk sac (giving rise to yolk sac tumour, otherwise known as Teilum's tumour, endodermal sinus tumour or embryonal carcinoma). Whereas teratomas are frequently well-differentiated, mature, benign tumours, choriocarcinomas and yolk sac tumours are highly malignant; yolk sac tumour is the most likely malignant component of a teratoma [12,24].

Pathology

Sacrococcygeal tumours can occur at any age, but are most commonly observed during the neonatal period. They have been observed in aborted fetuses, and nowadays are being diagnosed with increasing frequency *in utero* by maternal ultrasonography (Figure 14.1). A high proportion of these fetuses die *in utero* or at birth; Flake and colleagues [13] reported fetal death in 15 of 22 reported cases, from a variety of causes including preterm labour due to tumour mass and associated polyhydramnios, fetal exsanguination due to massive haemorrhage into the

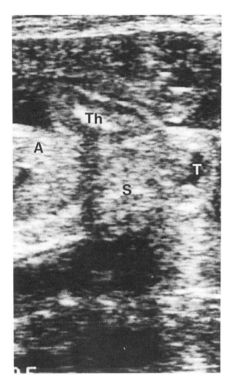

Figure 14.1 Prenatal ultrasound diagnosis of sacrococcygeal teratoma. A = fetal abdomen; Th = flexed thigh; S = sacrum; T = tumour with central cystic area

Type III: tumours which are apparent externally but have a mass which is predominantly pelvic and extends into the abdomen.
Type IV: presacral tumours with no external presentation.

In the survey, 47% of cases were type I and types I and II combined accounted for 81% of cases.

Histologically all three germ layers are represented. The differentiation can be made between mature teratomas with only well-differentiated components, immature teratomas in which the components show varying degrees of embryonic differentiation and malignant teratomas in which frankly

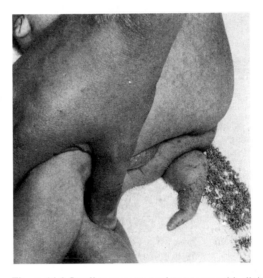

Figure 14.2 Small sacrococcygeal teratoma with digit growing from it

tumour either *in utero* or during labour and delivery, and tumour rupture during vaginal delivery or caesarean section. Placentomegaly with hydrops foetalis was observed in one-third of the cases and was a sign of imminent death *in utero*.

The tumour is usually rounded or lobulated, and well encapsulated. Very occasionally, appendages of grossly recognizable anatomical structures are observed; for example, in one of our cases a well-formed digit was seen growing from the mass of the tumour (Figure 14.2). The cut surfaces of teratomas are very variable in appearance; they may be predominantly cystic or solid, or a mixture of the two (Figure 14.3). Organs or parts of organs may sometimes be recognizable (Figure 4.4).

In the 1974 report of the American Academy of Pediatrics Surgical Sections (AAPSS) Survey of 405 cases of sacrococcygeal teratoma, Altmann and his colleagues [1] suggested the following classification of tumours according to anatomical site:

Type I: tumours which are predominantly external (sacrococcygeal) with only a minimal presacral component.
Type II: tumours presenting externally but with a significant intrapelvic extension.

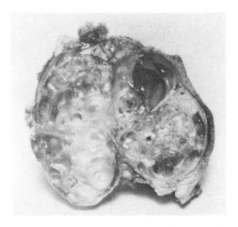

Figure 14.3 Cut surface of sacrococcygeal teratoma showing partly solid, partly cystic contents

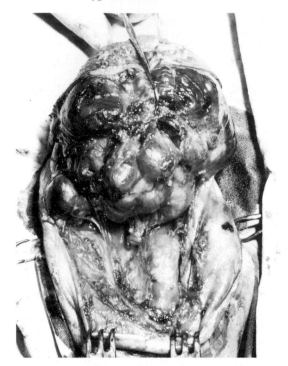

Figure 14.4 Benign sacrococcygeal teratoma in a female neonate, containing brain tissue which could be identified easily on naked-eye examination

The reason for the increased incidence of malignancy in presacral teratomas appears to be the fact that these tumours frequently go undiagnosed until they produce symptoms. Overall, approximately 18% of sacrococcygeal tumours are malignant [1,23]. The malignant teratoma will invade bone locally as well as the spinal cord and the rectum, and will metastasize, in particular to regional nodes, lungs, liver and vertebrae.

Incidence

Sacrococcygeal teratoma is regarded as being comparative rare; Riker and Potts [27] found fewer than 100 cases in the literature prior to 1948 and the overall incidence is generally quoted as being in the neighbourhood of 1 per 40 000 births [5,10]. However, the high proportion of intrauterine deaths observed in cases diagnosed antenatally [13] suggests that cases coming to surgery represent the 'tip of the iceberg' and that the true incidence must be considerably higher than the figure quoted above. From mid-1953 to 1985, 39 newborn infants with sacrococcygeal teratomas were treated in the Liverpool Neonatal Surgical Centre. Six of the 39 were admitted during the last year of the 32.5 year period. Eighty-one per cent were girls, a predominance which accords with other reports [1,9,11,31]. Only one of the 39 tumours was malignant.

neoplastic tissue is identified [10,31]. In some tumours the histological distinction between malignant and poorly differentiated embryonic tissue is difficult, and, especially in the case of very large tumours, a small focus of malignancy could easily be missed [12]. Raney and colleagues [25] have, in fact, reported a case in which a malignant area (in one of 22 sections) was found only on reviewing an apparently benign tumour after malignant recurrence. All sacrococcygeal teratomas have a malignant potential regardless of location [8]. In the newborn the great majority of the tumours are benign but with increasing age the number of teratomas with malignant degeneration increases rapidly [9,15,21,22,23,34]. In the AAPSS survey [1] the incidence of malignancy was 7% for neonatal tumours, 37% at 1 year of age and 50% at the age of 2 years. Billmire and Grosfeld [6], in an analysis of 84 cases, found 3% malignancy in patients under 1 month of age whereas the incidence in patients over the age of 1 month was 38%.

It has been noted that presacral teratomas have a higher incidence of malignancy than have sacrococcygeal ones [1,2,14,15,23], with the exception of the familial type described by Ashcraft and Holder [3] in which the incidence of malignancy is very low.

Clinical picture

Family, gestation and delivery history

Ashcraft and Holder [3] have reported an hereditary type of presacral teratoma associated with anal stenosis and sacral defects, with an autosomal dominant pattern of inheritance.

As mentioned previously, sacrococcygeal tumours are being diagnosed *in utero* with increasing frequency. In four of our cases a fetal mass was discovered on prenatal ultrasonography but the precise diagnosis was made in only one of these, at 20 weeks in a twin pregnancy. Bilateral hydronephrosis was noted in another of these fetuses.

In the AAPSS survey [1] more than 90% of the infants were full-term babies and were delivered normally; 9% were delivered by caesarean section, these being mainly infants with very large tumours which may have precluded vaginal delivery. Four of our infants were delivered by caesarean section, but for reasons other than the tumour in all but the one who was diagnosed prenatally; she was delivered by elective caesarean section. In two cases dystocia occurred; both infants were delivered vaginally, one after 'puncture' of the tumour (which weighed

1.55 kg) and the other only after the tumour (1.34 kg) had separated completely from the infant (1.73 kg), who later required removal of only a small remnant of tumour.

Presenting features

In about three-quarters of the cases (Altmann's types I and II) the infant is born with a rounded, often bossed cystic or solid mass overlying the sacrum and coccyx. The mass is usually in the midline but may be paramedian. Size ranges from a huge mass as big as the baby to a small inconspicuous mass in the buttock; the majority are large. The overlying skin is usually normal although in some there may be patches of port-wine staining and very occasionally the skin may be necrotic. We have seen a case in which the lesion was partially skin-covered and partially covered by patches of thin membrane overlying cysts, some of which had ruptured. Rupture of the teratoma is, however, rare in the newborn period, although it can occur during delivery as can haemorrhage into the tumour. If there is an intrapelvic extension the anus is pushed forward and on rectal examination the tumour can be palpated as a cystic or solid swelling lying presacrally. If there is an intra-abdominal extension, as in three of our cases, an abdominal mass can be palpated. Tumours which are entirely or almost entirely presacral in location (Altmann types III and IV) are not often encountered in the neonate, being diagnosed as a rule only at a later age when symptoms arise as a result of colonic or urinary tract obstruction [14,21]. Only one of our neonates had an entirely presacral tumour; she was admitted on the day after birth because of abdominal distension and a presacral mass was felt on rectal examination.

Associated anomalies

Associated anomalies can be expected in about one-fifth of the cases, the most common being musculo-skeletal anomalies with renal, CNS, cardiac and gastrointestinal tract anomalies occurring less frequently [1]. In our series spina bifida was found in eight cases, unstable hips in three (bilateral in two), and there was one instance each of hydrocolpos, cystic kidney, bifid penis, bilateral cryptorchidism, anal stenosis and pigmented naevus.

Radiology/imaging

Anteroposterior and lateral radiographs of pelvis and spine are taken routinely. Calcification is seen frequently and may be diffuse or in the form of recognizable structures, such as incompletely formed bones, or toothbuds (Figure 14.5); it was recorded in 44% of our cases. Calcification is a feature of both benign and malignant lesions [15]

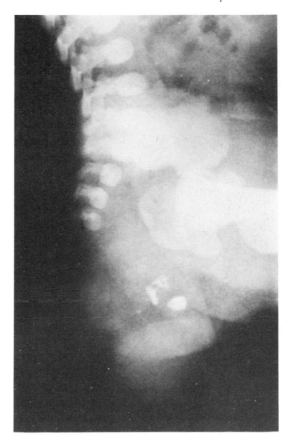

Figure 14.5 Showing densely calcified shadows in sacrococcygeal teratoma

but is less common in the malignant lesions [19]. The sacral spine is usually normal but may show developmental defects or destructive lesions [3,10]. Concave defects of the back of the vertebral bodies and neural arch defects are highly suggestive of intraspinal extension [10], but this is an unlikely finding in neonatal cases. Intrapelvic and abdominal extensions will be seen as soft tissue masses, with or without calcification, displacing the gas-containing bowel (Figures 14.6 and 14.7). Rectal gas should normally be seen directly against the sacrum on the lateral radiograph [10].

Ultrasonography (Figure 14.8) is of great value in determining whether the tumour is predominantly solid or cystic, in identifying the extent of pelvic or abdominal extensions and in identifying secondary obstructive uropathy. Kirk and Lister [20] found upper urinary tract dilatation pre-operatively in three of a series of 24 sacrococcygeal tumours and we have seen three such cases, all Altmann types III or IV

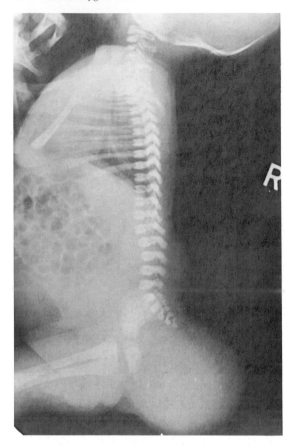

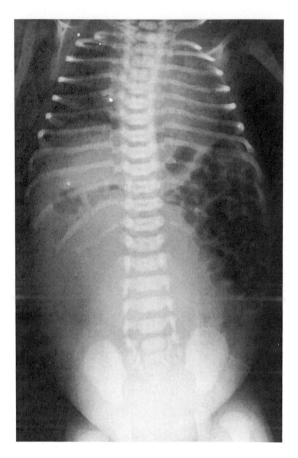

Figure 14.6 Showing slight calcification in a sacrococcygeal teratoma which has a large retroperitoneal extension displacing bowel forwards and upwards

Figure 14.7 Anteroposterior view of the same case as Figure 14.6. The retroperitoneal extension of the tumour is here seen to occupy most of the abdomen

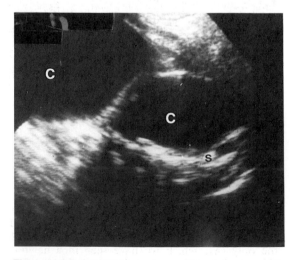

Figure 14.8 Sagittal ultrasound scan of an abdomino-pelvic sacrococcygeal teratoma shows it to be a bilocular cystic structure; this was confirmed at surgery. C = cyst; S = sacrum

On occasion, particularly if malignancy is suspected or if the diagnosis is in doubt, a CT scan will provide useful supplementary information about the extent of the mass within the pelvis, the integrity of the sacrum, the presence of intraspinal extension, etc.

Serum alpha-fetoprotein

Serum alpha-fetoprotein (AFP) is a very useful serum marker in sacrococcygeal teratoma, as an indicator of malignancy. The production of AFP by malignant sacrococcygeal teratomas conforms with the concept of these tumours being of yolk sac origin. Tsuchida and Hasegawa [33] collected 61 cases, from various centres in Japan, in which serum AFP levels had been studied in infants and children with teratomas from various sites. AFP levels were analysed in comparison with the distribution of normal serum AFP values in early infancy. Because these levels remain high for some months postnatally it was doubted whether it would be possible to use AFP as a tumour marker in the first few months of life. In fact, a clear correlation was made between the serum AFP level and the histological classification of the tumour; levels were above the normal range in 31 of 32 malignant teratomas, three of four 'immature' tumours and in only one of 24 mature tumours. Billmire and Grosfeld [6] reported similar findings in 29 patients; elevated AFP levels in 100% of malignant lesions, 50% of immature lesions and 6% of mature benign lesions. Eight of our patients, all with benign lesions, had serum AFPs within the normal range for age. One great value of the AFP marker lies in its use for serial postoperative monitoring for malignant recurrence; the early warning which it provides allows for commencement of treatment when the tumour bulk is small, thus increasing the chances of a successful outcome. This will be dealt with further, later in the chapter.

Differential diagnosis

The great majority of sacrococcygeal tumours presenting at birth can be diagnosed without any difficulty. Problems of diagnosis are most likely to arise with comparative small lesions and with Altmann types III and IV. The most important differential diagnoses are myelomeningoceles and chordomas.

Sacral myelomeningocele

Typically a myelomeningocele is membrane-covered, situated at a higher level than a sacrococcygeal teratoma and associated with neurological deficit. The distinction can be more difficult if the lesion is skin-covered. A simple clinical test is to press on the tumour; if the anterior fontanelle does not become distended the most likely diagnosis is sacrococcygeal teratoma [10]. The most important clue, however, is the fact that teratomas tend to displace the anus forwards (Figure 14.9). A lipomeningocele can present more difficulty but this also lies at a higher level, and in addition is a less circumscribed mass. Anterior myelomeningoceles are extremely rare; on clinical grounds the distinction from an Altmann type IV teratoma would be difficult; hence the value of CT scanning in such situations, especially in the neonate in whom radiological assessment of the sacrum may be difficult [18].

Chordoma

Chordoma, arising from remnants of the notochord, is very rare in newborn infants. It can occur anywhere along the spinal axis but is most common

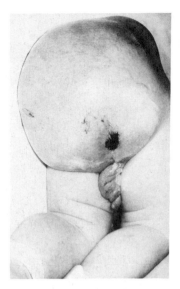

Figure 14.9 Sacrococcygeal teratoma displacing the anus forwards and downwards. In this case the anus was held open by a firm ring of encircling tumour

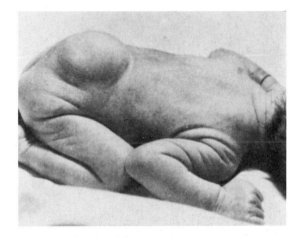

Figure 14.10 Infant with chordoma

in the sacrococcygeal region [26]. These tumours are typically situated in front of the sacrum, usually destroy bone and infiltrate into the spinal canal. In the only case which we have seen in a newborn (Figure 14.10) this was not the case and, apart from the fact that the anus was not displaced forwards, the clinical characteristics appeared to be identical with those of a teratoma.

Treatment

Pre-operative treatment

The newborn infant is prepared for operation according to the principles described in Chapter 6. A thoroughly reliable intravenous drip must be established (in an arm vein (Figure 14.11)) as blood loss can be copious; operative deaths resulting from haemorrhage have been recorded [1]. If blood has not already been taken for serum AFP estimation it can conveniently be taken by the anaesthetist.

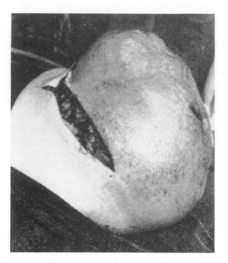

Figure 14.12 Lateral view of skin incision for removal of large sacrococcygeal teratoma. Note small vertical extension over midline of sacrum at the apex of the inverted V

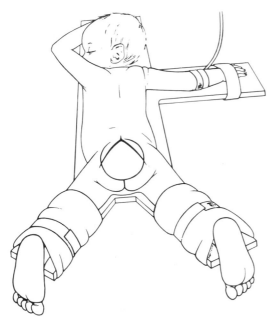

Figure 14.11 Position of the infant on the operating table for excision of sacrococcygeal tumour. The skin incision is outlined

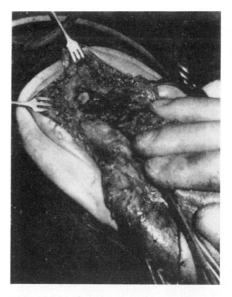

Figure 14.13 Excision of sacrococcygeal teratoma. The divided sacrum can be seen in the upper part of the wound. The tumour has been dissected free from lateral skin flaps and gluteal muscles which are seen being retracted laterally. The tumour mass is retracted downwards and dissected off the rectum from above downwards

Operation

The treatment of choice is complete operative removal of the tumour *en bloc* with the coccyx as soon as possible after diagnosis. As almost all teratomas are benign in the newborn period, and as the danger of malignancy increases rapidly with age, the operation should be done during the first 2 weeks of life and, if at all possible, during the first few days.

Sacrococcygeal operation

The child is placed in the prone position with the face turned sideways. The lower abdomen is raised

on a small sandbag or rolled-up towel and the legs are abducted (Figure 14.11). The rectum is packed with a generous amount of vaseline gauze to help in its identification during the operation. The skin incision is in the form of an inverted V ('chevron') with the apex placed at the upper limit of the base of the teratoma (Figure 14.11). It is helpful to make a small (1–2 cm long) incision from the apex of the V, running upwards in the midline over the lower segments of the sacrum (Figure 14.12). The junction between the fourth and fifth segments of the sacrum is identified and divided, leaving the coccyx and last sacral segment attached to the tumour. Removal of the coccyx is a very important step in the operation as it has been shown that if it is left behind, the danger of tumour recurrence and hence of malignancy is greatly increased [15,16,21]. The middle sacral vessels, which usually provide the main blood supply to the tumour, are ligated and divided.

The lateral skin flaps are now gradually raised and the tumour mass is dissected free from above downwards (Figure 14.13), commencing with any presacral extension. Care should be taken not to keep too close to the tumour; this is comparatively easy on its dorsal aspect, where the subcutaneous fat and splayed-out gluteal musculature can be divided with the diathermy needle at some distance from the tumour, but on its ventral aspect the tumour is often 'wrapped around' the rectum and even the anal canal (Figure 14.9) and has to be dissected off with scissors; numerous small bleeding vessels in the rectal wall need to be tied. Difficulty may also be encountered in removing extensions of tumour in the ischiorectal fat; here recognition of the transition from tumour to normal tissue can be particularly difficult.

When the tumour has finally been dissected completely free it is removed, together with the hinged triangular skin flap overlying it which is cut across, behind, and at a distance from, the anus. The greatly lengthened rectum will now be seen running down from the sacrum in an S-shaped curve to the anus (Figure 14.14).

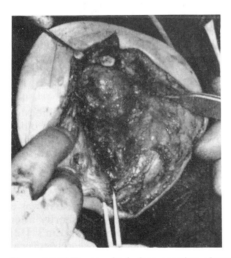

Figure 14.14 Tumour bed after resection of sacrococcygeal tumour. The divided sacrum is seen in the upper angle of the wound. The greatly lengthened S-shaped rectum can be seen running down the centre of the depth of the wound

The wound is now closed. Firstly, the levator ani is repaired as accurately as possible behind the rectum, and also hitched up to the presacral fascia with a few sutures, thus elevating the anus. The subcutaneous tissues are then repaired after any excess of skin has been trimmed away, and the skin is closed in the shape of an inverted Y. A glove-rubber drain down to the presacral space is left in. The rectal vaseline gauze pack is removed and a pressure dressing applied.

Abdominal operation

When the tumour extends into the abdomen it must be removed by a combined abdominosacral operation [17]. The abdomen is opened through a transverse subumbilical incision which, if necessary, can be extended upwards and laterally. The tumour is dissected free from the pelvic viscera and the middle sacral vessels are ligated and divided. The mass must be freed as far down into the pelvis as possible but its attachment to the coccyx must be left intact. The dissection can be difficult if the tumour

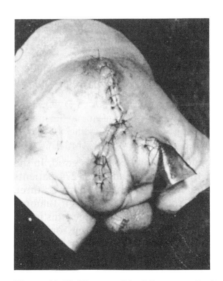

Figure 14.15 Closure of incision at end of operation for excision of sacrococcygeal teratoma

is impacted in the pelvis and if the tumour can be reduced in volume by aspiration of cyst or cysts this should be done, with precautions against spillage. The abdomen is now closed and the infant positioned, as described previously, for the sacrococcygeal operation. This proceeds as described, with transection of the lower sacrum. The mobilized intrapelvic mass is then delivered, whereupon the lower part of the tumour is dissected off rectum, gluteus muscles and levator ani, with closure as described. In one of our cases a very large solid

called mesonephroma ovarii (Schiller) and extra-embryonic (yolk sac – allantoic) structures of the rat's placenta. *Cancer*, **12**, 1092–1105

33. Tsuchida, Y. and Hasegawa, H. (1983) The diagnostic value of alpha-fetoprotein in infants and children with teratomas: a questionnaire survey in Japan. *J. Pediat. Surg.*, **18**, 152–155

34. Vaez-Zadeh, K., Sieber, W.K., Sherman, F.E. and Kiesewetter, W.B. (1972) Sacrococcygeal teratomas in children. *J. Pediat. Surg.*, **7**, 152–156

35. Willis, R.A. (1953) *Pathology of Tumours*. Butterworths, London

15

Conjoined twins

U.G. Stauffer

The birth of conjoined (Siamese) twins is even today generally received with emotion and fascination. The most famous twins were Chang and Eng Bunker, born in 1811 in Siam in a small community 30 miles from Bangkok, to a half-Chinese, half-Siamese mother and a Chinese father. These twins were united at the umbilicus by a bridge of tissue 17 cm in circumference, never underwent surgery and lived together for 63 years. They went to the USA, joining the P.T. Barnum side show, retired later to a farm near Mt Airy, North Carolina, married identical twin sisters and founded big families; Chang was the father of ten, Eng of nine children. They both died in 1874, within half an hour of each other. The fascinating historical and pathological facts of Chang and Eng are reported in detail by Luckhardt [30]. Since then, 'Siamese twins' is the best known term for conjoined twins all over the world. More than 600 cases have been described in the medical literature; however, most of these were based on autopsy reports and a successful surgical separation of conjoined twins is still a rare event.

Historical notes

The first attempt at surgical separation of conjoined twins was carried out as early as 1689 by Farius [2] but both children died. Only 1 year later, in 1690, König in Germany reported the first successful surgical separation of conjoined twins in the medical literature [46]; König's twins were united only by an abdominal skin bridge. During the next 250 years, only nine additional attempts to separate conjoined twins surgically could be recorded by Kiesewetter [26]. Undoubtedly, many other twins have undergone surgical separation, but they have not been

reported because the operation has been unsuccessful. The first partially successful operation with survival of one of conjoined twins sharing one organ was reported by Doyen in 1902. The twins were united at the abdomen by a bridge containing liver [46]. In 1972 Bankole and his co-workers [4] reviewed all operated cases from the world literature, from Farius in 1689 to 1971, and found 55 cases, 43 of them having been operated on after 1950. From 1972 to 1986, 27 additional surgical separations have been reported from various centres throughout the world. Excellent historical reviews of the entire subject of conjoined twins are found in the papers by Aird [2], Dragstedt [8], Kiesewetter [26] and Luckhardt [30].

Incidence

The general incidence of conjoined twins has been reported as ranging from 1 per 50 000 to 1 per 100 000 births [4,10,26,27,38,44,49]. In the USA 81 sets of conjoined twins out of 7 903 000 births were registered by the birth defects monitoring programme, a nationwide congenital malformation surveillance system that monitors discharge diagnosis associated with one-third of the births in the USA [10]. Conjoined twins are more common in females than in males by 2 or 3:1 [10,26,27,49]. Aird [3] speculated that six or more operable cases per year could be expected throughout the world if all cases were reported.

Classification

Many different classifications of conjoined twins have been suggested [4,11,12,19,21]. The classification derived by combining the anatomical area of

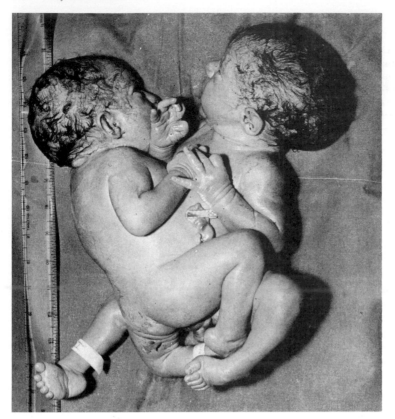

Figure 15.1 Conjoined twins born alive in Liverpool. They were joined from the lower chest wall to the perineum

tion derived by combining the anatomical area of union with the Greek root 'pagos', meaning 'that which is fixed', is convenient and informative for practical use [11,26,29,37,42,49]. The five types generally recognized are: thoracopagus, joined at the chest (40%); xipho- or omphalopagus, joined by the anterior abdominal wall from the xyphoid process to the level of the umbilicus or lower (34%) (Figure 15.1); pygopagus, joined at the buttocks (18%); ischiopagus, where the twins are joined in a linear fashion at the pelvis (6%); and the rarest type, craniopagus twins, those whose heads are joined (2%) [26,42]. Ischiopagus twins may be subdivided, according to the number of lower extremities present, as ischiopagus bipus, tripus and tetrapus (Figure 15.2). Of 81 conjoined twins registered by the birth defects monitoring programme in the USA from 1970 to 1977, the most common types were thoraco-omphalopagus (28%), thoracopagus (18%), and omphalopagus (10%) twins [10]. Of 117 conjoined twins collected by Tartuffi [42] 86 were either thoracopagus or xipho-pagus twins, 22 were pygopagus, seven ischiopagus and only two craniopagus twins.

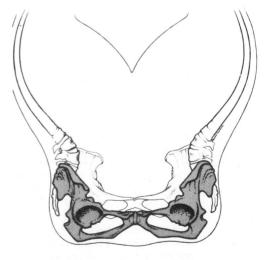

Figure 15.2 The same twins as in Figure 15.1. As well as being xipho- and omphalopagus they had a common pelvic ring and were therefore also ischiopagus tetrapus twins

Embryology

Conjoined twins arise from a single ovum within a single blastocyst, the outer trophoblastic shell of which forms the later chorionic sac or fetal portion of the developing placenta [11,52,59]. They are therefore monovular, monozygotic and monochorionic and have the same chromosomal pattern and the same sex. Duplication which leads to normal monovular twins occurs after the formation of the blastocyst and before the primary axis forms, probably after the fifth day, but before the 20th day after fertilization [6,52,53,59]. Conjoined twins result when this twinning process is incomplete. Various degrees of incomplete separation or axial duplication [9,49] result in the various types of conjoined twins. The embryology of monovular twins is well described in more detail by Corner [6], Filler [11], Streeter [52] and Zimmermann [59].

Aetiology

The cause of this incomplete separation is unknown. In most reported cases where a prenatal history was available, the pregnancy had been uneventful [10,31,42]. Conjoined twins have been induced in experimental animals with such diverse agents as butyric acid, acetone, manganese deficiency and radiation [19]. The cause of the striking female predominance in conjoined twins is still unknown.

Clinical picture

Most conjoined twins are born dead or die shortly after birth because of severe associated malformations incompatible with life. There is another group of conjoined twins who are severely injured by a traumatic delivery which may be the cause of death, as in one of the cases observed in the Zürich department. In a pair of omphalopagus twins the diagnosis was missed until the first of the twins had already passed partially into the vagina. Severe intrauterine asphyxia occurred and the obstetrician finally divided the bridge between the two twins blindly with scissors. The children, both of whom died, could probably have been saved by surgery. Antenatal diagnosis is therefore of prime importance: (1) to decide on the management of pregnancy; termination of pregnancy may be indicated if the diagnosis is made before the 20th, at the latest the 24th week but decisions concerning the management of pregnancy should always take into account survival chances following possible surgical separation; (2) to decide on the least traumatic route for delivery, if pregnancy goes to term; and (3) to alert paediatricians and surgical specialists to be prepared for the birth of a pair of conjoined twins

[13.23]. When the diagnosis is made intrapartum, caesarean section should be considered immediately unless the delivery proceeds in an orderly and atraumatic manner which is only possible with very small babies. Obstetricians should be aware that salvage of one or both twins is often possible; they should not, therefore, be sacrificed without thought.

Prenatal diagnosis and management

In recent years, ultrasonography has become the method used most commonly to diagnose and evaluate multiple pregnancies [28]. The first reported case of antenatal ultrasound diagnosis of conjoined twins in different presentations has been reported by Koontz *et al.* [28]. According to these authors the findings associated with conjoined twins are (1) lack of a separating membrane, (2) inability to separate the fetal bodies, (3) presence of fetal anomalies, (4) identification of more than three vessels in a single umbilical cord and (5) sonographic detection of any of the classic radiological signs stated earlier by Gray [18] and others: the twins may face each other; the fetal hands are at the same level and plane; the thoracic cages of the fetuses are together or in close proximity to each other; there may be an unusual backward flexion of the cervical spines; no change in the relative position of the fetuses is seen on repeated examinations. In case of

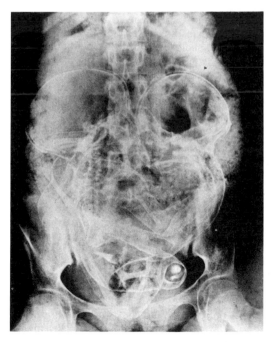

Figure 15.3 Amniography carried out by injecting radio-opaque dye into the amniotic sac by Mr H. Francis confirmed the antenatal diagnosis of conjoined twins

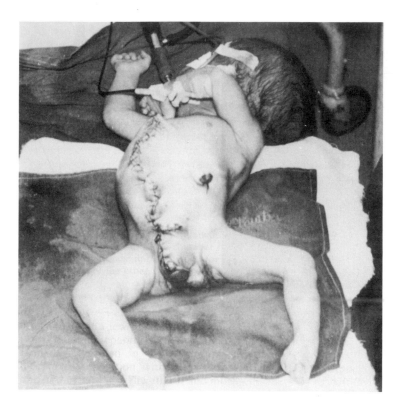

Figure 15.8 The viable twin at the end of the operation. The colon has been pulled through to the perineum. This child died 6 weeks later of severe recurrent pneumonia

successfully separated thoracopagus twins have been reported since 1972. Of the 25 well-documented cases of thoracopagus twins reported in the literature by Marin *et al.* [32] 75% had a conjoined heart with associated cardiovascular anomalies making them unsuitable for surgical separation even at the cost of the life of one of them. According to Schmaltz *et al.* [47] successful separation of thoracopagus twins has never been reported in twins with ventricular fusion and only once in twins with atrial fusion; the other survivors had a pericardial union only. Until 1972, 12 craniopagus twins were operated upon; four pairs survived, four pairs died and in four cases one infant survived [4]. In 1987, the Baltimore team reported for the first time the survival of both children after separation of craniopagus twins who had a common vena cerebri magna Galeni (Haller, personal communication). Of the four ischiopagus twins operated on before 1972, only one pair survived; two pairs died and in one case one twin had to be sacrificed [4]. At least seven partially successful separations of ischiopagus twins have been reported since then; however, many of these children have to live with considerable handicaps. It is obvious that these reported figures are necessarily selective and much too optimistic; probably a large number of unsuccessful operations are not reported in the literature.

References

1. Abrams, S.L., Callen, P.W. and Anderson, R.L. (1985) Anencephaly with encephalocele in craniopagus twins: prenatal diagnosis by ultrasonography and computed tomography. *J. Ultrasound Med.*, **4**, 485–488
2. Aird, I. (1954) The conjoined twins of Kano. *Br. Med. J.*, **1**, 831–837
3. Aird, I. (1959) Conjoined twins: further observation. *Br. Med. J.*, **1**, 1313–1320
4. Bankole, M.A., Odutan, S.A., Oluwasanmi, J.O. *et al.* (1972) The conjoined twins of Warri, Nigeria. *Arch. Surg.*, **104**, 294–301
5. Blum, E., Pearlman, M. and Graham, D. (1986) Early second-trimester sonographic diagnosis of thoracopagus twins. *JCU*, **14**, 207–208
6. Corner, G.W. (1922) The morphological theory of monochorionic twins as illustrated by a series of supposed early twin embryos of the pig. *Johns Hopkins Hosp. Bull.*, **33**, 389
7. Cywes, S. and Bloch, C.E. (1964) Conjoined twins: a review with a report of a case. *S. Afr. Med.*, **38**, 817–821
8. Dragstedt, L.R. (1957) Siamese twins. *Q. Bull. N.West Univ. Med. Sch.*, **31**, 359
9. Eades, J.W. and Thomas, C.G. (1966) Successful separation of ischiopagus tetrapus conjoined twins. *Ann. Surg.*, **164**, 1059–1072

10. Edmonds, L.D. and Layde, P.M. (1982) Conjoined twins in the United States, 1970–1977. *Teratology*, **25**, 301–308

11. Filler, R.M. (1986) Conjoined twins and their separation. *Semin. Perinatol.*, **10**, 82–91

12. Fischer, C.J. (1865–1868) Diploteratology; an essay on compound human monsters, comprising the history, literature, classification, description, and embryology of double and triple formation, including the so-called parasitic monsters, foetus in foetu, and supernumerary formation of parts or organs in man. *Trans. Med. Soc. St. N.Y.*, 1865, 232; 1866, 207; 1867, 396; 1868, 276

13. Gans, S.L., Morgenstern, L., Gettelman, E. *et al.* (1968) Separation of conjoined twins in the newborn period. *J. Pediat. Surg.*, **3**, 565–574

14. Gille, P., Aubert, D., Mourat, M. *et al.* (1983) Séparation de siamois pygopages. *Chir Pédiatr.*, **24**, 100–104

15. Golladay, E.S., Williams, G.D., Seibert, J.J. *et al.* (1982) Dicephalus dipus conjoined twins: A surgical separation and review of previously reported cases. *J. Pediat. Surg.*, **17**, 259–264

16. Grantzow, R., Hecker, W.Ch., Holschneider, A.M. *et al.* (1983) Zur Trennung eines symmetrischen Ischiopagenpaaares. *Z. Kinderchir.*, **39**, 204–210

17. Grantzow, R., Hecker, W.Ch., Holschneider, A.M. *et al.* (1985) Trennung eines asymmetrischen Xiphoomphalo-ischiopagus tripus. *Langenbecks Arch. Chir.*, **363**, 195–206

18. Gray, C.M., Nix, H.G. and Wallace, A.J. (1950) Thoracopagus twins: pre-natal diagnosis. *Radiology*, **54**, 398–399

19. Guttmacher, A.F. and Nichol, B.L. (1967) Teratology of conjoined twins. *Birth Defects*, **3**, 3

20. Herbert, W.N., Cefalo, R.C. and Koontz, W.L. (1983) Perinatal management of conjoined twins. *Am. J. Perinatol.*, **1**, 58–63

21. Hirst, B.C. and Piersol, G.A. (1891) *Human Monstrosities*, Lea, Philadelphia, Vol. 1, p. 17

22. Intody, Z., Palffy, J., Hajdu, K. *et al.* (1986) Pränatale Diagnostik eines Thoracopagus in der 19. Schwangerschaftswoche. *Zentralbl. Gynäkol.*, **108**, 57–61

23. Jones, P. (1975) Supplement to the 1975 Annual Report; Royal Children's Hospital, Melbourne

24. Meningsberg, K. and Harper, R.G. (1982) Separation of omphalopagus twins. *J. Pediat. Surg.*, **17**, 255–258

25. Kou, H., Gara, F. and Gueddana, F. *et al.* (1985) Diagnostic échographic anténatal d'un monstre double a 20 semaines d'aménorrhée. *J. Gynecol. Obstet. Biol. Reprod. (Paris)*, **14**, 883–887

26. Kiesewetter, W. (1966) Surgery on conjoined (Siamese) twins. *Surgery*, **59**, 860–871

27. Kling, S., Johnston, R.J., Michalyshyn, B. *et al.* (1975) Successful separation of xiophopagus-conjoined twins. *J. Pediat. Surg.*, **10**, 267–271

28. Koontz, W.L., Herbert, W.N., Seeds, J.W. *et al.* (1983) Ultrasonography in the antepartum diagnosis of conjoined twins. A report of two cases. *J. Reprod. Med.*, **28**, 627–630

29. Koop, C.E. (1974) Separating the siamese twins: the surgeon's story. *Med. Wld News*, **8**, 90

30. Luckhardt, A.B. (1941) Report of the autopsy of the siamese twins together with other interesting information concerning their life. A sketch of the life of Chang and Eng. *Surg. Gynec. Obstet.*, **72**, 116–125

31. Lu, T. and Lee, K.H. (1967) Obstetrical management of conjoined twins. *J. Obstet. Gynaec. Br. Commonw.*, **74**, 757–762

32. Marin-Padilla, M., Chin, A.J. and Marin-Padilla, T.M. (1981) Cardiovascular abnormalities in thoracopagus twins. *Teratology*, **23**, 101–113

33. Nicols, B.L., Blatner, R.J. and Rudolph, A.J. (1967) General clinical management of thoracopagus twins. *Birth Defects*, **3**, 38–51

34. Oberniedermayr, A., Buehlmeyer, K., Fendel, H. *et al.* (1968) Bericht über die Operation bei neugeborenen Thorakopagen und über einen weiteren, aber nicht lebensfähigen Thorakopagus. *Z. Kinderchir.*, **6**, 162–174

35. Pe-Nyun and Htut Saing (1972) Thoracoomphalopagus conjoined twins of Burma. *J. Pediat. Surg.*, **7**, 691–699

36. Pepper, C.K. (1967) Ethical and moral considerations in the separation of conjoined twins: summary of two dialogues between physicians and clergymen. *Birth Defects*, **3**, 128–134

37. Poradowska, W., Jaworska, M., Reszke, S. *et al.* (1969) Conjoined twins and twin parasite: clinical analysis of three examples. *J. Pediat. Surg.*, **4**, 688–693

38. Potter, E.L. (1952) *Pathology of the Fetus and Infants*, 2nd Edn. Year Book Medical Publishers, Chicago, p. 216

39. Reitman, H., Smith, E.E. and Geller, J.S. (1953) Separation and survival of xiphopagus twins. *J. Am. Med. Ass.*, **153**, 1360–1362

40. Ricketts, R.R. and Zubowicz, V.N. (1987) Use of tissue expansion for separation and primary closure of thoracopagus twins. *Pediat. Surg. Int.*, **2**, 365–368

41. Riker, W. and Traisman, H. (1964) Xiphopagus conjoined twins. *Am. J. Surg.*, **108**, 277–284

42. Robertson, E.G. (1953) Craniopagus parietalis. *Arch. Neurol. Psychiat.*, **70**, 189–205

43. Ross, A.J. III, O'Neill, J.A. Jr, Silverman, D.G. *et al.* (1985) A new technique for evaluating cutaneous vascularity in complicated conjoined twins. *J. Pediat. Surg.*, **20**, 743–746

44. Rudolph, A.J., Michaels, P.J. and Nichols, B.L. (1967) Obstetric management of conjoined twins. *Birth Defects*, **3**, 28–37

45. Rydnert, J., Holmgren, G. and Nielsen, K. (1985) Prenatal diagnosis of conjoined twins (diprosopus) with myelomeningocele. *Acta Obstet. Gynecol. Scand.*, **64**, 687–688

46. Scammon, R.E. (1926) Fetal malformations. In *Abt's Pediatrics*, W.B. Saunders, Philadelphia, p. 678

47. Schmaltz, A.A., Kemter, B.E. and Obladen, M. (1984) Kardiovaskuläre Diagnostik bei Thorakopagen. *Klin. Pädiatr.*, **196**, 264–270

48. She, Y.X., Li, Z.C., Song, L.C. *et al.* (1985) Successful separation of xiphoomphalopagus twins. *Z. Kinderchir.*, **40**, 237–240

49. Simpson, J.S. (1969) Separation of conjoined thoracopagus twins, with the report of an additional case. *Can. J. Surg.*, **12**, 89–96

50. Somasundaram, K. and Wong, K.S. (1986) Ischiopagus tetrapus conjoined twins. *Br. J. Surg.*, **73**, 738–741

51. Spencer, R. (1956) Surgical separation of siamese twins: case report. *Surgery*, **39**, 827–833

52. Streeter, G.L. (1919) Formation of single-ovum twins. *Bull. Johns Hopkins Hosp.*, **30**, 235

53. Streeter, G.L. (1920) A human embryo (mateer) of the presomite period. *Contr. Embryol.*, **9**, 389–424

54. Turner, R.J., Hankins, G.D., Weinreb, J.C. *et al.* (1986) Magnetic resonance imaging and ultrasonography in the antenatal evaluation of conjoined twins. *Am. J. Obstet. Gynecol.*, **155**, 645–649

55. Upadhyaya, P. (1971) Surgical separation of xiphoomphalopagus conjoined twins. *J. Pediat. Surg.*, **6**, 462–465

56. Wilson, H. and Storer, E.H. (1957) Surgery in 'siamese' twins: a report of three sets of conjoined twins treated surgically. *Ann. Surg.*, **145**, 718–725

57. Wong, T.J., Lyou, Y.T., Chee, C.P. *et al.* (1986) Management of xiphopagus conjoined twins with small bowel obstruction. *J. Pediat. Surg.*, **21**, 53–57

58. Woolley, M. and Joergenson, E. (1964) Xiphopagus conjoined twins. *Am. J. Surg.*, **108**, 277–284

59. Zimmermann, A.A. (1967) Embryologic and anatomic considerations of conjoined twins. *Birth Defects*, **3**, 18–27

Part III

Head and neck

16

The Pierre Robin syndrome

A.R. Green and D.O. Maisels

Terminology

In recent times there has been a dispute as to whether the term Pierre Robin syndrome should be changed to the term Robin anomalad. A syndrome is defined as a set of symptoms which occur together, or the sum of the signs of any morbid state [7]. An anomalad refers to a single malformation together with its subsequently derived structural changes [25]. Although possibly the more correct term, we feel that the latter is clumsy and leads to misunderstanding, and hence we have continued to use the older style of Pierre Robin syndrome.

Historical note

M. le Docteur Pierre Robin was medical stomatologist at L'Hôpital des Enfants-Malades in Paris. He wrote extensively, mostly in French, on the problems of glossoptosis, presenting the results of his research to the Parisian Medical Academy during the 1920s [19]. His first article in English on this subject was published in the *American Journal of Diseases of Children* in 1934 and entitled 'Glossoptosis due to atresia and hypotrophy of the mandible' [20].

Robin was by no means the first to have written about the condition, it having been reported by St Hilaire in 1822 [18], Fairbairn in 1846 [10], Virchow in 1864 [27] and Shukowsky in 1911 [24]: however, his description of, and emphasis on, the problems encountered by these children in maintaining an airway, feeding and their resultant failure to thrive has correctly resulted in this eponymous attribution.

Definition

Robin described the state of a small jaw (whether retrognathic, which, by retaining its growth potential, will revert in a matter of months, or micrognathic, which will not) as being the cause of a glossoptosis severe enough to result in an airway obstruction and in feeding difficulties (Figure 16.1). Because it was these difficulties which Robin stressed, we, like others, feel that the label of Pierre Robin syndrome should be given only to those cases in which these signs are present and that one should *not* include those children who have been born unaffected by the presence of a small jaw.

The place of the cleft palate within the syndrome is debated. Most writers feel that a cleft of the secondary palate is an essential part of the syndrome. They argue that there must be a large palatal defect for the tongue to fall backwards to such an extent as to obstruct the pharynx. It is interesting to note, however, that Robin made no mention of the presence of a cleft palate in his first paper in English in 1934. Rather it was Eley and Farber [9] who 4 years earlier had described a similar situation in four children with cleft palate. Latham [12], in his treatise on the pathogenesis of cleft palate associated with Pierre Robin syndrome, estimates that 80% of cases will have clefting of the palate. Burston, in the previous edition of this chapter, felt that there were in fact two separate entities. Firstly, there was the mandibular retrognathic child with an associated cleft palate in whom it was rare to find other abnormalities. Secondly, he described the micrognathic patient in whom the palate was not cleft, but frequently high arched. These latter cases commonly have other developmental anomalies and

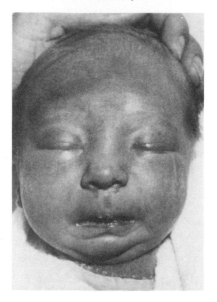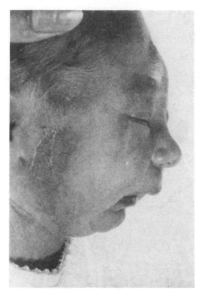

Figure 16.1 Neonate with marked mandibular retrognathia and cleft palate (see also Figure 16.3)

he suggested that where these children have associated cerebral impairment, they have a likely survival rate of under 50%. This group, however, accounted for only about 10% of children with the condition.

Associated conditions

The following conditions have been described as occurring with Pierre Robin syndrome.

Congenital heart disease (especially coarctation of the aorta and tetralogy of Fallot)
Stickler syndrome
Cerebrocostomandibular syndrome
Campomelic syndrome
Persistent left SVC syndrome
Spondyloepiphyseal dysplasia congenita
Congenital myotonic dystrophy
Diastrophic dwarfism
Beckwith–Wiedemann syndrome
Femoral hypoplasia
Radiohumoral synostosis syndrome
Fetal alcohol syndrome
Fetal hydantoin syndrome
Fetal trimethadione syndrome
Hyperphalangism
Congenital hepatic fibrosis

Aetiology

A single simple cause for Pierre Robin syndrome has not been proved. Mechanistic, genetic and teratogenic theories have been propounded.

Mechanical theory

The basic concept of the mechanical theory is that the syndrome can be completely explained by virtue of the development of a small jaw which is a direct result of restriction of intrauterine movement or abnormal uterine pressure. By not allowing fetal unfolding and extension of the neck, the jaw is entrapped firmly against the chest wall and retrognathia results. This in turn holds back the tongue, which becomes trapped between the developing palatal shelves, preventing their fusion, and causing a clefting of the secondary palate. This cleft has a recognizable 'U'-shape, conforming to the shape of the tongue, rather than the more usual V-shape seen in the non-Robin cleft palate. Latham [12] analysing a 17-week-old fetus has demonstrated tongue impaction between the palatal shelves (Figure 16.2).

Confirmatory evidence has been shown experimentally in rats, where the induction of oligohydramnios, either by cortisone administration [11] or by amniocentesis [16], at a suitable time in the rat's gestation period, prior to palatal fusion, will cause retrognathia and a cleft palate. The fact that a retrognathic jaw will in time grow to normal proportions (Figure 16.3), lends further weight to the argument that the initial factor is not one of defective germ plasm or lack of inherent growth potential.

Teratogenic theory

Edwards and Newal [8] feel that, although possibly rational in rats, the mechanistic theory cannot be

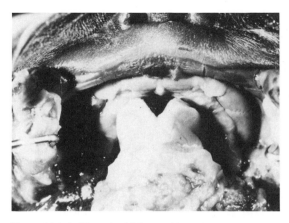

Figure 16.2 A 17-week-old fetus with cleft palate, showing the cleft in the tip of the tongue due to pressure on the nasal septum

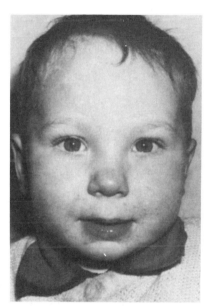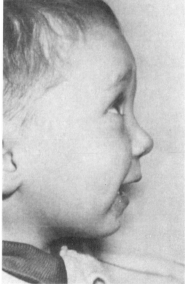

Figure 16.3 The child as in Figure 16.1 at 18 months, after palate repair: note the way in which the mandible has grown forward

Table 16.1 Experimental work on administration of teratogens

Agent	Animal	Reference	Abnormality
2-Deoxyguanosine	Duck yolk sac	[13]	Cleft palate and skeletal abnormalities
2-Deoxyguanosine	Duck yolk sac	[3]	Micrognathia + cleft palate
Hypervitaminosis A	Mouse	[23]	Retrognathia after palatal closure
6-Aminonicotinamide	Rat	[4]	Retrognathia + cleft palate (dose related)
Diazonorleucine	Rat	[6]	Cleft palate + inhibition Meckel's cartilage
ß-amino-propionitrate	Rat	[5]	Delayed elevation of palatal shelves related to retrognathia
Retinyl palmitate	Mouse	[14]	Spectrum of cleft palate malformations dependent on time of administration

tenable in humans. They feel that an inherent growth disorder must be present, and in keeping with other researchers [3–6,13,14,23] have been able to produce a variety of similar defects by the administration of teratogens (see Table 16.1).

Genetics

A truly inherited case of Pierre Robin syndrome is rare. The majority of cases occur as isolated incidents in families with a low risk of recurrence. There are children, however, with multiple defects where Pierre Robin syndrome is part of a wider condition in which a definite inherited trait is well recorded, e.g. Stickler syndrome.

Incidence

Estimates of the incidence of Pierre Robin syndrome vary markedly depending on the author's definition of the condition. Hence, reliable estimates are not readily available in standard texts. Bush and Williams [2] in their analysis of admissions to the Mersey Regional Cleft Palate Unit over the 23-year period 1960–82 (in a catchment area of 2.96 million inhabitants) demonstrated 110 cases which had been referred to the unit and which had fulfilled the following diagnostic criteria:

1. A typical 'U'-shaped cleft of the palate was present (Figure 16.4).

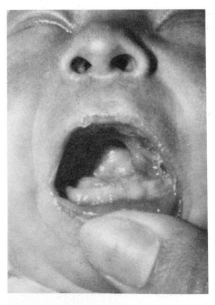

Figure 16.4 The neonate shown in Figure 16.1 to demonstrate the cleft palate and how easy it is for the tongue to fall back through the cleft

2. The cases had been hospitalized for at least 28 days with respiratory embarrassment and feeding problems, the majority of cases requiring to be nursed in the prone position on a cradle.
3. The diagnosis was confirmed by two orthodontists and a paediatrician. No case of mandibular retrognathia or micrognathia with an absence of cleft palate was included in the survey.

The combination of rigid selectivity of cases and the fact that the majority of cases occurring in the catchment area were being referred to the unit for assessment, led them to feel that their derived incidence figure of 1 per 8500 live births was a more realistic estimate than those of previous authors (1 in 2000, Poswillo [17], and 1 in 30 000, Rubin [22]. The mortality rate in this series was 21% (23 of 110), all deaths occurring in the first year of life.

Clinical presentation

The characteristic appearance of the undershot chin of the retrognathic child is unmistakable (Figure 16.1) and should alert the clinician to be wary of impending problems. Respiratory embarrassment occurs, especially when feeding. The classic clinical features of inspiratory distress, cyanosis, indrawing of the lower ribs and sternum and opisthotonos are all indicative of a severe degree of respiratory obstruction. Differential diagnosis must include other causes of acute neonatal respiratory embarrassment, especially choanal atresia and tracheo-oesophageal fistula. Milder degrees of the condition may, however, include subcyanotic attacks with restlessness and an airway obstruction occurring only if the child is lying on its back. These attacks can be of sinister significance, for they may initiate a vicious circle whereby the cerebral insult of a low oxygen tension can reduce the natural suck-swallow reflex (see below) and thus increase the likelihood of further attacks, the incoordinated swallow resulting in inhalation.

The tongue is usually of normal size, yet because of the small oral volume, may appear macroglossic. The degree of respiratory embarrassment is a direct correlation between the sizes of the tongue, cleft palate and oral cavity and the predilection for the tongue to fall backwards. The fact that the tongue has been involved in the aetiology of the condition is exhibited by the 'U'-shaped palate and the fact that the mucosal ulceration of the keel of the nasal septum, a common occurrence in the non-retrognathic cleft, is not seen in Pierre Robin syndrome children. The ulceration is caused by intrauterine tongue action and if the tongue has been trapped between palatal shelves, then this movement cannot occur. In addition, the tongue often has an anterior notch (Figure 16.2) which gives it a 'leaf-like' shape and results from the impingement of the tongue against the vomer.

Treatment

Burston emphasized that the true problem in patients with mandibular retrognathia was not purely the size and position of the tongue, but also the capacity of the infant to perform a properly coordinated suck–swallow mechanism. This can be hampered by surgical tethering of the tongue and hence the regimen used at the Regional Cleft Palate Unit at Alder Hey Hospital is based on a conservative non-surgical approach.

Conservative management

Early diagnosis of the condition at birth and recognition of the inherent dangers is important so that the child may be protected from, rather than require treatment for, serious cyanotic attacks. Transfer to a unit used to handling such cases is obviously an advantage and the child should be nursed on its front or side during transfer.

On admission, the child will, if its condition is severe enough, be nursed prone on a Burston frame (Figure 16.5) which constitutes a ventral plaster of Paris mould with adjustable head and arm pieces. Some care needs to be exerted to pad the plaster shell adequately and one needs to be aware of the possibility of damage to the facial nerve by pressure in the pretragal region and also of the danger of traction or pressure injuries to the brachial plexus. As the child grows the frame will require regular adjustment.

The advantage of the frame is that gravity will prevent the tongue from falling backwards and that regurgitation or vomitus will not be inhaled. Likewise, the excessive mucus formation which results from the inevitable rhinitis is neither ingested nor inhaled.

In some 50% of patients there is an element of head-moulding from the pressure of the frame on the forehead, causing the frontal bones to override the temporal bones. This condition is normally self-correcting, although several weeks may pass before complete reversion is achieved.

The child is initially kept on the frame continuously, except when feeding, at 3-h intervals, when it will be taken off. As time progresses, the child can be tried off the frame for 1 hour and then returned for a further 3 h. This type of regimen is required for at least the first 4 weeks and it may well take 3–4 months before an airway can adequately be maintained when off the frame. Discarding the frame is obviously a clinical decision to be taken individually for each patient. Monitoring when on the frame can be facilitated by use of a mirror situated beneath the face, so that nursing staff can see the facial colour. All children are nursed on an apnoea blanket.

Feeding

It cannot be stressed enough that the suck–swallow reflex must be stimulated early so that reliance on tube feeding is avoided. On admission a test feed with dextrose is given, so that should any feed be inhaled it will not cause harm. A 'grip tight' teat is usually adequate although a larger (lambs') teat has been required on occasions. The hole in the teat

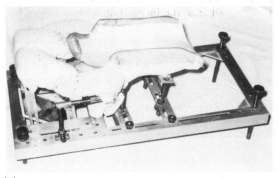

(a)

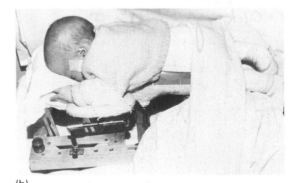

(b)

Figure 16.5 (a) The plaster shell set-up on the aluminium frame. The latter permits easy adjustment of the headboard, shell, and armrests. Screws are also provided to allow the frame as a whole to be tilted to the desired angle. (b) Infant lying on the cradle. Note the mirror beneath the face to allow easy observation of the jaw and tongue

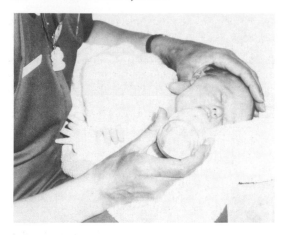

Figure 16.6 The feeding position recommended: note the sister's left thumb holding the mandible forward

normally requires enlargement until the delivery of food is adequate, but care not to exaggerate this is important as a flood of feed could easily be inhaled. The position when feeding is of paramount importance and the key to whether feeding will be successful (Figure 16.6).

The child should be laid on its side on the lap of the nurse, whose left hand supports the head and whose thumb is placed behind the angle of the jaw to project it forward, and so prevent the tongue blocking off the pharynx.

Should the child begin to cough or threaten to inhale, the nurse has only to allow her thigh to drop to put the child into a head-down position and so avert disaster. The feeding teat must be laid on the tongue and must not lie under the tongue, hence the nurse must be able to see and inspect the position of the teat.

Patience and time are required for a job that cannot and must not be rushed.

Supplementary tube feeds may be given during the night during sleep, not only in order to help weight gain, but also to prevent undue fatigue. It should be stressed, however, that the child will need to be hungry again the next morning if he is to resume an adequate oral intake. This regimen has now been in use at the Liverpool Unit for more than 20 years with an overall mortality rate of 21% [26]. Of 14 children who died in the years 1966–76 four children showed evidence of bronchopneumonia at necropsy although only one had a definite history of aspiration of feed [2].

Surgical management

Routledge [21] rightly felt that children with this condition required emergency treatment. He emphasized the necessity for anterior tongue fixation in Pierre Robin syndrome as the only way confidently to avoid the sequelae of glossoptosis. However, in those cases treated at Alder Hey Children's Hospital, it has been necessary to resort to surgery in only two cases, both of whom required just the insertion of a tongue stitch to help pull the tongue forward. We realize, however, that not all units will have the necessary time and resources at their disposal to pursue conservative management to a satisfactory conclusion. For those who want a detailed surgical description of tongue fixation, we would recommend the papers by Routledge [21], or of Parsons and Smith [15].

Tracheostomy has been advocated as a method of overcoming the respiratory difficulties. We can only say that in our experience of more than 100 cases, no child required tracheostomy. We would agree with the statement by Routledge [21] that 'a tracheostomy in so small a patient can be a most difficult procedure and the risk of permanent tracheal stenosis is high, when a tracheostomy has to be kept open for so long'. In addition, the bulk of the tracheostomy tube actively discourages oral feeding as it must rise and fall with each swallowing movement. It should be noted that when the time comes for formal cleft palate repair in these children, care must be taken in that narrowing of the airway may cause difficulty in safe extubation.

References

1. Bromley, D. and Burston, W.R. (1966) The Pierre Robin syndrome. *Nurs. Times*, **62**, 1717–1720
2. Bush, P.G. and Williams, A.J. (1983) The incidence of the Robin anomalad (Pierre Robin syndrome). *Br. J. Plastic Surg.*, **36**, 434–447
3. Cocke, W.M. (1966) Experimental production of micrognathia and glossoptosis associated with cleft palate (Pierre Robin syndrome). *Plastic Reconstr. Surg.*, **38**, 395–403
4. Diewert, V.M. (1979) A cephalometric study of orofacial structures during secondary palatal closure in the rat. *Arch. Oral Biol.*, **19**, 303–315
5. Diewert, V.M. (1981) Correlation between alterations in Meckel's cartilage and induction of cleft palate with beta aminoproprionitrate in the rat. *Teratology*, **24**, 43–52
6. Diewert, V.M. and Pratt, R.M. (1979) Selective inhibition of mandibular growth and induction of cleft palate by diazonorleucine (DON) in the rat. *Teratology*, **20**, 37–51
7. *Dorland's Medical Dictionary* (1965) W.B. Saunders, Philadelphia and London
8. Edwards, J.R.G. and Newall, D.R. (1985) The Pierre Robin syndrome reassessed in the light of recent research. *Br. J. Plastic Surg.*, **38** (3), 339–342

9. Eley, R.C. and Farber, S. (1930) Hypoplasia of the mandible (micrognathia) as a cause of cyanotic attacks in the newly born infant: report of four cases. *Am. J. Dis. Child.*, **39**, 1167–1176

10. Fairbairn, P. (1846) Suffocation of an infant from retraction of the base of the tongue connected with the defect of the phraenum. *Monthly J. Med. Sci.*, **6**, 280–282

11. Harris, J.W.S. (1964) Oligohydramnios and cortisone induced cleft palate. *Nature*, **203**, 533–534

12. Latham, R.A. (1966) Pathogenesis of cleft palate associated with the Pierre Robin syndrome and analysis of a seventeen week foetus. *Br. J. Plastic Surg.*, **19**, 205–214

13. Karnofsky, D.A. and Lacon, C.R. (1961) Effects of physiological purines on the development of the chick embryo. *Biochem. Pharmacol. (New York)*, **7**, 154–158

14. Newall, D.R. and Edwards, J.R.G. (1981) The effects of vitamin A on fusion of mouse palates. I. Retinyl palmitate and retinoic acid *in vivo*. *Teratology*, **23**, 115 124

15. Parsons, R.W. and Smith, B.J. (1980) A modified tongue-lip adhesion for Pierre Robin anomalad. *Cleft Palate J.*, **17** (2), 144–147

16. Poswillo, D.E. (1966) Observations of fetal posture and causal mechanism of congenital deformity of palate, mandible and limbs. *J. Dent. Res.*, **45** (Suppl.) 584–596

17. Poswillo, D.E. (1968) The aetiology and surgery of cleft palate with micrognathia. *Ann. Roy. Coll. Surg. Eng.*, **43**, 61–88

18. Randall, P. The Robin anomalad: micrognathia and glossoptosis with airway obstruction. In *Reconstructive Plastic Surgery*, (ed. J.M. Converse). W.B. Saunders Co., Philadelphia, pp. 2235–2245

19. Robin, P. (1923) Influence des dysmorphoses facio-cranio-vertebrals sur l'etat de sauté en général et leur rôle dans les cas de mortalité précoce. *Bull. Acad. Med.*, **39**, 647–649

20. Robin, P. (1934) Glossoptosis due to atresia and hypotrophy of the mandible. *Am. J. Dis. Child.*, **48**, 541–547

21. Routledge, R.T. (1960) The Pierre Robin syndrome: a surgical emergency in the neonatal period. *Br. J. Plastic Surg.*, **13**, 204–218

22. Rubin, A. (1967) *Handbook of Congenital Malformations*. W.B. Saunders, Philadelphia and London, pp. 145–146

23. Shih, L.Y., Trasler, D.G. and Fraser, F.C. (1974) Relation of mandibular growth to palate closure. *Teratology*, **9**, 191–203

24. Shukowsky, W.P. (1911) Zur Atiologie des Stridor Insspiratorius Congenitus. *Jahib. Kinderheilk. (Berlin)*, **73**, 459–474

25. Smith, D.W. (1975) Classification, nomenclature and naming of morphologic defects. *J. Paediat.*, **87**, 162–164

26. Williams, A.J., Williams, M.A., Walker, C.A. and Bush, P.G. (1981) The Robin anomalad (Pierre Robin syndrome). A follow-up study. *Arch. Dis. Child.*, **56** (9), 663–668

27. Virchow, R. (1864) Ueber Missbildung am Ohr und im Bereiche des ersten Kiemenbogens. *Virchows Arch Path, Anat. Physiol.*, **30**, 221 234

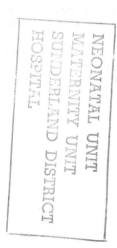

17

Neonatal surgery of the upper respiratory tract

J.H. Rogers

Introduction

The upper respiratory tract extends upwards from the laryngeal subglottis to include the pharynx, mouth, nose and Eustachian tube, in addition to the larynx itself. Congenital and early acquired problems may involve all these structures but their surgical treatment is often not required during the neonatal period. The neonatal problems encountered by the otolaryngologist are therefore limited; particularly as the relatively common problem of cleft palate is usually treated by the plastic surgeons and mandibular retrognathia by the orthodontists. The only significant neonatal conditions requiring early surgical treatment are choanal atresia and subglottic stenosis, and a tracheostomy may be necessary in any situation where obstruction or the threat of obstruction to the upper respiratory tract occurs.

Posterior choanal atresia

This congenital nasal abnormality is an obstruction to the normal opening between the nose and the nasopharynx. The obstruction usually occurs at the level of the posterior choana, although an associated partial obstruction often exists anteriorly in the nasal cavity itself. It is an important condition because the neonate instinctively breathes through the nose and in its bilateral form the condition causes severe respiratory distress. The atresia may also be unilateral and possibly incomplete, when it is known as choanal stenosis. The historical background is well reviewed by Pirsig [22] and summarized by Pracy [24].

Embryology

A knowledge of basic embryology is helpful for the discussion of choanal atresia. The early embryo is a bilaminar disc of ectoderm and endoderm and folds develop in the mid-line of the dorsal ectoderm to form a neural tube. Specialized cells adjacent to the neural tube are known as the neural crest and these, despite their ectodermal origin, make a major contribution to the mesoderm of the head, developing later into bone, muscle and cartilage. The embryonic disc folds upon itself to form the primitive gut whose anterior part, the pharynx, is separated from the exterior, the buccal cavity, by the buccopharyngeal membrane. The opening into the buccal cavity or primitive mouth is the stomodaeum (Figure 17.1) which is dominated by the overhanging forebrain and associated mesoderm. Rapid differential growth in this mesoderm causes grooves and folds to appear in the overlying ectoderm and this growth is responsible for the appearance of the facial 'processes' as described in traditional embryology.

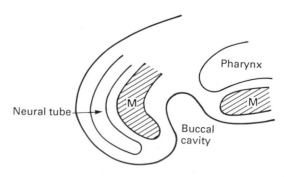

Figure 17.1 Anterior end of embryonic disc. M, mesoderm

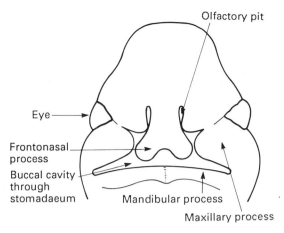

Eye

Olfactory pit

Frontonasal process

Buccal cavity through stomadaeum

Mandibular process

Maxillary process

Figure 17.2 'Face' of embryo

In the fourth week of intrauterine life, small areas of thickened ectoderm, the olfactory placodes, appear above the stomodaeum and rapidly become pits as the surrounding mesoderm proliferates. Differential growth of the mesoderm forms the lateral and medial folds, the latter fusing in the mid-line to form the frontonasal process (Figure 17.2). The olfactory pits 'burrow' into the mesoderm and come to lie in the roof of the buccal cavity and separated from it by the nasobuccal membrane. This ruptures to form the primitive nasal cavity. The face is formed by the medial growth of maxillary processes which have separated from the larger mandibular processes. The maxillary processes bypass the lateral nasal folds and fuse with the frontonasal process. The mesoderm between the primitive nasal cavities forms the anterior nasal septum while mesoderm cells which have migrated below the brain develop to form the ethmoid and sphenoid bones. The mid-line mass of the ethmoid projects downwards from the roof of the buccal cavity to form the posterior nasal septum whilst a shelf of mesoderm grows medially from each maxillary process to form the permanent palate.

It is important to realize that some of these changes occur within a few hours and that any change in the speed or direction of mesoderm migration may result in a congenital abnormality.

Pathology

The lesion in choanal atresia may be bilateral or unilateral but in either case it is not a well delineated localized obstruction to an otherwise normal nasal cavity. The abnormality involves all the structures embracing the posterior nasal cavities and there is a progressive circumferential narrowing of the cavity as it tapers posteriorly to the point of atresia at the posterior choana. This narrowing is caused by a thickening of the surrounding bones which encroach upon the lumen of the cavity. It is simplistic and confusing to categorize the obstruction as 'bony' or 'membranous' as the obstruction is always partially bony, but the terminal obstruction at the tip of the taper may be bony, cartilaginous or membranous. There is a tendency for the bony encroachment to be more marked laterally so that an exploring probe is deflected medially as it approaches the posterior choana.

Unilateral atresia is commoner than bilateral and the condition is commoner in females. The existence of choanal stenosis as a pathological entity is doubtful since the normal dimensions of the infantile choana have not been established and 'stenosis' may be a variation of the normal. Choanal atresia is said to occur in 1:7000 births and nearly half of these babies have congenital additional abnormalities, some of which may be fatal. These associated anomalies commonly affect the heart and the eyes as well as producing retarded mental and physical development. The main anomalies are summarized by the acronym CHARGE (coloboma, heart, atresia choanae, retardation, genitalia, ears) [18,21].

It has also been claimed that the normal development of the facial sinuses is impaired and that this is an acquired abnormality. However, this finding is infrequent and in any case is probably the result of earlier mis-direction of mesodermal migration.

Aetiology

Whereas it is agreed that the condition is the result of an early developmental abnormality, there is no agreement as to the exact embryological basis of it. Most traditional theories have been based on the persistence of a membrane which normally ruptures but these do not correlate with the clinical features of the condition. The three traditional theories with their criticisms may be summarized as follows:

1. A persistence of the nasobuccal membrane. Clinically, however, the atresia is maximal posteriorly near the definitive choana and not at the primitive choana which marks the site of the nasobuccal membrane.
2. A persistence of the buccopharyngeal membrane. This separates the stomodaeum from the primitive gut and lies posterior to the choana. A persistence of this membrane would produce an oropharyngeal stenosis and a stenosis in the nasopharynx itself. The latter is rare whilst the former is almost unheard of.
3. An abnormal persistence of mesodermal adhesions in the region of the choana. This has its attractions but it does not explain the commonly associated congenital abnormalities.

A more recent theory published by Hengerer and Strome [16] provides a useful practical embryological explanation based on an abnormality of mesodermal migration. The direction, speed and destination of this migration from the neural crest cells is controlled by genetic and environmental factors and various bony abnormalities can be caused in animals by an experimental interference with this mesodermal flow. Normally, the olfactory pits burrow dorsally into the burgeoning mesoderm and then turn caudally towards the roof of the stomodaeum.

An abnormality of mesoderm migration might prevent the caudal turn and cause the burrowing to continue in a dorsal direction. The pits may or may not reach the roof of the stomodaeum but in either case the abnormal nasobuccal membrane is likely to be thicker and more posterior. The mesoderm in this area eventually forms the nasal septum, the hard palate, the ethmoid and the sphenoid, structures which embrace the posterior choana and are seen to be involved clinically in the condition. The degree of over-migration would also determine the presence of bone, cartilage or membrane in the atretic area.

Clinical features

The presenting symptoms of bilateral choanal atresia are caused by the neonate's instinctive attempts to breathe through the nose although the degree of obligation varies. If the nose is blocked the baby will asphyxiate until the level of hypoxia is such that the baby cries, the mouth opens and a few rapid inspirations are taken. The cycle then repeats itself and the baby experiences recurrent episodes of anoxia which may ultimately result in cerebral damage and death. After 2 or 3 weeks the baby may begin to breathe through the mouth but it could be 6–8 weeks before this is achieved with ease. The condition is rare enough for it to be often misdiagnosed and the baby is frequently suspected of having a cardiac or pulmonary abnormality. The alert doctor will recognize the characteristic signs but even when the diagnosis has been made, any serious associated abnormality must be excluded.

Presenting signs

1. The condition is often suspected at birth or soon after it. The importance of the nasal airway is recognized by the midwife and suction of the nose to remove mucus and meconium is routine. An inability to pass a suction tube into the nasopharynx at this stage should arouse suspicion and the absence of a prolonged lusty cry may be noted.
2. The cycle of cyanosis and crying is seen. When the mouth is closed the baby becomes progressively more cyanosed while appearing to make violent efforts at inspiration. The chest and neck are indrawn and the face is contorted with effort. Eventually the baby gives a few cries and gasping inspirations through the mouth and the colour returns to normal. The cycle then repeats itself but the problem is solved by the introduction of an oral airway which keeps the mouth open and the tongue forward.
3. Any attempt to feed the baby is unsuccessful because sucking is impossible when the nose is blocked. Indeed, any attempt at feeding makes the symptoms worse as the oral route is now blocked and the hungry baby makes more frantic efforts to breathe.

Management

This includes the confirmation of the diagnosis and the treatment. Certain therapeutic steps may need to be taken before the diagnosis is confirmed and any other congenital abnormalities should be identified and assessed. To this end, the services of a neonatalogist should be obtained at the earliest opportunity.

Initial treatment

In bilateral atresia a reliable oral airway must be established as soon as possible. An oropharyngeal tube of suitable size is introduced and is taped to the side of the mouth for stability. A narrower gastric tube is introduced through the oral tube to allow feeding. Traditionally the McGovern nipple [19] has been employed for this purpose but it is no longer in common use. It is a long rubber nipple with lateral holes which permits sucking and breathing at the same time. Although sometimes helpful it is not as effective as the simpler oropharyngeal tube. This initial conservative treatment can be extended to cover the first 6–8 weeks of life when nasal breathing is instinctive. Benjamin has described a method [1] which is rather more stable. He passes a wide-bore tube through the mouth into the mid-oesophagus and a feeding tube is passed through it. This wide tube holds the mouth open and encourages oral breathing.

Confirmation and diagnosis

Good evidence for the diagnosis will already have been obtained by an inability to pass a catheter into the pharynx via the nose and the absence of frosting on a mirror held to the nostril. The former procedure is not foolproof since the catheter may coil up in the normal nose if it is misdirected or too rigid.

The obstruction can be examined directly in a variety of ways. Once the cavity has been cleared of mucus, vasoconstriction is achieved by the application of a dilute aqueous solution of cocaine. The obstruction may then be seen through the nostril with an aural speculum and suitable light source. The fibre-optic nasopharyngoscope will give a similar view [2] but can also be employed to provide a posterior view of the atretic area from the nasopharynx.

Traditionally, the attempted passage of a suitable fluid through the nose has been employed. Methylene blue can be identified in the pharynx or a radio-opaque dye can be observed as it passes backwards through the nasal passages. Both can be misleading as an enlarged turbinate can obstruct the fluid flow.

Computed tomography will identify the atretic plate with great clarity [2] and magnetic resonance imaging produces even better results. However, these methods, though attractive, are expensive and unnecessary.

In practice, the preliminary diagnosis can be made simply on the basis of the presenting signs and an inability to pass a catheter or malleable probe into the pharynx. Since surgery is now the treatment of choice for bilateral atresia, the diagnosis is confirmed by a direct visual examination under anaesthesia, prior to the operation.

Treatment

Once bilateral atresia has been confirmed and any associated congenital and medical problems treated, more permanent treatment is instituted. Conservative treatment, as described by Benjamin and noted above, will postpone surgery but it requires intensive nursing care and bonding between mother and baby is affected because of the baby's inability to suck.

Surgical treatment

Surgery is now the treatment of choice and advances in paediatric anaesthesia permit safe surgical intervention even in the very premature infant. However, general anaesthesia through an endotracheal tube must be administered by an experienced paediatric anaesthetist. Several routes of access have been described but the transnasal and transpalatal approaches are most commonly employed.

Transnasal approach

This was first used about two centuries ago when a sharp instrument would be passed blindly into the nose. This trocar would pierce the atretic plate but since the plate sometimes lies obliquely, the trocar could easily be deflected upwards and medially to enter the spinal cord or basisphenoid. Since the hole was always small and stenosis inevitable, the procedure would be oft-repeated with a consequent

increase in complications. The advent of the microscope allowed the operation site to be visualized and once seen, the plate can be pierced by a variety of devices [10] although the drill is still the commonest.

After achieving vasoconstriction with a suitably dilute aqueous solution of cocaine, the nostril is gently expanded by a nasal speculum or an aural speculum of adequate size. The microscope is directed through the speculum and the stenotic area covered in mucosa is visualized. If the obstruction is membranous, a blunt probe is all that is necessary to pierce the tissue and construct a suitable opening, but more commonly a combination of bone and soft tissue is found. In theory, microscopic otological instruments can be used to elevate the mucosa over the plate and flaps of this mucosa have been described. In practice, however, the raising of flaps is not feasible because of restricted access but every effort should be made to conserve as much mucosa as possible.

A hand-drill is used to pierce the plate and the initial opening is enlarged and smoothed until it will accept a 14–16 f.g. bougie. Two precautions are helpful during this drilling, which is directed inferiorly and medially to minimize potential damage. A retractor placed in the nasopharynx will hold the soft palate forwards and will protect the spinal cord. Similarly the index finger of the free hand can be placed against the palate and palpates and guides the drill-head when direct vision is impossible. When both openings have been completed, a suitable hollow stent is passed through them to prevent stenosis and the placing of this stent may consume considerable time.

Many forms of stent have been described but a Portex endotracheal anaesthetic tube is very suitable. An appropriate size is chosen so that it passes firmly but comfortably through the new opening. The tube will eventually be 'U'-shaped with the curve of the 'U' around the posterior border of the septum and the two free ends protruding from the nostrils. A window is cut in the side of the tube at a point which it is judged will be at the curve of the 'U'. Small holes are also cut in the sides of the tube to allow the suction of mucus accumulating in the nasal passages. At both ends of the tube, a mark is made which is equidistant from the window and this facilitates proper alignment after insertion. A piece of strong silk thread is passed through each nostril into the pharynx and the two pharyngeal ends are knotted together. The nasal end of one thread is then firmly sutured to the tube which is drawn into its final 'U'-position by traction on the second free nasal thread. The markers are then aligned so that the fenestrum is positioned correctly at the posterior septum and a fine catheter is passed in turn through each limb of the tube and identified in the pharynx. This demonstrates a correct position and a patent lumen. The free ends of the tube are sutured

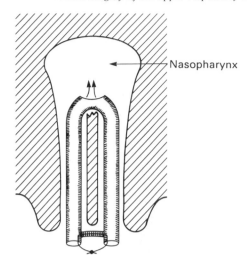

Nasopharynx

Figure 17.3 Diagram of transverse section through nose to show positioning of stent-tube after completion of operation

together to prevent slipping and malalignment of the fenestrum (Figure 17.3). The suture is conveniently placed through a short section of suction catheter, which acts as a strut and prevents damage to the columella. Before suturing them together, the free ends of the tube are cut as short as possible to avoid unnecessary projection from the face and the baby is thus able to suckle. Alternatively the tube can be placed the opposite way around with the fenestrum at the anterior columella and the free ends in the nasopharynx. Slipping is prevented by a piece of silk passed in a circle through the tube and around the posterior septum to be tied at the columella. This latter method is quicker, but problems tend to arise at the free ends of the tube and access to the nasopharynx is more difficult.

Transpalatal approach

This approach to the obstruction through the mouth was first described around the turn of the century. It should always be carried out under general endotracheal anaesthesia with the usual precautions taken to keep the infant warm. The head is extended by a pad under the shoulders and a Killian's mouth gag is suitable for keeping the mouth open. Since a palatal flap has to be raised, there is sometimes some blood loss and as the neonatal blood volume is small, it is wise to cross-match 1 unit of blood. The hard palate is infiltrated with 1:300 000 adrenaline and a 'U'-shaped incision is made just inside the line of the alveolus. Posteriorly the arms of the 'U' are extended laterally so that the palatine arteries are included in the flap. The convexity of the 'U' should lie as far forward as possible to allow comfortable suturing and a bony support for the

replaced flap. The mucoperiosteal flap, which is surprisingly thick and bulky, is raised by sharp and blunt dissection. It should be done quickly to avoid undue blood loss, but carefully to avoid tearing the flap and encouraging a future fistula. The elevation of the flap is continued posteriorly until the posterior border of the hard palate is reached. A suture passed through the convexity of the flap and tied to the gag support will retract the flap away from the operation site.

When the hard palate has been exposed, drilling is started with a small drill-head in the mid-line of the posterior border. The drilling is continued laterally and anteriorly until the atretic area, together with the posterior part of the normal septum, are seen and the nasal cavity mucosa exposed posteriorly. A blunt probe passed into the nasal cavity through the nostril, acts as a guide which can be seen as the bone is thinned. Some textbook descriptions of this operation now describe the elevation of nasal mucosal flaps which are later used to line the exposed bone of the new choanae but, in practice, such flaps are virtually impossible to construct. The nasal mucosa is elevated as carefully as possible from the atretic area, the vomer and the medial pterygoid plate and every effort is made to conserve it. An incision is made through the nasopharyngeal mucosa along the line of the posterior border of the hard palate and this gives visual access to the nasopharynx. At the same time, the nasopharyngeal mucosa, overlying the posterior surface of the atretic plate, is elevated.

The surgeon now has a good view of the obstruction, the nasopharynx and the posterior third of the nose. The nature and extent of the obstruction is assessed and an adequate opening is created by excising the fibrous tissue and drilling the bony projections which encroach upon the airway from the vomer and the pterygoid. Particular care must be taken laterally to avoid the palatine artery and since the posterior septum is nearly always thickened it should be removed. A thickening of the floor of the body of the sphenoid may have narrowed the opening from above and limited drilling will enlarge the choana superiorly. If the nasal mucosa is still intact, it is incised and the nasal probe is employed to identify any remaining bony obstruction which is removed. The probe also serves to protect sensitive tissues from the drill-head.

The new choana is made as large as is reasonably possible and a Portex tube stent is introduced as described above, although it is easier because of the improved visual access. When the stent has been correctly positioned, any mucosal 'flaps' worthy of that name are laid over areas of bare bone around the stent. The mucoperiosteal palatal flap is now sutured back into position with the help of a 5/8 circle needle and absorbable sutures. The flap heals very well and only four or five sutures are necessary.

Alternative surgical techniques

The laser has been used via the transnasal approach and it has the advantage of minimal bleeding and morbidity [15,20]. A trans-(nasal) septal access to the obstructed choana has also been described.

Postoperative care

If there are no other serious abnormalities and no complications, the infant recovers rapidly after the operation and is able to suckle after only 24 h. In the immediate postoperative period, intravenous fluids are continued for 12 h but nasogastric feeding should then be employed until suckling begins. Suckling is possible almost immediately after the transnasal operation has been done. The nasal stent behaves as a foreign body in the nose and it is advisable to cover the operation and early postoperative period with an antibiotic. The nasal mucosa is stimulated by the stent to produce increased quantities of mucus which seep from the nostril around the tube, and into the nasopharynx. Mucus also enters the tube through its side-holes and regular suction is necessary to keep the lumen clear. If the discharge becomes persistent it should be cultured and the relevant antibiotic given. Periods of between 1 week and 6 months have been recommended as the time for leaving the stent in position [3] and the author feels it should be left for as long as possible, up to 3 months. This allows the new choanae to become established and epithelialized and stenosis is less likely to occur. If the stent is removed after 1 or 2 weeks a suitably sized bougie needs to be passed daily. This procedure causes distress to both baby and parents and it traumatizes the healing area so that epithelialization is hindered and stenosis even encouraged. After 3 months in place the tube is best removed under general anaesthesia so that the nose, palate and nasopharynx can all be properly assessed. For the first few weeks a bougie should be passed weekly by the parents (after suitable instruction) and the intervals are then increased until bouginage can cease when there is no sign of stenosis. The parents are supplied with a suction machine, catheters and a bougie and the baby can return home once the parents feel competent to cope.

Complications

1. An oronasal fistula through the hard palate may rarely occur after the transpalatal operation. A small palatal flap or the removal of too much bone from the hard palate will predispose to this event and the one fistula in the author's experience was caused by the clumsy use of a drill-head which was too large. The small oronasal fistula will heal spontaneously but if it is persistent a flap of mucoperiosteum can be rotated to cover it.

2. The tube may become displaced or blocked and in the early stages it will be necessary to replace it.
3. Stenosis of the reconstructed choanae is an ever-present possibility and varying degrees of success are claimed for maintaining their patency. It is probable that a significant proportion become stenosed in spite of regular bouginage but many children seem remarkably unaffected by the continuous mucoid discharge. Others, however, become ridiculed by their peers and the surgeon will come under pressure to re-open the choanae. This may be achieved by a puncturing of the soft tissue stenosis with subsequent dilatation, but a more radical approach may be necessary. A repeat operation should be left as long as possible, until the child is in his teens, when a much larger choana can be constructed. Most surgeons would then advocate the transpalatal approach.

   It must be remembered that the baby learns to breathe through the mouth after the age of 2 months and so a re-stenosis is not usually a serious complication.

Unilateral choanal atresia

If the problem is unilateral there is no urgency in treatment although a temporary oral or nasopharyngeal tube will become necessary if the patent airway becomes blocked by oedema or mucus. A persistent mucoid discharge occurs from the obstructed side but a corrective operation should be postponed for as long as possible in order to create a choana of optimum size.

The choice of surgical approach

In practice, a surgeon will employ the surgical approach with which he has experience. There are, however, reasons for favouring one approach rather than the other.

The nasal approach is less destructive, quicker and involves less blood loss. It is the operation of choice when the obstruction is largely membranous or when the baby is very small or ill. It is probable that stenosis is more likely to occur when this method is used.

The transpalatal approach gives better access and is, therefore, safer and permits the creation of a choana of optimum size. It is the method of choice in most cases but particularly for a secondary operation following re-stenosis or for the correction of a unilateral atresia at a later age.

Choanal stenosis

There is a normal variation in the size of the posterior choana and those babies with the smaller openings may have difficulty immediately after birth. The stenosis may be aggravated by mucus and the symptoms and signs may mimic those of atresia. If the symptoms are significant they may be relieved by an oral airway or the passage of a nasopharyngeal tube. On those rare occasions where the symptoms are severe and persistent, a surgical enlargement of the choana becomes necessary.

Subglottic stenosis

The narrowest part of the infantile respiratory tract is the segment at the upper end of the trachea which is bound by the cricoid cartilage. It is known as the subglottic area and it is the only part of the respiratory tract to be enclosed in a complete ring of rigid tissue. Any further narrowing or stenosis at this point is likely to interfere with the airway and therefore threaten life. There is a considerable normal variation in the size of the neonatal subglottis and those with a normally small diameter are obviously more at risk.

Stenosis may be caused by a discrete swelling encroaching upon the lumen but more commonly it is caused by a more diffuse circumferential narrowing by soft or cartilaginous tissue. The stenosis may be temporary or permanent, congenital or acquired, and it is thought to have been first described by Rossi [28]. The adjacent glottis and trachea may also be involved in the stenotic process.

Pathology

The commonest cause of a localized discrete swelling is a cyst or haemangioma and both may be present at birth as well as appearing in the neonatal period and later in life.

The diffuse circumferential stenosis may be congenital or acquired. Congenital stenosis is caused by a cricoid cartilage of small diameter and it is often not severe.

Acquired stenosis always involves the soft tissues and sometimes the underlying cartilage. It may be temporary or permanent. A temporary stenosis is due to oedema which may be the result of infection, allergy or trauma and these are all of relevance to the neonate. The oedema is more marked laterally and a slit-like narrowing is therefore produced with the slit lying in an anteroposterior direction. However, it is the more permanent forms of stenosis which provide a severe challenge to the paediatric surgeon.

The exact nature of the pathological processes involved is not known but the commonest cause is protracted intubation [14] with its accompanying trauma. Mucosal damage is caused, with or without granulation formation and ulceration and eventually fibrous tissue is formed by the healing process. Chondritis or even necrosis of the underlying cricoid

may weaken and collapse the ring or it may become much thickened by scarring. Since intubation is very often necessary for the survival of the premature neonate, the problem is predominant in this clinical group and the numbers at risk become greater as neonatologists become more successful. However, better techniques and better tube materials are reducing the proportion of these babies who become affected. Similar trauma can be caused by over-enthusiastic dilatation of a slight stenosis but this form of treatment is becoming less popular.

Symptoms

Temporary oedema of the subglottis is characterized by stridor and a croupy cough and the stridor classically has an inspiratory and an expiratory component. These symptoms are typically found in acute laryngotracheobronchitis. An underlying congenital stenosis may only be recognized when such an acute infection supervenes. Similar symptoms with respiratory distress are found with a cyst or haemangioma.

The more serious forms of stenosis are typically recognized by a failure to extubate. The removal of the tube is rapidly followed by stridor, chest recession and eventually cyanosis as the soft tissues expand to occlude the lumen.

Treatment

The first line of treatment is to protect the airway and this is usually achieved by intubation although a tracheostomy may be necessary eventually. In order to prevent further trauma the tube should be as small as possible while providing an adequate airway and a leak around it. The obstruction should then be thoroughly assessed by a team of specialists comprised of a paediatrician, an anaesthetist and the surgeon.

Assessment

Radiological investigation in the form of a xerogram or a CT scan is helpful in assessing the length of the stenosis but in the author's experience it is not helpful in assessing the size of the residual lumen. This can only be done accurately by giving a general anaesthetic, a procedure which requires the services of an experienced paediatric anaesthetist. The stenosed area can be seen through the vocal cords and a series of endotracheal tubes of known diameter is passed through the stenosis until one tube is found to pass snugly but without force. The size of this tube is recorded. If possible a rigid telescope is then passed through the obstruction to assess the length of the stenosis and to confirm that there is no other abnormality in the trachea beyond. Sometimes the stenosis is so narrow that neither the smallest tube nor the bronchoscope can be passed through.

Treatment of acute subglottic stenosis

Although acute infections of the respiratory tract cause temporary subglottic stenosis they are not usually considered under this category and will therefore not be discussed further here.

Treatment of chronic subglottic stenosis

The first step in treatment is to decide whether intubation is necessary and, if so, how long it should be continued before carrying out a tracheostomy. There is no arbitrary rule for this and as neonatologists become more skilled in the use of tubes the period becomes longer. An improvement in the stenosis can be recognized by an increased leak of air around the tube and if this is progressive, the patient may be extubated without any further assistance. However, this is not the rule and there is a large battery of treatments available and a wide variety of opinion as to whether or when they should be used. Conservative treatment involves the use of steroids, dilatation and various endoscopic methods to remove soft tissue by forceps, the cryoprobe and now the carbon dioxide laser. A wait-and-see approach can also be adopted in the presence of a tracheostomy. Open surgical operations are carried out if the corrective measures fail but in all procedures a tracheostomy or stent may or may not be used. The choice of treatment depends on the lesion but also on the judgement of the surgeon, the skills or equipment available to him and the circumstances of the patient. The various forms of treatment will now be briefly described.

Steroids

These are widely used in the treatment of oedema and are, therefore, employed in acute infections. They have also been advocated for the treatment of chronic stenosis but, on practical grounds, most surgeons do not use them and on theoretical grounds they delay healing.

Dilatation

This is employed in mild degrees of stenosis and regular dilatation has been claimed to avoid a tracheostomy. Many feel, however, that the procedure provides additional trauma and may aggravate the situation. It is also felt that a stenosis which benefits from dilatation would probably have improved with no treatment at all. It should only be considered where there is soft tissue stenosis and of course would be quite useless for a small rigid

cricoid which is congenitally small or grossly thickened by infection.

Wait-and-see [4]

As the neonate grows the larynx grows with it and the diameter of the cricoid therefore increases. If the baby is provided with a tracheostomy and the parents are able to care for that tracheostomy at home it is an option to wait until the laryngeal airway is adequate. This course of action is best taken when the patient lives close to the hospital so that help can be given rapidly if necessary but it means that the baby can grow up at home without the long stay necessary in hospital when an open operation is carried out. The baby is admitted every 6 months to assess the airway and if there has been very little increase by the age of 2 years, other steps should be considered.

Endoscopic treatment

A soft tissue stenosis is most suitable for endoscopic treatment and it is most successful when the scar tissue is not too thick. Granulations can be removed with forceps and both diathermy and cryosurgery have been used in the past. However, both of them tend to produce scarring themselves and the carbon dioxide laser has become the instrument of choice over the past 15 years with very favourable results. The laser is also used for other soft tissue swellings such as the haemangioma and cyst.

In many cases, endoscopic treatment will avoid the necessity for a tracheostomy but any suspicion of a threat to the airway makes the operation mandatory.

Open surgery

A failure of conservative or endoscopic treatment will lead to open surgical intervention. It will also be the primary method of choice for a small thickened cricoid ring or where there is gross scarring with involvement of the adjacent trachea and glottis.

Open operations are aimed at splitting the cricoid and separating the cut ends to increase the size of the ring. In some operations the cut ends are held apart by an intraluminal stent as in the anterior cricoid split and the laryngotracheoplasty whereas, in others, autogenous tissue is interposed. The appropriate operation can only be decided after careful pre-operative assessment and after the lumen has been opened.

(1) Anterior cricoid split

This is usually advocated in the early stages of the problem and is particularly relevant to the neonate.

In the first 4 days the neonate is treated by intubation and if the smallest available tube has been used with no air leak around it, then an anterior cricoid split is considered. The soft cricoid ring and upper two tracheal rings are divided in the mid-line and a slightly larger endotracheal tube is introduced to separate the two ends and to splint them apart [7]. The tube acts as an airway and as a stent and a tracheostomy is unnecessary. The tube is usually left in place for 2 weeks and in many cases, extubation can then be accomplished.

(2) Laryngotracheoplasty [8]

This is probably the commonest open operation performed for subglottic stenosis in the UK and it is employed for a thickened cricoid with associated scar tissue. The thyroid cartilage and cricothyroid membrane are incised in the mid-line and a castellated incision is made through the cricoid and upper two or three tracheal rings (Figure 17.4). The larynx is opened up and as much scar tissue as possible is removed with great care while attempting to preserve the mucosa. Some cartilage may also be removed from the inner surface of the ring. A 'swiss roll' of Silastic sheeting is inserted and the castellations are sutured together while still partly displaced (Figure 17.5). This is difficult because the slivers of

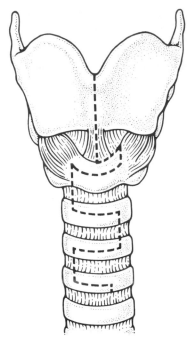

Figure 17.4 Castellated incision (Taken from *Scott-Brown's Otolaryngology*, 5th Edition, Butterworths, London)

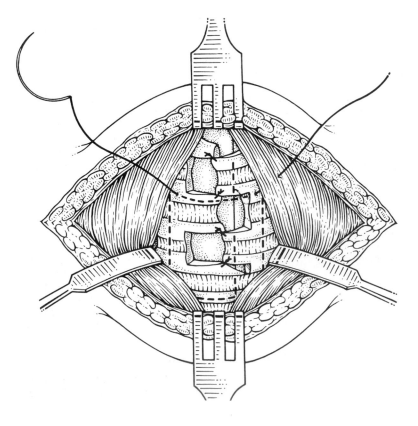

Figure 17.5 Insertion of transfixation suture to secure Silastic swiss roll (Taken from *Scott-Brown's Otolaryngology*, 5th Edition, Butterworths, London)

cartilage are flimsy and easily torn, but the operation is facilitated by the use of a microscope. The Silastic roll is transfixed by a suture which is buried subcutaneously and it is removed 6 weeks later. The operation obviously requires previous tracheostomy.

Interposition surgery

Many different forms of autogenous tissue have been employed to hold the cut ends of the cricoid apart and these include hyoid bone (either free or attached to muscle), and nasal septum. However, the commonest technique [6,32] is the interposition of shaped costal cartilage into the gap formed when the cricoid and upper tracheal cartilages are incised (Figure 17.6). If the scarring and thickening lie mainly anteriorly this procedure may suffice but a posterior problem can be similarly treated [25]. The posterior lamina is divided and a smaller piece of cartilage is interposed. A tracheostomy is necessary and stenting may or may not be employed. Various forms of stenting have been advocated [9] and the choice often depends on personal preference and availability.

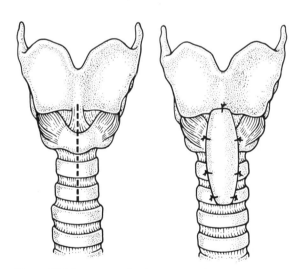

Figure 17.6 Laryngotracheal reconstruction showing the fixation of the anterior graft of costal cartilage (Taken from *Scott-Brown's Otolaryngology*, 5th Edition, Butterworths, London)

Tracheostomy

Introduction

Strictly speaking, a tracheostomy is a 'fistula' between the trachea and the skin surface of the neck. The operation is performed at all ages but the technique and care of the tracheostomy is rather different in the neonate because of the small structures involved and the degree of immaturity. The numbers of neonates requiring the operation are increasing as the neonatologists become more successful in preserving the smallest premature infants.

Historical

The operation has been attempted since prehistoric times and numerous descriptions are found in the earliest historical records [11,13].

The earliest indications were obstruction caused by an inhaled foreign body and drowning or trauma to the upper respiratory tract. The first successful tracheostomy in a child was reported in 1766 by Caron, a French surgeon who removed an inhaled bean from a 7-year-old boy. A later indication for the operation was 'croup', a label given by a Scottish physician, Francis Home [17], to the combination of sore throat and stridor. Some of these children would have had laryngotracheobronchitis but most would have suffered from diphtheria, which is still known as 'croup' in some parts of western Europe.

Tracheostomy became widespread in the treatment of diphtheria in the nineteenth century but latterly the O'Dwyer tube presented an attractive alternative and the discovery of an effective antitoxin in 1895 further reduced the numbers requiring surgery. The employment of a tracheostomy to remove bronchial secretions was first described for poliomyelitis before being used for chronic chest disease. The poliomyelitis epidemics of the 1950s stimulated the use of tracheostomy for positive pressure respiration which then became invaluable in the treatment of tetanus, severe burns and latterly the premature infant. Active immunization against diphtheria and poliomyelitis almost eliminated these diseases and left epiglottitis and laryngotracheobronchitis as the principal indications for paediatric tracheostomy. Intubation has now become the treatment of choice in these last two conditions and the incidence of tracheostomy has decreased dramatically in the developed world. In the last decade the skills of the neonatologist have improved the survival chances of the very premature infant with its multiple disabilities. The necessary prolonged intubation often results in subglottic stenosis and a failure to extubate necessitates tracheostomy. However, even in these infants, surgical interference is becoming less frequent as the neonatologist becomes more adept in avoiding subglottic trauma.

Anatomy and physiology

In the infant the air passages are both absolutely and relatively smaller than in the adult [30]. The length of the cervical trachea varies with the degree of extension but the distance from the cricoid to the suprasternal notch is only 2.5 cm in the neonate. The larynx is higher in the infant, where it lies at the level of the third cervical vertebra. Since there is no 'Adam's apple' in the infant the cricoid cartilage is often easier to palpate than the thyroid cartilage. The trachea lies closest to the skin surface at its upper end and the thyroid isthmus, though very variable in bulk, crosses the second, third and fourth tracheal rings (Figure 17.7).

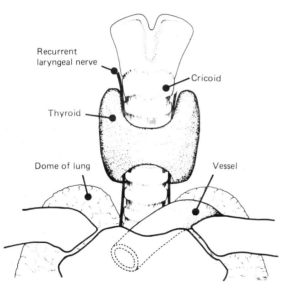

Figure 17.7 The essential anatomy of the cervical trachea (Taken from *Scott-Brown's Otolaryngology*, 5th Edition, Butterworths, London)

As in the adult, the recurrent laryngeal nerves lie laterally and posteriorly but a pretracheal pad of fat is often present in the suprasternal notch of infants. In extension, the mediastinal contents enter the neck so that the surgeon may encounter a high pleural dome, large vessels crossing the mid-line and, rarely, the thymus. The articulation between the head and neck is more mobile in infants and the chin may easily deviate from the mid-line during surgery.

The trachea is supported by incomplete cartilaginous rings which maintain the lumen and allow flexibility. It is lined by respiratory mucosa which warms and humidifies the inspired air and the cilia waft the mucous blanket upwards towards the larynx. The larynx is a valvular mechanism which allows the passage of air but normally denies access to solids and fluids. It also provides a defence mechanism in the form of the cough reflex and it has been adapted to a sophisticated degree for the production of sound.

Indications for tracheostomy

In general nowadays a tracheostomy is done where intubation is not possible or no longer feasible and the indications are the relief of airway obstruction, the provision of positive pressure respiration and the reduction of dead space and bronchial secretions. There have been several recent reviews of the indications for tracheostomy [5,29,31], but the statistics are variable because of different periods under review and the different patterns of referral to the centres concerned. The indications are summarized more specifically below.

Congenital laryngeal abnormalities

This group now accounts for the largest proportion of tracheostomies and bilateral vocal cord paralysis is the commonest single indication. Other indications are congenital subglottic stenosis, laryngeal webs, subglottic haemangiomas and laryngeal cyst. Laryngomalacia or supraglottic floppiness is by far the most common laryngeal abnormality but a tracheostomy is rarely required for its treatment. The cleft larynx which may be associated with a cleft trachea is a rare indication.

Acquired laryngeal abnormalities

Acquired subglottic stenosis is still the commonest acquired indication for tracheostomy and the details are discussed elsewhere in this chapter. Laryngeal papillomatosis is now better treated by the carbon dioxide laser and the decreased oedema and scarring means that tracheostomies are less frequently necessary.

Miscellaneous

Where ventilation needs to be prolonged and intubation is no longer feasible, a tracheostomy still plays its part. It also has a role in supralaryngeal obstruction as found in the Pierre Robin syndrome, severe sleep apnoea and craniofacial surgery. Intubation is now commonly employed for acute epiglottitis and laryngotracheobronchitis but a tracheostomy is sometimes necessary, particularly in less developed countries, where diphtheria may also necessitate the operation.

The operation of tracheostomy

The aim of the operation is to construct an airway into the trachea as safely as possible. It is more commonly done in males because of their increased susceptibility to congenital and acquired disorders.

There are rare occasions when an emergency tracheostomy is life-saving but if possible the operation should be done in an environment where there is complete control of the airway at all times. In the neonate it is essential that it should take place in a hospital or paediatric unit where staff are accustomed to such small infants. The operation should be performed electively in a sterile environment under a general anaesthetic administered through an endotracheal tube. The anaesthetic should be given by an experienced paediatric anaesthetist and the operation performed by, or supervised by, an experienced paediatric otolaryngologist.

Preparation

Antibiotics are only given prophylactically if there is a medical reason for doing so. A sample of sputum is cultured in readiness for a possible postoperative infection and 1 unit of blood is cross-matched.

The infant, suitably warmed, lies supine on the operating table. The head is extended to bring the trachea closer to the surface and to allow better access to the operation field (Figure 17.8). Extension is achieved by placing a roll of soft material under the head and lolling is controlled with a small head-ring. The extension should not be overemphasized as this may draw the mediastinal contents and lung apices into the neck and may tempt the surgeon to make a low tracheal incision which retreats into the neck on flexion.

The skin of the neck is cleaned with a suitable disinfectant and the chin is left uncovered in order that the surgeon can check the mid-line. A little local anaesthetic and adrenaline (1:100 000) is infiltrated subcutaneously between the cricoid and the sternal notch in order to produce vasoconstriction and to reduce postoperative discomfort. It is also wise to check that a suitably sized tracheostomy tube is at hand and that the proper connections are available.

Surgical techniques

Both the vertical and horizontal skin incisions are employed. The advantage of the vertical incision is that it runs in the line of the trachea and thus gives better access when the precise level of the proposed tracheostomy is difficult to judge pre-operatively. The mid-line is also less vascular. There is no cosmetic advantage in the neonate because both incisions are so small that they produce similar scars.

A vertical mid-line skin incision of 1.5 cm is made with the upper end at the level of the cricoid. The bleeding is usually minimal but diathermy should be employed if necessary. An assistant retracts the edges of the incision and blunt dissection is carried out in the mid-line with artery forceps or a small scissors. It is important not to open up tissue planes unnecessarily as this encourages surgical emphysema later. The strap muscles are separated and retracted and the trachea exposed. Even in the most difficult case, patient persistence in the mid-line will be rewarded and there is usually no bleeding. Although the tracheal rings are softer and less obvious than in the adult, it is difficult to mistake the trachea although it may be difficult to identify an individual tracheal ring. The tracheal rings are best numbered from the cricoid cartilage but the thyroid isthmus is another useful landmark. The isthmus varies greatly in width but it consistently overlies the second, third and fourth tracheal rings. The isthmus need not be cut and can be retracted superiorly or inferiorly to expose the relevant rings.

The fascia is cleared from the anterior surface of

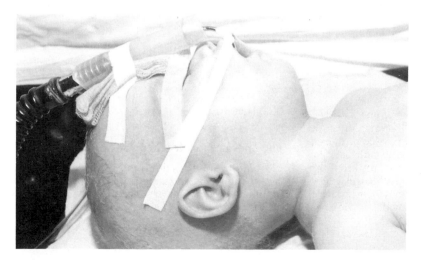

Figure 17.8 An infant in the tracheostomy position. Note the partial extension of the neck (Taken from *Scott-Brown's Otolaryngology*, 5th Edition, Butterworths, London)

the trachea without disturbing the recurrent laryngeal nerves posterolaterally. The trachea is now exposed in a small but bloodless field and the anaesthetist is alerted to the imminent incision of the trachea itself.

The tracheal incision

It is agreed that the vertical tracheal incision is best in the infant but it is important that it is made at the correct level. If it is too near the cricoid it will predispose to subglottic stenosis while if it is too low, the tip of the tracheostomy tube may enter the right main bronchus. The tracheal rings are identified again and a vertical incision is made through the second, third and fourth rings. Every effort is made to keep the first ring intact. The slit is made from below upwards to avoid damage to the mediastinal contents and it should be made in a controlled manner because a slip will extend the incision up to the cricoid. The tracheal wall is rather thicker than one would expect and although there is sometimes a little bleeding from the tracheal mucosa and the perichondrium, this is rarely significant. Any possible damage to the posterior wall of the trachea by the tip of the scalpel blade is prevented by the endotracheal tube.

Some surgeons feel that the procedure is assisted by the insertion of a silk suture to either side of the mid-line [12]. Before the vertical incision is made, a black silk suture is introduced to circle the third and fourth tracheal rings on either side. These are left

long and initially are held laterally in artery forceps but after the incision has been made between them, they are retracted to assist cannulation. Later they are taped to the chest wall for up to 1 week and may be used for recannulation if necessary. In the author's experience, these sutures are not mandatory since there is rarely any problem in introducing the tracheostomy tube and decannulation is prevented by other means. There is also a possibility that the sutures will weaken the tracheal wall and the threads become sodden and something of an obstacle during subsequent care of the tracheostomy.

The anaesthetist withdraws the endotracheal tube just proximal to the upper end of the incision under the guidance of the surgeon. A tracheostomy tube of suitable design and size is inserted under direct vision. This can be done in a calm unhurried way since the anaesthetist still has full control of the airway. The insertion may be difficult particularly if there is no bevel on the end of the tube and the following points may help. The incision should be enlarged if it is too small and stay sutures should be retracted if they have been placed. If the tube is metal its introducer should be in place while the ends of a plastic tube can be compressed in an artery forceps to facilitate insertion [23] (Figure 17.9). The tracheostomy tube can also be 'railroaded' over a fine catheter which has been passed through the tube and the tracheal incision.

A synthetic plastic or silicone tube is best used for the initial intubation and the models available are

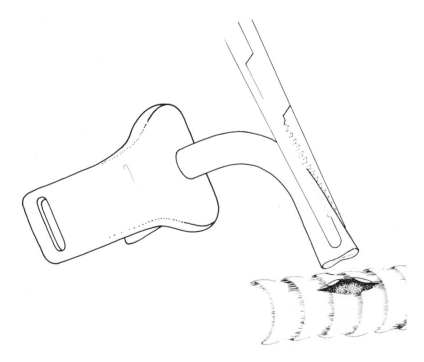

Figure 17.9 The tip of the tracheostomy tube is compressed by artery forceps to facilitate insertion (Taken from *Scott-Brown's Otolaryngology*, 5th Edition, Butterworths, London)

described below. The neonate will require the smallest size in terms of tube length and lumen diameter. The position of the tube is checked and the anaesthetist checks that both lungs are being ventilated and the endotracheal tube is withdrawn. No sutures are placed in the edges of the skin incision which usually sits comfortably around the tube and a tight fit is to be avoided since it predisposes to surgical emphysema.

The tube is now held in place by suturing the flange to the neck skin and by tying tapes around the neck. The importance of securing the tube cannot be overestimated since accidental decannulation is avoided if it is done properly. Silk sutures are placed through the flange and adjacent skin just lateral to the opening of the tube. This positioning prevents the substantial tube movement which can occur if the sutures are placed towards the tip of the flange. A tape is then tied from one side of the flange to the other around the back of the neck. One end of the tape is knotted to one side of the flange while the other is passed through a piece of endotracheal tubing of suitable length (Figure 17.10). This tubing conforms to the convexity of the baby's neck and protects the skin from rubbing of the tape. The free end of the tape is then knotted to the other end of the flange and is adjusted so that the tube is held firmly but not tightly in place. It is important that these adjustments to the tape are carried out while the neck is in slight flexion. If they are done in extension, the tube will loosen on subsequent flexion and accidental decannulation will be encouraged. It is, therefore, important that the tape adjustments are made by the surgeon or the anaesthetist and the task should not be delegated to an inexperienced member of the team. Older babies are given sedation but neonates are best left without so as to discourage apnoeic attacks. The baby is now moved from the operating table and care is taken to avoid traction on the tube while this is being done.

Postoperative care

The baby should return to a neonatal intensive care unit where there are adequate trained nursing and medical staff on duty for 24 h of the day. As soon as the infant arrives in that unit, an X-ray of the chest and neck is taken to confirm that the tip of the tracheostomy tube is not impinging on the carina or entering the right main bronchus. The X-ray may also demonstrate surgical emphysema in the superficial tissues or in the mediastinum. Feeding is given intravenously and adequate hydration is maintained to prevent tracheal crusting.

The details of neonatal intensive care will not be discussed here but positive end-expiration pressure (PEEP) may be necessary to maintain lung stability. The chin may also obstruct the stomal opening but this can be avoided by choosing a suitable tube or by inserting a segment of plastic tubing into the opening of the tracheostomy.

Since the tracheostomy has bypassed the nose, it is essential that humidified air is supplied to the neonate but care must be taken to avoid over-humidification. Particle size is not as important as was previously thought but cold humidity is probably best and an ultrasonic humidifier may be necessary to provide a sufficient volume. The glottis has also been bypassed and the cough reflex is lost. The trachea and bronchi respond by an increase in mucus secretion and regular aseptic suction is essential. The frequency of suction varies but the

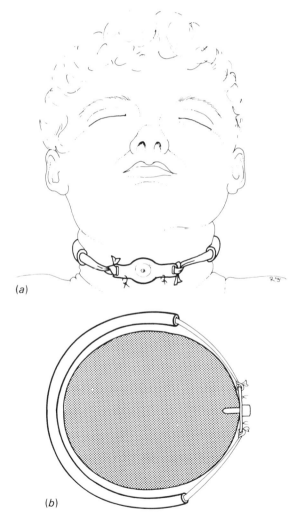

(a)

(b)

Figure 17.10 (a) The flanges are secured to the neck skin by a tape and by sutures adjacent to the collar of the tube. (b) A cross-section of the neck demonstrating the tape passing through protective tubing (Taken from *Scott-Brown's Otolaryngology*, 5th Edition, Butterworths, London)

catheter is introduced without suction while negative pressure is exerted on its withdrawal. The size of the catheter is most important. The external diameter should be less than half the internal diameter of the tracheostomy tube because, if not, hypoxia or lung collapse may occur.

A careful watch must be kept for surgical emphysema or pneumothorax but these are unlikely to occur after 12 h. A dressing is not necessary between the peristomal skin and the tube flange but a barrier cream is helpful if skin excoration threatens.

In the neonate, bonding is important and both parents are encouraged to take an active role in the routine care. Initially they should observe the tracheostomy care and should then be supervised in doing it themselves to overcome their natural fear. They should also be introduced to one of the parental organizations such as 'Aid for children with tracheostomies'.

One week after the operation the track is well formed and the tube can be changed. This is not mandatory and it can be left longer if it is clear and well positioned. The first change is best done in the intensive care unit of the operating theatre. An endotracheal tube, tracheal dilators and a spare tracheostomy tube must be immediately available and the change must be done by an experienced doctor. The tapes are again tied carefully and the tube position checked. Routine tracheostomy care is continued and if the baby is to return home, the necessary equipment is ordered for home care. Before the baby goes home both parents should be able to change the tracheostomy tube and the surgeon must be happy that they are confident about the daily care.

Complications

The tracheostomy is the main channel for respiration and any complication which interferes with it may be fatal. The mortality and morbidity following the operation is now much less than hitherto, which is attributed to the avoidance of emergency tracheostomies where possible and to the emphasis on a basic surgical technique and postoperative care. Complications are conveniently considered as being early or late, the dividing line being about 1 week into the postoperative period. Some problems, such as crusting and granulation formation, are so common that they may be regarded as normal consequences of the operation but if exaggerated they qualify as complications.

Early complications

Apnoea

Apnoeic attacks are most likely to occur in the neonate with chronic airway obstruction. Postoperative sedation should not be given and the dead space can be temporarily increased by a suitable attachment.

Air in the tissues

Surgical emphysema involving the tissue planes of the neck and the mediastinum is commonly seen and it resolves without treatment. A pneumothorax should be treated on its merits but a tight stoma and a low tracheostomy both predispose to it. Prevention is therefore the best form of treatment.

Accidental decannulation

This can be a serious complication, particularly in the first 2 or 3 days when the track has not formed. Prevention is again the best method to combat it but experienced staff should be able to recannulate the baby or pass an endotracheal tube.

Creation of a false passage

This is caused by changing the tube and is most liable to occur before the track is well formed. Changing the tube should be avoided in the first week and its position must be checked after recannulation.

Obstruction

Blockage of the tube by the baby's chin is prevented by a suitable attachment to the tracheostomy tube and the accumulation of mucus and crusts by adequate suction and humidification.

Haemorrhage

This is rare if blunt dissection is employed and the slight bleeding from skin edges or the tracheal mucosa will stop after an hour or two.

Chest infections

Pulmonary infection is more likely to occur with a tracheostomy and a history of previous lung problems may indicate the need for prophylactic antibiotics. A sample of tracheal aspirate is taken at operation and sent for culture and sensitivities.

Late complications

All the complications mentioned above may occur later but accidental decannulation and obstruction cause most fatalities and are very likely to happen at home. Serious haemorrhage from the erosion of a large vessel has also been described and is more likely with a low tracheostomy.

Once the track is formed, accidental decannulation is less serious but the track can stenose rapidly. Tracheal dilators should be easily available and at home the parents must learn to tie the tapes firmly.

Obstruction can be caused by a mucus plug or by a granuloma which commonly forms above the stoma on the anterior wall of the tracheal lumen. Adequate suction and humidification must be continued and a granuloma can be removed endoscopically or via the stoma. A heat-moisture exchanger is easily connected to the tracheostomy tube and this allows mobility for the baby without the encumbrance of a bulky humidifier.

Tracheostomy tubes

The tracheostomy tubes in use today are either made of metal or of flexible plastics such as polyvinylchloride and silicone rubber (Figure 17.11).

A typical metal tube is the Alder Hey tube and similar paediatric models are those of Jackson and Holinger. The Alder Hey tube has an inner and an outer tube and both may be fenestrated. The inner tube can be removed and cleaned without changing the outer tube and this obviously inspires confidence in the inexperienced parent. However, there are disadvantages because the edges of the fenestration and the shaft-tip are sharp and it is believed that they predispose to the formation of granulations. It is also difficult to site the fenestrum at a suitable point on the curvature of the tube. The fenestrum was designed for transglottic air flow but this can be equally achieved by using a tube of lesser diameter which allows a current of air to pass around it.

The synthetic tubes are now used almost exclusively in the treatment of neonates. Cosmetically they look better and the flanges sit more comfortably on the neck. Most now have a collar of international standard dimensions which means that standard anaesthetic or ventilation equipment is easily attached. Those without a fixed collar have attachments which achieve a similar purpose. All of these tubes can be found in varying sizes and are classified as 'paediatric' or 'neonatal'. The projecting collar acts as a chin restrainer and a phonation valve such as that made by Rusch can be attached to promote speech. The neonatal synthetic tubes commonly used in the UK are the Franklin tube of Great Ormond Street pattern, the Portex paediatric tube and the Shiley neonatal tube.

Decannulation

It is hoped that every baby with a tracheostomy will eventually be decannulated. The outcome obviously depends upon the original lesion but fortunately many resolve spontaneously or with medical and surgical treatment. The details of the assessment for decannulation are discussed elsewhere [27], but essentially the time comes when the airway appears to be adequate and it is felt that the patient will manage without a tracheostomy.

The airway is checked by direct endoscopy and if deemed adequate the tracheostomy is closed. This can be done by simply removing the tracheostomy tube and allowing the stoma to close but this technique is sometimes unsuccessful. The commonest causes for failure are the existence of a tracheal granuloma above the stoma and damage to the anterior tracheal wall around the stoma. These problems are solved by surgical decannulation whereby the tracheostomy track is excised and the tracheal stoma examined under direct vision [26]. The granuloma is removed and a small area of collapsed or fibrotic tracheal wall can be excised. The tracheal stoma is sutured and the skin incision closed to provide better healing, a more stable trachea and a more cosmetic skin scar.

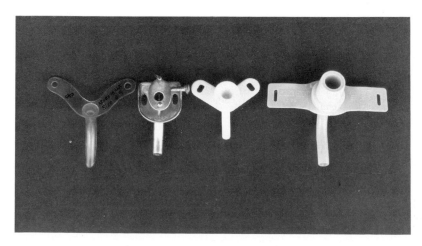

Figure 17.11 A selection of paediatric tracheostomy tubes in common use. From left to right: the Great Ormond Street tube (Franklin), the silver Alder Hey tube, the Shiley tube, and the Portex tube. Note the standardized collars on the latter two tubes (Taken from *Scott-Brown's Otolaryngology*, 5th Edition, Butterworths, London)

Conclusion

Tracheostomy in small babies is usually necessary when intubation has failed. The operation itself is relatively safe and the problems of decannulation have been largely solved. In the future, the aim should be to eliminate the need for tracheostomy, but with the advances in neonatal medicine, cranial and thoracic surgery and the increase in the numbers and speeds of motor vehicles and thus accidents, this is unlikely. There will be gradual changes in the types of tubes and their attachments and the operation itself may change as the age-old cricothyroidotomy and its successor, the minitracheostomy, are assessed more thoroughly.

References

1. Benjamin, B. (1977) Ten years' experience in congenital choanal atresia. *J. Otolaryngol. Soc. Australia*, **4**, 158

2. Benjamin, B. (1985) Evaluation of choanal atresia. *Ann. Otol. Rhinol. Laryngol.*, **94**, 429–432

3. Black, R.J., Pracy, R. and Evans, J.N.G. (1983) Congenital posterior choanal atresia. *Clin. Otol.*, **8**, 251–255

4. Bowdler, D.A. and Rogers, J.H. (1987) Subglottic stenosis in children; a conservative approach. *Clin. Otolaryngol.*, **12**, 383–388

5. Carter, P. and Benjamin, B. (1983) Ten year review of paediatric tracheotomy. *Ann. Otol. Rhinol. Laryngol.*, **92**, 398–400

6. Cotton, R. (1978) Management of subglottic stenosis in infancy and childhood. *Ann. Otol. Rhinol. Laryngol.*, **87**, 649–657

7. Cotton, R.T. and Seid, A.B. (1980) Management of the extubation problem in the premature child. Anterior cricoid split as an alternative to tracheotomy. *Ann. Otol. Rhinol. Laryngol.*, **89**, 508–511

8. Evans, J.N.G. and Todd, G.B. (1974) Laryngotracheoplasty. *J. Laryngol. Otol.*, **88**, 589–497

9. Evans, J.N.G. (1987) Stenosis of the larynx. In *Scott-Brown's Diseases of the Ear, Nose and Throat*, 5th Edn, Butterworths, London, Vol. 6, pp. 495–502

10. Fearon, B. and Dickson, J. (1968) Bilateral choanal atresia in the newborn: Plan of action. *Laryngoscope*, **78**, 1487–1499

11. Frost, E.A.M. (1976) Tracing the tracheostomy. *Ann. Otol. Rhinol. Laryngol.*, **85**, 618–624

12. Gerson, C.R. and Tucker, G.F. (1982) Infant tracheotomy. *Ann. Otol. Rhinol. Laryngol.*, **91**, 413–416

13. Goodall, E.W. (1934) The story of tracheostomy. *Br. J. Childh. Dis.*, **31**, 167–176

14. Gould, S.J. and Graham, J.M. (1985) Acquired subglottic stenosis in neonates. *Clin. Otolaryngol.*, **10**, 299–302

15. Healy, G.B., McGill, T., Jako, G.J., Strong, M.S. and Vaughan, C.W. (1978) Management of choanal atresia with the carbon dioxide laser. *Ann. Otol. Rhinol. Laryngol.*, **87**, 658–662

16. Hengerer, A.S. and Strome, M. (1982) Choanal atresia; a new embryologic theory and its influence on surgical management. *Laryngoscope*, **92**, 913–921

17. Home, F. (1765) *An Enquiry into the Natural Causes and Cure of Croup.* Kincaid and Bell, Edinburgh

18. Leclerc, J.E. and Fearon, B. (1987) Choanal atresia and associated anomalies. *Int. J. Pediat. Otorhinolaryngol.*, **13**, 265–272

19. McGovern, F.H. (1961) Bilateral choanal atresia in the newborn; A new method of medical management. *Laryngoscope*, **71**, 480–483

20. Muntz, H.R. (1987) Pitfalls to laser correction of choanal atresia. *Ann. Otol. Rhinol. Laryngol.*, **96**, 43–46

21. Pagon, R.A., Graham, J.M., Zonana, J. and Yong, S.L. (1981) Coloboma, congenital heart disease and choanal atresia with multiple anomalies; CHARGE association. *J. Pediat.*, **99**, 223–227

22. Pirsig, W. (1986) Surgery of choanal atresia in infants and children: historical notes and updated review. *Int. J. Pediat. Otorhinolaryngol.*, **11**, 153–170

23. Pracy, R. (1979) Intubation of the larynx, laryngotomy and tracheostomy. In *Scott-Brown's Diseases of the Ear, Nose and Throat*, 4th Edition, Vol 4, Butterworths, London, pp. 567–586

24. Pracy, R. (1978) Posterior choanal atresia. *Textbook of Neonatal Surgery*, 2nd Edn (ed. P.P. Rickham, J. Lister and I.M. Irving), Butterworths, London, pp. 143–147

25. Rethi, A. (1956) An operation for cicatricial stenosis of the larynx. *J. Laryngol. Otol.*, **70**, 283–293

26. Rogers, J.H. (1980) Decannulation by external exploration of the tracheostomy in children. *J. Laryngol. Otol.*, **94**, 563–567

27. Rogers, J.H. (1987) Tracheostomy and decannulation in children. In *Scott-Brown's Otolaryngology*, 5th Edn, Vol. 6, pp. 471–486. Butterworths, London

28. Rossi, F. (1826) De nonullis monstruositatibus in internis humani corporis partibus. Observationes. *Mem. R. Accad. Torino*, **30**, 155

29. Swift, A.C. and Rogers, J.H. (1987) The changing indications for tracheostomy in children. *J. Laryngol. Otol.*, **101**, 1258–1262

30. Tucker, J.A. and Tucker, G.F. (1979) A clinical perspective on the development and anatomical aspects of the infant larynx and trachea. In *Laryngo-Tracheal Problems in the Paediatric Patient* (ed. G.B. Healy and T.J. McGill), Charles Thomas, Springfield, Illinois, pp. 3–8

31. Wetmore, R.F., Handler, S.D. and Potsic, W.P. (1982) Paediatric tracheostomy experience during the past decade. *Ann. Otol. Rhinol. Laryngol.*, **91**, 628–632

32. Zalzal, G.H. and Cotton, R.T. (1986) How I do it – a new way of carving cartilage grafts to avoid prolapse into the tracheal lumen when used in subglottic reconstruction. *Laryngoscope*, **96**, 1039

Part IV

Rib cage, diaphragm and lungs

ninth gestational weeks. The severest form of cleft sternum is the combination of a total sternal cleft with ectopia cordis. According to Van Allen *et al.* [2] acute amniotic rupture in the third week of gestation may be the cause of these defects. Mechanical teratogenesis by tissue bands adherent to the heart may lead to ectopia cordis. Mechanical compression secondary to rupture of the amniotic sac at 3 weeks of gestation would interfere with normal cardiac descent and compress the chest, producing thoracic and pulmonary hypoplasia. Congenital heart defects associated with ectopia cordis may represent deformations secondary to mechanical distortion of the developing heart. The milder anomaly of cleft sternum, which is also associated with band disruptions, may occur later in development following rupture of the chorion, yolk sac or amnion [22].

Pathological anatomy and physiology

Congenital absence of ribs

Most of the thoracic cage defects described in the literature have been minor and have not given rise to any urgent symptoms during neonatal life. The affected ribs may be completely absent, including the costal cartilages, or may only be partially developed posteriorly. Associated hemivertebrae are very common (Figure 18.1). Most defects of the ribs lie parasternally in the region of the second to the fifth ribs and are often combined with a hypoplasia or aplasia of the breasts, an underdevelopment of the regional subcutaneous fat and partial or complete absence of the pectoralis major and minor muscles [7,13,32,33]. More rarely, the defects are situated more laterally and caudally [13,37]. Large laterocaudal defects are occasionally associated with an eventration of the diaphragm [7]. In an earlier series of 13 neonates reported by Rickham [33], four of the cases showed absence of the upper ribs, but the deficiency was usually between ribs numbers 6 and 12. The average number of absent ribs was five; in one infant eight ribs were missing. The condition appeared as frequently on the left side as on the right side. In one of the 13 cases both sides were affected.

A large rib defect will cause paradoxical respiration and life-threatening respiratory distress shortly after birth. With inspiration, the defect is sucked inwards because of the negative intrapleural pressure; with expiration, the lung protrudes outwards through the defect. With every breath this so-called lung hernia will empty the CO_2-rich air contained in it into the healthy lung on the opposite side. Paradoxical respiration will, in addition, cause a shift of the mediastinum, thus increasing the severity of the respiratory distress [13,16,33].

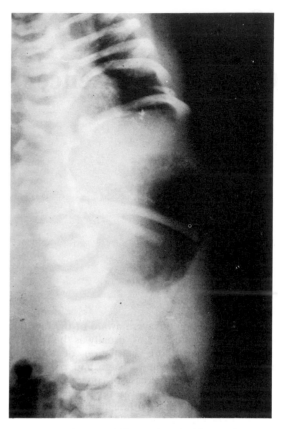

Figure 18.1 Absence of ribs on the left side associated with hemivertebra

Cleft sternum

Superior cleft of the sternum

This malformation involves only the upper half of the manubrium. If the defect is large enough, cardiac pulsation can be observed in the defect. Formerly, this malformation used to be called mistakenly a 'cervico-thoracic ectopia cordis'. The heart, however, is situated in its normal position and the soft tissues in the gap belong to the thoracic wall.

Inferior cleft of the sternum

The cleft is limited to the lower half of the sternum. These clefts are always associated with additional malformations. In addition to the cleft of the sternum, there is an anterior defect of the diaphragm, absence of the diaphragmatic part of the pericardium with a communication between abdominal cavity and pericardial cavity, and frequently also an exomphalos (see Chapter 27). Congenital malformations of the heart are nearly always present, the most frequent varieties being an isolated defect of the intraventricular septum or a tetralogy of Fallot.

Total cleft of the sternum

On clinical examination the diagnosis of total cleft of the sternum is occasionally made. At operation it is usually found, however, that the two sternal halves are still united in the region of the xyphoid process [32]. In these cases associated malformations do not occur. But if the cleft also includes the xyphoid process, associated malformations are practically always present in the region of the ventral part of the diaphragm and pericardium and frequently an exomphalos will also be present (see 'Inferior cleft of the sternum', above).

Cleft sternum and ectopia cordis

Occasionally, an ectopia cordis is found in association with total or partial sternal clefts [2,22]. There are usually associated malformations of the heart which is usually covered only by skin or pericardium and protrudes through the cleft.

Clinical picture

Congenital absence of ribs

In neonates with large defects, the deficiency of the chest wall, the bulging hernia and paradoxical

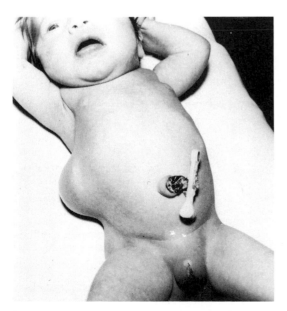

Figure 18.2 Bulging hernia of the chest wall with paradoxical respiration

respiration are obvious on inspection (Figure 18.2). In most of the cases in our series dyspnoea, tachypnoea, respiratory distress and cyanosis could at times be observed even when the infant was at rest. The symptoms increased dramatically on exertion when the baby was feeding or crying. In some infants prolonged feeding was impossible, as they became too exhausted by the exertion. If the infant survives without operation, the symptoms become less severe as he becomes older and the thoracic cage firmer, but in uncorrected cases gross thoracic and spinal deformities frequently develop later on [31].

Cleft sternum

It is easy to diagnose the presence of a cleft sternum with or without associated malformations. In cases of superior or inferior sternal clefts the thoracic cage remains stable. A respiratory distress syndrome does not, therefore, develop with these types of malformation. A total sternal cleft, however, will cause instability of the thoracic cage and may thus lead to a dramatic respiratory distress syndrome with severe dyspnoea, tachypnoea and cyanosis in the neonatal period. The unsupported part of the thoracic wall is sucked in with each inspiration, and during expiration the mediastinum bulges through the defect.

Cleft sternum and ectopia cordis

In this, fortunately, very rare anomaly, the heart lies totally or partially outside the thoracic cage. The condition is almost always associated with various severe cardiac anomalies and surgical correction is usually not possible. In recent years, ectopia cordis has been diagnosed several times by prenatal ultrasound [15,17,23,34,42]. Because of the poor prognosis, termination of pregnancy may be strongly considered in these cases if the diagnosis is made before the 20th to 24th week of gestation [23].

Treatment

Congenital absence of ribs

Treatment depends on the size of the defect, the localization of the defect and the patient's general state of health. If a large defect exists, resulting in a respiratory distress syndrome, an emergency operation has to be carried out [16,33]. Medium-sized and small defects should also be corrected as soon as possible because some show a tendency to grow in size and because correction is much more difficult in older children [13,32]. It is at times possible to minimize the paradoxical respiration and hence the constant shifting of the mediastinum by

(a)

(b)

(c)

(d)

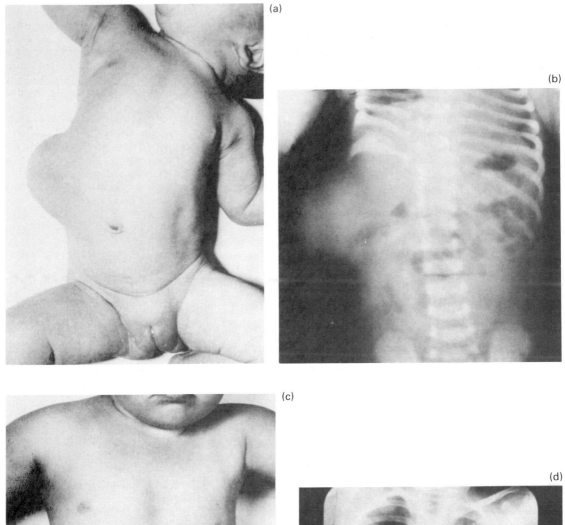

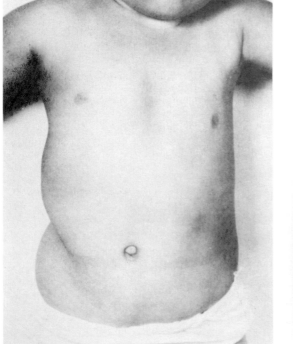

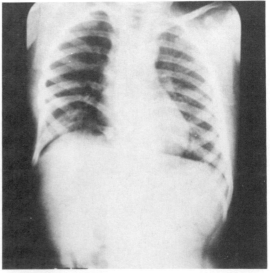

Figure 18.3 Deficiency of lower right ribs. (a and b) Clinical photograph and X-ray in neonatal period. (c and   d) Clinical photograph and X-ray of same child at 3 years. Treatment by strapping only

strapping the defect. This method of treatment was used successfully in one of our cases. Figure 18.3 shows clinical photographs and X-rays of a child with deficient lower right ribs at birth and at 3 years of age; this child had no treatment other than strapping of the defect, and had been free of respiratory troubles. Recurrent chest infection in a child treated by strapping is an indication for operative repair, whatever the size of the defect.

Operative treatment

Covering the defect with fascia lata grafts [1] is only of value in small defects. Bone graft operations have been advised, using bone either from other parts of the skeleton [30] or from adjacent or opposite ribs [14,16,18,26]. In large defects, longitudinal splitting of the ribs adjacent to the defect and the use of the lower free ribs to construct a new costal margin and to provide bony struts across the defect have been very successful [33] (Figure 18.4a–c). The covering of the defect is further strengthened by the external oblique muscle which is divided at its insertion into the rectus sheath, elevated, flapped backwards and upwards and then sutured across the defect (Figure 18.4d,e). Alternatively, a rotational latissimus dorsi muscle flap may be used to cover the defect [14]. The use of plastic material [13], for instance Silastic implants, is not advised because of the risk of infection [14] and because the material works loose with growth [16].

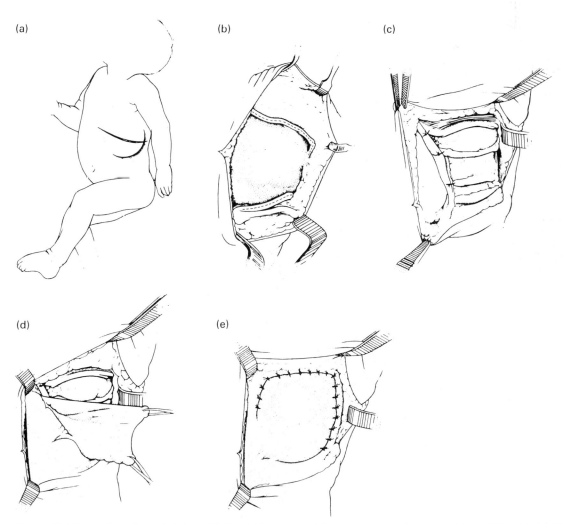

(a) (b) (c)

(d) (e)

Figure 18.4 Correction of costal defect. (a) Skin incision. (b) Exposure of defect. Note dashed line for splitting of ribs. (c) Suturing of split ribs across defect. (d) Raising of flap of external oblique muscle. (e) Suturing of flap across defect

Cleft sternum

Surgical correction of a total cleft sternum should be performed in the neonatal period whether the infant is symptomatic or not. Simple closure of the defect, as for a median sternotomy, is possible during the first month of life and this avoids the more complex reconstructions necessary in older children [3,8,19,36,38]. A longitudinal incision is made and the cleft is defined. The two margins of the cleft sternum are freshened and united with sutures. If there is a residual gap in the jugular region, this can be covered by suturing the straight muscles of the neck and sternomastoid muscles together [18]. This will prevent the occurrence of mediastinal or lung hernias. A superior cleft of the sternum should also be corrected as early as possible. The earlier the correction, the easier it is to perform and the better are the results [3,32,36]. If operation is postponed for several months or even years, the leverage of the shoulder girdles will increase the size of the defect. In addition, the thorax will become less and less elastic. A longitudinal skin incision is made over the defect and the 'U'-shaped margins of the cleft sternum are dissected free. Hecker [18] advises extending the split in the sternum caudally so as to convert the partial cleft into a total cleft which can then be repaired (Figure 18.5a,b). Ravitch [32] advises cutting through the longitudinal limbs of the 'U' and suturing these limbs together in the midline. If the correction is not carried out during the first weeks of life, the parasternal costal cartilages usually have to be resected because of the decreasing elasticity of the thoracic wall [16]. Treatment of an inferior cleft of the sternum depends on the severity of the associated malformations. Total correction of all the malformations in a number of sittings may be possible [28,29,32].

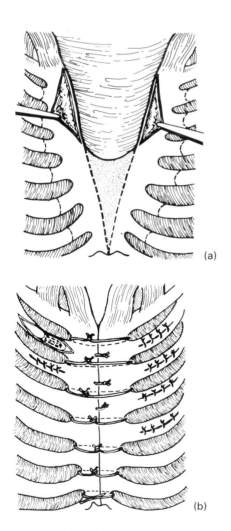

(a)

(b)

Figure 18.5 Hecker's operation for superior sternal cleft. (a) The 'U'-shaped margins of the cleft sternum are dissected free. (b) The sternum is split caudally and the whole sternum is sutured together

Prognosis

Congenital absence of ribs

If there are no associated malformations and provided the operation is carried out early, the prognosis is good. Recurrences are rarely observed. If there are severe associated malformations, as for instance congenital malformation of the heart, myelomeningoceles etc., the future of the patient depends more on the associated malformations than on the absence of ribs. The frequently associated scoliosis can become progressively worse and may need early corrective treatment.

Cleft sternum

The prognosis depends on the severity of the case and especially on the absence or presence of associated malformations (see above). If the associated malformations are not endangering life and provided correction of the cleft is done early, the prognosis is good and perfectly normal later development can be expected. Surgical correction of ectopia cordis has been attempted several times but was unsuccessful in all but two cases up to 1982 [5,6].

References

1. d'Abreu, A.L. (1958) *A Practice of Thoracic Surgery*, 2nd Edn, Edward Arnold, London
2. Von Allen, M.J. and Myhre, S. (1985) Ectopia cordis thoracalis with craniofacial defects resulting from early amnion rupture. *Teratology*, **32**, 19–24

3. Chappuis, J.P., Takvorian, P. and Philibert, M. (1984) A propos de deux cas de fissure sternale congénitale. *Pédiatrie*, **39**, 195–202

4. de Chauliac, G. (1619) *La Grande Chirurgie* (ed. M. Laurence Joubert), C. Michel, Tournon

5. Dahl, M., Viljanto, J. and Merikanto, J. (1981) Ectopia cordis. *Ann. Chir. Gynaecol.*, **70**, 128–132

6. Dobell, A.R., Williams, H.B.U. and Long, R.W. (1982) Staged repair of ectopia cordis. *J. Pediat. Surg.*, **17**, 353–358

7. Fevre, M. and Hannouche, D. (1968) Les brèches thoraciques par aplasie ou par anomalies costales. *Ann. Chir. Infant.*, **9**, 152–164

8. Firmin, R.K., Fragomeni, L.S. and Lennox, S.C. (1980) Complete cleft sternum. *Thorax*, **35**, 303–306

9. Garcia-Cruz, D., Vaca, G., Ibarra, B. *et al.* (1982) Tetrasomy 9p: clinical aspects and enzymatic gene dosage expression. *Ann. Genet. (Paris)*, **25**, 237–242

10. Garcia-Cruz, D., Rivera, H., Barajas, L.O. *et al.* (1985) Monosomy 20p due to a de novo del (20) (p.12.2). Clinical radiological delineation of the syndrome. *Ann. Genet. (Paris)*, **28**, 231–234

11. Gaziel, Y., Hoek, B.B. and van Niekerk, C.H. (1983) Agenesis of the right lung associated with hypoplasia of the fourth right rib. A case report. *S. Afr. Med. J.*, **64**, 871–872

12. Goodman, H.I. (1933) Hernia of the lung. *J. Thorac. Surg.*, **2**, 368–379

13. Gubern Salisachs, L., Carbonel Estrany, M. and Gubern, P.I.L. (1974) Les hernies pulmonaires. *Ann. Chir. Infant.*, **15**, 493–501

14. Haller, J.A. Jr., Colombani, P.M., Miller, D. *et al.* (1984) Early reconstruction of Poland's syndrome using autologous rib grafts combined with a latissimus muscle flap. *J. Pediat. Surg.*, **17**, 64–66

15. Harrison, M.R., Filly, R.A., Stanger, P. *et al.* (1982) Prenatal diagnosis and management of omphalocele and ectopia cordis. *J. Pediat. Surg.*, **17**, 64–66

16. Hartl, H. (1973) In *Operationen im Kindesalter* (ed. by H. Kunz), Georg Thieme, Stuttgart, p. 296

17. Haynor, D.R., Shuman, W.P., Brewer, D.K. *et al.* (1984) Imaging of fetal ectopia cordis: roles of sonography and computed tomography. *J. Ultrasound Med.*, **3**, 25–27

18. Hecker, W.Ch., Daum, R. and Maier, W.A. (1970) Die Eingriffe im Säuglings- und Kindesalter. In *Chirurgische Operationslehre*, Vol. II, Suppl. edition of Breitner, Urban and Schwarzenberg, München

19. Helardot, P., Mouzard, A. and Bienayme, J. (1980) Fissure sternale congénitale totale. A propos d'un traité précocement. *Chir. Pédiatr.*, **21**, 41–43

20. Hernandez, A., Garcia-Cruz, D., Plascencia, L. *et al.* (1979) Some clinical and cytogenetic observations on a ring chromosome 13. *Ann. Genet.*, **22**, 221–224

21. Hersh, J.H., Waterfill, D., Rutledge, J. *et al.* (1985) Sternal malformation/vascular dysplasia association. *Am. J. Med. Genet.*, **21**, 177–186

22. Kaplan, L.C., Matsuoka, R., Gilbert, E.F. *et al.* (1985) Ectopia cordis and cleft sternum: evidence for mechanical teratogenesis following rupture of the chorion or yolk sac. *Am. J. Med. Genet.*, **21**, 187–202

23. Kraat, H., Aarnoudse, J.G., Meuboom, E.J. *et al.* (1985) Prenatal ultrasonic diagnosis and management of ectopia cordis. *Eur. J. Obstet. Gynecol. Reprod. Biol.*, **20**, 177–180

24. Krauss, C.M., Hassell, L.A. and Gang, D.L. (1985) Anomalies in an infant with Nager acrofacial dysostosis. *Am. J. Med. Genet.*, **21**, 761–764

25. Marquis, J.R. and Lee, J.K. (1976) Extensive central nervous system calcification in a stillborn male infant due to cytomegalovirus infection. *Am. J. Roent.*, **127**, 665–667

26. Montgomery, J.G. and Lutz, H. (1925) Hernia of the lung. *Ann. Surg.*, **82**, 220–231

27. Morel-Lavallee, V.A.F. (1847) Hernies du poumon. *Mem. Soc. Chir., Paris*, **1**, 75

28. Mulder, D.G., Crittenden, I.H. and Adams, F.H. (1960) Complete repair of a syndrome of congenital defects involving the abdominal wall, sternum, pericardium and heart: excision of left ventricular diverticulum. *Ann. Surg.*, **151**, 113–122

29. Murphy, D.A., Aberdeen, E., Dobbs, R.H. *et al.* (1968) The surgical treatment of a syndrome consisting of thoracoabdominal wall, diaphragmatic, pericardial and ventricular septal defects and a left ventricular diverticulum. *Ann. Thorac. Surg.*, **6**, 528–534

30. Peraesalo, O. and Laustela, E. (1956) Congenital anomaly of the bony thorax. *Ann. Chir. Gynaec. Fenn.*, **45**, 303–310

31. Ravitch, M. (1962) Congenital absence of ribs. In *Pediatric Surgery* (ed. W.T. Mustard, M.M. Ravitch, W.H. Snyder, K.J. Welch and C.D. Benson), Year Book Medical Publishers, Chicago

32. Ravitch, M. (1971) The forms of congenital deformities of the chest and their treatment. *Progr. Pediat. Surg.*, **3**, 1–12

33. Rickham, P.P. (1959) Lung hernia secondary to congenital absence of ribs. *Arch. Dis. Child.*, **34**, 14–17

34. de Rochambeau, B., Coicaud, C., Bernard, M. *et al.* (1986) Ectopie cardiaque: dépistage échographique précoce in utero. *J. Gynecol. Obstet. Biol. Reprod. (Paris)*, **15**, 99–103

35. Saka, K., Oki, T. and Nogami, H. (1984) Agenesis of bilateral iliac bone. A case report. *Clin. Orthop.*, **182**, 190–192

36. Salley, R.K. and Stewart, S. (1985) Superior sternal cleft: repair in the newborn. *Ann. Thorac. Surg.*, **39**, 582–583

37. Salmon, M. (1968) Discussion de la communication de Fèvre et Hannouche. *Ann. Chir. Infant.*, **9**, 166

38. Samarrai, A.A., Charmockly, H.A. and Attra, A.A. (1985) Complete cleft sternum: classification and surgical repair. *Int. Surg.*, **70**, 71–73

39. Schinzel, A. and Schmid, W. (1980) Interstitial deletion of the long arm of chromosome 1, del (1) (q21 leads to q25) in a profoundly retarded 8-year-old girl with multiple anomalies. *Clin. Genet.*, **18**, 305–313

40. Schubert, W., Stoba, C. and Pinter, A. (1981) Beitrag zur Sternumspalte. *Z. Kinderchir.*, **32**, 208–213

41. Urschel, H.C. Jr, Byrd, H.S., Sethi, S.M. *et al.* (1984) Poland's syndrome: improved surgical management. *Ann. Thorac. Surg.*, **37**, 204–211

42. Wicks, J.D., Levine, M.D., Mettler, F.A. Jr (1981) Intrauterine sonography of thoracic ectopia cordis. *Am. J. Roent.*, **137**, 619–621

19

Congenital diaphragmatic hernia and eventration of the diaphragm

Irene M. Irving and P.D. Booker

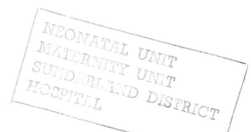

Historical notes

The first description of diaphragmatic hernia in adults was given by Ambroise Paré in 1575 [89,104]. The pathology of the malformation was discussed in some detail by Morgagni [82] in 1761, and in 1789 Sir Astley Cooper [30] not only described the pathology and clinical features of the condition in some detail, but also gave a classification of the various diaphragmatic hernias which is still valid today. In 1848 Bochdalek [15] described the embryology of the malformation and the foramen which still carries his name; however, his concept of the pathogenesis of diaphragmatic hernia has not been confirmed by modern embryological studies [83,129].

The first adult to recover from an operation for traumatic diaphragmatic hernia was reported by Walker [121] in 1889. During the first 30 years of this century the treatment for neonates with diaphragmatic hernias was conservative [42,72] and inevitably the mortality was very high. In 1931 Hedblom [53] drew attention to the high mortality associated with conservative treatment and suggested early operation as the only way to decrease it. Although isolated successes following operative repair of diaphragmatic hernia in neonates were reported during the 1930s [10,34,88,117], operation as the treatment of choice did not become generally accepted until Ladd and Gross [65] published their successful series in 1940.

Congenital diaphragmatic hernia

Embryology: normal development of the diaphragm

The development of the diaphragm is a highly complex process. The most important phases of its formation occur during the fourth to sixth weeks of embryonic life, by the end of which time there is complete partition between the primitive thoracic and abdominal cavities. Subsequently, formation of the periphery of the diaphragm continues up to the twelfth week of intrauterine life. The diaphragm forms by the fusion of the septum transversum, the pleuroperitoneal membranes and the dorsal mesentery of the oesophagus, with a later contribution from the body wall.

At about the 10 somite stage the pericardial cavity is relatively large and communicates freely caudally with the peritoneal cavity by way of the two pericardioperitoneal canals. After the formation of the head fold of the embryo during the fourth week the septum transversum, in which the liver develops, forms an incomplete ventral partition between the pericardial and peritoneal cavities. Dorsolaterally, paired crescentic pleuroperitoneal membranes are formed, mainly as a result of the invasion of the body wall by the developing lungs, and their free edges project into the caudal ends of the pericardioperitoneal canals which become the future pleural cavities (Figure 19.1b). During the sixth week the free edges of the pleuroperitoneal membranes fuse with the dorsal mesentery of the oesophagus medially and the septum transversum ventrally (Figure 19.1c). Closure of the pleuroperitoneal openings is assisted by the ingrowth of myoblasts into the pleuroperitoneal membranes. The opening on the right side closes slightly before the one on the left [81]. During the ninth to twelfth weeks the growing lungs and pleural cavities split the body wall into an outer layer which forms the body wall and an inner layer which contributes to the periphery of the diaphragm posterolaterally (Figure 19.1d). In the fully developed diaphragm the septum transversum is represented by the central tendon, the dorsal mesentery of the oesophagus by the median portion of the diaphragm and the crura, whilst the greater

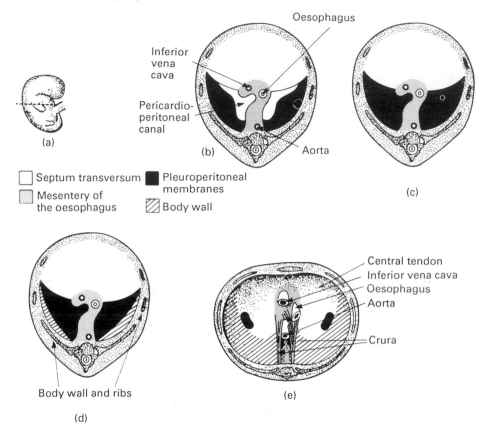

Septum transversum ☐   Pleuroperitoneal membranes ■

Mesentery of the oesophagus ▦

Body wall ▨

Figure 19.1 Drawings illustrating development of the diaphragm. (a) Sketch of a lateral view of an embryo at the end of the fifth week (actual size) indicating the level of section, (b)–(e) show the diaphragm as viewed from below. (b) Transverse section showing the unfused pleuroperitoneal membranes. (c) Similar section at the end of the sixth week after fusion of the pleuroperitoneal membranes with the other two diaphragmatic components. (d) Transverse section through a 12-week embryo after ingrowth of the fourth diaphragmatic component from the body wall. (e) View of the diaphragm of a newborn infant, indicating the probable embryological origin of its components. (From Moore, K.L. (1988) *The Developing Human: Clinically Oriented Embryology*, 4th edition, W.B. Saunders Co., Philadelphia, by courtesy of the author and publishers)

part of the remainder has formed from body wall; the pleuroperitoneal membrane contribution corresponds to a relatively small intermediate part (Figure 19.1e).

Pathological anatomy

Congenital hernias of the diaphragm have been classified by various authors; they differ slightly [83,129] but most are in broad agreement [36,48,56] (Figures 19.2 and 19.3).

Hernia through the 'foramen of Bochdalek'

In 1848 Bochdalek published his description of congenital posterolateral diaphragmatic hernia; this type of hernia still bears his name but strictly

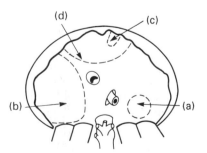

Figure 19.2 The diaphragmatic defects through which hernias occur in the neonate. (a) Posterolateral (Bochdalek) hernia. (b) Unilateral agenesis of diaphragm. (c) Morgagni (parasternal) defect. (d) Ventral (septum transversum) defect

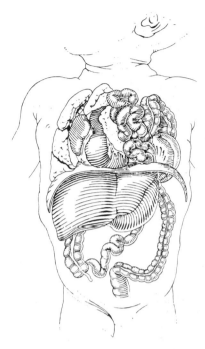

Figure 19.3 Typical displacement of abdominal viscera in a case of left-sided diaphragmatic hernia

by Bochdalek is not the anatomical site of closure of the pleuroperitoneal canal. Hence, although it is reasonable, and time-honoured, to speak of a 'Bochdalek's hernia' it is inaccurate to refer to a 'hernia through the foramen of Bochdalek', and in fact the most accurate and descriptive term is 'congenital posterolateral diaphragmatic hernia' [129]. These constitute the great majority of congenital diaphragmatic defects, of which a high proportion are left-sided. From mid 1953 to 1985, 153 neonates with congenital diaphragmatic hernia were treated in the Liverpool Regional Neonatal Surgical Centre or in the intensive care unit of Alder Hey Hospital. Of these, 146 were posterolateral hernias, 129 (88%) being left-sided. The preponderance of left-sided lesions may well be related to the earlier closure of the right pleuroperitoneal opening [81] but the protective effect of the liver is probably more important, and it is difficult to say whether in fact right-sided defects do not occur more frequently than we suspect, with the liver shielding the defect and preventing herniation.

Posterolateral defects vary in size from comparatively small triangular or oval defects with well-developed diaphragmatic muscle anteriorly and a rim of muscle posteriorly (Figure 19.2a) to huge deficiencies (Figure 19.2b), classified by Harrington [48] as congenital partial absence of the diaphragm, in which there is no remnant of diaphragm posterolaterally and which, in its extreme form, is best described as unilateral agenesis of the diaphragm.

The contents of the chest vary; on the left side the pleural cavity usually contains stomach, small intestine and colon, spleen and left lobe of liver, whilst a hernia on the right side contains liver and variable amounts of small and large intestine. The majority of the posterolateral hernias have no true peritoneal sac because the abdominal organs enter the pleural cavity before the pleuroperitoneal canal is completely obliterated [129]. In our series, only 20% of cases had a hernial sac.

Hernia through the foramen of Morgagni

The foramen of Morgagni (Figure 19.2c) is a gap, or potential gap, lying between the sternal and costal attachments of the diaphragm and transmitting the internal mammary artery. Herniation through the foramen of Morgagni, sometimes referred to as a parasternal hernia, is uncommon in neonates and there were only four such cases in this series; these were reported by Thomas and Clitherow in 1977 [115]. These hernias are more common on the right than the left and a membranous sac is almost invariably present. Those presenting in infancy, in contrast to those presenting in adult life, are often associated with additional anomalies, especially congenital heart lesions [77,92].

speaking this is a misnomer [129]. In his original paper [15] he described the herniation of abdominal contents into the thorax through a dorsal split in the diaphragm. In his diagram of the diaphragm he indicates two openings through which, he postulated, the hernia could develop; one of these is the lumbocostal triangle, which is a gap between the vertebral and costal attachments of the diaphragm above the lateral part of the last rib behind the kidney; the other appears to be a gap between the lateral arcuate ligament and the quadratus lumborum. He postulated that posterolateral congenital hernia was acquired *in utero* as a result of bowel being forced through the weak lumbocostal triangles into the chest and suggested that the abdominal contents were initially covered by a membrane which could later rupture and disappear. This concept is no longer valid. According to more recent understanding of the development of the diaphragm, posterolateral defects result from defective formation and/or fusion of the pleuroperitoneal membrane [81]. If fusion has not occurred by the tenth week, when the intestines return to the abdomen from the umbilical cord, or if the bowel returns prematurely, herniation into the chest can occur.

Furthermore, the lumbocostal triangle described

Ventral diaphragmatic (septum transversum) defect

Failure of development of the septum transversum results in a semilunar defect of the ventral diaphragm extending dorsally almost to the vena caval opening and anterolaterally to the rib cage in the mid-clavicular line (Figure 19.2d). Such defects are typically associated with an underlying pericardial defect as well as with a lower sternal defect, upper abdominal wall deficiency and intracardiac anomalies (Cantrell's pentalogy [24]). Less extensive defects, resulting from partial failure of septum transversum development, may be associated with some but not all of the features of the pentalogy; for instance, eight cases reported by Wesselhoeft and DeLuca [127] (who use the term 'central diaphragmatic herniation') include one infant with the full pentalogy, and two with diaphragmatic and pericardial defects and large epigastric omphaloceles but no sternal or cardiac anomalies. Robinson and colleagues [96] use the term 'bilateral anteriomedial defect' for what seems to have been a median septum transversum defect in four cases, all with associated cardiac anomalies.

Comments

1. A certain amount of confusion appears to exist in the literature between Morgagni hernias and septum transversum defects and the author suspects that some so-called Morgagni hernias in neonates have been septum transversum defects.
2. Our series includes three cases with pericardial deficiencies but none conformed with the Cantrell pentalogy type of defect. All were unilateral extensive left-sided deficiencies, presenting clinically as typical Bochdalek hernias, and in each case there was a deficiency of the left side of the pericardium. A detailed diagram in one case shows absence of all but a narrow posterolateral rim of the left hemidiaphragm, suggesting a combined septum transversum/pleuroperitoneal fold deficiency.

Bilateral congenital diaphragmatic hernia

Morgagni hernias are bilateral in 15–30% of cases [4,90]. In the case of posterolateral hernias bilaterality is exceedingly rare; a recent report of such a case [40] was only the eleventh on record. There were no bilateral hernias in our series.

Associated anomalies

Apart from pulmonary hypoplasia, which will be discussed separately, the commonest anomaly associated with congenital diaphragmatic hernia is malrotation of the midgut. Anomalies of intestinal

Table 19.1 Congenital diaphragmatic hernia. Associated anomalies in 153 cases (excluding pulmonary hypoplasia)

Malrotation		63
Congenital heart lesions		
Patent ductus arteriosus	3	
Hypoplastic left heart	2	
VSD	1	8
ASD + coarctation of aorta	1	
Pulmonary stenosis	1	
Undescended testes		8
Meckel's diverticulum		7
Skeletal anomalies		
Minor deformites of hands	3	
Talipes	2	7
Multiple hemivertebrae	1	
Craniostenosis	1	
Myelomeningocele		3
Renal anomalies		
Ectopic (thoracic) kidney	1	
Ectopic (pelvic) kidney	1	3
PUJ obstruction	1	
Inguinal hernia		2
Extralobar pulmonary sequestration		2
Cystic adenomatoid malformation of lung		1
Duodenal atresia		1
Hirschsprung's disease		1
Oesophageal atresia		1
Choanal atresia		1

rotation or fixation were recorded in 63 of our cases but this is certainly an underestimate as the presence of bowel in the chest is incompatible with its normal fixation to the posterior abdominal wall. Other anomalies, shown in order of frequency in Table 19.1, were comparatively uncommon. Since the development of the heart is so closely associated with that of the diaphragm one would expect diaphragmatic hernia to be associated frequently with anomalies of the heart and great vessels. There is, however, little mention of this association in the literature, and even in a collected series of 94 cases of congenital diaphragmatic hernia diagnosed *in utero*, only five (5%) had cardiac anomalies [1]. The association however, between left ventricular hypoplasia and congenital diaphragmatic hernia has been studied by Siebert, Haas and Beckwith [103] who found significantly decreased cardiac mass, due to hypoplasia of the left atrium and ventricle and interventricular septum, in eight infants who had died of the complications of left-sided congenital diaphragmatic hernias; they suggest that *in utero* compression of the mediastinum may interfere with left-sided cardiac development and that the myocardial underdevelopment may be an important factor in the pathogenesis of cardiac insufficiency in patients with left-sided hernias. Of the eight patients in our series with cardiac anomalies none survived; all died soon after birth, with or without surgery.

Pulmonary hypoplasia

The most important factor determining survival in an infant with congenital diaphragmatic hernia is the degree of associated pulmonary hypoplasia. There is little doubt that the cause of this condition is compression of the developing lungs, by the herniated viscera on the ipsilateral side and by the displaced mediastinum on the contralateral side although it should be mentioned that Iritani [58] has recently proposed the interesting theory, based on experimental findings, that it may be the failure of the lung to develop that causes the hernia, rather than vice versa. Ipsilateral hypoplasia is more severe than contralateral and the lower lobes are more involved than the remainder of the lungs [9]. The degree of hypoplasia varies from severe bilateral hypoplasia, which is incompatible with life, through intermediate degrees of severity to comparatively mild compromise of lung development. The place of any individual case in this spectrum appears to depend upon the timing and degree of compression of the lungs during development [50]; in other words on when the viscera herniate into the chest, and on the volume of the hernia. This has been demonstrated both by experimental work [32,46,51,60,87,108,110] and by clinical ultrasound data [1]. If a large hernia occupies the chest during the phase of bronchial tree development (before 16 weeks' gestation) [57] the number of bronchial divisions will be permanently reduced and although, if the baby survives, there is the potential for alveolar development until at least 8 years of age [57], the final number of alveoli is limited by the reduced number of conducting airways and the lung is therefore permanently hypoplastic. Pulmonary hypoplasia affects not only the airways but also the vasculature; there is a reduction in the total cross-sectional area of the pulmonary vascular bed [49] and also an increase in arterial medial wall thickness, as well as peripheral extension of muscle into intra-acinar arteries [71]; the functional results of these features will be discussed later. It has been shown by Harrison and colleagues that in a lamb experimental model the lung made hypoplastic by balloon compression *in utero* can continue to grow and develop before birth if the compression is relieved *in utero* [49].

The hypoplastic lung is excessively fragile and hence susceptible to barotrauma, resulting in alveolar rupture, with progression to pulmonary interstitial emphysema, pneumomediastinum and pneumothorax and even, on rare occasions, culminating in pneumopericardium, surgical emphysema and air embolism [109].

Aetiology

The cause of congenital diaphragmatic hernia is unknown. Anderson [3] and Warkany and colleagues [123] were able to produce the condition in rat offspring by depriving the mothers of vitamin A but there is no evidence of any clinical parallel to this observation. Although the great majority of cases are sporadic, the possibility of the presence of a genetic factor exists since multiple familial occurrence is well documented; Mishalany and Gordo [78], in 1986 reported the third instance of identical twins each with left-sided posterolateral congenital diaphragmatic hernia, bringing the number of reported familial cases to 58 in 29 families, 54 of the cases occurring in siblings. Our series includes a pair of identical twins, both affected, and a binovular twin, the other twin being normal in this case.

Incidence

It is difficult to estimate the true incidence of congenital diaphragmatic hernia, firstly because a considerable proportion of affected infants die either prenatally or very shortly after birth without surgery [1], and secondly because a few will not have symptoms during the neonatal period and will be diagnosed later in life [31]. The most accurate estimates of birth prevalence are to be obtained from malformation registries. During the period 1979–83 the Liverpool registry recorded congenital diaphragmatic hernia in 1 in 4500 live and stillbirths (0.22 per 1000). Comparison of these registered cases with admissions to the Liverpool Neonatal Surgical Centre shows that one-third of these babies were either stillborn or died without having been transferred for surgery. A higher incidence (1 in 2200 of all births) was reported by Butler and Claireaux [22] in 1962 based on the British Mortality Survey, which showed that the majority of children with congenital diaphragmatic hernia never reached a surgical centre and that many of the infants who did not come to operation were grossly premature. Diaphragmatic hernia accounted for 8% of all fatal congenital anomalies. Ninety-five per cent of the stillbirths and 24% of the live births had major associated malformations such as abnormalities of the central nervous system (anencephaly, Arnold–Chiari malformation, hydrocephalus, etc.), congenital heart disease and exomphalos.

Clinical features

Prenatal diagnosis

Prenatal diagnosis of congenital diaphragmatic hernia can be obtained reliably by maternal ultrasonography. During the last decade the criteria for prenatal diagnosis have become well established. Definitive diagnosis rests upon the demonstration of abdominal viscera within the thorax. This is not easy to detect on routine sonography but three features which are more readily detectable – polyhydramnios, mediastinal displacement and absence of an intra-abdominal stomach bubble – should prompt a careful examination of the fetal chest for herniated organs [27]. Important differential diagnoses include mediastinal cysts and cystic adenomatoid malformation of the lung, but in these cases the upper abdominal anatomy is normal [27,85].

The high incidence of polyhydramnios in cases diagnosed prenatally (76% in Adzick's collected series of 94 cases [1], is in marked contrast to the incidence of 7% in our clinical series. Prenatal diagnosis is also associated with a very high mortality rate – 100% in Nakayama's series of nine cases [85] and 80% in the collected series referred to above. In our own series, 35 cases treated during the years 1981–85 included five prenatally diagnosed infants, none of whom survived. These considerations suggest that prenatal diagnosis selects out the worst cases. Prognosis needs to be very guarded, therefore, despite the fact that forewarning of the diagnosis allows for optimal perinatal care, including transfer of the baby *in utero* to the most suitable neonatal centre, planned delivery and immediate resuscitation.

Presenting symptoms and signs

In neonates with congenital diaphragmatic hernia respiratory symptoms are predominant and in the majority of cases these will date from birth and will become worse as swallowed air, or feed, increases the volume of herniated stomach and bowel. Cyanosis, present in three-quarters of our cases, is associated with dyspnoea but sometimes dyspnoea alone is the presenting symptom. (Cyanosis without dyspnoea is more likely to be due to a congenital heart lesion.)

The onset and severity of the respiratory symptoms have prognostic significance. We have found that babies who are apnoeic from birth do not survive. All of our fatal cases had severe respiratory symptoms during the first 48 h of life and had been cyanosed and dyspnoeic. On the other hand, absence of respiratory symptoms (5% of our series) is a uniformly good prognostic sign.

Vomiting is an uncommon symptom and was recorded in only seven of our cases. One was a case of hernia through the foramen of Morgagni, with neither cyanosis nor dyspnoea. In the others the vomiting was indicative of an underlying complication such as malrotation of the midgut, ruptured stomach (in two infants, one of whom vomited blood) and a single rare case of strangulated diaphragmatic hernia [95]; this infant presented with vomiting and also passed blood per rectum.

Physical examination

The most reliable physical sign is apparent dextrocardia and any newborn with respiratory distress and a displaced apex beat must be regarded as having a diaphragmatic hernia until proved otherwise. We have seen four cases in which a displaced apex beat was found on routine examination of asymptomatic babies who were subsequently X-rayed and diagnosed. The other classic signs of prominence and decreased movement of the affected side of the chest, a scaphoid abdomen and bowel sounds heard on auscultation of the chest are less reliable, but diminution of breath sounds on the affected side of the chest will almost always be found. In our experience resonance rather than dullness is the rule on percussion of the chest, but stony dullness was found in the infant mentioned previously who had a strangulated diaphragmatic hernia.

Radiological investigation

A single straight X-ray of chest and abdomen is usually all that is required. The typical picture is that

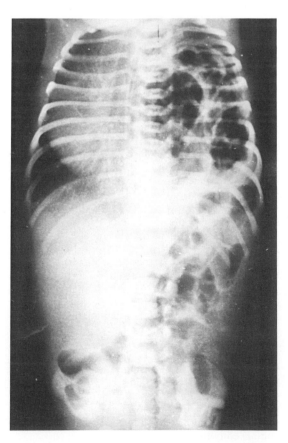

Figure 19.4 Radiograph of chest and abdomen of infant with diaphragmatic hernia, showing gas-filled intestinal loops in the left pleural cavity and gross shifting of the mediastinum to the right. The abdominal gas pattern is abnormal

of gas-filled intestinal loops on the affected side of the chest with compression of the lung into a small area at the apex of the pleural cavity, displacement of the mediastinum to the opposite side and compression of the opposite lung (Figure 19.4). Herniated spleen or liver may be seen as dense shadows. It is very important to include the abdomen in the X-ray as a normal bowel gas pattern casts considerable doubt on the diagnosis (see Differential diagnosis). The gas shadows in the abdomen are typically reduced in number and/or displaced (Figures 19.4 and 19.5) and can often be seen to be in continuity with the gas shadows in the chest (Figure 19.4). The X-ray may be difficult to interpret if it has been taken before the herniated bowel has filled with gas. Such a case is illustrated in Figure 19.5. In the difficult case the diagnosis may sometimes be confirmed by passing a nasogastric tube and observing its thoracic position on X-ray, but this is not always helpful as it may not pass into the herniated stomach. In cases where doubt persists a small amount of non-ionic contrast medium can be given by mouth and/or rectally, but this should be

necessary only on very rare occasions in the neonate.

Differential diagnosis

Conditions which produce the appearance of multiple air-filled circular areas in the lung fields on radiography may, if unilateral, be mistaken for diaphragmatic hernia, especially if associated with cyanosis and dyspnoea. The condition which mimics it most closely is cystic adenomatoid malformation of the lung [23]; the appearance of the chest X-ray may be totally misleading and it is only the fact that the abdominal gas pattern is normal which allows the correct diagnosis to be made (see Chapter 22). Staphylococcal cysts in one lung caused us once to operate in error many years ago, but this is a condition which we no longer see, and one which would not require consideration in the very young baby. A loculated haemopneumothorax secondary to haemorrhagic disease of the newborn has also been reported as leading to the wrong diagnosis [18]. We know of two cases of diaphragmatic hernia

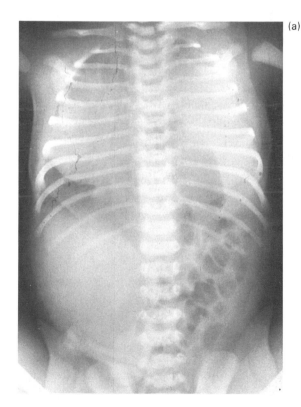

(a)

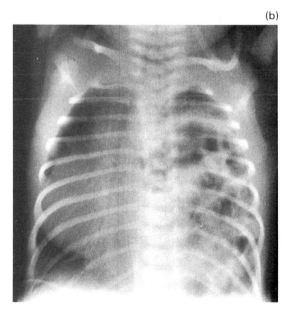

(b)

Figure 19.5 Radiographs of infant with a left-sided diaphragmatic hernia (a) taken shortly after birth showing gas-filled bowel in abdomen, a displaced heart shadow, a solitary gas shadow in the left hemithorax (stomach) and an otherwise opaque left hemithorax. (b) Repeat chest film after transfer of baby showing a more typical appearance of gas-filled intestinal loops; these proved to be distal small intestine and colon, which had filled with gas between (a) and (b)

mistakenly diagnosed as pneumothorax in which chest aspiration was performed with disastrous results. In all of these conditions the important radiological clue is the normal abdominal gas pattern. The features of eventration of the diaphragm will be described separately.

Peri-operative management

Most of the literature concerning the peri-operative management of neonates with congenital diaphragmatic hernia classifies affected babies into various groups. Unfortunately, although the need for some form of classification seems generally agreed, the precise method of grouping varies with each centre. The classification used by the authors in this chapter is similar to that proposed by workers in Toronto [37], and is based on the degree of pulmonary hypoplasia, the time of presentation and blood gas analysis:

Group 1:
 insignificant pulmonary hypoplasia
 usually asymptomatic for first 6 h after birth
 have near-normal blood gas values
 insignificant right-to-left shunting postoperatively
 pharmacological intervention usually not needed
 mortality rate <5% [74,99]

Group 2:
 significant degree of pulmonary hypoplasia
 usually symptomatic within 6 h of birth
 highest possible pre-ductal P_{aO_2} >80 mmHg
 lowest possible P_{aCO_2} <40 mmHg
 prone to episodes of pulmonary hypertension
 mortality rate about 30% [68,99]

Group 3:
 severe bilateral pulmonary hypoplasia
 always symptomatic within 6 h of birth
 highest preductal P_{aO_2} <60 mmHg
 lowest possible P_{aCO_2} >40 mmHg
 intractable pulmonary hypertension
 100% mortality rate [16,37,114,118]

The treatment to be outlined is essentially the peri-operative management of group 2 neonates, as these potentially salvageable babies provide us with the majority of our problems. The basic principles of therapy, however, are applicable to all affected neonates to some degree or other.

The pulmonary hypoplasia associated with congenital diaphragmatic hernia not only results in a reduced surface area for gas exchange but also in a proportionately small pulmonary vascular bed [41,63,71]. The number of blood vessels per unit of lung is also disproportionately reduced. These anatomical factors inevitably lead to a 'fixed' increase in pulmonary vascular resistance (PVR). In addition, babies with pulmonary hypoplasia have an increased thickness of pulmonary arterial smooth muscle and demonstrate severe hyperreactivity of the pulmonary vascular bed. Peri-operative management of group 2 babies is aimed at avoidance of any stimulus that has an adverse effect on PVR and aggressive treatment of pulmonary hypertension (PHT) and right-to-left shunting if and when it occurs.

All babies who have had a congenital diaphragmatic hernia diagnosed within a few hours of birth should be paralysed, intubated and artificially ventilated with 100% oxygen. Muscle relaxation is essential to prevent swallowing and non-compliance with ventilation. The pressure required to fully inflate a hypoplastic lung is often higher than the rupture pressure not only of the hypoplastic lung itself but also of the more normal lung. A pneumothorax on either side (or both!) is therefore a relatively common and potentially life-threatening complication. Sudden deterioration of the baby at any time in the peri-operative period always requires exclusion of a pneumothorax as a precipitating cause. A low inflating pressure (less than 25 cmH$_2$O) is therefore desirable. A blood pH above 7.4 reduces the severity of pulmonary hypoxic vasoconstriction, however, and a respiratory alkalosis is certainly beneficial if it can be achieved without compromising cardiac output or producing a pneumothorax. In order to hyperventilate affected babies, whilst at the same time keeping mean intrathoracic pressures to a minimum, very high respiratory rates and small tidal volumes may be needed. However, if despite these measures it proves impossible to reduce the P_{aCO_2} below 40 mmHg, the prognosis is poor. A recent study by Bohn *et al.* [16] analysed the peri-operative respiratory indices of 66 affected neonates to determine whether outcome was related to pulmonary hypoplasia as predicted by pre-operative P_{aCO_2}. They found a mortality of 77% in babies with a P_{aCO_2} >40 mmHg. In babies where P_{aCO_2} could only be corrected using high frequency ventilation, mortality was still more than 50%. (Postoperatively, the ability to hyperventilate to a P_{aCO_2} <40 mmHg proved to be an important predictor of survival; only one out of 31 died, whereas only two out of 27 babies with a P_{aCO_2} >40 mmHg survived).

The gut within the hernia should be kept decompressed by continuous or frequent intermittent suction on a nasogastric tube. The value of tilting the baby towards the side of the hernia, although commonly advised, is somewhat questionable in the paralysed, ventilated patient. (In group 1 patients, however, such posturing of the patient may help to reduce hernia size and allow maximum movements of the diaphragm on the normal side.) An intravenous cannula should be inserted and, because of the adverse effect that pH has on PVR, full correction of the inevitable metabolic acidosis is advised. A sample of arterial blood for blood gas analysis should be taken from the right arm and the FiO_2

adjusted to ensure a P_{aO_2} of 100 ± 20 mmHg, as pulmonary artery P_{aO_2} levels below 60 mmHg may profoundly increase PVR [20]. Samples taken from the left arm or lower limbs can be misleading due to right-to-left shunting through the ductus arteriosus. If, despite the above measures, the P_{aO_2} is below 80 mmHg then vasodilator treatment should be considered (see below). Failure of hyperventilation with 100% oxygen to improve the patient's condition often indicates that the severity of lung hypoplasia is too great for long-term survival.

Once at the referral centre, babies may require further treatment to optimize oxygenation and perfusion. In the presence of an elevated right ventricular (RV) afterload produced by pulmonary hypertension, the right atrial pressure increases and the mean pressure in the systemic venous system must be elevated to maintain an adequate venous return and RV preload. Although vasodilatation and artificial ventilation may help to reduce right-to-left shunting and improve oxygenation, they may also significantly reduce RV preload such that RV function is seriously impaired. Thus, fluid management is critical in these patients and monitoring of central venous pressure (CVP) will be essential to optimize RV pre-load. In addition, a CVP line will enable safe and reliable administration of other vasoactive drugs that may be needed; many babies will require further cardiovascular support with inotropic agents such as dopamine or dobutamine. Fentanyl, in a single dose of 25 µg/kg [54], or by infusion at 3 µg/kg per h [118], has been shown to reduce the vasoconstrictor response of the pulmonary circulation to various stressful stimuli. The hyperreactivity of the pulmonary vascular bed in these babies makes even routine endotracheal suction a potentially life-threatening procedure, and an opioid infusion may help to reduce the frequency and severity of pulmonary hypertensive crises.

The intubated, ventilated baby should be taken to theatre with acid/base status, perfusion and oxygenation optimized and thus in the best possible condition to undergo major surgery. There is no advantage to be gained by rushing into theatre with a poorly perfused, cold, acidotic, hypoxic baby. Surgery is not going to improve the patient's condition unless there is strangulation of the bowel or some other rare complication such as rupture of the stomach, which we have seen in two patients. The presence of gut or liver in the chest is not, by itself, a life-threatening condition in the paralysed, ventilated baby. The replacement of hernia contents back into the abdomen does not usually result in any immediate expansion of the lung, since it is hypoplastic rather than atelectatic. In fact, Sakai *et al.* [98] have demonstrated that respiratory mechanics in these babies, far from improving, will frequently deteriorate following hernia repair. The determination of the optimum timing for surgery in severely

affected babies is still the subject of some debate, but on the basis of available evidence, a period of pre-operative stabilization of 24–48 h may be advisable [25,98].

Operation

The majority of paediatric surgeons agree that in neonates the abdominal approach is the method of choice for dealing with diaphragmatic hernia as it is associated with fewer postoperative complications than the thoracic approach [43,61,120]. Repair of the diaphragm from above, although favoured by many surgeons for older infants and children, should not be used in neonates as reduction of the intestine into the underdeveloped peritoneal cavity can be an extremely difficult and traumatizing procedure. Furthermore, the correction of associated malrotation of the midgut and division of Ladd's bands is much easier via the abdominal approach, as is the actual repair of the defect in the diaphragm, at least on the left side. With one exception, a 3-week-old infant with a right-sided hernia, we have used the abdominal route, and this will be the only method described.

The infant is placed flat on his back on the operating table and the abdomen is opened through an oblique incision, starting about 2 cm above the middle of the costal margin and running in a gently curved line to just above the umbilicus (Figure 19.6a). In our experience, this incision gives a better exposure of the undersurface of the diaphragm than the paramedian incision [61,65] or the subcostal incision [76], and it cuts through fewer of the nerves of the anterior abdominal wall. The herniated viscera (Figure 19.6b) are then gently pulled out of the chest. Stomach and bowel can usually be delivered easily but some difficulty may be experienced in returning part of the liver, or the spleen, through a relatively small defect. With patience, however, it is possible to deliver all the displaced abdominal organs from the chest (Figure 19.7). The intestine should then be covered with moist, warm packs. In dealing with a right-sided hernia with herniated liver, attempts should not be made to withdraw the liver first, even though it lies anteriorly, as it will be found that there is insufficient room to pull the liver down without damaging it; it is essential to deliver small intestine and colon first and finally the liver [43].

The diaphragmatic defect is now inspected; in the usual left-sided posterolateral defect exposure is facilitated by division of the left triangular ligament and retraction of the left lobe of the liver. The pleural cavity can be viewed through the defect and the lung inspected; it is usually seen to be very small and compressed into the apex of the pleural cavity. The anaesthetist must not attempt to inflate the lung as alveolar rupture, causing pneumothorax, can

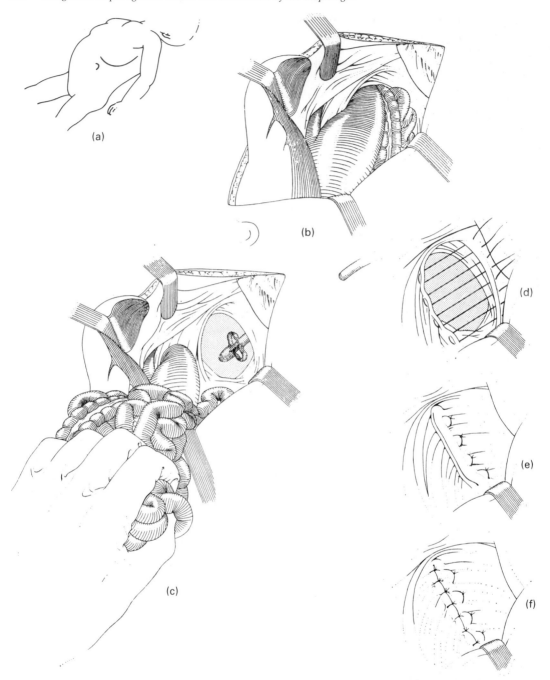

Figure 19.6 Operative repair of left-sided diaphragmatic hernia through an abdominal incision (see text)

easily result. Lack of movement in the lung and difficulty in seeing it clearly should prompt a careful look for a sac which can easily be overlooked as it is a thin membrane closely adherent to the lung and the parietal pleura. It should be picked up with forceps at the apex of the pleural cavity and gently everted through the hernial opening. A sac which billows out of the wound is a sure indication of an air leak from the ipsilateral lung. Preferably the sac should be excised but occasionally, in the case of a large defect, it can be retained and plicated as part of the repair [59].

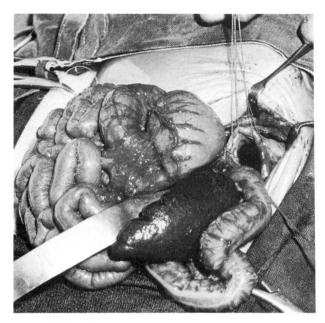

Figure 19.7 Small intestine, colon and spleen have been withdrawn from the chest through a relatively small posterolateral defect. The muscular margins of the defect are held up with stay sutures

Sudden deterioration of the child's condition during operation may well be due to the development of a pneumothorax on the other side; this can be decompressed immediately by passing a cannula through the anterior mediastinum from the ipsilateral pleural cavity.

The rim of the defect is now carefully defined. It is usually triangular in shape, the base of the triangle lying above the adrenal gland (Figure 19.6c). Although at first sight it may appear that there is no posterior rim to the defect, it is usually possible to find and dissect free a flattened-out rim of muscle by incising the posterior parietal peritoneum where it runs into the parietal pleura in the posterior margin of the defect.

Whether or not the ipsilateral pleural cavity should be drained is debatable (see Postoperative management). If it is to be drained, the pleural catheter is inserted before closure of the diaphragmatic defect, through the ninth intercostal space in the mid-axillary line (Figure 19.6c). The hernial opening is now closed in two layers using 3/0 or 2/0 non-absorbable suture material. A row of interrupted mattress sutures is first inserted about 5 mm away from the edge in such a way that when they are tied the edges of the defect are overlapping (Figure 19.6d,e). After these sutures have been tied the remaining free flap is sutured down with

interrupted 3/0 sutures [38] (Figure 19.6f). Cook and colleagues stress that care must be taken not to injure the adrenal gland during this repair; out of 17 of their cases of diaphragmatic hernia examined at autopsy, 15 were found to have extensive adrenal haemorrhage [29].

If the defect is too large, or if the posterior rim is absent, simple closure may be impossible and more complicated procedures will have to be used.

If the posterior part of the diaphragm is completely missing, it may be possible to suture the anterior rim of the defect to the lower ribs with either periosteal or pericostal sutures, or alternatively to the intercostal muscles. The perinephric fat and fascia have also occasionally been used for this purpose [126] but this is not, in our experience, very satisfactory.

In cases where the above procedures are not possible the defect must be patched. This can be done by using a hinged flap of muscle (transversus abdominis and internal oblique) from the anterior abdominal wall [106]; this is a comparatively simple procedure which we have used successfully. The latissimus dorsi flap [11] is a time-consuming operation best reserved for secondary repairs. Other options include free fascial grafts [107], preserved dura [5] and various synthetic materials including Dacron-reinforced Silastic [64,116], Marlex mesh

[8], expanded polytetrafluoroethylene [86] and Dacron, which Valente and Brereton recommend in the light of their experience with ten cases of unilateral agenesis of the diaphragm [119]. Bax and Collins [5] recommend the use of a synthetic patch in all cases, even those with small defects, so as to reconstruct the dome of the diaphragm, which they regard as being of great functional importance.

When the diaphragmatic defect is closed, the intestines are inspected and any malrotation is corrected. The abdominal organs are then returned to the peritoneal cavity, but in a number of cases this will be difficult, or even impossible, because of the reduced capacity of the abdomen. It is unwise to close the abdominal wall under tension as the increased intra-abdominal pressure will not only interfere with diaphragmatic movements but may also predispose to recurrence of the hernia as well as possibly compromising the blood supply to the bowel. In such cases thorough digital stretching of the abdominal wall will often permit satisfactory closure but if not, it will be necessary on rare occasions to create a ventral hernia, either by undermining the abdominal skin and closing it directly over the bowel [43] or by using a Silastic pouch to create an artificial ventral hernia [105]. In either event the abdominal wall can be closed secondarily within 7–10 days.

Morgagni hernias and ventral (septum transversum) defects should be corrected transabdominally in the neonate. In the case of the latter type, Cantrell and colleagues [24] found that even the largest defect could be repaired in the newborn by bringing the remaining diaphragm anteriorly and suturing it to the anterior thoracic wall and costal margin; this manoeuvre simultaneously obliterates the pericardial defect.

Postoperative management

No attempt should be made at the end of the operation to expand the ipsilateral lung, as this manoeuvre may cause a pneumothorax. There have been reports [28,100] that increases in survival rate are possible if pleural drainage can be avoided in the postoperative period. Although a pneumothorax may be one consequence of the efforts made to oxygenate these patients, it has been suggested that the maximum inspiratory pressure is not the only factor determining the incidence of pulmonary barotrauma and that the transpulmonary pressure gradient (TPG) may be more important. An experimental study using lambs [33] has supported the concept that chest drainage of the ipsilateral pleural cavity may promote pulmonary barotrauma in hypoplastic lungs because it increases the TPG. These authors recommended that, to reduce TPG to a minimum, it is necessary to keep ventilatory pressures as low as possible, by employing high rates

and small tidal volumes, and on the other hand, to avoid draining the pleural cavity. The remaining intrapleural air protects the lungs from overdistension by allowing them to expand slowly against a slightly positive pleural pressure. This intrapleural air pocket reabsorbs spontaneously, usually over a few days. Evidence of mediastinal shift due to accumulating fluid and/or air under tension will, however, require immediate drainage, though applying negative pressure to the drain is probably best avoided.

If the baby has required pre-operative artificial ventilation (IPPV) or if the operation has been performed within 24 h of birth, postoperative IPPV should be continued for at least a further 24 h, before weaning is considered. During this time the $P_{a\text{CO}_2}$ should, if possible, be kept between 30 and 35 mmHg, the arterial pH >7.4 and the $P_{a\text{O}_2}$ between 80 and 100 mmHg. Monitoring of pre- and postductal oxygen saturations using oximeters can give a rapid and accurate guide to the extent of right-to-left shunting, as long as peripheral perfusion remains good.

Evidence of significant right-to-left shunting, indicating increasing pulmonary vascular resistance, and resulting in falls in postductal arterial oxygen saturation, should be treated aggressively. Immediate steps to obtund this vicious circle of increasing hypoxia and acidosis include hyperventilation with 100% oxygen, systemic alkalinization using a sodium bicarbonate infusion, and if necessary, consideration of vasodilator and extracorporeal membrane oxygenation (ECMO) therapy. Maintenance of cardiac output may require the use of inotropic support. Isoprenaline is the only inotropic agent to directly decrease the pulmonary vascular resistance, though its use is limited by its relatively modest effect on contractility and its pronounced chronotropic activity. Dopamine or dobutamine both have little direct effect on PVR in doses less than 10 μg/kg per min (20,35,55,66,113,130].

Monitoring of CVP is useful as a means of assessing fluid requirements, particularly if there is excessive transudate loss of protein-rich fluid into the pleural cavity, or if vasodilator therapy is required; human albumin solution or blood should be used as the replacement fluid in these cases, depending on the haematocrit. Crystalloid (10% dextrose) intake should be restricted to half normal requirements, i.e. 2 ml/kg per h, for the first 48 h, after which it can be gradually increased, on condition that the urine output is >1 ml/kg per h. Sodium intake should be monitored carefully, particularly if a bicarbonate infusion is being administered. Diuretic therapy (e.g. frusemide 1 mg/kg) may be needed to maintain a negative fluid balance, after due allowance for insensible losses, in babies with heart failure.

Recent work with high frequency ventilation and

ECMO therapy has shown encouraging results in selected patients. ECMO is not a therapy that will quickly become a routine, in view of its high cost in staff time and the relatively limited number of centres with the necessary expertise. It should probably only be considered for babies in group 2 who are severely ill, failing to respond to more conventional treatment, but who have shown the potential for extrauterine survival. Hypoplastic lungs probably do not grow or develop significantly on ECMO, which provides only a period of 'lung rest', removing the lungs from the traumas of high airway pressures and inspired oxygen content. Survival rates for selected babies receiving ECMO have been dramatically good; up to 86% [68,69,114,125].

Vasodilator therapy

The only specific pulmonary vasodilator is oxygen. All drugs currently in use for the purpose of reducing PVR also have similar effects on systemic vascular resistance (SVR). One of the commonest drugs to be used in babies with PHT is tolazoline. This drug acts as an antagonist at alpha-adrenergic and histamine receptors; it may also have a direct action on vascular smooth muscle and on the myocardium [122]. Tolazoline also inhibits prostanoid synthesis [38]; this action may be of particular value, as it has been shown experimentally that pharmacological blockade of thromboxane synthesis leads to a significant reduction in the pulmonary hypoxic vasoconstrictor response in newborn lambs [2]. Further studies in the human population using specific thromboxane inhibitors are awaited with interest. Nevertheless, the use of tolazoline is not without risk; side effects include gastrointestinal haemorrhage and cardiac and renal toxicity. The elimination half-life of tolazoline is between 5 and 13 h in neonates and when given by continuous infusion is likely to accumulate [79,80]. Monin and colleagues have recently questioned the rationale for using such a drug in this manner; they suggested that intermittent doses of 0.5 mg/kg may be equally effective and safer than the higher doses usually proposed [79].

Many other drugs having vasodilator properties, such as nitroprusside, nitroglycerine and phenoxybenzamine have been used successfully in this condition, but none have any significant advantages over any other agent. One drug which does have some theoretical advantages, however, is epoprostenol (prostacyclin). It is a short-acting drug, its activity only lasting a few minutes. It is given by continuous infusion at a dose of 5–20 ng/kg per min. It is a powerful vasodilator and a potent inhibitor of platelet aggregation. In clinical use it seems remarkably free of troublesome side-effects and may prove to be a useful addition to our therapeutic armamentarium [21,73]. The outstanding disadvantage of epoprostenol, at least at the present time, is its high cost.

The rationale for vasodilator therapy in neonates with CDH has recently been questioned by Vacanti and colleagues [118], who point out that an expansion of vascular capacitance necessitates additional intravenous fluid. This may result in an increase in lung water; higher inflation pressures may then be required for adequate ventilation with consequent reduced cardiac output and an increased risk of pneumothorax.

Results and follow-up

The results of surgical repair of diaphragmatic hernia depend to a large degree on the type of case admitted to the hospital. In hospitals to which patients are admitted from widely scattered places of origin the diaphragmatic defects tend to be small, the infants of adequate weight and with few serious associated abnormalities. The results should, therefore, be good [18]. In centres where great efforts are made to admit as many cases as possible the case material will be less favourable and will approach the type of case reported by Butler and Claireaux in the British Perinatal Mortality Survey [22]. The experience of the San Francisco team [85] suggests that the highest mortality may be expected from centres dealing with a high proportion of prenatally diagnosed cases.

In individual institutions changing referral patterns have affected mortality rates over the last half century. Gross [43] reported an 11% mortality rate at the Boston Children's Hospital for the period 1940–50, during which time 91% of the patients were over 24 h old on admission [44]. In 1964 he reported [44] that the overall mortality rate had reached 32% because much younger neonates with a poorer survival rate were being admitted; by this stage only 52% were more than 24 h old.

Our own case material and results over the years show a comparable trend; during the first decade of the Liverpool Neonatal Surgical Centre (1953–62) 30 cases, of which 60% were more than 24 h of age, all came to surgery, with a mortality of 40%. During the last decade of the series (1976–85) 64 admissions included only five (8%) over the age of 24 h; six died without surgery and the mortality amongst the operated cases was 48%. We consider that the most important factor affecting the mortality figures adversely has been the admission of an increasing proportion of babies who formerly would have died shortly after birth but who are now diagnosed early, resuscitated, intubated and transported by a 'flying squad', but who finally prove to have insufficient lung tissue for survival.

Although the great majority of babies who become symptomatic after the age of 24 h survive, many authors report a mortality of about 50% for patients who require ventilatory assistance during the first 18–24 h of life [17,50,94,109]. In recent years, however, there have been some encouraging reports of improving survival amongst the 'critical' patients. It is difficult to compare different series closely because of varying criteria. Results attributable to the use of ECMO have already been mentioned. Langham and colleagues [68] have analysed the results in 93 neonates reported to the neonatal ECMO registry and report a 42% mortality, the majority of deaths being due to bleeding complications and renal insufficiency. These results represent a significant advance in treatment since ECMO was used only for neonates who met criteria predictive of death in individual centres, but this technique is expensive and is available in only a small number of centres.

Other authors, in reporting improved results, lay emphasis on various aspects of pre- and postoperative cardiorespiratory care. Cloutier [28], for example, stresses the importance of avoiding lung damage by rapid over-expansion and records a marked improvement in survival in a small group treated without aspiration or drainage of the ipsilateral pleural cavity. Hansen and colleagues [47] also emphasize the importance of a decreased incidence of pneumothorax as a factor responsible for an improvement in survival from 45 to 82% over two consecutive 3-year periods. Reynolds [94] reports improved survival of 'critical' infants (defined as those who develop distress in the first hour of life, require resuscitation and cannot be stabilized before operation), following improvements in respiratory care. Marshall and Sumner [74] reports a survival rate of 71% in 62 babies treated at Great Ormond Street and attributed their improved results to close cooperation between surgeons and anaesthetist both in immediate management and in postoperative care. An outstanding, albeit small, series of cases was reported from Leeds by Nair and colleagues [84] who achieved 92% survival in 13 babies all presenting within 12 h of birth and all severely acidotic and hypoxic. All were repaired by the transthoracic route; four diaphragms required patching. The authors attribute their excellent results to their management of acidosis and hypoxia by dopamine infusion and prolonged respiratory support.

There is a significant morbidity following diaphragmatic hernia repair. Most authors mention recurrence. In our series there were seven recurrences, diagnosed at intervals ranging from 3 to 21 months after the initial repair. One child died, having shown a clinical picture of malabsorption. The remainder were repaired, two requiring a prosthetic patch; one of these two children, who had had an agenesis of the left hemidiaphragm extending to the oesophagus, required a fundoplication at the same operation for intractable gastro-oesophageal reflux. Another child required a fundoplication at 3 weeks of age for the same reason. More frequent use of patching, as advocated by Bax and Collins [5] would probably reduce the recurrence rate.

Although the great majority of children with repaired diaphragmatic hernia enjoy normal exercise tolerance, follow-up studies show that evidence of pulmonary hypoplasia persists. Berdon and colleagues [9] noted the development of lower lobe emphysema in serial studies of a case of severe hypoplasia of the right lung. Chatrath, El Shafie and Jones [26] studied ventilatory function in 14 of our survivors between the ages of 6 and 12 years and found evidence of impaired ventilatory function, especially in those noted at operation to have marked pulmonary hypoplasia, even though lung volume measurements were within normal limits. Their results showed that although the hypoplastic lung had expanded to fill the thoracic cavity it had not grown normally. A similar follow-up was performed in Sydney by Reid and Hutcherson [93] on 30 patients up to the age of 21 years. Lungs that were hypoplastic at birth remained underdeveloped as judged by pulmonary function tests and hypoperfusion on lung scan, and there was some suggestion of a pre-emphysematous state in the older patients, although this was asymptomatic. During the last 10 years we have followed up survivors with marked ipsilateral hypoplasia by doing serial ventilation/ perfusion scans which show persistent diminished perfusion, but not ventilation, of the ipsilateral lung.

The future: fetal surgery?

Despite the advances in peri-operative management which have been made in recent years there remains a substantial group of babies with congenital diaphragmatic hernia who are non-viable because of pulmonary insufficiency.

In lamb experiments it has been shown that the fetal lung made hypoplastic by balloon compression can, if the compression is relieved *in utero*, continue to grow and develop before birth [49]. It has also been shown that *in utero* correction of diaphragmatic hernia is physiologically sound and technically feasible in the lamb [52]. We are a long way, however, from applying this knowledge to the clinical situation. Despite the fact that prenatal diagnosis is becoming almost commonplace, it is still not possible to identify with complete accuracy those fetuses who would be potential candidates for intrauterine surgery, namely, those with diaphragmatic hernia causing very severe pulmonary hypoplasia but without other lethal anomalies. Furthermore, there remains the unsolved problem of the sensitivity of the human uterus and the threat of inducing premature labour by hysterotomy [52].

Even if these problems were to be solved, there remains the considerable burden on the mother of two operations: hysterotomy and caesarean section, as well as the risk to the fetus. Further developments in this very challenging area will be awaited with interest.

Eventration of the diaphragm and diaphragmatic paralysis

Historical notes

The first description of a congenital eventration due to hypoplasia of the diaphragm was given by Petit in 1774 [91] and the first successful operation on an infant with this condition was reported by Bisgard [13] in 1947. Successful surgical treatment for eventration due to phrenic nerve palsy was first reported by Bingham [12] in 1954.

Aetiology

Eventrations can be classified into two groups: congenital (non-paralytic) and acquired (paralytic).

Congenital eventration is the result of incomplete development of the muscular portion of the diaphragm. The cause of this failure is not known, but it has been found in cases of fetal rubella [19] and cytomegalovirus infection [7,124] and in babies with trisomic chromosomal abnormalities [128]. Familial incidence is extremely rare [112].

Acquired eventration in the neonate is usually the result of a traction injury to the roots of the phrenic nerve during traumatic breech delivery [111], resulting, in severe cases, in actual tearing of the roots [39]. Paralysis caused by direct pressure on the phrenic nerve by forceps applied to the neck carries a better prognosis [112]. In older infants and children the commonest cause of phrenic nerve palsy is injury during cardiac surgery [67].

So as to differentiate clearly between the two conditions the term phrenic nerve palsy will be used for the acquired lesions and the term eventration restricted to the congenital lesions.

Pathological anatomy and physiology

Eventration may be partial or total. A localized area of muscular hypoplasia produces a characteristic 'hump', most commonly situated anteromedially. Such lesions are unlikely to cause problems in the neonatal period. We have encountered them in the EMG syndrome (see Chapter 27). The whole hemidiaphragm may be affected by varying degrees of hypoplasia, from a moderate degree of thinning of the muscle to complete absence of muscle fibres, the diaphragm being reduced to a thin, often transparent, membrane of connective tissue [70]. This extreme variety may be difficult to distinguish

from a diaphragmatic hernia with a sac. Eventration is said to be much more common on the left than the right but in our series of nine neonatal cases five were right-sided. Bilateral congenital eventration is rare; Rodgers and Hawks reported three cases in 1986 and could find only 25 previous cases in the English literature [97].

The functional effects of severe muscular hypoplasia are the same as those of complete phrenic nerve paralysis; the affected diaphragm is not only elevated, with compression of the ipsilateral lung, but also moves paradoxically; this prevents air entry into the ipsilateral lung and also causes a marked shift of the very mobile mediastinum which jeopardizes function of the contralateral lung.

Associated anomalies

A variety of additional malformations have been recorded in cases of eventration; as well as the related pulmonary hypoplasia, these include defects of the ribs, cardiac anomalies, renal ectopia, cerebral agencis, hydrocephalus and exomphalos [97,112]. Table 19.2 lists the additional anomalies recorded in nine neonatal cases of eventration treated in Liverpool during 1953–85. In two babies no additional malformations were recorded and in one malrotation was the only associated problem.

Incidence

The incidence of eventration is very difficult to determine since there is a tendency to include figures for congenital eventrations with diaphragmatic hernias, whilst asymptomatic lesions will not be included in such series. Conversely, figures derived from surveys of adult radiographs will not do justice to the neonatal incidence. The figure generally quoted for adult incidence is approximately 1:10 000 [62]. Our own figures (nine cases in neonates as against 153 diaphragmatic hernias) provide only a

Table 19.2 Eventration of diaphragm. Associated anomalies in nine cases (excluding pulmonary hypoplasia)

Malrotation		4
Cardiac anomalies		
Coarctation of aorta	1	
VSD	1	3
Partial anomalous pulmonary venous drainage	1	
Renal anomalies		
Thoracic kidney	1	
Pelvic kidney	1	3
Solitary dysplastic pelvic kidney	1	
Deformities of pinna		2
Meckel's diverticulum		1
Perineal anus		1
Single umbilical artery		1
Undescended testis		1
Vertebral anomalies		1
Down's syndrome		1

crude estimate of prevalence and the finding of evidence of 'diaphragmatic weakness' in 4% of 2500 newborn chest radiographs reviewed by Beck and Motsay [6] must be an overestimate. Their criteria are not given.

The incidence of phrenic nerve palsy secondary to birth trauma is generally considered to be lower than that of eventration [14,70] but evidently varies widely from centre to centre. In Liverpool we do not see such cases whereas in the University Children's Hospital, Zurich, 12 cases were treated between 1960 and 1975, compared with two neonatal cases of eventration [112].

Clinical picture

Symptoms and signs

Eventration

Babies with eventration present in the same way as diaphragmatic hernia but in our experience they tend to have less severe symptoms. In seven of our nine cases cyanosis or dyspnoea or both were noted on the day of birth but only three were admitted during the first 24 h of life and only two required emergency intubation. Three were admitted between 24 and 48 h, the remainder at 3, 6 and 14 days. Physical signs were indistinguishable from those of diaphragmatic hernia.

Phrenic nerve palsy

Neonates suffering from a severe degree of phrenic nerve palsy due to birth trauma present with dyspnoea, tachypnoea and cyanosis. Symptoms may develop on the day of birth but may be delayed for days or weeks and the severity of the paralysis does not always correspond with the severity of the symptoms [111]. Typically the infant will have had a difficult breech birth and will have an Erb's palsy [111].

Radiological findings

Radiography of the chest and abdomen in the upright position usually shows the elevated hemidiaphragm clearly (Figures 19.8 and 19.9). It must

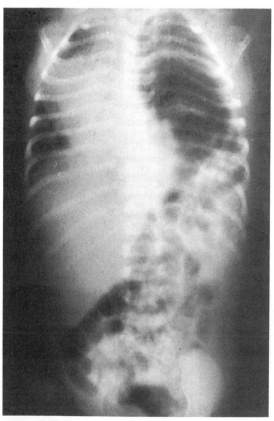

(a)

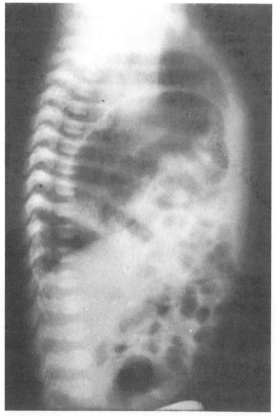

(b)

Figure 19.8 (a) Anteroposterior and (b) lateral chest and abdominal radiographs of a left-sided congenital eventration. On the AP view the thickness of the structure limiting the bowel in the upper chest suggests that it is not merely a hernial sac; the lateral view shows that the entire leaf of the diaphragm is elevated

be remembered, however, that the diaphragm may be displaced to a normal position by positive pressure ventilation [97,101] and that a totally different picture may emerge when the child is allowed to breathe spontaneously. In all cases of phrenic nerve palsy fluoroscopy is indicated to show whether or not there is paradoxical movement of the diaphragm as this is of prime importance in prognosis [111]. In the majority of cases of eventration presenting in the neonatal period the child's condition and chest radiograph (Figure 19.8) provide ample evidence that surgery is required, but fluoroscopy will help in the assessment of less severe degrees of eventration.

Treatment

The choice between conservative and surgical management rests on clinical assessment, radiography, fluoroscopy and blood gas analysis. In the case of incomplete phrenic nerve palsy, as evidenced by absence of paradoxical movement, conservative management will often tide the child over until normal function returns. Paradoxical movement, however, is a strong indication for surgery. Plication of the diaphragm is now a well accepted technique both for eventration and phrenic nerve palsy. There is, however, some controversy about the appropriate timing in the latter group of patients, some authors advocating early plication [75,102,111] whilst others prefer a trial of mechanical ventilation for 2 or 3 weeks [67,101] or even up to 3–6 weeks

[45]. In our opinion the hazards of prolonged ventilation outweigh both the risks of surgery (which are negligible) and the possibility of damaging a diaphragm which would have recovered spontaneously.

Surgical technique

In the case of eventration an abdominal approach is preferable for the reasons given in the case of diaphragmatic hernia. The operation is basically the same apart from the fact that the diaphragm is plicated rather than repaired. In the case of phrenic nerve palsy the diaphragm can be approached from above or below but in the case of right-sided paralysis the thoracic approach is recommended [101]. Several forms of 'plication' have been described. Schwartz and Filler [101] review the various techniques and describe their method of pleating the diaphragm without injury to the phrenic nerve. The technique used by Stauffer and Rickham [111] is illustrated in Figure 19.10. Non-absorbable sutures are used and the diaphragm is flattened as much as possible. In the case of eventration the plication can be reinforced by a flap of transversus abdominis [97].

Results

Of our nine neonatal cases of eventration only four survived. Two babies, both with multiple anomalies including congenital heart lesions, died without

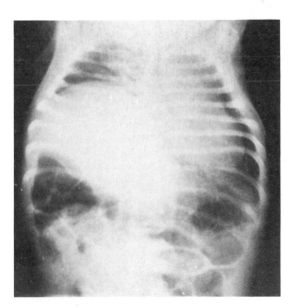

Figure 19.9 Radiograph of a 2-day-old newborn with acquired eventration of the right diaphragm. There is a shift of the mediastinum and the heart to the left. Paradoxical movement was seen on fluoroscopy.

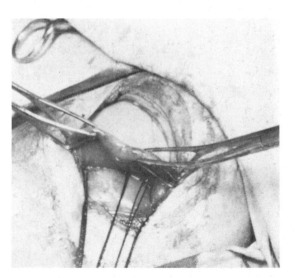

Figure 19.10 Plication of the right diaphragm by transthoracic approach. A row of non-absorbable mattress sutures is placed at the base of the plication. The plication will then be fixed anteriorly to the abdominal wall and the ribs

having had surgery. There were three postoperative deaths, two as a result of pulmonary hypoplasia and one due to renal insufficiency. Of the four survivors one has a recurrent right-sided eventration but has not required further surgery. Better results can be expected in cases of eventration presenting in older infants [112] and the prognosis is also more favourable in phrenic nerve palsy due to birth injury; Stauffer and Rickham [111] reported 100% recovery in eight neonates treated by plication of the diaphragm, but one death occurred amongst four cases managed conservatively.

References

1. Adzick, N.S., Harrison, M.R., Glick, P.L., Nakayama, D.K., Manning, F.A. and deLorimier, A.A. (1985) Diaphragmatic hernia in the fetus; prenatal diagnosis and outcome in 94 cases. *J. Pediat. Surg.*, **20**, 357–361
2. Alexander, F., Manny, J., Lelcuk, S., Shepro, D. and Hechtman, H.B. (1986) Cyclo-oxygenase products mediate hypoxic pulmonary hypertension. *J. Pediat. Surg.*, **21**, 1101–1107
3. Anderson, D.H. (1949) Effect of diet during pregnancy upon the incidence of congenital diaphragmatic hernia in the rat. *Am. J. Path.*, **25**, 163
4. Baran, E.M., Houston, H.E., Lynn, H.B. and O'Connell, E.J. (1967) Foramen of Morgagni hernia in children. *Surgery*, **62**, 1076–1081
5. Bax, N.M.A. and Collins, D.L. (1984) The advantages of reconstruction of the dome of the diaphragm in congenital posterolateral diaphragmatic defects. *J. Pediat. Surg.*, **19**, 484–487
6. Beck, W.C. and Motsay, D.S. (1952) Eventration of the diaphragm. *Arch. Surg.*, **65**, 557–563
7. Becroft, D.M.O. (1979) Prenatal cytomegalovirus infection and muscular deficiency (eventration) of the diaphragm. *J. Pediat.*, **94**, 74–75
8. Benjamin, H.B. (1963) Agenesis of the left hemidiaphragm. *J. Thorac. Cardiovasc. Surg.*, **46**, 265–270
9. Berdon, W.E., Baker, D.H. and Amoury, R. (1968) The role of pulmonary hypoplasia in the prognosis of newborn infants with diaphragmatic hernia and eventration. *Am. J. Roent.*, **103**, 413–421
10. Bettman, R.B. and Hess, J.H. (1929) Incarcerated diaphragmatic hernia in an infant. *J. Am. Med. Ass.*, **92**, 2014–2016
11. Bianchi, A., Doig, C.M. and Cohen, S.J. (1983) The reverse latissimus dorsi flap for congenital diaphragmatic hernia repair. *J. Pediat. Surg.*, **18**, 560–563
12. Bingham, J.A.W. (1954) Two cases of unilateral paralysis of the diaphragm in the newborn treated surgically. *Thorax*, **9**, 248–252
13. Bisgard, J.D. (1947) Congenital eventration of the diaphragm. *J. Thorac. Surg.*, **16**, 484–491
14. Bishop, H.C. and Koop, C.E. (1958) Acquired eventration of the diaphragm in infancy. *Pediatrics*, **22**, 1088–1096
15. Bochdalek, V. (1848) Einige Betrachtungen ueber die Einstellung des angeborenen Zwerchfellbruches als Beitrag zur pathologischen Anatomie der Hernien. *Viertelijahrs. Prakt. Heilk.*, **19**, 89
16. Bohn, D., Tamura, M., Perrin, D., Barker, G. and Rabinovitch, M. (1987) Ventilatory predictors of pulmonary hypoplasia in congenital diaphragmatic hernia, confirmed by morphological assessment. *J. Pediat.*, **111**, 423–431
17. Boix-Ochoa, J., Peguero, G., Seijo, G., Natal, A. and Canals, J. (1974) Acid-base balance and blood gases in prognosis and therapy of congenital diaphragmatic hernia. *J. Pediat. Surg.*, **9**, 49–57
18. Bonham-Carter, R.E., Waterston, D.J. and Aberdeen, E. (1962) Hernia and eventration of the diaphragm in childhood. *Lancet*, **i**, 656–659
19. Briggs, V.A., Reilly, B.J. and Loewig, K. (1973) Lung hypoplasia and membranous diaphragm in the congenital rubella syndrome: A rare case. *J. Can. Ass. Radiol.*, **24**, 126–127
20. Burrows, F.A., Klinck, J.R., Rabinovitch, M. and Bohn, D. (1986) Pulmonary hypertension in children; perioperative management. *Can. Anaesth. Soc. J.*, **33**, 606–628
21. Bush, A., Busset, C., Knight, W.B. and Shinebourne, E.A. (1987) Modification of pulmonary hypertension secondary to congenital heart disease by prostacyclin therapy. *Am. Rev. Resp. Dis.*, **136**, 773–776
22. Butler, N. and Claireaux, A.E. (1962) Congenital diaphragmatic hernia as a cause of perinatal mortality. *Lancet*, **i**, 659–663
23. Campbell, D.P. and Raffensperger, J.G. (1972) Congenital cystic disease of the lung masquerading as diaphragmatic hernia. *J. Thorac. Cardiovasc. Surg.*, **64**, 592–595
24. Cantrell, J.R., Haller, J.A. and Ravitch, M.M. (1958) A syndrome of congenital defects involving the abdominal wall, sternum, diaphragm, pericardium, and heart. *Surg. Gynec. Obstet.*, **107**, 602–614
25. Cartlidge, P.H.T., Mann, N.P. and Kapila, L. (1986) Preoperative stabilisation in congenital diaphragmatic hernia. *Arch. Dis. Child.*, **61**, 1226–1228
26. Chatrath, R.R., El Shafie, M. and Jones, R.S. (1971) Fate of hypoplastic lungs after repair of congenital diaphragmatic hernia. *Arch. Dis. Child.*, **46**, 633–635
27. Chinn, D.H., Filly, R.A., Callen, P.W., Nakayama, D.K. and Harrison, M.R. (1983) Congenital diaphragmatic hernia diagnosed prenatally by ultrasound. *Radiology*, **148**, 119–123
28. Cloutier, R., Fournier, L. and Levasseur, L. (1983) Reversion to fetal circulation in congenital diaphragmatic hernia: a preventable postoperative complication. *J. Pediat. Surg.*, **18**, 551–554
29. Cook, R.C.M. and Beckwith, J.B. (1971) Adrenal

injury during repair of diaphragmatic hernia in infants. *Surgery*, **69**, 251–255

30. Cooper, Sir Astley P. (1827) *The Anatomy and Surgical Treatment of Abdominal Hernia*, Longman, Rees, Orme, Brown and Green, London

31. Day, B. (1972) Late appearance of Bochdalek hernia. *Br. Med. J.*, **i**, 786

32. DeLorimier, A.A., Tierney, D.F. and Parker, H.R. (1967) Hypoplastic lungs in fetal lambs with surgically produced congenital diaphragmatic hernia. *Surgery*, **62**, 12–16

33. De Luca, U., Cloutier, R., Laberge, J.M., Fournier, L., Prendt, H. and Major, D. (1987) Pulmonary barotrauma in congenital diaphragmatic hernia: experimental study in lambs. *J. Pediat. Surg.*, **22**, 311–316

34. Donovan, E.J. (1938) Congenital diaphragmatic hernia. *Ann. Surg.*, **108**, 374–388

35. Driscoll, D.J., Gillette, P.C., Duff, D.F., Nihill, M.R., Gutgesell, H.P., Vargo, T.A. *et al.* (1979) Hemodynamic effects of dobutamine in children. *Am. J. Cardiol.*, **43**, 581–585

36. Dunhill, T. (1935) Diaphragmatic hernia. *Br. J. Surg.*, **22**, 475–503

37. Ein, S.E. and Barker, G. (1987) The pharmacological treatment of newborn diaphragmatic hernia – update 1987. *Pediat. Surg. Int.*, **2**, 341–345

38. Ford, W.D.A., James, M.J. and Walsh, J.A. (1984) Congenital diaphragmatic hernia; association between pulmonary vascular resistance and plasma thromboxane concentration. *Arch. Dis. Child.*, **59**, 143–146

39. France, N.E. (1954) Unilateral diaphragmatic paralysis and Erb's palsy in the newborn. *Arch. Dis. Child.*, **29**, 357–359

40. Furuta, Y., Nakamura, Y. and Miyamoto, K. (1987) Bilateral congenital posterolateral diaphragmatic hernia. *J. Pediat. Surg.*, **22**, 182–183

41. Geggel, R.L., Murphy, J.D., Langleben, D., Crone, R.K., Vacanyi, J.P. and Reid, L.M. (1985) Congenital diaphragmatic hernia; arterial structural changes and persistent hypertension after surgical repair. *J. Pediat.*, **7**, 457–459

42. Greenwald, H.M. and Steiner, M. (1929) Diaphragmatic hernia in infancy and childhood. *Am. J. Dis. Child.*, **38**, 361–392

43. Gross, R.E. (1953) *The Surgery of Infancy and Childhood*. W.B. Saunders, Philadelphia, pp. 428–444

44. Gross, R.E. (1964) Thoracic surgery for infants. *J. Thorac. Cardiovasc. Surg.*, **48**, 152–176

45. Haller, J.A. Jr, Pickard, L.R., Tepas, J.J., Rogers, M.C., Robotham, J.L., Shorter, N. *et al.* (1979) Management of diaphragmatic paralysis in infants with special emphasis on selection of patients for operative plication. *J. Pediat. Surg.*, **14**, 779–785

46. Haller, J.A. Jr, Signer, R.D., Gollady, E.S., Inon, A.E., Harrington, D.P. and Shermeta, D.W. (1976) Pulmonary and ductal hemodynamics in studies of simulated diaphragmatic hernia of fetal and newborn lambs. *J. Pediat. Surg.*, **11**, 675–680

47. Hansen, J., James, S., Burrington, J. and Whitfield, J. (1984) The decreasing incidence of pneumothorax and improving survival of infants with congenital diaphragmatic hernia. *J. Pediat. Surg.*, **19**, 385–388

48. Harrington, S.W. (1948) Various types of diaphragmatic hernia treated surgically. *Surg. Gynec. Obstet.*, **86**, 735–755

49. Harrison, M.R., Bressack, M.A., Churg, A.M. and deLorimier, A.A. (1980) Correction of congenital diaphragmatic hernia in utero. II. Simulated correction permits fetal lung growth with survival at birth. *Surgery*, **88**, 260–268

50. Harrison, M.R. and deLorimier, A.A. (1981) Congenital diaphragmatic hernia. *Surg. Clin. N. Am.*, **61**, 1023–1035

51. Harrison, M.R., Jester, J.A. and Ross, N.A. (1980) Correction of congenital diaphragmatic hernia in utero. I. The Model: Intrathoracic balloon produces fatal pulmonary hypoplasia. *Surgery*, **88**, 174–182

52. Harrison, M.R., Ross, N.A. and deLorimier, A.A. (1981) Correction of congenital diaphragmatic hernia in utero. III. Development of a successful surgical technique using abdominoplasty to avoid compromise of umbilical blood flow. *J. Pediat. Surg.*, **16**, 934–942

53. Hedblom, C.A. (1931) Diaphragmatic hernia. *J. Am. Med. Ass.*, **85**, 947–952

54. Hickey, P.R., Hansen, D.D., Wessel, D.L., Lang, P., Jonas, R.A. and Elixson, E.M. (1985) Blunting of stress responses in the pulmonary circulation of infants by fentanyl. *Anesth. Anal.*, **64**, 1137–1142

55. Holloway, E.L., Polumbo, R.A. and Harrison, D.C. (1975) Acute circulatory effects of dopamine in patients with pulmonary hypertension. *Br. Heart J.*, **37**, 483–485

56. Hume, J.B. (1932) Diaphragmatic hernia. *Br. J. Surg.*, **19**, 527–538

57. Inselman, L.S. and Mellins, R.B. (1981) Growth and development of the lung. *J. Pediat.*, **98**, 1–15

58. Iritani, I. (1984) Experimental study on embryogenesis of congenital diaphragmatic hernia. *Anat. Embryol.*, **169**, 133–139

59. Kenigsberg, K. and Gwinn, J.L. (1965) The retained sac in repair of postero-lateral diaphragmatic hernia in the newborn. *Surgery*, **57**, 894–897

60. Kent, G.M., Olley, P.M., Creighton, R.E., Dobbinson, T., Bryan, M.H., Symchych, P. *et al.* (1972) Hemodynamic and pulmonary changes following surgical creation of a diaphragmatic hernia in fetal lambs. *Surgery*, **72**, 427–433

61. Kiesewetter, W.B., Gutierrez, I.Z. and Sieber, W.K. (1961) Diaphragmatic hernia in infants under one year of age. *Arch. Surg.*, **83**, 560–572

62. Kinzer, R.E. and Cook, J.C. (1944) Lesions of diaphragm with special reference to eventration and a report of three cases. *Am. J. Roent.*, **52**, 611–614

63. Kitewaga, M., Hislop, A., Boyden, E.A. and Reid, L. (1971) Lung hypoplasia in congenital diaphragmatic hernia. A quantitative study of airway, artery and alveolar development. *Br. J. Surg.*, **58**, 342–345

64. Lacey, S.R., Goldthorn, J.F. and Kosloske, A.M. (1983) Repair of agenesis of the hemidiaphragm by prosthetic materials. *Surg. Gynec. Obstet.*, **156**, 310–312

65. Ladd, W.E. and Gross, R.F. (1940) Congenital diaphragmatic hernia. *New Engl. J. Med.*, **223**, 917–925

66. Lang, P., Williams, R.G., Norwood, W.I. and Casteneda, A.R. (1980) The hemodynamic effects of dopamine in infants after corrective cardiac surgery. *J. Pediat.*, **96**, 630–634

67. Langer, J.C., Filler, R.M., Coles, J. and Edmonds, J.F. (1988) Plication of the diaphragm for infants and young children with phrenic nerve palsy. *J. Pediat. Surg.*, **23**, 749–751

68. Langham, M.R. Jr, Krummel, T.M., Bartlett, R.H., Drucker, D.E.M., Tracy, T.F., Toomasian, J.M. *et al.* (1987) Mortality with extracorporeal membrane oxygenation following repair of congenital diaphragmatic hernia in 93 infants. *J. Pediat. Surg.*, **22**, 1150–1154

69. Langham, M.R., Krummel, T.M., Greenfield, L.J., Drucker, D.E.M., Tracy, T.F., Mueller, D.G. *et al.* (1987) Extracorporeal membrane oxygenation following repair of congenital diaphragmatic hernias. *Ann. Thorac. Surg.*, **44**, 247–252

70. Laxdal, O.E., McDougall, H. and Mellin, G.W. (1954) Congenital eventration of the diaphragm. *New Engl. J. Med.*, **250**, 401–408

71. Levin, D.L. (1978) Morphological analysis of the pulmonary vascular bed in congenital left-sided diaphragmatic hernia. *J. Pediat.*, **92**, 805–809

72. Liepmann, W. (1903) Die Aetiologie der congenitalen Zwerchfellhernien. *Arch. Gynaekol.*, **68**, 780–800

73. Long, W.A. and Rubin, L.J. (1987) Prostacyclin and PGE1 treatment of pulmonary hypertension. *Am. Rev. Resp. Dis.*, **136**, 773–776

74. Marshall, A. and Sumner, E. (1982) Improved prognosis in congenital diaphragmatic hernis: experience of 62 cases over 2-year period. *J. Roy. Soc. Med.*, **75**, 607–612

75. Mearns, A.J. (1977) Iatrogenic injury to the phrenic nerve in infants and young children. *Ann. Thorac. Surg.*, **32**, 251–259

76. Meeker, I.A. and Snyder, W.H. (1962) Surgical managment of diaphragmatic defects in the newborn infant. *Am. J. Surg.*, **104**, 196–203

77. Merten, D.F., Bowie, J.D., Kirks, D.R. and Grossman, H. (1981) Anteromedial diaphragmatic defects in infancy: current approaches to diagnostic imaging. *Radiology*, **142**, 361–365

78. Mishalany, H. and Gordo, J. (1986) Congenital diaphragmatic hernia in monozygotic twins. *J. Pediat. Surg.*, **21**, 372–374

79. Monin, P., Dubruc, C., Vert, P. and Morselli, P.L. (1987) Treatment of persistent fetal circulation syndrome of the newborn – comparison of different doses of tolazoline. *Eur. J. Clin. Pharmacol.*, **31**, 569–573

80. Monin, P., Vert, P. and Morselli, P.L. (1982) A pharmacodynamic and pharmacokinetic study of tolazoline in the neonate. *Develop. Pharmacol. Therap.*, **4**(Suppl.), 124–128

81. Moore, K.L. (1982) *The Developing Human*, 3rd edn, W.B. Saunders Company, Philadelphia, pp. 170–178

82. Morgagni, J.B. (1769) *The Seats and Causes of Diseases Investigated by Anatomy*, Millar and Cadell, London

83. Müntener, M. (1968) Beitrag zur Kenntnis der Entwicklung des menschlichen Zwerchfells. *Z. Kinderchir.*, **5**, 350

84. Nair, U.R., Entress, A. and Walker, D.R. (1983) Management of neonatal posterolateral diaphragmatic hernia. *Thorax*, **38**, 254–257

85. Nakayama, D.K., Harrison, M.R., Chinn, D.H., Callen, P.W., Filly, R.A., Golbus, M.S. *et al.* (1985) Prenatal diagnosis and natural history of the fetus with a congenital diaphragmatic hernia; Initial clinical experience. *J. Pediat. Surg.*, **20**, 118–124

86. Newman, B.M., Jewett, T.C., Lewis, A., Cerny, F., Khan, A., Karp, M. *et al.* (1985) Prosthetic materials and muscle flaps in the repair of extensive diaphragmatic defects: an experimental study. *J. Pediat. Surg.*, **20**, 362–367

87. Ohi, R., Suzuki, H., Kato, T. and Kasai, M. (1986) Development of the lung in fetal rabbits with experimental diaphragmatic hernia. *J. Pediat. Surg.*, **11**, 955–959

88. Orr, T.G. and Neff, F.C. (1935) Diaphragmatic hernia in infants under one year of age treated by operation. *J. Thorac. Surg.*, **5**, 434–440

89. Paré, A. (1575) *Les Oeuvres*, Buon, Paris

90. Paris, F., Tarazoni, V., Casillas, M., Blasco, E., Canto, A., Pastor, J. *et al.* (1973) Hernia of Morgagni. *Thorax*, **28**, 631–636

91. Petit, J.L. (1774) *Traité des Maladies Chirurgicales*, Vol. 2, T.F. Didot jeune, Paris, p. 226

92. Pokorny, W.J., McGill, C.W. and Harberg, F.J. (1984) Morgagni hernias during infancy: Presentation and associated anomalies. *J. Pediat. Surg.*, **19**, 394–397

93. Reid, I.S. and Hutcherson, R.J. (1976) Long-term follow-up of patients with congenital diaphragmatic hernia. *J. Pediat. Surg.*, **11**, 939–942

94. Reynolds, M., Luck, S.R. and Lappen, R. (1984) The 'critical' neonate with diaphragmatic hernia. A 21-year perspective. *J. Pediat. Surg.*, **19**, 364–369

95. Rickham, P.P. (1955) Strangulated diaphragmatic hernia in the newborn period. *Thorax*, **10**, 104–106

96. Robinson, A.E., Gooneratne, N.S., Blackburn, W.R. and Brogdon, B.G. (1980) Bilateral anterome-

dial defect of the diaphragm in children. *Am. J. Roent.*, **135**, 301–306

97. Rodgers, B.M. and Hawks, P. (1986) Bilateral congenital eventrations of the diaphragms: successful surgical management. *J. Pediat. Surg.*, **21**, 858–864

98. Sakai, H., Tamura, M., Hosakawa, Y., Bryan, A.C., Barker, G.A. and Bohn, D.J. (1987) Effect of surgical repair on respiratory mechanics in congenital diaphragmatic hernia. *J. Pediat.*, **111**, 432–438

99. Sawyer, S.F., Falterman, K.W., Goldsmith, J.P. and Arensman, R.M. (1986) Improving survival in the treatment of congenital diaphragmatic hernia. *Ann. Thorac. Surg.*, **41**, 75–78

100. Schmitt, M., Pierre, E., Prévot, J., Lotte, E. and Droulle, P. (1985) Les hernies diaphramatiques congénitales. Diagnostique anténatal. Drainage thoracique. Ventilation à haute fréquence. *Chirurg. Pédiat.*, **26**, 8–12

101. Schwartz, M.Z. and Filler, R.M. (1978) Plication of the diaphragm for symptomatic phrenic nerve paralysis. *J. Pediat. Surg.*, **13**, 259–263

102. Shoemaker, R., Palmer, G., Brown, J.W. and King, H. (1981) Aggressive treatment of acquired phrenic paralysis in infants and small children. *Ann. Thorac. Surg.*, **32**, 250–259

103. Siebert, J.R., Haas, J.E. and Beckwith, J.B. (1984) Left ventricular hypoplasia in congenital diaphragmatic hernia. *J. Pediat. Surg.*, **19**, 567–571

104. Sigerist, H.E. (1951) *A History of Medicine*, Oxford University Press, New York and London

105. Simpson, J.S. (1969) Ventral silon pouch: Method of repairing congenital diaphragmatic hernias in neonates without increasing intra-abdominal pressure. *Surgery*, **66**, 798–801

106. Simpson, J.S. and Gossage, J.D. (1971) Use of abdominal wall muscle flap in repair of large congenital diaphragmatic hernia. *J. Pediat. Surg.*, **6**, 42–44

107. Singleton, A.O. and Stehonwer, O.W. (1945) The fascia-patch transplant in the repair of hernia. *Surg. Gynec. Obstet.*, **80**, 243–249

108. Soper, R.T., Pringle, K.C. and Scofield, J.C. (1984) Creation and repair of diaphragmatic hernia in the fetal lamb: techniques and survival. *J. Pediat. Surg.*, **19**, 33–40

109. Srouji, M.N., Buck, B. and Downes, J.J. (1981) Congenital diaphragmatic hernia. Deleterious effects of pulmonary interstitial emphysema and tension extrapulmonary air. *J. Pediat. Surg.*, **16**, 45–54

110. Starrett, R.W. and deLorimier, A.A. (1975) Congenital diaphragmatic hernia in lambs. Hemodynamic and ventilatory changes with breathing. *J. Pediat. Surg.*, **10**, 575–582

111. Stauffer, U.G. and Rickham, P.P. (1972) Acquired eventration of the diaphragm in the newborn. *J. Pediat. Surg.*, **7**, 635–643

112. Stauffer, U.G. and Rickham, P.P. (1978) Congenital diaphragmatic hernia and eventration of the diaphragm. In *Neonatal Surgery* (eds P.P. Rickham,

J. Lister and I.M. Irving), 2nd edition, Butterworths, London, pp. 163–178

113. Stephenson, L.W., Edmunds, L.H., Raphaely, R., Morrison, D.F., Hoffman, W.S. and Rubis, L.J. (1979) Effects of nitroprusside and dopamine on pulmonary arterial vasculature in children after cardiac surgery. *Circulation*, **60**, 104–110

114. Stolar, C., Dillon, P. and Reyes, C. (1988) Selective use of extracorporeal membrane oxygenation in the management of congenital diaphragmatic hernia. *J. Pediat. Surg.*, **23**, 207–211

115. Thomas, G.G. and Clitherow, N.R. (1977) Herniation through the foramen of Morgagni in children. *Br. J. Surg.*, **64**, 215–217

116. Touloukian, R.J. (1978) A 'new' diaphragm following prosthetic repair of experimental hemidiaphragmatic defects in the pup. *Ann. Surg.*, **187**, 47–51

117. Truesdale, P.E. (1935) Diaphragmatic hernia in children. *New Engl. J. Med.*, **213**, 1159–1172

118. Vacanti, J.P., Crone, R.K., Murphy, J.D., Smith, S.D., Black, P.R., Reid, L. *et al.* (1984) The pulmonary hemodynamic response to peri-operative anaesthesia in the treatment of high-risk infants with congenital diaphragmatic hernia. *J. Pediat. Surg.*, **19**, 672–679

119. Valente, A. and Brereton, R.J. (1987) Unilateral agenesis of the diaphragm. *J. Pediat. Surg.*, **22**, 848–850

120. Vos, L.J.M., Eijgelaar, A. and Kuijjer, P.J. (1971) Congenital posterolateral diaphragmatic hernia. *Z. Kinderchir.*, **10**, 147

121. Walker, E.W. (1900) Diaphragmatic hernia. *J. Am. Med. Ass.*, **35**, 778

122. Ward, R.M. (1984) Pharmacology of tolazoline. *Clin. Perinatol.*, **113**, 703–713

123. Warkany, J., Roth, C.B. and Wilson, J.G. (1948) Multiple congenital malformations: A consideration of etiologic factors. *Pediatrics*, **1**, 462–471

124. Wayne, E.R., Burrington, J.D., Myers, D.N., Cotton, E.N. and Block, W. (1973) Bilateral eventration of the diaphragm in a neonate with congenital cytomegalic inclusion disease. *J. Pediat.*, **83**, 164–165

125. Weber, T.R. Connors, R.H., Pennington, G., Westfall, S., Keenan, W., Kotagal, S. *et al.* (1987) Neonatal diaphragmatic hernia; an improving outlook with extracorporeal membrane oxygenation. *Arch. Surg.*, **122**, 615–618

126. Weinberg, J. (1938) Diaphragmatic hernia in infants: surgical treatment with use of renal fascia. *Surgery*, **3**, 78–86

127. Wesselhoeft, C.W. and De Luca, F.G. (1984) Neonatal septum transversum diaphragmatic defects. *Am. J. Surg.*, **147**, 481–485

128. Wexler, H.A. and Poole, C.A. (1976) Neonatal diaphragmatic dysfunction. *Am. J. Roent.*, **127**, 617–622

129. White, J.J. and Suzuki, H. (1972) Hernia through the foramen of Bochdalek: a misnomer. *J. Pediat. Surg.*,

7, 60–61

130. Williams, D.B., Kiernan, P.D., Schaff, H.V., Marsh, H.M. and Danielson, G.K. (1982) The hemodynamic response to dopamine and nitroprusside following right atrium-pulmonary artery bypass (Fontan procedure). *Ann. Thorac. Surg.*, **34**, 51–57

20

Gastro-oesophageal reflux and hiatus hernia

James Lister

Surgery in the newborn period is very rarely indicated in the treatment of hiatus hernia and practically never in the treatment of chalasia of the cardia. Symptoms and signs of gastro-oesophageal reflux, however, usually date from birth and many of these infants present considerable management difficulties in the first few weeks of life, sufficient to warrant their admission to hospital and possibly to a neonatal surgical unit: a short discussion is therefore justified in this book.

Historical notes

The condition of hiatus hernia was first described in an adult by Bright in 1836 [6]. Findley and Kelly [16] recognized that the condition was either present at birth or developed soon afterwards.

Neuhauser and Berenburg [32] in 1947 reported 12 newborns with frequent vomiting which they believed to be due to 'chalasia' or a neuromuscular dysfunction of the lower oesophagus; they did not find hiatus hernias in these children, though Carre [9] in reporting his series of 117 children in 1952 believed that when vomiting was persistent and no hiatus hernia could be demonstrated radiologically, it was still likely that there was a minor degree of what he described as 'partial thoracic stomach'.

Although as long ago as 1950 it was shown experimentally [15] that regurgitated gastric contents caused distal oesophagitis, and later that the degree of oesophagitis depended on the acidity and peptic content of the regurgitated fluid [3] and the duration of exposure [27], it was not until the 1970s that management was concentrated on control of reflux rather than treatment of hiatus hernia.

Whilst in the 1970s it was recognized that gastro-oesophageal reflux was responsible for a wide variety of complications and that the condition could be quite simply controlled by operation, it was also demonstrated that in the vast majority of cases the natural history of the condition was one of spontaneous correction. Boix-Ochoa and Canals [5] in 1976 reported the results of 4026 monometric studies in 680 children with ages ranging from 1 day to 6 months. Although gastro-oesophageal reflux was common in the first few days of life, at 6–7 weeks all their patients had developed an effective anti-reflux barrier. There has thus been an increasing reluctance by surgeons to operate on these children in the first few weeks of life.

Anatomy and pathophysiology

The anti-reflux mechanism at the gastro-oesophageal junction depends on a number of factors, each one of which on its own appears to offer rather poor control.

1. Although the anatomy of the oesophageal hiatus varies considerably from person to person, it does form a short muscular tunnel and the lasso-like winding of the fibres of the right crus around the oesophagus has a 'pinch cock' action [21,24] (Figure 20.1).

2. The oblique entrance of the oesophagus into the cardia forming the acute angle of His provides a valve-like mechanism discouraging reflux. In addition to the right crus holding the oesophagus this configuration at the cardia is further secured by the attachment of the prolongation of the fascia transversalis on the undersurface of the diaphragm – the so-called 'phreno-oesophageal ligament'.

3. The mucous membrane of the lower oesophagus

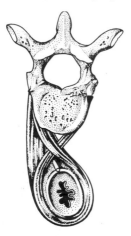

Figure 20.1 The arrangement of right crural muscle fibres around the oesophagus

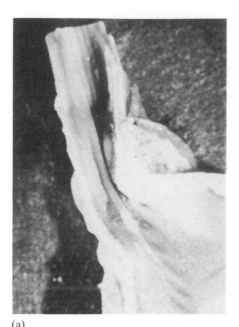

(a)

(b)

Figure 20.2 Lower oesophagus appearances in 22-week fetus: (a) longitudinal folds; (b) rosette formed at opening into stomach

is raised into longitudinal folds and appears as a rosette from within the stomach (Figure 20.2). This mucosal 'choke' may contribute to the formation of an anti-reflux barrier [13].

4. The closing of the distal oesophagus by positive intra-abdominal pressure is believed to be a major factor in the anti-reflux mechanism.

5. Although there is a rather weak sling of gastric muscle around the lower oesophagus and our studies of the developing fetus showed the muscular wall of the oesophagus to be thickened at its lower end, there is no clearly demonstrable lower oesophageal sphincter in the developed oesophagus. There is manometric evidence, however, of a high pressure zone in the distal oesophagus [23,37,39] where the pressure cannot be entirely attributed to raised intraperitoneal pressure.

The anti-reflux barrier depends on a delicate balance between intra-oesophageal and intragastric pressures. Failure of one or more of the mechanical factors listed above may lead to breaking of the barrier, whilst a pathological increase in intra-gastric pressure (for example as a result of pyloric stenosis) may have the same result. Jewett and Waterston [22] in a study of 602 children with hiatus hernia, found that 25% had central nervous system disorders, such as mental retardation, hydrocephalus, spasticity and myelomeningocele and, of 52 cases adequately studied, ten (19%) showed pylorospasm; there were, in addition, three children with pyloric stenosis, two with duodenal stenosis and one with midgut malrotation. In our own series of 114 cases, three had a diaphragmatic hernia, ten had pyloric hypertrophy, three had midgut malrotation and one had a patent omphalomesenteric duct.

In hiatus hernia a part of the stomach protrudes through the oesophageal hiatus of the diaphragm into the chest. Three types of hernia were described by Allison [1] (Figure 20.3). In the sliding hernia, where the lower oesophagus with the gastro-oesophageal junction is displaced upwards into the thorax to a greater or lesser extent, there will clearly

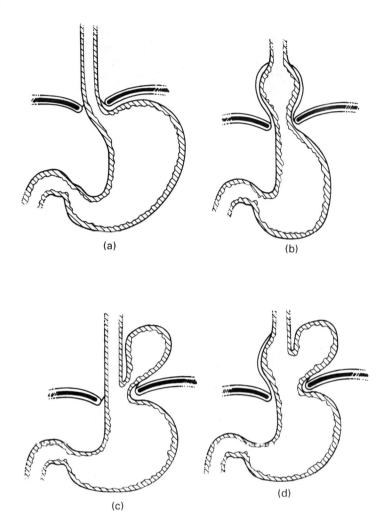

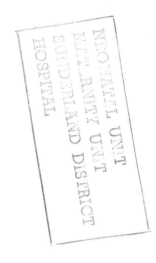

Figure 20.3 Varieties of hiatus hernia, (a) normal anatomy; (b) sliding hernia with gastro-oesophageal junction above diaphragm; (c) para-oesophageal or rolling hernia; (d) combined type – sliding plus rolling

be mechanical disruption of at least some of the anti-reflux mechanisms; such interference will also occur in the combined type of hernia. In the rolling or para-oesophageal hernia, however, where the fundus of the stomach has protruded upwards into the chest, the gastro-oesophageal junction and distal part of the oesophagus usually remains intra-abdominal and reflux is unlikely.

Once the anti-reflux barrier has failed then the oesophagus will be exposed to gastric acid regurgitation. Gastric acidity is high in the first few days of life [30] but normally falls thereafter. Oesophagitis may be slow in onset and indolent or may be fulminant with rapid ulceration, bleeding and stricture formation; there has been no clear explanation why this variation should occur though the stripping action of oesophageal peristalsis is likely to play a part. In older children with reflux, those who

formed strictures tended to be those with high gastric acidity levels, though not always [25], and in younger children Casasa and Boix-Ochoa, who measured maximum acid output in 250 children, found it to be high in most cases of failed conservative management [11].

In addition to oesophagitis, anaemia as a result of continuing minor blood loss, and failure to thrive, repeated reflux may cause respiratory problems. A relationship to the sudden infant death syndrome has been shown [26].

The complications of a sliding hiatus hernia are those of gastro-oesophageal reflux, but the para-oesophageal hernia presents different problems: the herniated stomach is liable to congestion with considerable bleeding and even to volvulus and in addition forms a space occupying lesion in the chest with associated complications.

Incidence

It is impossible to be sure of the incidence of these conditions, as many of the less severe cases are never referred to the surgeon or even investigated by radiography. It appears, however, that these conditions are more common in the UK than in the USA. Boys seem to be more commonly affected than girls and there is frequently a familial incidence of the condition [7].

In our own series of neonates admitted with gastro-oesophageal reflux from 1954 to 1985 there were 114 cases, in 41 of which a hiatus hernia was proved. Many less severe cases will never reach hospital to be referred to a surgeon or even to have contrast studies of the oesophagus and stomach. There is a remarkable difference in the incidence of the condition between the UK and the USA which has been attributed to differing radiological interpretation [17] and to the tendency in North America to nurse babies prone, in which position there is rapid emptying of the stomach [19]. Although there is a tendency for boys to be affected more commonly than girls this was not true of our neonatal series in which there were almost equal numbers: 55 males and 59 females.

It is of some interest that in the first 21 years of the series 86 infants were admitted whilst only 28 were admitted in the 10 years from 1976 to 1985, suggesting that latterly paediatricians tended to have more confidence in medical management.

Clinical picture

Presenting symptoms and signs

In the newborn the presenting symptom is almost invariably the vomiting of stomach contents. This usually starts shortly after birth; 13 of our cases were admitted during the first 24 h of life, 61 from the second to eighth day and 40 over 8 days. Vomiting is often projectile in nature so that it may resemble that of pyloric stenosis except for the time of onset; it may be severe enough to result in weight loss, dehydration and electrolyte upset, and it typically occurs when the child is laid flat in his cot after a feed [18]. Twelve of our cases – four with hiatus hernia – had haematemesis, but in only one had blood loss been sufficient to require transfusion. In 27 cases the vomitus was bile-stained, an incidence of nearly 25% – differing markedly from experience in pyloric stenosis (see Chapter 29).

Dysphagia is a late sign, usually suggesting severe oesophagitis with spasm or even stricture formation [38]. It may also occur in the very rare cases of rolling hiatus hernia.

Associated anomalies

In addition to the 17 cases mentioned above with anomalies which could cause gastric outlet obstruction, six other associated anomalies were found in individuals – micrognathia, Pierre Robin syndrome, cleft lip, laryngomalacia, angioma of liver and hypospadias. Three children had Moncrieff's syndrome of hiatus hernia, mental deficiency and sucrosuria [31].

Radiological appearances

A barium swallow will be diagnostic. Cardio-oesophageal incompetence is best demonstrated by screening the infant in the prone position with the foot end of the examination table elevated (Figure 20.4). Occasionally, repeated examinations are

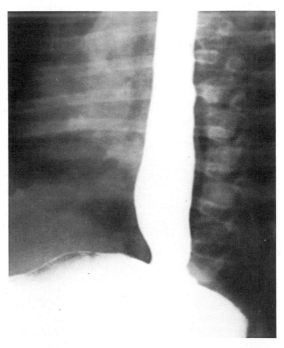

Figure 20.4 Cardio-oesophageal incompetence demonstrated by taking a radiograph of the infant in the head-down position after barium meal

necessary before the characteristic picture of the reflux is obtained. In hiatus hernia the knuckle of stomach above the diaphragm will be demonstrated (Figure 20.5), the gastric mucosal rugae often showing on the radiogram as characteristic ridges; the mucosa of the lower oesophagus in the normal neonate, however, shows marked longitudinal folds (Figure 20.2a) which must not be confused with the

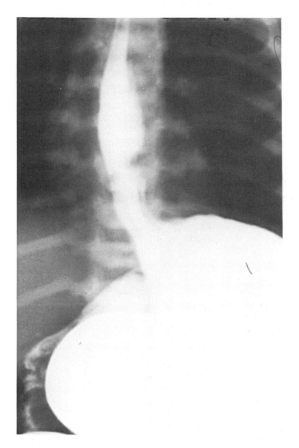

Figure 20.5 Barium swallow in a neonate with free reflux and probable hiatus hernia. A knuckle of stomach lies above the diaphragm. The longitudinal folds clearly visible are often described as gastric mucosa but are more likely to be the mucosal folds of the lower oesophagus (Figure 20.2a)

of oesophagitis; in such cases a bright red, easily traumatized and, at times, already ulcerated lower oesophagus will be observed.

Treatment

Management of these infants during the neonatal period consists first in combating their fluid and electrolyte depletion, if necessary in the severe cases by intravenous infusions, and, secondly, in preventing vomiting by feeding and nursing these children continuously in the sitting-up position.

In the ill newborn who has to be nursed in an incubator, facilities should exist to allow the infant to be nursed in a sitting position whilst in the incubator (Figure 20.6). Otherwise, the infant is best nursed in the sitting position in a special 'oesophageal box'. Many types of chairs into which babies may be strapped are now produced commercially (Figure 20.7).

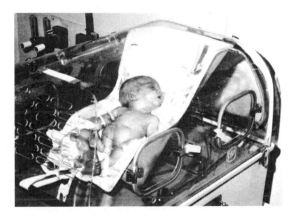

Figure 20.6 Infant with gastro-oesophageal reflux nursed in the semi-sitting position

wider lumen and rugae of the herniated stomach. Also in the newborn some oesophageal regurgitation is not uncommon because, by and large, the angle of His is less acute in early infancy, especially when the child is crying or the stomach is full of air, but free regurgitation and a wide cardiac orifice are very suggestive of hiatus hernia.

The experienced radiologist will also recognize alterations in the swallowing mechanism and abnormalities in oesophageal motility and gastric emptying.

Technetium sulphacolloid feeds with isotope scanning may be of help in the very young child, particularly for demonstrating lung contamination.

Oesophagoscopy

This investigation is not essential for diagnosis and should be carried out only to confirm the presence

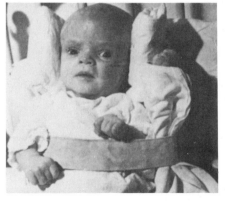

Figure 20.7 Neonate with gastro-oesophageal reflux nursed in sitting up position in oesophageal box

Prevention of vomiting is helped by thickening the feeds. In the milder cases, Benger's feed is adequate for this purpose. In the severe cases, thickening of the feeds with a commercial preparation of ceratonia, such as Nestargel, has proved to be very useful. (A 0.5% solution will thicken a milk feed so that it can just be fed through a teat with a large hole, whilst a 1% solution becomes so thick that it can only be fed with a spoon.) Sodium alginate (Gaviscon) 5 ml added to 120 ml feeds has also proved of value. Small frequent feeds are indicated, not only to reduce the bulk of gastric content but also to stimulate oesophageal peristalsis and stripping waves [27]. If the baby vomits in spite of all these precautions then refeeding is necessary.

Alkali may also be added to feeds whenever there is suspicion of oesophagitis. Mist. Alum. Hydrox. (BNF), 3–5 ml per feed, is suitable for those infants who tend to have loose stools, whilst in those who tend to be constipated Mist. Mag. Trisil. (BPC), in similar doses, is suitable. These antacids are for symptomatic management and no other drugs have been shown to be useful.

The natural history of this disease is that it is self-limiting and vomiting decreases as the child grows older, especially when he goes on to a weaning diet. Early medical management is said to result in a 96% cure rate [9], and repeat X-rays at 2 years may show that a hiatus hernia has completely disappeared

(Figures 20.8a and b). In a long-term follow-up of hiatus hernia in infants and children, Prinsen [34] showed that all successfully medically treated children were symptom-free within 2 weeks and that no children developed strictures whilst on treatment – if there was any stenosis it was present at the time of diagnosis.

We have had experience [29] outside this series of a child who presented at 10 days of age with complete occlusion of the lower oesophagus due to a stricture later shown to be secondary to a hiatus hernia; this child required urgent surgical intervention, as did a 3-day-old child in Cahill's series [8].

Positive indications for operative treatment in gastro-oesophageal reflux with or without sliding hiatus hernia are complications from oesophagitis such as stenosis, as in the above child, or severe anaemia; but failure to thrive in spite of medical management presents a rather more vague indication in the neonatal period. Only one case in this series was operated on in the neonatal period, as an incidental procedure during repair of a diaphragmatic hernia, but three others had repairs later – one at 5 months and two at 12 months. A Nissen fundoplication [33] (Figure 20.9) achieves an excellent result in these cases; X-rays of a case outside this series [28], treated at 3 weeks of age, are shown in Figure 20.10.

The rolling or para-oesophageal hernia should be

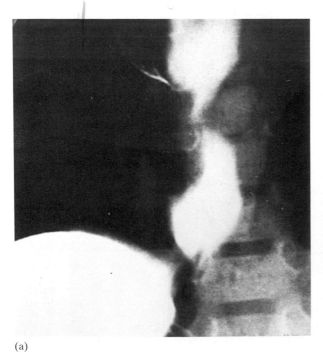

(a)

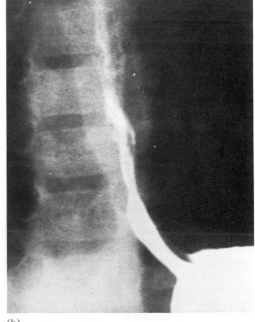

(b)

Figure 20.8 (a) Hiatus hernia with apparent oesophageal stricture and proximal dilatation in an infant 2 weeks old. (b) Barium swallow in the same child as in Figure 20.8(a) at 3 years of age. The hiatus hernia together with the narrowing of the oesophagus have disappeared with conservative treatment only

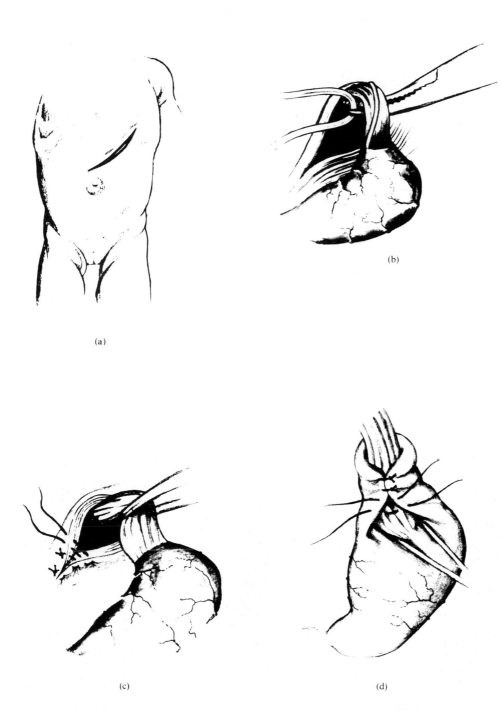

(a)

(b)

(c)

(d)

Figure 20.9 Nissen fundoplication. The abdomen is opened through a left upper oblique incision (a) and after division of the triangular ligament the abdominal oesophagus is mobilized and retracted with a sling (b). The oesophageal hiatus is tightened with a few non-absorbable sutures placed posteriorly (c) and the fundus plicated around the lower oesophagus with similar sutures (d). Over-tightening of this plication is avoided in the newborn by the presence of an FG24 tube passed down the oesophagus

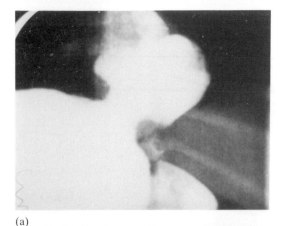

(a)

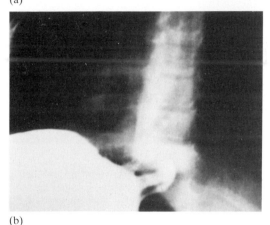

(b)

Figure 20.10 Sliding hiatus hernia in the newborn. Contrast studies (a) before and (b) after Nissen fundoplication

regarded in the same way as any other abdominal hernia: the risk of severe complication such as volvulus or serious bleeding is significant and early operation is indicated. A Nissen fundoplication is the operation of choice [28] (Figure 20.11) and should be undertaken without delay. Randolph found one massive hernia requiring operation at the age of 3 days [35].

Results

Apart from the three children operated on after the neonatal period, our remaining 110 patients were free of symptoms when discharged and remained so. It was not our experience that large numbers came to surgery later [14], though some series suggest [36] that more than 80% of children undergoing surgery for hiatus hernia have had symptoms dating from the first month of life.

In general, our experience is that only one-third of all children with hiatus hernia are referred to surgeons and, of those, not more than one-third

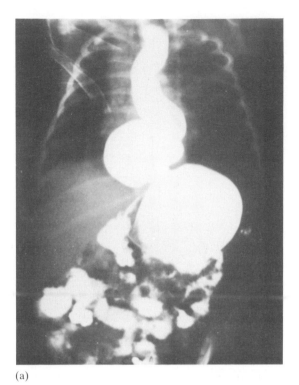

(a)

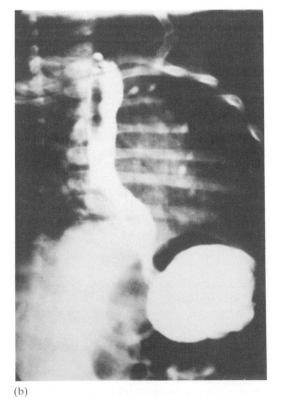

(b)

Figure 20.11 Rolling hiatus hernia in newborn. Contrast studies (a) before and (b) after Nissen fundoplication

(11% of the total diagnosed) will require an operative procedure [25,28]. This figure is somewhat lower than the 15% operated on in Toronto [36]. Of those who reach the surgeon in the first 4 weeks of life, the number requiring surgery is, in our experience, even less – three out of 86, or under 4%.

References

1. Allison, P.R. (1951) Reflux oesophagitis, hiatus hernia and the anatomy of repair. *Surg. Gynec. Obstet.*, **92**, 419–431

2. Astley, R. (1952) *Radiology of the Alimentary Tract in Infancy*, Edward Arnold, London

3. Belsey, R.H.R. (1962) The surgery of the diaphragm. In *Surgery of Childhood* (ed. J.J. Mason Brown), Edward Arnold, London

4. Berenberg, W. and Neuhauser, E.B.D. (1950) Cardio-oesophageal relaxation (chalasia). *Pediatrics, Springfield*, **5**, 414–419

5. Boix-Ochoa, J. and Canals, J. (1976) Maturation of the lower oesophageal sphincter. *J. Pediat. Surg.*, **11**, 749–756

6. Bright, R. (1836) Account of a remarkable displacement of the stomach. *Guy's Hosp. Rep.*, **1**, 398

7. Burke, J.B. (1952) Partial thoracic stomach in childhood. *Br. med. J.*, **1**, 1150

8. Cahill, J.L., Aberdeen, E. and Waterston, D.J. (1969) Results of surgical treatment in esophageal hiatal hernia in infancy and childhood. *Surgery*, **66**, 597–602

9. Carre, I.J. (1972) Clinical features and natural history of partial thoracic stomach (hiatus hernia). *Acta Paediat. Scand.*, **61**, 491

10. Carre, I.J., Astley, R. and Smellie, J.M. (1952) Minor degree of partial thoracic stomach in childhood. *Lancet*, **ii**, 1150–1153

11. Casasa, J.M. and Boix-Ochoa, J. (1977) Surgical or conservative treatment in hiatal hernia in children: a new decisive parameter. *Surgery*, **82**, 573–575

12. Chrispin, A.R. and Friedland, G.W. (1966) A radiological study of the neural control of oesophageal vestibular function. *Thorax*, **21**, 422–427

13. Chrispin, A.R., Friedland, G.W. and Wright, D.E. (1967) Some functional characteristics of the oesophageal vestibule in infants and children. *Thorax*, **22**, 188–192

14. Coupland, G.A.E. and Rickham, P.P. (1968) Vagotomy and pyloroplasty in the surgical treatment of hiatus hernia in children. *Aust. N.Z. J. Surg.*, **37**, 121–124

15. Ferguson, D.J., Palonera, E.S., Sako, Y., Clatworthy, H.W. Jr, Toon, R.W. and Wangensteem, O.H. (1950) Studies on experimental oesophagitis. *Surgery*, **28**, 1022–1039

16. Findley, C. and Kelly, A.B. (1931) Congenital shortening of the oesophagus and the thoracic stomach resulting therefrom. *J. Laryng. Otol.*, **46**, 797

17. Friedland, G.W., Dodds, W.J., Sunshine, P. and Zboralske, F. (1974) The apparent disparity in incidence of hiatal herniae in infants and children in Britain and the United States. *Am. J. Roentgen.*, **120**, 305–314

18. Gross, R.E. (1953) *The Surgery of Infancy and Childhood*, W.B. Saunders, Philadelphia

19. Guttman, F.M. (1972) On the incidence of hiatal hernia in infants. *Pediatrics*, **50**, 325–328

20. Hurst, A.F. and Stewart, M.J. (1929) *Gastric and Duodenal Ulcer*, Oxford University Press, London

21. Jackson, C. (1922) The diaphragmatic pinch-cock. *Laryngoscope*, **32**, 139

22. Jewett, T.C. and Waterston, D.J. (1975) Surgical management of hiatal hernia in children. *J. Pediat. Surg.*, **10**, 757–761

23. Kehrer, B., Oesch, A. and Bettex, M. (1972) Manometric studies of esophageal motility in infants with hiatus hernia. *J. Pediat. Surg.*, **7**, 499–503

24. Koncz, J. (1959) Chalasia oder Relaxatio cardio-oesophagea. In *Lehrbuch der Chirurgie und Orthopadie des Kindesalters* (ed. A. Oberniedermayer), Springer Verlag, Berlin

25. Lari, J. and Lister, J. (1972) Some problems in the surgical management of children with hiatus hernia. *Arch. Dis. Childh.*, **47**, 201–206

26. Leape, L.A., Holder, T.M. and Franklin, J. *et al.* (1977) Respiratory arrests in infants secondary to gastro-oesophageal reflux. *Pediatrics*, **60**, 924–928

27. Lichter, I. (1974) Measurement of gastro-oesophageal acid reflux; its significance in hiatus hernia. *Br. J. Surg.*, **61**, 253–258

28. Lister, J. (1972) Hiatus hernia in children. *Postgrad. Med. J.*, **48**, 501–506

29. Lister, J. and Wright, T. (1967) Oesophageal stricture in the neonatal period. *Proc. R. Soc. Med.*, **60**, 449–450

30. Miller, R.A. (1941) Observations on the gastric acidity during the first weeks of life. *Arch. Dis. Childh.*, **16**, 22–30

31. Moncrieff, A. and Wilkinson, R.H. (1954) Sucrosuria with mental defect and hiatus hernia. *Acta Paediat. Scand.*, **43**, 495–516

32. Neuhauser, E.B.D. and Berenburgh, W. (1947) Cardio-esophageal relaxation as a cause of vomiting in infants. *Radiology*, **48**, 480–483

33. Nissen, R. and Rosette, M. (1959) *Die Behandlung von Hiatus Herniau und Reflux Oesophagitis mit Gastropexie und Fundoplicatio*, Georg Thieme Verlag, Stuttgart

34. Prinsen, J.E. (1975) Hiatus hernia in infants and children; a long-term follow-up of medical therapy. *J. Pediat. Surg.*, **10**, 97–102

35. Randolph, J.G., Lilly, J.R. and Anderson, K.D. (1974) Surgical treatment of gastroesophageal reflux in infants. *Ann. Surg.*, **180**, 479–486

36. Rohatgi, M., Shandling, B. and Stephens, C.A. (1971) Hiatal hernia in infants and children: results of surgical treatment. *Surgery*, **69**, 456–462

37. Strawczynski, H., Beck, I.T., McKenna, R.D. and Nickerson, G.H. (1964) The behavior of the lower oesophageal sphincter in infants and its relationship to gastroesophageal regurgitation. *J. Pediat.*, **64**, 17–23

38. Waterston, D. (1969) Hiatus hernia. In *Pediatric Surgery*, 2nd Edn, (ed. W.T. Mustard, M.M. Ravitch, W.H. Snyder, K.J. Welch and C.D. Benson), Year Book Medical Publishers, Chicago

39. Willich, E. (1971) The function of the cardia in childhood. *Progr. Pediat. Surg.*, **3**, 141–167

21

Oesophageal atresia and tracheo-oesophageal fistula

R. E. Cudmore

Historical notes

The first known description of oesophageal atresia with the common form of tracheo-oesophageal fistula was by Thomas Gibson [98], son-in-law of Richard Cromwell, who gave an account in 1697 of a baby with this condition who died at the age of 2 days. He performed a postmortem to show the typical and now well-known defect.

More than a century passed before a further case, often quoted as the first, was recorded by Martin [224] in 1821. Others such as Scholler [297] in 1838, Levy [195] in 1845, Hirschsprung [131] in 1861 and de Bary [56] in 1864 described various cases. H-type fistula was first described by Lamb [187] in 1873. By 1884, Mackenzie [214,215] was able to collect 63 cases from the literature. Plass [259] in 1919 published a comprehensive review of 136 cases whilst by 1931 [288] a world total of 225 cases had been reported. In early years, interest in the anomaly focused on its embryology and pathological anatomy but occasional attempts at correction were made. Notable amongst these were reports by Holmes [146] in 1869 and Steele [323] in 1888.

Hoffman [134] attempted a cervical repair and, having failed, he resorted to gastrostomy, probably the first ever performed for this condition. The first serious attempt at ligation of the fistula with oesophagostomy and gastrostomy was described by Richter [280] in 1913, whilst Mathieu [225] in 1933 had commented that 'surgery must be held forth as the only optimistic procedure for lessening what is now inevitable death' [317]. Shaw [305] in 1939 and Lanman [189] in 1940 were the first to report attempted primary anastomosis of the oesophagus. The first two patients to survive a multiple staged procedure were treated by Ladd [184] and Leven [192–194] in 1939. Although Richter [280] had

suggested a method of primary anastomosis, the first survival of a primary procedure was described by Haight and Towsley [115] in 1941. Imperatori [149] is credited with the first successful closure of an H-type fistula. In England, the first successful operation for oesophageal atresia was performed by Franklin [88] in 1947 at the Hammersmith Hospital, London. Colon was first used for reconstruction of the oesophagus by Sandblom [292] in 1948 but prior to this date, various methods of reconstruction had been tried [216].

Staged repair for critically ill and premature babies was described by Holder, McDonald and Woolley in 1962 [140], since which time many others have written in support of this approach, including Koop [176]. In recent years, interest has focused on the delayed primary anastomosis and varying techniques of stretching the upper pouch as advocated by Howard [147], Rehbein [276], Hasse [121] and Hendren [127] but to a large extent these have been abandoned in favour of myotomy. A masterly review of the history of tracheo-oesophageal fistula has been written by Myers [234] who in surveying the 300 years since the condition was first described, divides the period into pre-survival, survival and salvage eras.

Engel [70] in 1970 reported the first case of a mother with a successfully treated fistula giving birth to a child with tracheo-oesophageal fistula.

Anatomy

In a full-term neonate, the oesophagus is 9–10 cm in length with a lumen of 3–4 mm. The muscular wall is thick and consists of an outer longitudinal coat which superiorly forms two longitudinal condensations that come to lie more anteriorly and pass deep to the constrictor muscles. The V-shaped space between these two condensations is filled by circular muscle and the overlapping edge of the inferior pharyngeal constrictor muscle. Striated muscle is found in the upper third of the organ which then gradually changes so that the lower third consists entirely of smooth muscle. The inferior thyroid artery supplies the upper third of the oesophagus whilst the lower third is well supplied by the left gastric and phrenic arteries, but the middle portion receives a more tenuous supply both from bronchial arteries and directly from the aorta. On account of this, extensive mobilization of the lower pouch may jeopardize its viability. The arterial supply in the neonate has been demonstrated by Lister [201], using barium/gelatine injections to outline the vessels for dissection and X-rays.

Pathological anatomy

Atresia with or without fistula can occur in many forms and numerous variations have been described [172]. The best known classification is that of Vogt [345], modified by Ladd [184] and further modified by Roberts [286]. However, it has now become customary to describe each anomaly as it is found and to group babies by weight and associated anomalies, since these factors influence the choice of surgical therapy more than does the anatomical variation [350]. The most common abnormality is Vogt Type 3 in which there is a blind upper pouch with a fistula to the trachea or bronchus from the lower oesophagus; this occurs in about 87% of patients. Pure oesophageal atresia occurs in approximately 8% of patients whilst fistula without atresia occurs in approximately 4%. Of the remaining rare varieties the commonest is that in which the upper pouch opens into the trachea and the lower pouch is blind.

Wide variation is found in the distance between the two ends of the oesophagus, depending upon the extension of the upper pouch into the chest as well as the position of the distal fistula. The average distance is a little over 1.0 cm, the range being 0.5–5.0 cm [283,326]. Not infrequently the pouches are contiguous so that there is an overlap and a common wall which may give the impression at first sight that the oesophagus is normal. When there is no fistula from distal oesophagus to trachea, as in atresia without fistula, or an upper pouch fistula, the distal pouch is not held high and usually extends only a short distance upwards above the diaphragm.

The site of entry of the lower fistula into the trachea is variable; it may enter at any point from 2.0 cm above the carina to the proximal centimetre of either bronchus. The commonest site however, is 0.5–1.0 cm above the carina [285]. The fistula from the lower pouch to the trachea is always end to side but in the rare cases where there is a fistula from the upper pouch to the trachea, it is side to side, arising just proximal to the fundus of the upper pouch. Indeed, the presence of an upper pouch fistula may not be suspected until operation when the upper pouch is mobilized. The upper pouch is invariably thick-walled due to hypertrophy of the muscle, presumably from constant swallowing and regurgitating of the amniotic fluid by the fetus *in utero*.

The distal segment of the oesophagus is always hypoplastic; Koop and Hamilton [176] found in 1.5% of cases that air did not flow into the stomach because the lumen from the fistula to the lower oesophagus was so small.

In the so-called H-type fistula, the oesophagus is in continuity and there is a connection between the trachea and the oesophagus usually at a level above the thoracic inlet. Insertion into the trachea is at a higher level than insertion into the oesophagus: the fistula therefore runs obliquely downwards from trachea to oesophagus and thus resembles an N rather than an H [160].

As a result of the connection between the airway and the gullet, two problems arise. First, air passes freely into the stomach causing dilatation and abdominal distension with subsequent diaphragmatic elevation and splinting. Second, the pressure of air within the stomach causes acid to pass freely back into the respiratory tract producing a peptic pneumonitis. Lung complications are a frequent pre-operative problem: together with the maturity and weight of the baby and any associated anomalies they will influence survival rates and must be taken into account when planning surgical therapy. To give some meaningful comparison in discussion of management and results, Waterston, Bonham-Carter and Aberdeen [350] proposed a classification based on these factors. This has become internationally accepted and is as follows.

Group A Babies of over 2.5 kg birth weight and well.
Group B₁ Babies of 1.8–2.5 kg birth weight and well.
Group B₂ Babies of over 2.5 kg birth weight with moderate pneumonia or congenital anomaly.
Group C₁ Babies of birth weight under 1.8 kg.
Group C₂ Babies of any birth weight with severe pneumonia and severe congenital anomaly.

Embryology

The normal development of the trachea and oesophagus begins at about the fourth week when a median laryngotracheal groove appears in the ventral wall of the foregut. As this groove deepens and the foregut elongates, ridges appear on the lateral walls and beginning at the caudal end, they fuse to separate the laryngotracheal tube from the oesophagus.

The lung buds develop at the caudal end of the primordial trachea. Both oesophagus and trachea elongate so that separation is not complete until about 5 weeks when the bifurcation of the trachea comes to lie opposite the fourth thoracic vertebra. The stomach can be recognized as a dilatation in the foregut by the end of the fourth week and it is carried below the forming diaphragm by elongation of the oesophagus and the cranial growth of the body away from the septum transversum.

The varied tracheo-oesophageal anomalies cannot all be explained by one mechanism and various theories have been postulated to explain tracheo-oesophageal fistula [336]. Gruenwald [107], examining a 9-mm embryo, thought the normal laryngo-tracheal tube grew faster than the oesophagus so that if separation of the oesophagus and trachea was slightly delayed, the faster growing trachea would separate the proximal and distal oesophagus, giving rise to the classic deformity. The mid part of the oesophagus would be incorporated into the dorsal trachea, explaining the presence of squamous epithelium in the trachea [110].

Smith [314], examining the Carnegie collection of embryos, argued that the anomaly was the result of hyperplasia of the lateral epithelial ridges of the developing foregut combined with the rapid tracheal elongation. He discounted the theory of Ingalls and Prindle [150], which postulated pinching off of the oesophagus by external pressure from the developing pneumoenteric processes and also condemned the theory of abnormal subclavian vessels causing local pressure [86,188].

Vascular insufficiency [201], inflammation [209] and ulceration [292] and deficiency of material [170,260] for development have all been postulated. The current best explanation for the embryogenesis of oesophageal atresia is that of de Lorimier and Harrison [206]. Whilst Ruano Gil [291] has studied extensively the embryology of oesophageal atresia in a Carnegie Stage 16 embryo, Kleckner, Pringle and Clark [171] maintain that little is known about the embryology of tracheo-oesophageal fistula. Investigating the proposal that the anomaly results from hyperflexion of the foregut during a critical stage of fetal development which results in a disturbance of alignment when the trachea and oesophagus are separating they were, in an elegant series of experiments, unable to confirm the theory and came to the conclusion that it was still not understood why oesophageal atresia should occur. It is clear that failure of separation of pharynx and trachea will lead either to a fistula or to webbing between the two parts, or atresia. Grafting of tracheo-bronchial elements into the oesophagus can

also occur [33]. Hokama [136] showed in his histological study of atretic specimens that there were tracheo-bronchial elements [246,251] in most of the cases examined. This could account for stenosis or abnormality of motility following an apparently successful anastomosis. Other reports of intrathoracic foregut duplication cysts associated with atresia indicate a failure of adequate separation of the oesophagus from the lung buds.

Aetiology

This is unknown and no true genetic influence has been demonstrated but there must be multiple factors influencing the embryo at a vulnerable period. Embryos at 5 weeks [327] post-conception have been demonstrated to have the complete lesion whilst anomalies of other systems associated with oesophageal atresia may be dated at this time. Szendry and his colleagues [328] carried out an aetiological study of pure oesophageal atresia whilst Kirillova [166] has postulated an origin for duplications of the intestinal tract together with atresias and stenoses which may have some bearing on oesophageal anomalies with fistulas. There is as yet no animal experimental model for the study of this anomaly.

Familial cases were reported as early as 1936 [46,103,313]. A family with three affected siblings was reported by Hausmann [122] but the children were from three different wives of the same father. Dennis [60] reported oesophageal atresia occurring in three generations. Monozygous twins with only one twin affected have been recorded on several occasions [150] and Woolley [357] reported monozygotic twins who were both affected and were successfully treated by Gross [104]. Identical affected twins were also described by Blank [25]. Haight [113] recorded the largest series of twins in which only one of each pair had atresia and of his ten patients, at least one was definitely monozygotic. The incidence of twinning does seem to be exceptionally high in oesophageal atresia [212]. As more successfully treated children have grown to adult life, it is becoming clear that there can be a familial incidence [11] although the risk rates of oesophageal atresia in families is not yet fully understood [72,343]. Oesophageal atresia in father and daughter has been described by Lipson [200] in 1984 and father and son by Kashuk [162] in 1983. Further familial incidences have been described and in our series a child recently presenting with an 'H' type fistula at the age of 10 years had two cousins with the fistulous anomaly.

Associated anomalies

More than half the babies presenting with tracheo-oesophageal fistula have associated anomalies and

Table 21.1 Overall numbers of associated anomalies in Liverpool series 1953–85

	1953–70 (248 cases)	1971–85 (199 cases)	1953–85 (447 cases)
Palate and larynx	16 (6.5%)	20 (10%)	36 (8%)
Cardiac	48 (19.5%)	68 (34.1%)	116 (26%)
Gastrointestinal	20 (8%)	18 (9%)	38 (8.5%)
Anorectal	29 (11.7%)	22 (11%)	51 (11.4%)
Urogenital	35 (14.1%)	47 (23.6%)	82 (18%)
Vertebral	20 (8%)	26 (13.1%)	46 (10.3%)
Skeletal	21 (8.4%)	27 (13.6%)	48 (10.7%)

The increase in incidence in cardiac and urogenital anomalies is presumably related to increased survival of severe congenital heart lesions and more intensive investigation of the urinary tract

many large series [97,141,349] confirm this, including the Liverpool cases (Table 21.1). Cardiac and rectal anomalies have been known for many years to be associated with oesophageal atresia but as abnormalities of other systems became identified, the acronym VATER [266,267] was coined to describe this non-random association of anomalies [14,15,352].

VATER originally stood for Vertebral, Anal, Tracheo-Esophageal, Radial and Renal anomalies but further associations allowed it to be extended to VACTERL [53] adding cardiac and limb problems to the others associated with oesophageal atresia and fistula [333]. A similar acronym, CHARGE (coloboma, heart disease, choanal atresia, retarded growth, genital hypoplasia and ear(deafness)) has also been described in association with tracheo-oesophageal fistula by Lillquist [196]. Hence, any anomaly can be found in association [52] with oesophageal atresia and needs to be actively sought though, in reality, cardiac [51,226], renal, genitourinary and gastrointestinal anomalies [270] are the most commonly encountered, together with those of the skeleton [26,51,269,339]. Muraji [231], in discussing the surgical problems in patients with the VATER anomaly, concludes that 70% of babies demonstrating such stigmata are preterm or of low birth weight. There seems to be axial mesodermal dysplasia arising at about the 35th day postconception though there is controversy over whether this is random or non-random [332].

Apart from obvious anorectal anomalies, associated anomalies of the gastrointestinal tract may be unseen but lethal. Antenatal ultrasound scans may alert the obstetrician to their presence [41]. Spitz [318] in a review of 18 patients with associated duodenal atresia emphasizes that these babies are a high risk group; all his patients fell into Waterston group C_2 [350]. Mollitt [228] in reviewing 12 associated gastrointestinal anomalies found malrotation of the gut to be the most common and duodenal atresia second. Duplication cysts have also been

reported [126,169,250] and we had three in our series. Pyloric stenosis occurs [3,54,101] and, whilst this may be a random association, there is some evidence that there is a higher than normal relationship [91,268].

Renal anomalies were critically analysed by Atwell and Beard [10] who found that half the infants studied had a notable renal tract anomaly, 40% significant enough to influence management and prognosis. Warman [348] has also reviewed renal tract anomalies in oesophageal atresia whilst Sofatzis [316] has described malformation of the female genitalia in the VATER association.

Although cardiac anomalies are well documented with between 30 and 40% incidence in various series, it should be remembered that there is also a variety of bronchopulmonary anomalies [19,32,299] from pulmonary agenesis to sequestered lobes and that these may well complicate anaesthesia or mitigate against a successful outcome. In a review of the literature Black found only 15 cases of oesophageal atresia associated with pulmonary agenesis [24] and all were fatal; he described a treatment strategy to preserve lung function. Tracheal [294] and laryngeal anomalies have been described [190].

In reviewing 411 cases of oesophageal atresia admitted between 1954 and 1983 we found more respiratory anomalies than expected [202]; there were 51 (12%) cases, 15 with laryngeal stenosis, 18 with tracheomalacia and 18 with bronchopulmonary anomalies. This is a rather higher incidence than in other reported series, possibly because of more frequent recognition in recent years. The lung anomalies included two foregut cysts, two cases of cystic adenomatoid malformation, four patients with lung agenesis and nine with lung hypoplasia.

Tracheomalacia, even of a minor degree, plays an important part in lung complications [341], as does the presence of non-ciliated epithelium in the respiratory tree, a not uncommon finding [69].

Vertebral and skeletal abnormalities (Table 21.2) which range from phocomelia, sacral agenesis and absent radius to hemivertebrae and rib anomalies, have an incidence of 20–50% overall; limb anomalies should alert the surgeon to the possibility of a trisomy 18 [269] form of chromosome abnormality.

Table 21.2 The variety of skeletal malformations associated with 339 consecutive cases of oesophageal atresia

Skeletal malformation	No. of cases
Anomaly of spine and/or ribs	30 (9%)
Anomaly of fingers	21 (6%)
Absence of radius	9 (3%)
Major anomaly of lower limb	4 (1%)
Phocomelia	2 (<1%)

Incidence

Most authors agree that the incidence of this condition is approximately 1 per 3000–3500 live births [173], though Myers [232] gives an incidence of 1:4500. A total of 323 cases have been treated in Liverpool over the last 21 years. These cases were drawn from a wide area (see Chapter 2); in Liverpool and Bootle, where an accurate record of congenital deformities is kept (see Chapter 1), there were 30 cases of oesophageal atresia out of a total of 98 065 births during the years 1967–75. This indicates an incidence of 0.30 per 1000 (1 in 3300). Sex incidence is almost equal [351].

Clinical picture and diagnosis

Maternal hydramnios [155] should alert the paediatrician to the possibility of an infant being affected with oesophageal atresia. Waterston [350] found an 85% incidence of hydramnios in oesophageal atresia alone and 32% in those with atresia and tracheo-oesophageal fistula.

Amniocentesis performed on the hydramniotic uterus may allow a prenatal diagnosis [74] to be made by intra-amniotic injection of contrast medium. It has been noted that the alpha-fetoprotein [303] of the amniotic fluid may be raised together with raised acetylcholinesterase which may also act as a marker. However, prenatal ultrasonography [263,271,363] (see Chapter 7) has added to the accuracy of the diagnosis, is non invasive and prepares both parents and surgeon for the appropriate therapy after birth. The classic sign after delivery is of a baby who froths at the mouth in spite of oropharyngeal suction, because he cannot swallow his saliva. There may also be choking, coughing, dyspnoea and cyanosis, especially if attempts are made to feed the baby. But frothing alone should make the nursing attendant suspicious and in such children oesophageal continuity must be confirmed before any attempt at feeding is made. Similarly, if hydramnios [85] is present then it is an inviolable rule that a tube should be passed to ensure patency of the oesophagus. In some centres, a soft plastic nasogastric tube is passed routinely on every baby in order to exclude oesophageal atresia; any aspirate should be tested with litmus paper to confirm that it contains acid gastric juice. There is a theoretical objection to the passage of a tube in that it may curl in the upper pouch (Figure 21.1) and give the impression of oesophageal patency. More rarely, and this has only occurred once in our series, a tube may go down the trachea, through the fistula and down into the stomach. If a firm tube is passed, it will not curl; it should be of at least no. 10 or 12 FG calibre and passed through the mouth; it will then be unlikely to be passed accidentally into the trachea. Acid secretions may collect in the pouch

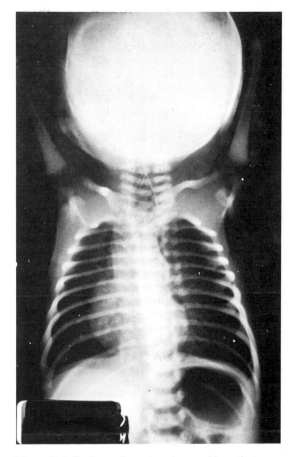

Figure 21.1 Radiograph to show how a thin catheter may curl in the upper pouch

from reflux through the fistula and give the impression on testing with litmus that the tube is in the stomach, but the quantity of fluid should be a guide to whether or not the tube is in the stomach. In all suspected cases, radiology should be carried out but not before a general examination for skeletal abnormalities presence of a heart murmur and patency of the anus.

Radiology

It is sufficient for diagnosis to take one good erect film of the whole baby with a radio-opaque no. 10 or 12 FG catheter passed through the mouth so that firm pressure can be exerted to push down the upper pouch. There is a characteristic feel of the tube at the base of the pouch and the nurse or doctor should push firmly. Hence, one may gauge on the film the pouch length in relation to the vertebral bodies. A red rubber catheter is best for this purpose as the whole tube shows up, though a plastic catheter with a radio-opaque strip will show reasonably well (Figure 21.2).

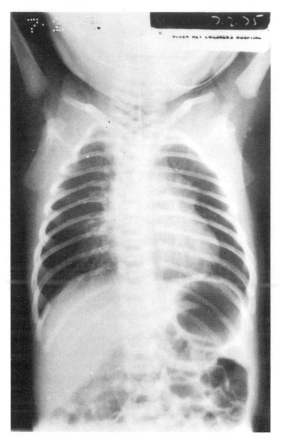

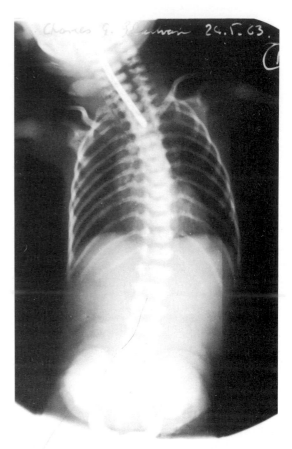

Figure 21.2 X-ray to show the tube in the upper pouch. Gas in the abdomen indicates the presence of a fistula. A thicker catheter gives a better contrast

Figure 21.3 Chest radiograph with a wider tube to delineate the upper pouch. Absence of abdominal air suggests atresia only

The X-ray will reveal the presence or absence of air in the stomach and bowel, indicating the presence of a fistula or atresia alone (Figure 21.3). Very rarely in tracheo-oesophageal fistula (about 1% of cases) there is no air in the intestine [57]. Occasionally, a lateral X-ray will demonstrate air in the fistula but it is not our practice to take such a film routinely. A careful note should be made of vertebral and rib anomalies. Limb deformities are usually obvious on clinical examination but adequate X-rays of these can be obtained later.

The possible presence of associated duodenal atresia must be remembered and the intestinal gas pattern should be noted. Ultrasound studies have also been used to identify associated gastrointestinal anomalies [123] (see Chapter 8). The chest portion of the X-ray should also be studied carefully for evidence of enlarged heart or lung plethora indicating congenital heart disease, whilst this first X-ray will also give an indication of pneumonitis.

Tam [331] has described the use of CT scanning for the accurate delineation of the site and size of any fistula present and of the size of the oesophageal gap, and scanning may also be helpful in diagnosing cardiac lesions as well as other gut anomalies. The baby has to be placed longitudinally in the head of the scanner but with experienced staff it is a very useful adjunct to routine X-rays in diagnosis. The chest X-ray may well suggest the presence of a right-sided aorta [55] and either ultrasonography [152] or CT scanning should help to resolve this problem. Though a right-sided aorta does not make repair of the oesophagus through the right chest impossible [261], it often makes it more difficult [120] and it is an advantage to approach the oesophagus through a thoracotomy on the opposite side to the aorta [180].

We do not advocate the use of opaque contrast media to delineate the upper pouch size, believing with others that air is the best contrast medium; this can be injected through the tube if necessary.

Shaw [306] in 1920 was the first to use barium sulphate to outline the upper pouch. Fatalities were reported because of aspiration and the method fell into disfavour, but since then various proprietary preparations have been used: Lipiodol (iodized oil viscous injection) is oily and can cause a lipid pneumonitis whilst Hypaque (sodium diatrizoate) and Gastrografin (sodium and meglumine diatrizoates), being hypertonic solutions, can cause lethal pulmonary oedema if spillage occurs. Micropaque (micromized barium sulphate suspended in methylcellulose and autoclaved) can be safely used in small (0.5 ml) amounts and is non-irritative if spillage occurs [242]. Koop [176] condemns the use of opaque media in the upper pouch but Myers [233] is a firm advocate of the procedure provided it is done by experienced personnel in an adequately equipped department and provided the pouch is aspirated as soon as the examination is completed. All his patients have routine contrast studies.

Differential diagnosis

Pharyngeal pseudodiverticulum

An unusual condition which may be confused with tracheo-oesophageal fistula is a pseudodiverticulum [8] of the pharynx which prevents passage of a nasogastric tube and gives the impression of an atresia [87]. Because of this confusion some of these babies have had a thoractomy and no chest lesion has been found. The cause is obscure but most writers feel it is associated with trauma from too vigorous nasogastric suction during resuscitation procedures at birth [210]. In these cases barium studies are advocated and treatment is easily instituted by gastrostomy with drainage of the neck or mediastinum [29,65,353].

Oesophageal perforations occurring in neonates have been reported. These usually occur in babies with severe respiratory distress who have been vigorously resuscitated and nasogastric tubes subsequently passed have gone into abnormal positions [364]. As a result, both pneumothorax and pneumomediastinum have resulted. Vigorous supportive therapy is indicated [29,65,353] and aggressive surgery with drainage and even thoracotomy may be necessary. Fleming [84] points out that oesophageal perforation can occur spontaneously. A true diverticulum of the oesophagus can occur; it is very rare and usually occurs posteriorly at the pharyngo-oesophageal junction [240]. Severe respiratory difficulty is likely to be the presenting sign in a child 10–14 days old [302].

Fistula without atresia

Tracheo-oesophageal fistula without atresia is even more difficult to diagnose and rarely presents in the neonatal period [175]. One of our cases was referred on the first day of life. The condition must be suspected in any baby with paroxysms of coughing and choking especially during feeds [77,211]. A distended tympanitic abdomen is a typical feature sometimes suggesting Hirschsprung's disease and the child has frequent attacks of pneumonitis [175,230] with right upper lobe collapse.

Numerous techniques to demonstrate the fistula have been described [9]. The simplest is by passing a nasogastric tube, placing the open end under water and then withdrawing the tube slowly. Air bubbles in the water may be seen as the catheter tip passes the fistula. Alternatively, an air leak may be heard through an oesophageal stethoscope during anaesthesia [16]. Methylene blue [89] can be injected into the oesophagus or trachea and its egress through the fistula viewed by bronchoscope or oesophagoscope [163,355]. Bronchoscopy and oesophagoscopy are mandatory in the diagnosis of this condition [62]. Benjamin [18] emphasizes the need for bronchoscopy in all congenital tracheal anomalies as does Gans [94], who affirms that endoscopy is vital for the diagnosis of this condition and is superior to any dye studies. Wang [347] describes two cases safely diagnosed by metrizamide though others have used barium paste in the past. All those with extensive knowledge and experience of this problem, however, emphasize the need for fibreoptic tracheobronchoscopy and the passage of a stent through the fistula at the time of operation. On no account should the neck or chest be explored for an 'H-type' fistula unless the opening has been demonstrated. Exploration on suspicion will inevitably lead to vagal nerve damage as the oesophagus and trachea are stripped apart, and some deaths have been reported.

Laryngotracheo-oesophageal cleft

This rare but important anomaly must be considered in the tracheo-oesophageal differential diagnosis for a tube may in fact not pass down the oesophagus but into the trachea giving the impression of a blind upper pouch. These clefts may be divided into three groups: involving the larynx only, larynx and proximal trachea up to the fourth ring or a complete cleft to or close to the carina [254]. Ogawa [244] has described a child with a cleft into the main bronchus. Often, the cleft is seen by the neonatologist at the time of initial resuscitation and intubation of a compromised or obstructed baby, but minor clefts may be missed for a considerable time. There is no doubt that a major cleft is a problem of airway management [165] and repair is urgent [262], unless the airway can be protected until any pneumonitis can be controlled [21]. Donohoe [63] describes a special tube for this purpose and with excellent illustrations explains the best method of closure. Our only recent case of a total cleft was successfully closed in a child who also had duodenal obstruction, but the child died some 3 months later from respiratory infection.

Pre-operative care

Pre-operative care begins from the moment of diagnosis at the place of delivery and referring hospitals must be issued with clear instructions on how best to transport the child [142]. The safest way, of course, is for a hospital team to collect the baby [178] by road or air [283] (see Chapter 4). The baby must at least be accompanied by a competent nurse who can regularly suck out the pharynx with a portable sucker or by syringe. The baby is best transported in the lateral position or prone and horizontal rather than with the head up or down.

On arrival at the surgical unit, the baby should be carefully examined and routine X-rays taken [55]. It is important to keep the baby warm while these manipulations take place. The usual pre-operative blood samples should be taken, including a cross-match although it is rarely necessary to transfuse blood at operation.

The upper pouch must be kept empty of saliva and this can be done by intermittent suction using a soft plastic catheter passed nasally or orally [2,326]. Some of this aspirate should be sent for culture [191]. The frequency of such aspiration depends on the rate at which secretions accumulate.

Continuous suction was suggested by Gross [104]. Damage to the oesophageal mucosa [194] can be avoided by the use of a double lumen plastic catheter designed by Replogle [278] which allows air to be drawn into the pouch as the secretions are aspirated. Talbert and Haller [330] found that such a tube could best be secured in the pouch by introducing it through a lateral pharyngostomy – a technique which was used by us some years ago but which has now been abandoned as it seemed to confer no advantage to management. Upper pouch suction is not without its problems and has to be supervised carefully by experienced nurses. Noblett and Wright [243] and later Bar-Moar [13] described patients who became cyanotic when suction was applied to the Replogle catheter. It is assumed that the high negative pressure in the pharynx prevented the baby from having effective inspiration.

The infant's position must be changed regularly, at least every 1–3 h, but if there is pulmonary collapse or pneumonia then the baby should be placed with the affected side uppermost. Gentle physiotherapy with chest percussion to the affected side is a useful adjunct to therapy and will often encourage re-expansion of a lobe blocked by mucus.

Tracheal intubation and positive pressure ventilation gives the advantage of easy access for regular aspiration of the bronchial tree. However, ventilatory therapy is usually reserved for babies in respiratory distress since it carries with it its own problems: the leak through the tracheo-oesophageal fistula makes ventilation difficult and too high ventilatory pressure can cause gastric perforation.

Jones and others [156] describe four babies with oesophageal atresia and tracheo-oesophageal fistula who developed pneumo-peritoneum whilst being ventilated. Three of these died from a perforation at the lesser curve of the stomach. To avoid this complication in the high risk patient with pneumonia or respiratory distress syndrome, Filston [82] recommends occluding the fistula with a Fogarty balloon catheter. Kadowaki [158] blocked off the lower oesophagus and hence the fistula with a transgastric balloon inserted at the time of surgery for other intra-abdominal anomalies; this was designed to facilitate delayed thoracotomy for repair of the oesophagus.

In the uncomplicated case, there is some debate about the best position for nursing the baby pre-operatively [38]. The Trendelenburg (head-down) position advocated by some [184,285] has the disadvantage that it allows free reflux [324] and spill over of acid secretions into the lungs. The head-up or even half-sitting position [42,138,325] discourages reflux but also discourages drainage of saliva from the mouth. We, like others, have found a compromise – nursing the baby horizontal and semiprone – to be perfectly satisfactory. Bar-Moar [12] proposed the use of cimetidine intravenously pre-operatively to reduce the acidity of any refluxing gastric juice; this seems a logical step and cimetidine should be continued postoperatively until the anastomosis is healed.

In addition, to aid aspiration of the secretions, humid air from a suitable humidifier is led into the incubator.

Surgical repair

In all babies, the principle to be observed is that ligation of the fistula with an attempt at primary anastomosis should be undertaken at the earliest possible opportunity [142,143,282]. For all but Group C_2 babies, this will be within the first 24 h after birth [255]. To delay unduly puts the baby at risk from acid pneumonitis [50].

For the ill, low birthweight baby with pneumonia or respiratory distress syndrome, a staging procedure had been advocated in the past [284]; gastrostomy followed by ligation and division of the fistula and a delayed primary anastomosis later was considered to be the safest management [75,76,116,137,176,221]. Cozzi and Wilkinson in 1967 [49] found no advantage in the staged management – a view supported by Templeton [332] who argues that the best early treatment is fistula ligation. Gastrostomy [36] alone allows air to blow off down the fistula but this also decreases ventilatory pressure so that even in a mechanically ventilated baby, it is difficult to ventilate the child adequately [82,321]. Primary gastrostomy [161] is also advocated as a means of preventing acid reflux but the main problem in fistula with associated respiratory distress syndrome [332] is not acid reflux but decreased lung compliance [130]. Ito [151], however, as a proponent of staged procedures reported 92% survival in a series of 12 babies operated upon up to 150 days after birth. He emphasizes the importance of aspirating the upper pouch, trachea and gastrostomy and employs enteral feeding. In an attempt to prevent reflux, temporary banding of the gastro-oesophageal junction [73] and balloon occlusion of the lower oesophagus, via trachea [82] or gastrostomy have been employed. A side-effect of the balloon method [236] is that the lower pouch dilates and improves the chances of repair. This is known as pressure induced growth (PIG) [256]. Similarly gastric transection has been postulated but is no longer used. It is a much more difficult procedure than gastrostomy [92,124,272].

Should it not be possible to anastomose the two ends of the oesophagus, it was customary for some years to perform a gastrostomy and oesophagostomy after ligation and division of the fistula with the intention of a later colon transplant. It became clear however, that if left *in situ*, the upper pouch could elongate and a delayed primary anastomosis could be achieved [111]. Howard and Myers in 1965 [147] first proposed a delayed primary anastomosis, stating, 'It is our firm conviction that the best oesophagus possible is one which is constructed entirely from the elements originally developed for its formation'. At the first operation the fistula was divided, a gastrostomy performed and bougies were then passed orally to elongate the upper pouch. This technique, with elongation of the upper pouch apparently enhanced by bouginage, prompted the development of numerous other methods of encouraging upper pouch elongation [58]. Apart from using pressure catheters [358], mercury filled bougies [217,335] or dilators [59,135,361], other intriguing methods have been used. Rehbein [276,277] introduced the 'thread and olive' technique as a means of joining upper and lower segments by fistulization; others [296,310] have reported their experience of this method and Booss [27,28] developed it further by inserting the perlon thread endoscopically. Shafer's [301,304] method also relies on the creation of a fistula, achieved in his cases by means of a silk structure. Hendren [127] has had some success with a very sophisticated electromagnetic method.

Whether or not bouginage of the blind pouch helps is still controversial [34]. There is no doubt that the repeated trauma of bouginage irritates the mucosa of the blind pouch, stimulates excessive mucus production and may encourage bacterial overgrowth which may cause trouble at the time of delayed anastomosis. Puri [264] argues that the two ends grow together anyway, with or without bouginage and would prefer to perform a gastrostomy and await events; we share his view.

Lividatis [203,204] offered an alternative method of elongating the upper pouch; he described the use of a circular myotomy to the upper pouch which allows it to be stretched without compromising its vascularity and hence its viability [174,311]. Animal experiments [329] confirmed that this technique reduces tension on the anastomosis. The technique has now been widely used [71,300]; the myotomy may be performed in the chest, but when the upper pouch is short it is easier to commence mobilization in the chest and then continue through a separate cervical incision, performing the myotomy and returning the pouch to the chest for completion of the anastomosis [133]. Myotomy does not add to the complications of oesophageal surgery such as leakage and stricture nor does it necessarily decrease them either [125,153]: there may, however, especially in the presence of distal obstruction, be some ballooning of the mucosa giving rise to a diverticulum [249] or a mediastinal pseudocyst [308]. Rossello [290] in a series of dog experiments found that a series of partial stepladder-type myotomies gave greater elongation to the normal oesophagus than a single myotomy, and one, two or three myotomies may be safely used. Long-term follow-up has not revealed significant deficiencies in oesophageal motility following myotomy.

Whilst circular myotomy has been a major advance in bridging long gaps, improved operative and anaesthetic techniques have also reduced the number of patients in whom a primary anastomosis is impossible. Thus the number of children needing colon [197,205,307,349], gastric [44,293,322] or bowel interposition [118,218] is also decreasing [4,5,20,319].

Careful consideration must also be given not only to the timing of chest surgery for poor risk patients but also the timing of surgery for other anomalies [143]. For example, if imperforate anus is present, it may be wiser to perform a colostomy a day or two after the chest surgery, whilst the presence of duodenal atresia would indicate the need for an early gastrostomy. Each problem needs to be carefully assessed and a planned programme of management established [295].

Operative techniques

The approach to the fistula in the common anomaly through the right side of the chest can be intra- or extrapleural [23]. Controversy surrounds these two approaches [137,178] but a survey by the surgical section of the American Academy of Pediatrics [141] showed a better survival from an extrapleural route and this is now generally preferred.

The opponents of the extrapleural approach claim that it is a more tedious and difficult dissection with tearing of the pleura and inevitable pneumothorax. However, once the extrapleural approach is mastered it is relatively easy to perform and pleural tears are rare and can be immediately oversewn. The technique does not unduly prolong the operation and the lung is never completely collapsed as it is in the intrapleural approach. The overwhelming advantage is that an anastomotic leak remains extrapleural and will drain saliva or air without contaminating the pleural cavity. In the transpleural approach a leak will lead to a pyopneumothorax often under tension. In the last 10 years, we have used the extrapleural approach exclusively.

Management of the fistula varies widely. Ligation in continuity carries a high rate of recurrence but simple ligation and division or division and suturing seem to be very satisfactory. Insertion of a piece of intercostal muscle or suturing pleura over the ligated end have been described as methods of discouraging fistula recurrence [227,362], and more recently myoosseus flaps have been recommended especially in recurrent cases [108].

Anastomotic technique varies [179,213]. The actual technique is probably not so important, as is avoidance of interference with the blood supply to the two ends by excessive mobilization [219] of the lower segment or the insertion of too many sutures at the anastomotic line [164]. Various methods of two-layered anastomosis have been described, by Haight [112,113], ten Kate [334] and Swenson [327], but most would agree with Koop [177] that a simple one-layered anastomosis, using silk, is sufficient. More recently, there has been a move to the use of polyglycolic acid sutures instead of silk [241]. Carachi [37], in an experimental pig model, studied the healing of the transected oesophagus and came to the conclusion that 4/0 silk was still the best suture, with knots on the inside for the back wall and on the outside for the front. In a similar investigation, Kullendorf, also using pigs, [182,183] compared silk with supramid and found no difference but recommended a traction suture between the oesophagus and the prevertebral fascia as a means of reducing longitudinal stress on the anastomosis. Rickham [283] advocated 7/0 silk with no transanastomotic feeding tube but performed a gastrostomy.

The use of a transanastomotic tube continues to cause controversy. Carachi [37] thought it made no difference though we prefer to use it, believing that it takes some tension off the anastomosis by keeping the stomach decompressed.

Clearly the distance between the two ends of the oesophagus is a critical factor as tension will embarrass the circulation. However, a certain amount of tension in itself does not seem to cause breakdown and indeed it is probably better to attempt an oesophageal anastomosis under some tension rather than abandon the attempt: a gap of up to 2.0–2.5 cm can usually be overcome by local mobilization alone. To lessen tension, various techniques have been described including myotomy as described above [181,229].

Sulamaa [198,325,326] and, later, Beardmore [258,340] used a method whereby the fistula is tied in continuity and the proximal blind pouch anastomosed end to side to the lower end; a similar technique was described by Gross and colleagues [106]: by this method the lower pouch is held up by the fistula and tension on the anastomosis may be reduced. Touloukian [337,338] reported a similar series with three fistula recurrences in the first 18 patients but none since. Many surgeons remain unconvinced because of the concern regarding recurrent fistula [22,68,338]; we have no experience with this technique. Gough [102] described a flap technique to lengthen the upper pouch but this does not seem to have been widely used.

Operation

'To anastomose the ends of an infant's oesophagus, the surgeon must be as delicate and precise as a skilled watchmaker. No other operation offers a greater opportunity for pure technical artistry.' (Potts quoted by Cloud [43])

The upper pouch is already being aspirated via a Replogle tube and this is replaced by a Jacques rubber catheter split along its length with a 4F (1.3 mm) feeding tube threaded through if a transanastomotic tube is to be used (Figure 21.4). Prior to this, it is our practice to bronchoscope the baby in order to demonstrate the site of the fistula and to exclude the presence of an unexpected upper pouch fistula, which could interfere with the freeing of the upper pouch [81]. If need be, a very fine catheter can be passed through the fistula for identification purposes [145,168].

The infant is placed in the left lateral position with the right arm over the face [105,273]. Position is maintained by tape placed over the baby's pelvis. A transverse incision in the line of the fourth or fifth rib is usual although Freeman [90] described a deformity of the scapula from division of nerves to serratus anterior with this incision; it is not a constant finding. The classic Denis Browne midaxillary vertical incision obviates nerve damage but gives, in our opinion, less than adequate exposure of the ribs and access to the chest. It is not our custom to remove a rib [67,100] but rather to divide the intercostal muscles in the 4/5 space very carefully so that the pleura is not opened. The pleura can best be reflected by using wet pledgelets and as it is stripped away so more intercostal muscle can be cut until the costochondral junction is approached small Finochietto retractor can be inserted and gently opened until the ribs are separated sufficiently. Once the chest is opened better illumination can be obtained by a fibre light source taped to the retractor though some may prefer a head light source. The vena azygos is divided and ligated as it joins the superior vena cava. This may be done with 2/0 silk but Liga clips (Figure 21.6) are an acceptable and useful alternative. Once the vein is divided it is relatively simple to identify the trachea and the vagus nerve which clearly stands out posterior to it and leads to the fistula. Care must be taken if a right-sided aorta is encountered as this may militate against a successful anastomosis, although it does not prevent closure of the fistula.

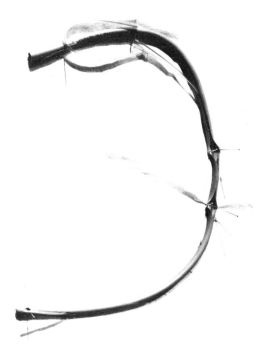

Figure 21.4 The thin transanastomotic tube is threaded inside a Jaques catheter split along its length in order to facilitate removal once the fine tube is in place

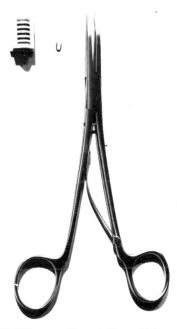

Figure 21.6 The use of metal clips, which are placed using a special applicator, facilitates control of the vena azygos

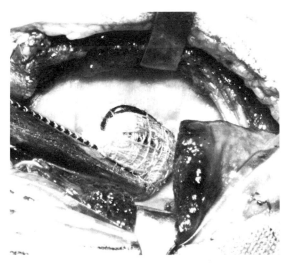

Figure 21.5 The lung and pleura are stripped away from the ribs by using wet cotton pledgelets held in a forceps

anteriorly (Figure 21.5). If the pleura is inadvertently torn, it should be repaired immediately with 4/0 catgut [253]. The pleura is then stripped away posteriorly and superiorly to expose the azygos vein and the posterior mediastinum. It is important to free the pleura inferiorly so that retractors do not tear it; initially, 1–2 cm wide copper strips are used, bent at an angle and held over packs, but later a

The fistula is freed with right-angled forceps and a tape can be passed around it to provide traction and allow the angle between trachea and fistula to be identified (Figure 21.7). Tenuous adhesions are carefully divided. Care must be taken not to enter the trachea but, with careful dissection, several millimetres of extra length can be obtained which may make the difference between success and failure of the primary anastomosis and prevent formation of a tracheal diverticulum. The fistula is generally ligated though it may be oversewn after transfixion ligation with 2/0 silk.

gastrostomy tube after 48 h have elapsed; they should be done under gravity and not forced into the stomach by syringe or under pressure. As adhesion between stomach and peritoneum is rapid feeds are usually safe after this period of time. Sometimes there is concern that the feeds are not passing into the stomach properly and if so it is wise to pass some barium contrast medium down the tube to see whether it is in the right place. Occasionally the tube falls out in the early stages. Should this occur it must be replaced under direct vision at a re-laparotomy. It is unwise to insert a new tube via the gastrostomy hole in the first week to 10 days after the gastrostomy has been made as the stomach may be pushed away from the peritoneum and subsequent feeds are then intraperitoneal; this obviously causes a rapid deterioration in the baby's condition.

Other complications that have been described are gastrocolic fistula and intestinal obstruction. Provided the anatomy is clearly defined, these complications should not arise. Finally, it should be noted that an abdominal gastrostomy opening closes very rapidly after removal of the tube. Advantage can be taken of this if the gastrostomy stoma is leaking a great deal. Removal of the tube for several hours allows the hole to heal in and a more snug fitting catheter can be inserted.

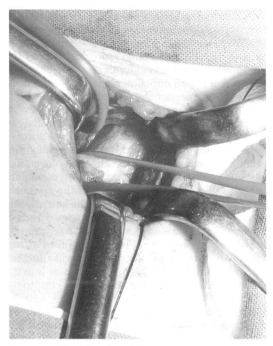

Figure 21.9 Mobilization of the H type fistula. Preliminary catheterization of the fistula is essential. Note the 'sloops' to identify oesophagus and fistula

H fistula

H (or N) fistula rarely presents in the neonatal period but should it do so, as at any age, it is vital to see the position of the fistula endoscopically and to pass a catheter through for identification purposes.

Although some authors [16] report up to 30% H fistulas occurring in the chest, this has not been our experience: our cases were all in the neck. The approach is therefore transcervical, usually from the right side as for oesophagostomy described above and the tube through the fistula should make identification relatively easy (Figure 21.9). There should be little surrounding fibrosis in the small baby and the surgeon should aim to mobilize and protect with slings the oesophagus above and below the fistula [6]. By slight traction on these, the oesophagus can be pulled away from the trachea and the fistula identified and doubly ligated with heavy gauge non-absorbable material or divided and over-sewn [186,360]. Provided dissection stays close to the oesophagus, the recurrent laryngeal nerve is not unduly at risk. On the right side, the recurrent nerve can usually be seen and protected. The left is more vulnerable but with care should not be harmed. Drainage of the wound is not necessary but the vocal cords should be inspected at the end of the operation.

Delayed primary anastomosis

Some advances have been made in the management of pure oesophageal atresia with a wide gap, and the same principles of management can be applied to cases of atresia with a tracheo-oesophageal fistula, unsuitable for early correction because of the width of the gap or because of multiple anomalies, low birth weight, pheumonia, etc. It is becoming more obvious that colonic or stomach interposition is not necessarily the correct surgery for wide-gap cases [154]. Delayed primary anastomosis offers better long-term results [79] and the immediate treatment is to close the fistula if there is one, make a feeding gastrostomy or establish parenteral nutrition, and deal with other life-threatening anomalies such as anorectal or duodenal atresia. Once these measures have been established surgery for the oesophageal atresia can be safely delayed for several weeks. Skilled nursing can usually keep the upper pouch empty; regular X-rays with opaque catheters or bougies passed through the mouth and through the gastrostomy into the distal oesophagus will demonstrate any diminution of the gap between the two ends of the oesophagus. Each case has to be assessed on its own merits but from 6 to 8 weeks after the gastrostomy we attempt an anastomosis – Puri [264] suggests 8–10 weeks. Various techniques for this have been described but we follow that described by Gough [102] and attributed to ten Kate (see Figure 21.10). When accompanied by initial myotomy [99,281], the gap can invariably be bridged, though there is a high incidence of reflux and oesophagitis later [31].

Postoperative management

Pulmonary complications and leakage from the anastomosis leading on to stricture formation are the main problems postoperatively [43,306]. In theory, they are preventable though their incidence must be affected by the management of associated anomalies such as congenital heart disease or duodenal obstruction.

The baby is received back from theatre into his prewarmed, humid environment and must be observed constantly by both nursing and medical staff, watching for change of colour or respirations, tracheal tugging or intercostal recession. Nursed on its side the child must be turned every hour [38], though in the presence of pneumonia or atelectasis the affected side should be kept uppermost for a longer period [208]. Handling must be very gentle and should be kept to a minimum so, ideally, investigations should be arranged to coincide with nursing procedures.

Even in the presence of an adequate primary anastomosis, the baby often cannot cope with saliva, so it is important that suction of the pharynx be continued as frequently as pre-operatively. To avoid inadvertent damage to the anastomosis, the length of the catheter which can safely be inserted is marked on a tape attached to the incubator.

In the ideal situation, the fluid level in the chest drain stops moving at 24 h and chest X-rays show no change or minimal collapse or pneumonitis which rapidly clears with movement, physiotherapy and antibiotics. The latter, however, are not given routinely. The chest drain can be removed in 4–5 days though some prefer to keep it in longer [178]. Daily chest X-rays are necessary until the tube is removed.

Small nasogastric feeds are given by the feeding tube on the second day, starting with glucose saline and building up slowly to normal so that by the fourth or fifth day full feeds are being given. Occasionally, the transanastomotic tube is pulled out by a vigorous baby. With caution it can be replaced but the nervous can leave it out. Usually no harm is done.

Complications

Pulmonary

In the ill baby, of any weight, with pulmonary changes pre-operatively, postoperative respiratory problems must be anticipated and even in the seemingly straightforward case, pulmonary complications may occur [40] – usually as a result of an anstomotic leak. Daily X-rays of the chest are essential until the chest drain is removed (see above) but more frequent X-rays may be deemed necessary, particularly if there is any sudden change in the baby's condition.

Some babies will not breathe on their own postoperatively and require ventilation, and others who appear to manage well at first may need reintubation and bronchial lavage [275]. Tracheal tugging, subcostal recession and cyanosis are signs to be watched for and are indicative of the need for

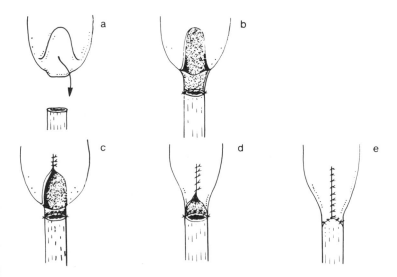

Figure 21.10 To show the formation of a tube for reconstruction of oesophageal atresia. (See Gough [102] and text)

anaesthetic intervention. Indeed, it has been suggested that all babies should be nursed routinely for the first 24–48 h postoperatively with an endotracheal tube in place. Extubation is performed only when the child's clinical condition is stable and the chest X-ray is clear [220].

Anastomotic leak

Leakage is not necessarily the result of careless surgery as suggested by Drainer [64]. Leaks occur even after the most carefully constructed anastomoses and are presumably due to a combination of a number of factors, including tension on the anastomosis, a poor blood supply and a degree of hypoxia [202]. Spitz and colleagues [321] advocate a period of 5 days elective ventilation for infants with a very tense anastomosis; they attribute the success of the policy to the elimination of swallowing and the maintenance of neck flexion. An extrapleural leak may only be demonstrated by a collection of saliva and air from the chest drain [70]. With the chest drain *in situ*, manoeuvring the tube, washing it out and applying low grade suction may be sufficient to encourage saliva to drain. As most leaks manifest themselves on the third to fifth day, it is wise to keep the chest drain in until this time. Small leaks often close spontaneously and an expectant approach should be adopted (Figure 21.11). Feeds must be stopped and intravenous alimentation instituted [83]. Supportive respiratory care may be necessary at this stage [306,359]. Some have advocated resuturing of early anastomotic leaks [207,321] but this is a hazardous procedure which is more likely to result in complete dehiscence of the anastomosis then a closure of the leak. Most leaks are in fact due to partial dehiscence only and an expectant policy can confidently be instituted [344]. Repositioning of the chest drains and possibly insertion of extra drains is usually all that is required. A contrast swallow [51] will help in the estimation of how severe any leak has been whilst a distally placed transanastomotic tube may help the leak to heal more quickly [95].

When there has been a major intrapleural leak there may well be a tension pneumothorax with quite severe respiratory distress; in these cases it will almost certainly be necessary to abandon the anastomosis, close the ends and make an oesophagostomy and gastrostomy. This situation is rare however. Most smaller leaks close and may not necessarily be followed by stricture. Leakage does not necessarily indicate that a stricture will occur later.

Recurrent fistula

This complication is easily overlooked and, even when suspected, it may be difficult to demonstrate [112,116,148]. It should be suspected in the presence

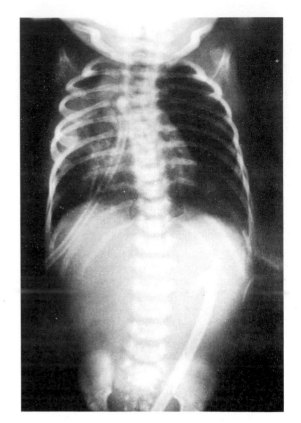

Figure 21.11 Anastomotic dehiscence. There is an extrapleural leak with collapse of the right upper lobe. Note that the mediastinuan is central. Treated by low grade suction to the pleural drain

of a persistent cough with choking and cyanosis at the time of feeding [80]. Alternatively, there may be repeated pneumonic episodes with right upper lobe consolidation on X-ray or failure to thrive [309]. The incidence of recurrent fistula varies but is probably within the range of 5–15% of all cases [140,148,306,32]. It is presumably caused by abscess formation from a suture line leak or spillage of tracheal contents due to inadequate ligation of the fistula [159]. If a recurrent fistula is suspected it should be searched for very carefully and repeated investigation may be necessary. Endoscopy is mandatory if recurrence is suspected and the fistula may not necessarily be seen on the first examination and may need repeat endoscopy. Once the recurrent fistula has been identified it must be closed: in three out of four of our patients obliteration was achieved successfully by diathermy fulguration through a bronchoscope [274,346]: in the fourth re-exploration was necessary. Fulguration is worth attempting since operative repair is difficult through dense adhesions [312]. A catheter through the fistula certainly helps with identification at the time of re-operation and a transpleural right sided approach is necessary. It is wise to mobilize the trachea and oesophagus widely and even then, a second re-exploration may be necessary. Up to a 50% mortality was recorded in early reports [252] but in our hands, no child has succumbed after a recurrent fistula repair. Insertion of a pericardial flap [30], free muscle, or muscle graft are all methods of trying to prevent further recurrence. For the severe problem, a transtracheal approach has been advocated by Martin [223].

Postoperative respiratory distress

A characteristic brassy cough almost always persists following repair of oesophageal atresia. Nerve damage may occasionally be responsible for this [144] but bronchoscopy usually shows a degree of trachomalacia [17]: in most cases this cough has disappeared in a year or 18 months as the trachea becomes less pliable. However, a distended proximal pouch pressing on the back of the trachea as well as anterior vascular compression may produce severe respiratory distress and life-threatening apnoeic spells [78]. Gastro-oesophageal reflux with aspiration may also cause severe respiratory distress [9].

The symptoms of tracheomalacia are dramatically relieved by aortopexy [78], a procedure normally carried out through an incision in the second left intercostal space: by hitching the aorta to the manubrium the anterior vascular compression is relieved and the trachea is pulled forward from the dilated upper pouch as well as being held open [287]. Variations of the operation have been reported: Spitz has described a dacron patch aortopexy [320] and Vaishnav and MacKinnon [342] believe a cervical approach to be simpler. Long-term deficits in pulmonary function have been described by Dudley [66] and by Couriel [48].

Anastomotic stricture

There is invariably some narrowing at the anastomotic site, which may be mild or severe [144,298]. Gross [104] divided strictures into (1) early, occurring in the first 3–4 weeks postoperatively; (2) late, from 1 to 5 months; and (3) later, occurring some 10–12 months after the original surgery.

The incidence varies but seems to occur in one-third to one-half of cases at some time [109,112]. In a long-term follow-up of cases treated in Alder Hey between 1965 and 1974 [202] we found a 26% incidence of stricture significant enough to require dilatation. Some departments recommend a barium

swallow 7 days after a successful anastomosis and repeated dilatation if there is any narrowing [51]. In our experience narrowing is almost always present but not all babies have symptoms of hold-up [315]. Therefore it is our practice to investigate only those babies who have symptoms at whatever age they develop, and others would agree with this. Dilatation is not difficult; with a rigid oesophagoscope graded gum elastic bougies are passed through the stricture, stopping at the first sign of bleeding. We have not perforated the oesophagus using this technique. Gans [93] recommends the use of a Fogarty or balloon catheter [230] to dilate the stricture and if a gastrostomy is present, Tucker's dilators are useful. Steroid injections [139] may have a place in the occasional patient who does not respond to simple dilatations.

It should be remembered that incompetence of the cardia is not unusual following repair of oesophageal atresia and acid reflux may contribute to stricture formation: anti-reflux procedures may be indicated [132,257]. Gautier and his colleagues [96] found gastro-oesophageal reflux in half their babies with oesophageal atresia at 10 days of age and an increased rate of stricture formation in that group.

Gastro-oesophageal reflux after oesophageal atresia repair may also cause recurrent vomiting [48], and poor weight gain [132]. Twenty-four hour pH studies for gastro-oesophageal reflux have demonstrated its frequent presence [245]; up to two-thirds of children following repair of tracheo-oesophageal fistula have been shown to have reflux up to 6 years after surgery [7,157]. Symptomatic gastro-oesophageal reflux is found in up to a quarter of all cases: with the serious consequences of stricture formation and respiratory complications it must be treated aggressively – if necessary by surgical antireflux procedures: operative intervention is, however, rarely indicated in the neonatal period. In 57 survivors with a primary anastomosis reviewed at 5–15 years of age, we found 17% had persistent troublesome reflux and one-third of these had fundal plication [202].

Oesophageal motility after successful anastomosis is often abnormal [112,167,185,199]. This can be demonstrated in video barium studies [35,61,117] when the normal oesophageal stripping wave can be seen to be held up at the anastomosis [248,265]. The cause of this is obscure: vagal denervation might be considered an operational hazard but rarely occurs, and the condition has been reported in H fistula. Nakazato [237] has investigated the myenteric plexus in the oesophagus and stomach of a patient with atresia. He suggests there is an abnormality in that plexus which leads to a functional impairment of motility. Our own studies of biopsies of the proximal oesophageal pouch showed aganglionosis in some cases.

Results

In assessing results, the use of Waterston's classification is a convenient method of comparison between various centres [279].

There are many notable reviews of results from the major survey by the American Academy of Pediatrics [141] in 1964 up until the present time [64, 283,321]. Comparison over the years is not strictly reliable because of changing factors contributing to improved survival. Rickham [283] attributes the main improvement in results to care in transport and improvement in intensive care, including skilled anaesthetic supervision with intubation and controlled respiration even before surgery. Connolly and Guiney [45] in a review of 139 patients seen in 10 years between 1974 and 1983 reported an increase in the infants weighing less than 1.8 kg from 7% before 1979 to 18% after, yet in the same time the mortality rate in these infants fell from 50% to zero. A Group A baby should certainly survive and live a normal life though he may have some swallowing or reflux problems [207,247]. Most Group B and C patients should also survive [129] given modern techniques of respiratory and nutritional support though the long-term growth of some patients may be less than adequate [7,284,289,354,356].

Of 124 cases admitted to Alder Hey between 1975 and 1985, 30 (24%) died. This unsatisfactorily high death rate reflects, to a certain extent, the changing nature of the patients admitted: only 28 of the 124 patients were in Waterston classification Group A, 36 were in Group B, of whom two died, but 10 were in Group C_1 and 50 in Group C_2 and most of the deaths were amongst these (four in Group C_1 and 24 in Group C_2). The majority of the Group C deaths were related to their associated anomalies: one of the Group B deaths was from pneumonia at 15 days of age, probably related to gastro-oesophageal reflux and the other was the result of an anastomotic breakdown.

Even though some deaths are inevitable in Group C babies with very low birth weights and multiple anomalies [1], aggressive treatment by neonatologists and intensive surgical therapy has led to increased survival in this group [39,222]. These babies may have an oesophagus in continuity or a functioning oesophageal replacement [119] but they may have problems attributable to their other anomalies and/or mental retardation consequent upon their prematurity: they are thus severely handicapped.

Like the neonatologist, the paediatric surgeon may find himself in the position of expecting the survival of the very small infant with multiple abnormalities but being concerned as to whether survival should be encouraged in a child whose quality of life will be very poor. Fortunately, such cases represent only a minute proportion of babies with oesophageal atresia.

'Oesophageal atresia is the epitome of modern surgery.'

References

1. Abrahamson, J. and Shandling, B. (1972) Esophageal atresia in the underweight baby. A challenge. *J. Pediat. Surg.*, **7**, 608–613
2. Adler, D. (1958) Congenital tracheo-oesophageal fistula. *S. Afr. med. J.*, **32**, 958–963
3. Ahmed, S. (1970) Infantile pyloric stenosis associated with major anomalies of the alimentary tract. *J. Pediat. Surg.*, **5**, 660–666
4. Anderson, K.D. (1984) Oesophageal substitution. *Aust. N.Z. J. Surg.*, **54**, 447–449
5. Anderson, K.D. (1986) Gastric tube esophagoplasty. *Prog. Pediat. Surg.*, **19**, 55–61
6. Andrassy, R.J., Ko, P. and Hanson, B.A. Congenital tracheo-esophageal fistula without esophageal atresia. A 22-year experience. *Am. J. Surg.*, **140**, 731–733
7. Andrassy, R.J., Patterson, R.S., Ashley, J., Patrissi, G. and Mahour, G.H. (1983) Long-term nutritional assessment of patients with esophageal atresia and/or tracheoesophageal fistula. *J. Pediat. Surg.*, **18** (4), 431–435
8. Armstrong, R.G., Lindberg, E.F. and Stanford, W. (1970) Traumatic pseudo-diverticulum of the esophagus in the newborn infant. *Surgery*, **67**, 844–846
9. Ashcraft, K.W., Goodwin, C.D., Amoury, R.A. *et al.* (1977) Early recognition and aggressive treatment of gastro-esophageal reflux following repair of esophageal atresia. *J. Pediat. Surg.*, **12**, 317–321
10. Atwell, J.D. and Beard, R.C. (1974) Congenital anomalies of the upper urinary tract associated with esophageal atresia and tracheo-esophageal fistula. *J. Pediat. Surg.*, **9**, 825–831
11. Auchterlonie, I.A. and White, M.P. (1982) Recurrence of the VATER association within a sibship. *Clin. Genet.*, **21**, 122–124
12. Bar-Maor, J.A., Shoshany, G. and Mories-Chass, I. (1981) Use of Cimetidine in esophageal atresia with lower tracheo-esophageal fistula. *J. Pediat. Surg.*, **16**, 8–11
13. Bar-Maor, J.A. and Simon, K. (1981) Another complication of continuous upper pouch suction in esophageal atresia. *J. Pediat. Surg.*, **16**, 730
14. Barnes, J.C. and Smith, W.L. (1978) The VATER association. *Radiology*, **126**, 445–449
15. Barry, J.E. and Auldist, A.W. (1974) The VATER association. *Am. J. Dis. Child.*, **128**, 769–771
16. Bedard, P., Girvan, D.P. and Shandling, B. (1974) Congenital H type tracheo-esophageal fistula. *J. Pediat. Surg.*, **9**, 663–668

17. Benjamin, B., Cohen, D. and Glasson, M. (1976) Tracheomalacia in association with congenital tracheoesophageal fistula. *Surgery*, **79**, 504–508

18. Benjamin, B. (1980) Endoscopy in congenital tracheal anomalies. *J. Pediat. Surg.*, **15**, 164–171

19. Benson, J.E., Olsen, M.M. and Fletcher, B.D. (1985) A spectrum of bronchopulmonary anomalies associated with tracheoesophageal malformations. *Pediat. Radiol.*, **15**, 377–380

20. Bentley, I.F.R. (1965) Primary colonic substitution for atresia of the esophagus. *Surgery*, **58**, 731–736

21. Berkovits, R.N., Bax, N.M.A. and van der Schans, E.J. (1987) Surgical treatment of congenital laryngo-tracheo-oesophageal cleft. *Prog. Pediat. Surg.*, **21**, 34–46

22. Berman, J.K. and Berman, E.K. (1953) Congenital atresia of the esophagus with T.E.F.–a simplified technique of restoring continuity. *Am. J. Surg.*, **86**, 436–442

23. Bishop, P.J., Klein, M.D. and Philippart, A.I. (1985) Transpleural repair of esophageal atresia without a primary gastrostomy: 240 patients treated between 1951 and 1983. *J. Pediat. Surg.*, **20**, 823–828

24. Black, P.R. and Welch, K.J. (1986) Pulmonary agenesis (aplasia). Esophageal atresia and tracheoesophageal fistula: a different treatment strategy. *J. Paediat. Surg.*, **21**, 936–938

25. Blank, R.H. *et al.* (1967) Congenital esophageal atresia with T.O.F. occurring in identical twins. *J. Thorac. Cardiovasc. Surg.*, **58**, 192–196

26. Bond-Taylor, W., Starer, F. and Atwell, J.D. (1923) Vertebral anomalies associated with oesophageal atresia with reference to the initial operative mortality. *J. Pediat. Surg.*, **8**, 9–13

27. Booss, D., Hollwarth, M. and Sauer, H. (1982) Endoscopic esophageal anastomosis. *J. Pediat. Surg.*, **17**, 138–143

28. Booss, D. and Kolarkski, J. (1986) Current surgical strategies in long-gap esophageal atresia with regard to endoscopic anastomosis. *Prog. Pediat. Surg.*, **19**, 1–7

29. Borde, J., Mitrofanoff, P. and Walton, P. (1976) False neonatal pharyngo-oesophageal diverticula. *Ann. Chir. Infant.*, **17**, 35

30. Botham, M.J. and Coran, A.G. (1986) The use of pericardium for the management of recurrent tracheo-oesophageal fistula. *J. Pediat. Surg.*, **21**, 164–166

31. Brereton, R.J., Zachary, R.B. and Spitz, L. (1978) Preventable death in oesophageal atresia. *Arch. Dis. Child.*, **53**, 276–283

32. Brereton, R.J. and Rickwood, A.M. (1983) Esophageal atresia with pulmonary agenesis. *J. Pediat. Surg.*, **18**, 618–620

33. Briceno, L.I., Grases, P.J. and Gallego, S. (1981) Tracheobronchial and pancreatic remnants causing esophageal stenosis. *J. Pediat. Surg.*, **16**, 731–732

34. Brown, S. and Nixon, H.H. (1983) Spontaneous anastomosis of the esophagus in esophageal atresia. *J. Pediat. Surg.*, **18**, 293–296

35. Burgess, J.N., Carlson, H.C. and Ellis, F.H. (1968) Esophageal function after successful repair of esophageal atresia with tracheo-esophageal fistula. *J. Thorac. Cardiovasc. Surg.*, **56**, 667–673

36. Campbell, J.R. and Sasakin, T.M. (1974) Gastrostomy in infants and children. An analysis of complications and techniques. *Am. Surg.*, **40**, 505–508

37. Carachi, R., Stokes, K.B. and Brown, T.C.K. (1984) Esophageal anastomosis – an experimental model to study the anastomotic lumen and the influence of a transanastomotic tube. *J. Pediat. Surg.*, **19**, 9–93

38. Castilla, P., Irving, I.M., Rees, G.J. and Rickham, P.P. (1971) Posture in the management of esophageal atresia. Variations on a theme by Dr E.B. Neuhauser. *J. Pediat. Surg.*, **6**, 709–714

39. Chavrier, Y. and Revillon, Y. (1984) Tracheo-oesophageal fistula in children. *Chir. Pediat.*, **25**, 228–233

40. Chrispin, A.R., Friedland, G.W. and Waterston, D.J. (1966) Aspiration pneumonia and dysphagia after technically successful repair of esophageal atresia. *Thorax.*, **21**, 104–110

41. Claiborne, A.K., Blocker, S.H. and Martin, C.M. (1986) Prenatal and postnatal sonographic delineation of gastrointestinal abnormalities in a case of the VATER syndrome. *J. Ultrasound Med.*, **5**, 45–47

42. Clatworthy, H.W. Jr (1955) Esophageal atresia. Importance of early diagnosis and adequate treatment illustrated by a series of patients. *Pediatrics*, **16**, 122–128

43. Cloud, D.T. (1968) Anastomotic techniques in esophageal atresia. *J. Pediat. Surg.*, **3**, 561–564

44. Cohen, D.H., Middleton, A. and Fletcher, J. (1974) Gastric tube esophagoplasty. *J. Pediat. Surg.*, **9**, 451–460

45. Connolly, B. and Guiney, E.J. (1987) Trends in tracheo-oesophageal fistula. *Surg. Gynecol. Obstet.*, **164**, 308–312

46. Copleman, B., Cannata, B.V. and London, W. (1950) Tracheo-oesophageal anomalies in siblings. *J. Med. Soc. N.J.*, **47**, 415

47. Coran, A.G. (1973) Pericardio-esophagoplasty. A new operation for partial oesophageal replacement. *Am. J. Surg.*, **125**, 294–299

48. Couriel, J.M., Hibbert, M., Olinsky, A. and Phelan, P.D. (1982) Long term pulmonary consequences of oesophageal atresia with tracheoesophageal fistula. *Acta Paediat. Scand.*, **71**, 973–978

49. Cozzi, F. and Wilkinson, A.W. (1967) Oesophageal atresia. *Lancet*, **ii**, 1222–1225

50. Cozzi, F. and Wilkinson, A.W. (1975) Low birth-weight babies with oesophageal atresia or tracheo-oesophageal fistula. *Arch. Dis. Child.*, **50**, 791–795

51. Cumming, W.A. (1975) Esophageal atresia and congenital tracheo-esophageal atresia. *Pediat. Clins N. Am.*, **13**, 277

52. Czeizel, A. (1981) SCHISIS association. *Am. J. Med. Gen.*, **10**, 25–35

53. Czeizel, A. and Ludanyi, I. (1984) VACTERL association. *Acta Morphol. Hungary*, **32**, 75–96

54. Czernik, J. and Raine, P.A. (1982) Oesophageal atresia and pyloric stenosis – an association. *Z. Kinderchir.*, **35**, 18–20

55. Day, D.L. (1985) Aortic arch in neonates with esophageal atresia: preoperative assessment using CT. *Radiology*, **155**, 99–100

56. de Bary, J. (1864) Atresie des Oesophagus mit vollstandiger Transpositio viscerum. *Virchows Arch. Path. Anat.*, **31**, 430–434

57. de Beaufen, M.J., Mollard, P. and Campo-Paysaa, A. (1972) Reconstruction of the oesophagus by Howard's method. *Annls Chir. Infant.*, **13**, 65

58. de Lorimier, A. (1966) Treatment of esophageal atresia with a short proximal oesophageal segment. *J. Am. Med. Ass.*, **195**, 697–698

59. de Lorimier, A.A. and Harrison, M.R. (1980) 'Long gap' esophageal atresia; primary anastomosis after oesophageal elongation by bouginage and esophagomyotomy. *J. Thorac. Cardiol. Surg.*, **79**, 138–141

60. Dennis, N.R., Nicholas, J.L. and Kovar, I. (1973) Oesophageal atresia – 3 cases in 2 generations. *Arch Dis. Child.*, **48**, 980–982

61. Desjardins, J.G., Stephens, C.A. and Moes, C.A.F. (1964) Results of surgical treatment of congenital T.O.F. with a note of cineflurographic findings. *Ann. Surg.*, **160**, 141–145

62. Djupesland, G. (1980) A technique for the demonstration and surgical localization of congenital H-type tracheo-esophageal fistula. *J. Laryngol. Otol.*, **94**, 1065–1068

63. Donohoe, P.K. and Gee, P.E. (1984) Complete laryngotracheoesophageal cleft: Management and repair. *J. Pediat. Surg.*, **19**, 143–148

64. Drainer, I.K. and Dow, G.R. (1975) Oesophageal atresia in the western region of Scotland. *J.R. Coll. Surg. Edinb.*, **19**, 276–281

65. Ducharme, J.C., Betrand, R. and Debie, J. (1971) Three cases of pharyngeal perforation, mimicking tracheo-oesophageal fistula. *Can. Med. Ass. J.*, **104**, 785–787

66. Dudley, N.E. and Phelan, P.D. (1976) Respiratory complications in long-term survivors of oesophageal atresia. *Arch. Dis. Child.*, **51**, 279–282

67. Durning, R.P., Scoles, P.V. and Fox, O.D. (1980) Scoliosis after thoracotomy in tracheoesophageal fistula patients. A follow-up study. *J. Bone Joint Surg.*, **62A**, 1156–1159

68. Ein, H.E. and Thaman, T.E. (1973) A comparison of results of primary repair of esophageal atresia and tracheo-esophageal fistulae using end to side and end to end anastomosis. *J. Pediat. Surg.*, **8**, 641–645

69. Emery, J.L. and Haddadin, A.J. (1971) Squamous epithelium in respiratory tract of children with tracheo-oesophageal fistula. *Arch. Dis. Child.*, **46**, 236–242

70. Engel, P.M., Vos, L.J. and de Vries, J.A. (1970) Esophageal atresia with tracheo-esophageal fistula in mother and child. *J. Pediat. Surg.*, **5**, 564–565

71. Eraklis, A.J., Rossello, P.J. and Ballantine, T.V. (1976) Circular myotomy of the upper pouch in primary repair of long segment esophageal atresia. *J. Pediat. Surg.*, **11**, 709–712

72. Erichsen, G., Hauge, M. and Madsen, C.M. (1981) Two-generation transmission of oesophageal atresia with tracheo-oesophageal fistula. *Acta Paediat. Scand.*, **70**, 253–254

73. Fagelman, K.M. and Boyarsky, A. (1985) Temporary banding of the gastroesophageal junction in the critically ill neonate with esophageal atresia and tracheoesophageal fistula. *Surgery*, **98**, 594–597

74. Farrant, P. (1980) The antenatal diagnosis of oesophageal atresia by ultrasound. *Br. J. Radiol.*, **53**, 1202–1209

75. Farris, J.M. and Smith, G.K. (1956) The evaluation of temporary gastrostomy. *Ann. Surg.*, **144**, 475–486

76. Ferguson, C.C. (1970) Management of infants with oesophageal atresia and tracheo-oesophageal fistula. *Ann. Surg.*, **172**, 750–754

77. Ferguson, C.F. (1951) Congenital tracheo-esophageal fistula not associated with atresia of the esophagus. *Laryngoscope*, **61**, 718–766

78. Filler, R.M., Rossello, P.J. and Lebowitz, R.L. (1976) Life-threatening anoxic spells caused by tracheal compression after repair of esophageal atresia: Correction by surgery. *J. Pediat. Surg.*, **11**, 739–748

79. Filston, H.C., Merten, D.F. and Kirks, D.R. (1981) Initial care of esophageal atresia to facilitate potential primary anastomosis. *South Med. J.*, **74**, 1530–1533

80. Filston, H.C., Rankin, J.S. and Kirks, D.R. (1982) The diagnosis of primary and recurrent tracheo-esophageal fistulae. Value of selective catherisation. *J. Paediat. Surg.*, **17**, 144–148

81. Filston, H.C., Rankin, J.S. and Grimm, J.K. (1984) Esophageal atresia. Prognostic factors and contribution of preoperative telescopic endoscopy. *Ann. Surg.*, **199**, 532–537

82. Filston, H.C., Chitwood, W.R., Schkolne, B. *et al.* (1982) The Fogarty balloon catheter as an aid to management of the infant with esophageal atresia and tracheo-esophageal fistula complicated by severe RDS or pneumonia. *J. Pediat. Surg.*, **17**, 149–151

83. Firor, H.V., Pildes, R. and Vidyasagar, J. (1973) Delayed repair of esophageal fistula. Use of a jejunostomy as an alternative to intravenous alimentation. *J. Thorac. Cardiovasc. Surg.*, **66**, 828–832

84. Fleming, P.J., Venugopal, S., Lewins, M.D., Martin, D.J. and Simpson, J.S. (1980), Esophageal perforation into the right pleural cavity in a neonate. *J. Pediat. Surg.*, **15**, 335–336

85. Flowers, W.K. (1983) Hydramnios and gastrointestinal atresias: a review. *Obstet. Gynec. Surv.*, **38**, 685–688

86. Fluss, Z. and Poppen, K.J. (1951) Embryogenesis of tracheo-oesophageal atresia. *Arch. Path.*, **52**, 1968

87. Fossa, S., Podesta, E. and Venzano, G. (1976) Pseudodiverticuli esofegi neonatali di origine traumatica. *Minerva Paed.*, **28**, 30–39

88. Franklin, R.H. (1947) Congenital atresia of the oesophagus. *Lancet*, **ii**, 243–244

89. Freeman, N.V. (1973) Clinical evaluation of the fibreoptic bronchoscope for pediatric endoscopy. *J. Pediat. Surg.*, **8**, 213–220

90. Freeman, N.V. and Walkden, J. (1969) Previously unreported shoulder deformity following right lateral thoracotomy for esophageal atresia. *J. Pediat. Surg.*, **4**, 627–636

91. Friedman, A.P., Velcek, F.T. and Ergin, M.A. (1980) Oesophageal atresia associated with pyloric atresia. *Br. J. Radiol.*, **53**, 1009–1011

92. Gamble, H.A. (1938) Tracheo-oesophageal fistula – description of a new operative procedure. *Ann. Surg.*, **107**, 701–707

93. Gans, S.L. and Berci, G. (1973) Inside tracheo-esophageal fistula. New endoscopic approaches. *J. Pediat. Surg.*, **8**, 205–211

94. Gans, S.L. and Johnson, R.O. (1977) Diagnosis and surgical management of H type tracheo-esophageal fistula. *J. Pediat. Surg.*, **12**, 233–236

95. Gauderer, M.W. and Izant, R.J. (1983) Distally placed trans-anastomotic drainage tube in the management of the severely leaking esophageal anastomosis. *J. Pediat. Surg.*, **18**, 829–822

96. Gauthier, F., Gaudiche, O. and Baux, O. (1980) Atresia of the oesophagus and gastrointestinal reflux. *Chir. Paed.*, **21**, 253–256

97. German, J.C., Mahour, G.H. and Woolley, M.M. (1976) Esophageal atresia and associated anomalies. *J. Pediat. Surg.*, **11**, 299–306

98. Gibson, T. (1697) *The Anatomy of Human Bodies Epitomised*, Awnsham and Churchill, London

99. Gigiotti, G.L., Domini, R., Cacciari, A. *et al.* (1975) Circular esophageal myotomy for primary correction of esophageal atresia. *Rev. Chir. Pediat.*, **18**, 308–313

100. Gilsanz, V., Boechat, I.M. and Birnberg, F.A. (1983) Scoliosis after thoracotomy for esophageal atresia. *Am. J. Roent.*, **141**, 457–460

101. Glasson, M.J., Bandrevics, V. and Cohen, D.H. (1973) Pyloric stenosis complicating esophageal atresia. *Surgery*, **74**, 530–535

102. Gough, M.H. (1980) Oesophageal atresia: Use of an anterior flap in the difficult anastomosis. *J. Pediat. Surg.*, **15**, 310

103. Grieve, J.G. and McDermott, J.G. (1939) Congenital atresia of the oesophagus in two brothers. *Can. Med. Ass. J.*, **41**, 185–186

104. Gross, R.E. (1953) *The Surgery of Infancy and Childhood*, W.B. Saunders, Philadelphia

105. Gross, R.E. (1970) *An Atlas of Children's Surgery*, W.B. Saunders, Philadelphia

106. Gross, R.E. and Scott, H.W. (1946) Correction of esophageal atresia and tracheoesophageal fistula by closure of the fistula and oblique anastomosis of the esophageal segments. *Surg. Gynec. Obstet.*, **82**, 518–526

107. Gruenwald, P. (1940) A case of atresia of the oesophagus combined with tracheo-oesophageal fistula in 9 mm human embryo. *Anat. Rec.*, **78**, 293–302

108. Gustafson, R.A. and Hrabovsky, E.E. (1986) Intercostal muscle and myo-osseous flaps in difficult paediatric thoracic problems. *J. Pediat. Surg.*, **17**, 541–545

109. Haas, L. and Sturridge, M.F. (1961) Congenital tracheo-oesophageal fistula. *Proc. R. Soc. Med.*, **54**, 329–330

110. Haddadin, A.J. and Emery, J.L. (1971) Pulmonary retention simulating pneumonia as a cause of death in children with tracheo-esophageal fistula. *Surgery*, **70**, 311–315

111. Hagberg, S., Rubenson, A. and Sillen, U. (1986) Management of long-gap esophagus: experience with end-to-end anastomosis under maximal tension. *Prog. Pediat. Surg.*, **19**, 88–92

112. Haight, C. (1948) Congenital tracheoesophageal fistula with esophageal atresia. *J. Thorac. Surg.*, **17**, 600–612

113. Haight, C. (1957) Some observations on esophageal atresia and T.O.F. of congenital origin. *J. Thorac. Surg.*, **34**, 141–172

114. Haight, C. (1962) The esophagus. In *Pediatric Surgery* (eds W.T. Mustard, M.M. Ravitch, W.H. Snyder, K.J. Welch and C.D. Benson) Year Book Medical Publishers, Chicago

115. Haight, C. and Towsley, H.A. (1943) Congenital atresia of the esophagus with tracheo-esophageal fistula: extrapleural ligation of fistula and end to end anastomosis of oesophageal segments. *Surg. Gynec. Obstet.*, **76**, 672–688

116. Haight, C. and Towsley, H.A. (1944) Congenital atresia of the esophagus and tracheo-esophageal fistula. Reconstruction of the esophagus by primary anastomosis. *Ann. Surg.*, **120**, 623–655

117. Haller, J.A., Brooker, A. and Talbert, J. (1966) Esophageal function following resection. *Ann. Thorac. Surg.*, **2**, 180–187

118. Halsband, H. (1986) Esophagus replacement by free, autologous jejunal mucosa transplantation in long-gap esophageal atresia. *Prog. Pediat. Surg.*, **19**, 22–36

119. Hands, L.J. and Dudley, N.E. (1986) A comparison between gap-length and Waterston classification as guides to mortality and morbidity after surgery for esophageal atresia. *J. Pediat. Surg.*, **21**, 404–406

120. Harrison, M.R., Weitzman, J.J. and de Lorimier, A.A. (1980) Localisation of the aortic arch prior to repair of esophageal atresia. *J. Pediat. Surg.*, **15**, 312

121. Hasse, W. (1975) Bougierung des oberen and unteren Oesophagussegumentes bei der oesophagusatresie. *Z. Kinderchir.*, **17**, 170

122. Hausmann, P.F., Close, A.S. and Williams, L.P. (1957) Occurrence of tracheo-esophageal fistula in 3 consecutive siblings. *Surgery*, **41**, 542–543

123. Hayden, C.K. Jr., Schwartz, M.Z. and Davis, M. (1983) Combined esophageal and duodenal atresia: sonographic findings. *Am. J. Roent*, **140**, 225–226

124. Heatley, C.A. (1936) Some problems in oesophageal atresia. *Ann. Otol. Rhinol. Laryngol.*, **45**, 1122–1132

125. Hecker, W.C. (1986) Long-gap esophageal atresia: experience with Kato's instrumental anastomosis,

with cervicothoracic procedure and primary anastomosis, and with retrosternal colonic interposition.
Prog. Pediat. Surg., **19**, 9–21

126. Hemalatha, V., Batcup, G. and Brereton, R.J.
(1980) Intrathoracic foregut cyst (foregut duplication) associated with esophageal atresia. *J. Pediat.
Surg.*, **15**, 178–180

127. Hendren, W.H. and Hale, J.R. (1975) Electromagnetic
bouginage to lengthen esophageal segments in congenital esophageal atresia. *New Engl. J. Med.*, **293**, 428

128. Hertzler, J.H. (1965) Congenital esophageal atresia
problem and management. *Am. J. Surg.*, **109**, 780–
787

129. Hicks, L.M. and Mansfield, P.B. (1981) Esophageal
atresia and tracheoesophageal fistula. Review of
thirteen years' experience. *J. Thorac. Cardiovasc.
Surg.*, **81**, 358–363

130. Hight, D.W., McGowan, G., Smith, J. *et al.* (1987)
Atresia of the oesophagus – new trends in the
management of high risk neonates. *Arch. Surg.*, **122**,
421–423

131. Hirschsprung, H. (1862) Den midfodte tillukning af
Spiseroret samt Bidrag til Kundskab om den Med-
fodte Ryndtarmstillukning. *Medico-Chirurg. Rev.*,
30, 437

132. Hoffer, F.A. (1987) The treatment of post-operative
and peptic esophageal stricture after esophageal
atresia repair. *Pediat. Radiol.*, **17**, 454–458

133. Hoffman, D.G. and Moazam, F. (1984) Transcervical myotomy for wide-gap esophageal atresia. *J.
Pediat. Surg.*, **19**, 680–682

134. Hoffman, W. (1899) *Atresia oesophagi congenita et
communicatio inter oesophagum et tracheum*, Inaugural dissertation, Julius Abel, Greifswald

135. Hofmann, S. (1975) Ösophagusatresie – Notoper-
ationen bei grosser Distanz zwischen den Ösophagus-
segmenten. *Z. Kinderchir.*, **16**, 205

136. Hokama, A., Myers, N.A., Kent, M. *et al.* (1986)
Oesophageal atresia with tracheo-oesophageal fistula: a histopathological study. *Paed. Surg. Int.*, **1**,
117–121

137. Holder, T.M. (1964) Trans-pleural versus retro-
pleural approach for repair of tracheo-esophageal
fistula. *Surg. Clins N. Am.*, **44**, 1433–1439

138. Holder, T.M. and Ashcraft, K.W. (1966) Esophageal
atresia and tracheo-esophageal fistula. In *Current
Problems in Surgery*. Year Book Medical Publishers,
Chicago

139. Holder, T.M., Ashcraft, K.W. and Leape, L. (1969)
The treatment of patients with esophageal strictures
by local steroid injections. *J. Pediat. Surg.*, **4**, 646–
653

140. Holder, T.M., McDonald, V.G. Jr and Woolley,
M.M. (1962) The premature or critically ill patients
with oesophageal atresia. Increased success with a
staged approach. *J. Thorac. Cardiovasc. Surg.*, **44**,
344–358

141. Holder, T.M., Cloud, D.J., Lewis, E. and Pilling,
G.P. (1964) Esophageal atresia and tracheo-

esophageal fistula. A survey of its members by the
Surgical Section of the American Academy of Pediatrics. *Pediatrics*, **34**, 542–549

142. Holder, T.M. (1978) Current trends in the management of oesophageal atresia and tracheo-esophageal
fistula. *Ann. Surg.*, **44**, 31

143. Holder, T.M. and Ashcraft, K.W. (1981) Developments in the care of patients with esophageal atresia
and tracheoesophageal fistula. *Surg. Clin. N. Am.*,
51, 1051–1061

144. Holinger, P.H. and Johnston, K.C. (1963) Post-
surgical endoscopic problems of congenital espha-
geal atresia. *Ann. Otolar.*, **72**, 1035–1049

145. Holinger, P.H., Brown, W.T. and Maurizi, D.G.
(1966) Endoscopic aspects of post surgical managment of congenital esophageal atresia and fistula. *J.
Thorac. Cardiovasc. Surg.*, **49**, 22–30

146. Holmes, T. (1869) *The Surgical Treatment of the
Diseases of Infancy and Childhood*, Lindsay and
Blakenstow, Philadelphia

147. Howard, R. and Myers, W.A. (1965) Esophageal
atresia. A technique for elongation of the upper
pouch. *Surgery*, **58**, 725–727

148. Humphreys, G.H., Hogg, B.M. and Ferrer, J. (1956)
Congenital atresia of the esophagus. *J. Thorac.
Surg.*, **32**, 332–346

149. Imperatori, C.J. (1939) Congenital tracheoesophageal fistula without atresia of the esophagus – Report
of a case with plastic closure and cure. *Arch.
Otorhinolaryngol.*, **30**, 352–359

150. Ingalls, T.H. and Prindle, R.A. (1949) Esophageal
atresia with tracheo-esophageal fistula. Epidemiologic and teratologic implications. *New Engl. J. Med.*,
240, 987–995

151. Ito, T., Sugito, T. and Nagaya, M. (1984) Delayed
primary anastomosis in poor risk patients with
oesophageal atresia associated with tracheo-
oesophageal fistula. *J. Pediat. Surg.*, **19**, 243–247

152. Jackson, G.H., Yiu-Chiu, V.S., Smith, W.L. and
Chiu, L.C. (1983) Sonography of combined esophageal and duodenal atresia. *J. Ultrasound Med.*, **2**,
473–474

153. Janik, J.S., Filler, R.M. and Ein, S.H. (1981) Long
term follow up of circular myotomy for esophageal
atresia. *J. Pediat. Surg.*, **16**, 835–840

154. Janik, J.S., Simpson, J.S. and Filler, R.M. (1981)
Wide gap esophageal atresia with inaccessible upper
pouch. *J. Thorac. Cardiovasc. Surg.*, **82**, 198–202

155. Johnston, P.W. and Hastings, N. (1966) Congenital
tracheo-esophageal fistula with esophageal atresia.
Am. J. Surg., **112**, 233–240

156. Jones, T.B., Kirchner, S.G. and Lee, F.A. (1980)
Stomach rupture associated with esophageal atresia,
tracheoesophageal fistula, and ventilatory assistance.
Am. J. Roent., **134**, 675–677

157. Jolley, S.G., Johnson, D.G., Roberts, C.C. *et al.* (1981)
Patterns of gastro-esophageal reflux in children following
repair esophageal atresia and distal tracheoesophageal
fistula. *J. Pediat. Surg.*, **16**, 857–861–862

158. Kadowaki, H., Nakahira, M. and Umeda, K. (1986) A method of delayed esophageal anastomosis for high risk congenital atresia with additional intra-abdominal anomalies; Transgastric balloon 'fistulectomy'. *J. Pediat. Surg.*, **17**, 230–233

159. Kafrouni, G., Brick, C.H. and Woolley, M.M. (1970) Recurrent tracheo-esophageal fistula. A diagnostic problem. *Surgery*, **68**, 889–894

160. Kappelman, M.M., Dorst, J., Haller, J.A. and Stambler, A. (1969) A review of H-type fistula with case report. *Am. J. Dis. Child.*, **118**, 568–575

161. Karl, H.W. (1985) Control of life-threatening air leak after gastrostomy in an infant with respiratory distress syndrome and tracheoesophageal fistula. *Anesthesiology*, **62**, 670–672

162. Kashuk, J.L. and Lilly, J.R. (1988) Esophageal atresia in father and son. *J. Pediat. Surg.*, **18**, 621–628

163. Killen, D.A. (1964) Endoscopic catherization of H-type tracheo-esophageal fistula. *Surgery*, **55**, 317–320

164. Killendorf, C.M., Okmian, L. and Jonsson, N. (1981) Technical considerations of experimental oesophageal anastomosis. *J. Pediat. Surg.*, **16**, 979–982

165. Kingston, H.G., Harrison, M.W. and Smith, J.D. (1983) Laryngo-tracheoesophageal cleft – a problem of airway management. *Anesth. Analg.*, **62**, 1041–1043

166. Kirillova, I.A., Kulazhenko, V.P. and Lurie, I.W. (1984) Atresia, stenosis and duplication of the gastrointestinal tract: consideration of their origin. *Acta Morphol. Hung.*, **32**, 9–21

167. Kirkpatric, I.A., Gregson, S.L. and Pilling, G.P. (1961) The motor activity of the esophagus in association with esophageal atresia and tracheoesophageal fistula. *Am. J. Roent.*, **86**, 884–887

168. Kirks, D.R. (1979) Selective catheterisation of tracheo-esophageal fistula. *Am. J. Roent.*, **133**, 763–764

169. Kirks, D.R. and Filston, H.C. (1981) The association of esophageal duplication cyst with esophageal atresia. *Pediat. Radiol.*, **11**, 214–216

170. Klebs, E. (1869) *Handbuch der Pathologie and Anatomie*, Berlin

171. Kleckner, S.C., Pringle, K.C. and Clark, E.B. (1984) The effect of chick embryo hyperflexion in tracheoesophageal development. *J. Pediat. Surg.*, **19**, 340–344

172. Kluth, D. (1976) Atlas of esophageal atresia. *J. Pediat. Surg.*, **11**, 901–919

173. Koch, A., Rohr, S. and Plaschkes, J. (1986) Incidence of gastroesophageal atresia. *Prog. Pediat. Surg.*, **19**, 103–113

174. Kontor, E.J. (1976) Esophageal atresia with wide gap: primary anastomosis following Livaditis procedure. *J. Pediat. Surg.*, **11**, 583–584

175. Konrad, R. and Ratthoff, F. (1958) Kritische Gedanken: Zum Problem der Oesophagus atresie. *Zentbl. Chir.*, **83**, 1902–1916

176. Koop, C.E. and Hamilton, J.P. (1965) Atresia of the esophagus. Increased survival with staged procedures in the poor risk infant. *Ann. Surg.*, **162**, 389–401

177. Koop, C.E., Kiesewetter, W.B. and Johnson, J. (1954) The treatment of atresia of the esophagus by the trans-pleural approach. *Surgery Gynec. Obstet.*, **98**, 687–692

178. Koop, C.E., Schnaufer, L. and Broenule, A.M. (1974) Esophageal atresia and tracheo-esophageal fistula: supportive measures that affect survival. *Pediatrics*, **54**, 558–564

179. Kort, J. (1966) Closure of the oesophagus without sutures. *Chirurg.*, **37**, 155

180. Kraeft, H. and Hecker, W. (1987) Oesophageal atresia with fistula to the cervical trachea with descending right aorta and other malformation. *Z. Kinderchir.*, **32**, 371–375

181. Krnfalt, S.A., Okmian, L. and Jonsson, N. (1973) Healing of oesophageal anastomosis after release of tension by myotomy. *Z. Kinderchir.*, **12**, 444–456

182. Kullendorf, C.M. and Jonsson, N. (1981) Two anastomotic widening procedures for the repair of oesophageal atresia. An experimental evaluation. *Scand. J. Thorac. Cardiovas. Surg.*, **15**, 329–335

183. Kullendorf, F., Okmian, L. and Jonsson, N. (1981) Technical considerations of experimental esophageal anastomosis. *J. Pediat. Surg.*, **16**, 979–982

184. Ladd, W.E. (1944) The surgical treatment of esophageal atresia and tracheo-esophageal fistulas. *New Engl. J. Med.*, **230**, 625–637

185. Laks, H., Wilkinson, R.H. and Schuster, S. (1972) Long term results following correction of esophageal atresia and tracheo-esophageal fistula. A clinical and cinefluorographic study. *J. Pediat. Surg.*, **7**, 591–597

186. Lam, C.R. (1979) Diagnosis and surgical treatment of 'H' type fistula. *World J. Surg.*, **3**, 365–371

187. Lamb, D.S. (1873) A fatal case of congenital tracheo-esophageal fistula. *Philad. Med. Times*, **3**, 705

188. Langman, J. (1952) Oesophageal atresia accompanied by a remarkable vessel anomaly. *Archvm Chir. Neerl.*, **4**, 39–42

189. Lanman, T.H. (1940) Congenital atresia of the oesophagus. A study of 32 cases. *Arch. Surg.*, **41**, 1060–1083

190. Leiberman, A., Bar-Ziv, J. and Karplus, M. (1985) Subglottic laryngeal atresia associated with tracheoesophageal fistula. Long term survival. *Clin. Pediat.*, **24**, 523–525

191. Leung, T.S., Bayston, R. and Spitz, L. (1986) Bacterial colonisation of the upper pouch in neonates with oesophageal atresia. *Z. Kinderchir.*, **41**, 78–80

192. Leven, N.L. (1936) Surgical management of congenital atresia of the oesophagus with tracheo-oesophageal fistula. Report of two cases. *J. Thorac. Surg.*, **6**, 30–39

193. Leven, N.L. (1941) Congenital atresia of the oesophagus with tracheo-oesophageal fistula. Report of successful retro-pleural ligation of fistulous communication and cervical oesophagostomy. *J. Thorac. Surg.*, **10**, 648–657

194. Leven, N.L. (1952) The surgical management of congenital atresia of the esophagus and tracheo-esophageal fistula. *Ann. Surg.*, **136**, 701–719

195. Levy, C. (1845) Zwei Falle von sackformiger Verschliessung des oberen Theils der Speiserohre mit Einmundung des unteren Theils in die Luftrohre. *Neue Ztschr.*, **18**, 436

196. Lillquist, K., Warburg, M. and Andersen, S.R. (1980) Colobomata of the iris, ciliary body and choroid in an infant with oesophagotracheal fistula and congenital heart defects. An unknown malformation complex. *Acta Paediat. Scand.*, **69**, 427–430

197. Lindahl, H., Louhimo, I. and Virkola, K. (1983) Colon interposition or gastric tube? Follow-up study of colon-esophagus and gastric tube-esophagus patients. *J. Pediat. Surg.*, **18**, 58–63

198. Lindahl, H., Louhimo, I. and Virkola, K. (1983) 30-year follow-up of the original Sulamaa (end-to-side) operation for oesophageal atresia. *Z. Kinderchir.*, **38**, 152–154

199. Lind, J.F., Blanchard, R.J. and Guyda, H. (1966) Oesophageal motility in tracheo-oesophageal fistula and atresia. *Surg. Gynec. Obstet.*, **123**, 557–564

200. Lipson, A.H. and Berry, A.B. (1984) Oesophageal atresia in father and daughter. *Aust. Paediat. J.*, **20**, 329

201. Lister, J. (1964) The blood supply of the oesophagus in relation to oesophageal atresia. *Arch. Dis. Child.*, **39**, 131–137

202. Lister, J. (1985) Oesophageal atresia and respiratory complications. *Ann. Chir. Gyn.*, **74**, 53–59

203. Livaditis, A. (1973) Oesophageal atresia: A method for overbridging a large segmental gap. *Z. Kinderchir.*, **13**, 298–306

204. Livaditis, A. (1975) Long gap between oesophageal segments. *Z. Kinderchir.*, Suppl., **17**, 67

205. Longino, L.A., Woolley, M.M. and Gross, E.E. (1959) Esophageal replacement in infants with usage of a segment of colon. *J. Am. Med. Ass.*, **171**, 1187–1192

206. Lorimier, de A.A. and Harrison, M.R. (1985) Oesophageal atresia; Embryogenesis and management. *World J. Surg.*, **9**, 250–257

207. Louhimo, I. and Lindahl, H. (1983) Esophageal atresia: primary results of 500 consecutively treated patients. *J. Pediat. Surg.*, **18**, 217–229

208. Louhimo, I., Sulamaa, M. and Suutarinin, T. (1970) Postoperative intensive care of oesophageal atresia patients. *J. Pediat. Surg.*, **5**, 633–640

209. Luschka, H.J. (1869) Blinde Endigung des Halsteiles der Speiserohre und Kommunikation ihres Pars. Thoracica und des Luftrohre. *Virchows Arch. path. Anat.*, **47**, 378–381

210. Lynch, F.P., Coran, A.G. and Cohen, S.R. (1974) Traumatic esophageal pseudo-diverticulum in the newborn. *J. Pediat. Surg.*, **9**, 675–680

211. Lynn, H.B.J. and Davies, L.A. (1961) Tracheo-esophageal fistula without atresia of the esophagus. *Surg. Clins N. Am.*, **41**, 871–882

212. McConnell, R.B. (1966) *The Genetics of Gastrointestinal Disorders*, Oxford University Press, London

213. Mackenzie, M. (1884) *A Manual of Diseases of the Throat and Nose*. Wood, New York

214. Mackenzie, M. (1860) Malformations of the oesophagus. *Arch. Laryngol.*, **1**, 301

215. McKneally, M.F., Britton, L.W., Scott, J.R. and Kausel, H.W. (1984) Surgical treatment of congenital esophageal atresia. *Ann. Thorac. Surg.*, **38**, 606–610

216. Mahoney, E.B. and Sherman, C.D. (1954) Total esophagoplasty using intra-thoracic right colon. *Surgery*, **35**, 937–946

217. Mahour, G.H., Woolley, M.M. and Gwinn, J.L. (1974) Elongation of the upper pouch and delayed anastomotic reconstruction in esophageal atresia. *J. Pediat. Surg.*, **9**, 373–383

218. Malmfors, G., Holmin, T. and Okmian, L. (1981) Reconstruction of the thoracic oesophagus using autotransplanted small intestine. An experimental study in the piglet. *Scand. J. Thorac. Cardiovasc. Surg.*, **15**, 337–342

219. Malmfors, G. and Okmian, L. (1985) End-to-end anastomosis in oesophageal atresia – clinical application of experimental experiences. *Z. Kinderchir.*, **40**, 67–70

220. Man, D., Wheildon, M.H. and Eckstein, H.B. (1982) Paralysis of the right hemidiaphragm following primary anastomosis for oesophageal atresia and tracheoesophageal fistula. *Z. Kinderchir.*, **37**, 32–33

221. Martin, L.W. (1965) Management of esophageal anomalies. *Pediatrics*, **36**, 342–350

222. Martin, L.W. and Alexander, F. (1985) Esophageal atresia. *Surg. Clin. N. Am.*, **65**, 1099–1113

223. Martin, L.W., Cox, J.A., Cotton, R. and Oldham, K.T. (1986) Transtracheal repair of recurrent tracheo-esophageal fistula. *J. Pediat. Surg.*, **21**, 402–403

224. Martin, M. (1821) Report in *Exposé des travaux de la société royale de médicin de Marseilles*

225. Mathieu, A. and Goldsmith, H.E. (1933) Congenital atresia of the esophagus with tracheo-esophageal fistula. *Am. J. Surg.*, **22**, 233–238

226. Mellins, R.B. and Blumental, S. (1964) Cardiovascular anomalies and esophageal atresia. *Am. J. Dis. Child.*, **107**, 160–164

227. Middleton, C.J. and Foster, J.H. (1972) Visceral pleural patch for support of oesophageal anastomosis. *Arch. Surg.*, **104**, 87–89

228. Mollit, D.L. and Golladay, S. (1983) Management of the newborn with gastro-intestinal anomalies and tracheo-esophageal fistula. *Am. J. Surg.*, **146**, 792–795

229. Muangsombut, J., Hankins, J.R. and Mason, J.R. (1974) The use of circular myotomy to facilitate resection and end to end anastomosis of the esophagus. *J. Thorac. Cardiovasc. Surg.*, **68**, 522–529

230. Mullard, K.G. (1954) Congenital tracheo-esophageal atresia without atresia of the esophagus. *J. Thorac. Surg.*, **28**, 39–54

231. Muraji, T. and Mahour, G.H. (1984) Surgical problems in patients with VATER associated anomalies. *J. Pediat. Surg.*, **19**, 550–554

232. Myers, N.A. (1974) Oesophageal atresia: the epitome of modern surgery. *Ann. R. Coll. Surg. Engl.*, **54**, 277–287

233. Myers, N.A. (1975) Oesophageal atresia: diagnosis and treatment. *Z. Kinderchir.*, Suppl., **17**, 18

234. Myers, N.A. (1986) The history of oesophageal atresia and tracheoesophageal fistula 1670–1984. *Prog. Paediat. Surg.*, **20**, 106–157

235. Nagaraj, H.S., Mullen, P. and Groff, D.B. (1979) Iatrogenic perforation of the oesophagus in premature infants. *Surgery*, **86**, 583–589

236. Nakahira, M., Takenchi, S. and Tamati, S. (1980) Transgastric balloon fistulectomy. *Jap. J. Ped. Surg.*, **12**, 97–103

237. Nakazato, Y., Landing, B.H. and Wells, T.R. (1986) Abnormal Auerbach plexus in the esophagus and stomach of patient with esophageal atresia and tracheo-esophageal fistula. *J. Pediat. Surg.*, **21**, 831–837

238. Narasimharao, K.L., Sachdeva, S. and Narang, A. (1985) Perforation of pharynx mimicking esophageal atresia. *Ind. Pediat.*, **22**, 538–540

239. Navarro, F.A. Jr, Menasha, M. and Benjamin, S.B. (1985) Transluminal dilation of esophageal strictures in infants following atresia repair. *Gastrointest. Endosc.*, **31**, 200–202

240. Nelson, A.R. (1956) Congenital true oesophageal diverticulum: report of a case. *Ann. Surg.*, **145**, 258–264

241. Nelson, O. and Okmian, L. (1976) Polyglycolic acid sutures in oesophageal anastomosis. *Z. Kinderchir.*, **18**, 253

242. Nice, C.M. (1964) Bronchography in infants and children with barium sulphate as contrast agent. *Am. J. Roent.*, **91**, 564–570

243. Noblett, H.R. and Wright, E.M. (1978) A complication of continuous upper pouch suction in esophageal atresia. *J. Pediat. Surg.*, **13**, 369–370

244. Ogawa, T., Morita, T., Tsuchiyah *et al.* (1985) A new type laryngo-tracheoesophageal cleft with extended broncho-esophageal cleft. *J. Pediat. Surg.*, **20**, 164–166

245. Ogita, S., Goto, Y., Hashimoto, K., Iwai, N., Nishioka, B. and Majima, S. (1983) Prevention of gastroesophageal reflux using Nissen fundoplication in the staged repair of esophageal atresia with distal tracheoesophageal fistula. *Jpn J. Surg.*, **13**, 554–556

246. Ohkawa, H., Takahashi, H., Hoshino, Y. and Sato, H. (1975) Lower esophageal stenosis in association with tracheobronchial remnants. *J. Pediat. Surg.*, **10**, 453

247. O'Neill, J.A Jr., Holcomb, G.W. Jr. and Neblett, W.W. (1982) Recent experience with esophageal atresia. *Ann. Surg.*, **195**, 739–745

248. Orringer, M.B., Kirsch, M.M. and Sloan, H. (1977) Long-term oesophageal function following repair of oesophageal atresia. *Ann. Surg.*, **186**, 436–483

249. Otte, J.B., Gianell, P., Wese, F.X. *et al.* (1984) Diverticulum formation after circular myotomy for esophageal atresia. *J. Pediat. Surg.*, **19**, 68–70

250. Parker, A.F., Christie, D.L. and Cahill, J.L. (1979) Incidence and significance of gastroesophageal reflux following repair of esophageal atresia and tracheoesophageal fistula and the need for anti-reflux procedures. *J. Pediat. Surg.*, **14**, 5–8

250. Patti, G., Marrocco, G., Mazzoni, G. and Catarci, A. (1985) Esophageal and duodenal atresia with preduodenal common bile duct and portal vein in a newborn. *J. Pediat. Surg.*, **20**, 167–168

251. Paulino, F., Roselli, A. and Aprigliana, F. (1963) Congenital esophageal stricture due to tracheobronchial remnants. *Surgery*, **53**, 547–550

252. Penton, R.S. and Brantigan, O.C. (1951) A viable pedicle graft for repairing intrathoracic structures. A preliminary report. *Bull. Sch. M. Univ. Maryland*, **36**, 152–155

253. Pettersson, G. (1962) Experiences in esophageal reconstruction. *Arch. Dis. Child.*, **37**, 184–189

254. Pettit, P.N., Butcher, R.B., Bethea, M.C. and King, T.D. (1979) Surgical correction of complete tracheo-oesophageal cleft. *Laryngoscope*, **89**, 804–811

255. Petrovsky, B.V. *et al.* (1969) Palliative and radical operations for acquired oesophagotracheal and esophagobronchial fistulae. *Surgery*, **66**, 463–470

256. Pieper, W.M., Hofmann-von Kap-Herr S. and nii-Amon-Kotei, D. (1986) Pressure-induced growth (PIG) of atretic esophagus: a contiugent management for high-risk esophagus atresia. *Prog. Pediatr. Surg.*, **19**, 114–116

257. Pieretti, R., Shandling, B. and Stephens, C.A. (1974) Resistant esophageal stenosis associated with reflux after repair of esophageal atresia. *J. Pediat. Surg.*, **9**, 355–357

258. Pietsch, J.B., Stokes, K.B. and Beardmore, H.G. (1978) Esophageal atresia with tracheo-esophageal fistula. End-to-end versus end-to-side repair. *J. Pediat. Surg.*, **13**, 677–681

259. Plass, E.D. (1919) Congenital atresia of the esophagus with tracheo-esophageal fistula associated with a fused kidney. *Johns Hopkins Rep.*, **18**, 259–286

260. Politzer, G. and Portele, K. (1954) Die formale Genese Kongenitaler Oesophagusatresie. *Beitr. Path. Anat.*, **114**, 355–371

261. Potts, S.R. (1982) Right sided aorta associated with tracheo-oesophageal fistula and oesophageal atresia. *Ulster Med. J.*, **51**, 125–126

262. Pracy, R. and Stell, P.M. (1974) Laryngeal cleft, diagnosis and management. *J. Laryngol. Otol.*, **88**, 483–486

263. Pretorius, D.H., Meier, P.R. and Johnson, M.L. (1983) Diagnosis of esophageal atresia *in utero*. *J. Ultrasound Med.*, **2**, 475

264. Puri, P., Blake, N., O'Donnell, B. and Guiney, E.J. (1981) Delayed primary anastomosis following spontaneous growth of esophageal segments in esophageal atresia. *J. Pediat. Surg.*, **61**, 180–184

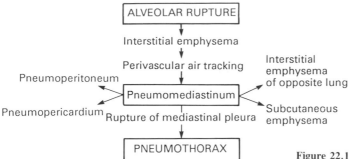

Figure 22.1 Pneumothorax: the usual sequence of events

Although an emphysematous bulla may rupture directly through the visceral pleura of the lung, causing pneumothorax, the air is usually extravasated into the lung substance (pulmonary interstitial emphysema) and along the perivascular sheaths [43,90,107] to the mediastinum, where it may accumulate under considerable pressure. If the mediastinum is not decompressed, either spontaneously or therapeutically, serious circulatory embarrassment occurs due to compression of the venae cavae and also of the pulmonary veins at the hila ('air block syndrome') [43,91,116]. Pneumopericardium may complicate the picture by causing tamponade. Rupture of the mediastinal pleura with resultant pneumothorax may relieve the situation [60] by improving the circulation and, by splinting the lung, halting the air leak. If, however, a tension pneumothorax develops (Figure 22.2), severe respiratory distress develops due to complete collapse of the ipsilateral lung and compression of the contralateral lung by mediastinal displacement. In extreme cases the baby may 'blow-up'; air tracks into the neck, axillae and chest wall and retroperitoneally down as far as the groins. Occasionally air accumulates in the peritoneal cavity [4,42,82].

The three groups of babies who are particularly likely to develop spontaneous (or iatrogenic) pneumomediastinum and pneumothorax shortly after birth are as follows:

(1) Babies who have suffered from fetal distress or birth trauma [43,116,127] especially those who are meconium-stained [25,117]. In such cases, aspiration of blood, mucus, meconium, amniotic debris, etc. [105] leads to uneven and incomplete lung expansion with sustained high transpulmonary pressures causing damage to the opened alveoli and air leakage.

(2) Preterm infants suffering from respiratory distress syndrome, especially if positive pressure ventilation has been necessary [3,12,57,102]. This is the most common cause of pneumothorax occurring later than the immediate postnatal period.

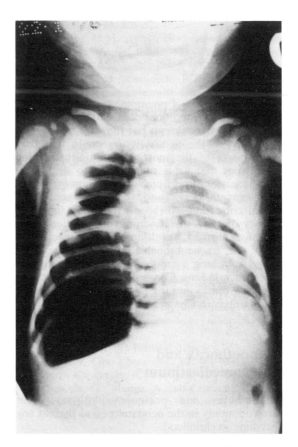

Figure 22.2 Tension pneumothorax (see text)

(3) Babies with pulmonary hypoplasia. This is associated most commonly with diaphragmatic hernia and has been discussed in Chapter 19. Also well documented is the association between renal agenesis, 'Potter facies' [107] and hypoplastic lungs [7]; in such cases both the lung condition and the facial features are believed to be due to oligohydramnios, a theory which is borne out by the finding of similar facies as well

as pulmonary hypoplasia and, sometimes, pneumothorax in infants born after prolonged leakage of amniotic fluid [104]. Other severe renal malformations, notably polycystic disease, may also be associated with pulmonary dysplasia [8,35,80,84], often complicated by pneumothorax and pneumomediastinum; these babies do not necessarily have 'Potter facies' [7,35,84].

Pneumonia, especially staphylococcal pneumonia with lung cysts, used to be an important cause of pneumothorax but has become a relatively rare cause in recent years. Pneumothorax secondary to perforation of segmental bronchi by suction catheters has been recorded [3] in the newborn and another rare but potentially lethal cause is spontaneous perforation of the oesophagus [28,136].

Excluding infants with pneumothorax complicating diaphragmatic hernia, 29 infants with pneumothorax and/or pneumomediastinum were admitted to the Liverpool Neonatal Surgical Centre during the period 1953–85. Twenty-one babies were less than 24 h old, 14 having had symptoms from birth. These 'surgical' cases constitute a selected group, as evidenced by the following data:

(1) Seven infants had gross renal anomalies incompatible with life (one case each of renal agenesis, polycystic kidneys and bilateral multicystic kidneys and four cases of bilateral hypoplastic/dysplastic kidneys). All these babies had additional severe anomalies.

(2) One baby with a huge exomphalos had bilateral tension pneumothorax.

(3) One infant had a rare type of vascular sling [115], an aberrant left pulmonary artery which encircled and obstructed the right main bronchus, causing gross interstitial and alveolar emphysema of the right lung and rupture of the right lower lobe.

(4) In one infant a spontaneous perforation of the lower oesophagus was the cause of a right pneumothorax.

(5) There was one case of pneumothorax secondary to streptococcal pneumonia, one in a low birthweight baby with respiratory distress syndrome and one in a child known to have inhaled meconium.

(6) In 16 cases the aetiology was less obvious. Four, however, had been delivered by emergency caesarean section for fetal distress, two had had difficult forceps deliveries and a further two had been 'mucusy' from birth and were admitted with suspected oesophageal atresia. The only child who died in this group of 16 showed evidence at autopsy of massive aspiration of amniotic debris. In seven cases the cause of the pneumothorax remained obscure.

Clinical picture

Presenting symptoms and signs

As noted in our own series, the infant frequently shows signs of respiratory distress within minutes or hours of birth [25]. The severity of the symptoms depends on whether or not the air in the pleura or mediastinum is under tension and also on the presence or otherwise of underlying serious lung pathology. A small pneumothorax may produce no symptoms at all and may be an incidental X-ray finding; alternatively, the infant may simply be irritable and restless [88]. When, however, a tension pneumothorax is building up (Figure 22.2) the baby's condition can deteriorate with alarming rapidity, with increasing cyanosis, grunting or gasping respirations up to 120/min and sometimes periodic breathing. In tension pneumomediastinum the clinical picture is that of circulatory embarrassment as well as respiratory embarrassment [19,60].

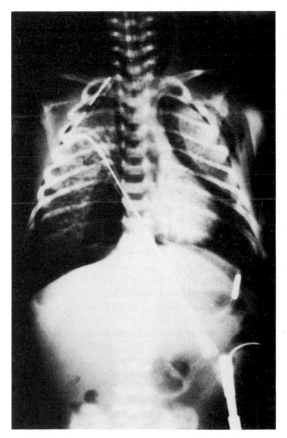

Figure 22.3 Gross pneumomediastinum. Mediastinal air outlines the heart. A right-sided pneumothorax has been drained. There is evidence of pulmonary interstitial emphysema in both lungs

On examination of the chest, marked displacement of the cardiac impulse will be noted if a unilateral tension pneumothorax is present and the affected side will be hyper-resonant on percussion, with diminished or absent breath sounds. If bilateral tension pneumothoraces are present these helpful lateralizing signs will not be present; the infant, who is likely to be in extremis, will, however, be noted to have an overinflated chest, with bilateral depression of breath sounds. In pneumomediastinum a marked anterior bulge of the sternum is characteristic, and in such cases the heart sounds may be inaudible. Subcutaneous emphysema in the neck, axillae, chest wall or groins is indicative of a decompressing pneumomediastinum, and in such an infant the presence of a pneumothorax or pneumothoraces is highly likely.

The diagnosis of neonatal pneumothorax and pneumomediastinum by transillumination with a fibre-optic 'cold light' was reported by Kuhns and colleagues in 1975 [76]. The principal benefits of this technique are in the detection of sudden, life-threatening situations which require immediate therapy, in serial examinations of neonates at high risk of developing pneumothorax and in following the resolution of a small pneumomediastinum.

The maximal risk situation is that of an infant with pulmonary hypoplasia or respiratory distress syndrome who is receiving positive pressure ventilation. Pneumothorax should be suspected immediately if a sudden deterioration occurs, or if continuously-monitored P_{aO_2} suddenly drops. The presence of pulmonary interstitial emphysema on the chest X-ray is an important predictive factor [54,113] (Figure 22.3).

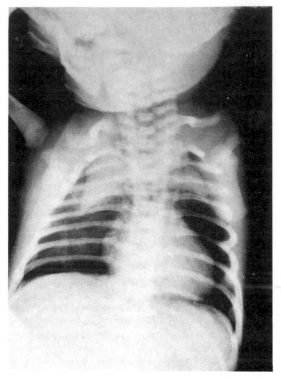

Figure 22.4 Pneumomediastinum. The thymus is raised

Radiography

An emergency chest radiograph must be obtained on any neonate who is suffering from respiratory distress. The features of tension pneumothorax are characteristic (Figure 22.2); the affected side of the chest is radiolucent and lung markings are absent, the collapsed lung is seen at the hilus, the intercostal spaces are widened, the diaphragm is depressed and the mediastinum is shifted, often markedly, to the opposite side. In smaller pneumothoraces the lung outline is visible peripherally, provided the film has been taken with the infant in the erect position. Care must be taken, however, not to mistake an axillary skin fold or the margin of the scapula for the edge of a partially collapsed lung [64].

The radiographic features of pneumomediastinum can be confusing, but a sizeable collection of air will outline the cardiac shadow (Figure 22.3). Other characteristic features are a raised thymus with an isthmus of air separating it from the heart [84] (Figures 22.4 and 22.5). A lateral view should

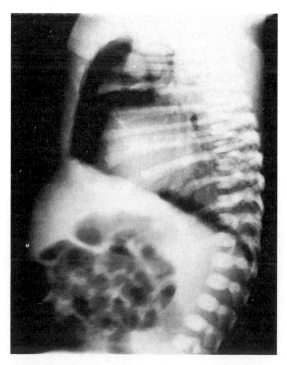

Figure 22.5 Pneumomediastinum. There is a large collection of air retrosternally. A strip of air separates the thymic shadow from the cardiac shadow

always be taken; a retrosternal air bubble is pathognomonic (Figure 22.5).

Treatment

Minor degrees of pneumothorax or pneumomediastinum in a baby with no symptoms or with minimal respiratory embarrassment can be treated conservatively provided the infant is kept under constant close observation. Seven of our 19 cases were so treated and recovered uneventfully. Oxygen administration will hasten the reabsorption of the air [25,108]. In a baby with severe underlying lung pathology even a small pneumothorax can add considerably to the existing respiratory embarrassment and will therefore require active treatment.

Aspiration of a pneumothorax is performed through the second interspace in the mid-clavicular line using an intravenous cannula attached to a 20-ml syringe and a three-way tap. This simple procedure can be life-saving in a desperately ill child with a tension pneumothorax, and in such a case must be followed by tube drainage. Occasionally, as in three of our 29 cases, a single aspiration is all that is required to treat a moderate sized spontaneous pneumothorax when there is no evidence of a persistent air leak; the infant must, however, be watched very carefully for signs of recurring respiratory embarrassment and the chest X-ray must be repeated shortly after aspiration to ensure that the lung has re-expanded, and again thereafter if there is any deterioration in the child's condition. If the air re-accumulates, tube thoracostomy is indicated.

Tube thoracostomy is required in the majority of cases of symptomatic pneumothorax and is mandatory when a persistent air leak has been demonstrated by aspiration, in seriously ill infants and in infants who have developed a pneumothorax while being ventilated. A no. 10 FG pleural drain (Argyle) is used, and is inserted through a small incision overlying the second or third intercostal space anteriorly. The trochar should be removed from the drain because of the danger of piercing the lung if it is used. A tunnel is made through the muscle layers by blunt dissection with a pair of mosquito forceps and the pleura is pierced; the tip of the catheter is then held in the forceps and inserted into the pleural cavity. It is good practice to insert a purse-string stitch in the skin around the site of catheter insertion; this is left loose under the dressing and is tied at the time of removal of the catheter. The catheter must be anchored firmly to the chest wall by a skin suture as well as adhesive, and connected to an underwater-seal drain. Low-grade suction (not more than 10–15 cmH$_2$O) can be applied to the open tube of the drainage bottle if there is a continuous air leak [127]. It is unusual for air to drain for more than 1 or 2 days, although in one of our cases an air leak persisted for 10 days before closing spontaneously.

Pneumomediastinum usually decompresses itself, as described previously, but in the rare instances when a sizeable collection of air under tension is causing circulatory embarrassment, this can be aspirated through an intravenous cannula inserted close to the sternum in the right or left third intercostal space, with dramatic relief of symptoms [60]. Aspiration may have to be repeated two or three times if air re-accumulates.

Results

Pneumothorax and pneumomediastinum per se should not prove fatal if diagnosis and treatment are prompt and efficient. The outcome depends on the nature of the underlying lung pathology and on the presence or otherwise of congenital anomalies or other complicating factors. Ogata and colleagues [102] reported a significantly higher mortality rate (52%) in babies with RDS complicated by pneumothorax than in those without pneumothorax (27%), but other factors, lower birth weight, for example, were contributory. Lipscomb and colleagues [87] have observed a significant association between pneumothorax in babies with RDS and the development of intraventricular haemorrhage. In our own 'surgical' series, 12 of 29 infants died (41%) but, as noted previously, this was a selected group with a high proportion of severe malformations.

Chylothorax in the neonatal period

Chylothorax was first described by Asellius in 1627 [5]. It is a rare condition and is especially uncommon in newborn infants but is the most frequent cause of pleural effusion in the newborn [26]. Some neonatal cases of chylothorax have a known aetiology; we have seen several chylous effusions following diaphragmatic hernia repair and one case following oesophageal atresia repair in a child with a right-sided aorta; it is also a well recognized complication of PDA ligation and other cardiac surgery [132]. In recent years it has become recognized as a complication of superior vena cava thrombosis complicating central venous parenteral nutrition [33,95,132]. In other cases chylothorax in infants has been associated with lymphangiomatosis [11].

Many cases of neonatal chylothorax lack any known aetiology and are then labelled 'congenital' or 'spontaneous'. The section which follows is devoted to those cases but the principles of treatment are applicable also to the cases of acquired chylothorax.

Congenital chylothorax (spontaneous neonatal pleural effusion)

The first case of this condition was reported in 1926 by Stewart and Linner [128]; this infant died but in

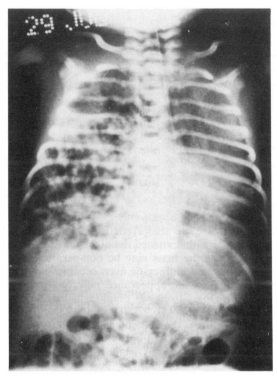

Figure 22.16 Congenital cystic adenomatoid malformation of right lower lobe. The position of the oesophageal tube indicates the degree of mediastinal shift. Almost the whole of the right upper and middle lobes are compressed into the apex of the pleural cavity

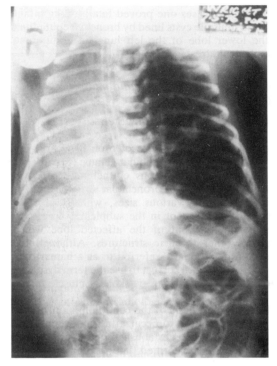

Figure 22.17 Congenital cystic adenomatoid malformation of the left lower lobe. The oesophageal tube indicates the degree of mediastinal displacement. The appearance of the left side of the chest mimics diaphragmatic hernia but the normal abdominal gas pattern should lead to the correct diagnosis

appearance and feel of the lung at surgery were indistinguishable from lobar emphysema. The whole of the right lung was grossly affected and pneumonectomy was performed. Histology showed CCAM affecting all three lobes. The baby survived for 3 weeks on ventilation but with progressive respiratory insufficiency. Autopsy revealed widespread changes of CCAM in the remaining lung. Our other patients recovered without incident; this is the usual course of events.

Intralobar pulmonary sequestration

This condition is included for the sake of completeness as it is a well-recognized cause of localized pulmonary cyst formation [40]. It rarely, if ever, produces problems during the neonatal period [21], but causes problems in later life as a result of infection. It occurs almost exclusively in the posterior basal segment of one of the lower lobes and by definition is partly surrounded by normal lung within the visceral pleura. The segment in question develops without any communication with the tracheobronchial tree or pulmonary artery. Its blood

supply is derived from the aorta above, or occasionally below, the diaphragm. Treatment is by lobectomy.

Extralobar pulmonary sequestration

This condition, also known as lower accessory lung [29], cannot be classified with its intralobar counterpart as a cause of pulmonary cystic disease because, as its name implies, it is an extrapulmonary lesion. It is completely separate from the lung, invested by its own visceral pleura and residing in 90% of cases in the posterior left costophrenic sulcus adjacent to the oesophagus [40]. Its arterial supply is derived from the lower thoracic or upper abdominal aorta and its venous drainage is to the systemic or portal system [40]. Although there is no connection between the sequestered lobe and the tracheobronchial tree, there may be rudimentary bronchial connections arising from the oesophagus or stomach [50,52]. Although there have been many theories of origin of pulmonary sequestrations, the most feasible is the view that both intra- and extralobar sequestrations arise from an accessory bronchopulmonary bud of the foregut; this theory explains the variations in blood supply as well as the occasional communications with the foregut [21,52,123].

More than 50% of the reported cases have had an associated diaphragmatic hernia on the left side [40] which may lead to discovery of the sequestration in the neonatal period; on occasions the sequestrated lobe may be found below the diaphragm. Cases are on record in which the mass itself has caused respiratory distress shortly after birth [16,40,72] but this is unusual. More frequently, as the infant grows older, repeated pulmonary infections and other chronic respiratory problems arise. The radiographic appearance in the typical case consists of a triangular or oval-shaped basal, posterior lung mass. A barium swallow should always be performed in suspected extralobar sequestration so as to identify patent gastrointestinal communication. Angiography is also indicated to demonstrate the anomalous systemic blood supply; this is not only a diagnostic procedure but also a safeguard against operative injury of an unsuspected anomalous vessel, which may have fatal results [114]. Surgical resection is indicated in symptomatic cases and when the sequestrated lobe is discovered during diaphragmatic hernia repair, but an asymptomatic extralobar lesion is probably best left alone as the risk of infection in such cases is slight [114,133].

Acquired pulmonary cysts: localized pulmonary interstitial emphysema

As mentioned in the section on pneumothorax, pulmonary interstitial emphysema (PIE) is one of the sequelae of alveolar rupture. It is extremely common in babies with RDS who require ventilation, and usually resolves [133]. In a small fraction of these babies (<2%) the development of relatively large discrete cystic areas which (1) significantly decrease effective lung volume and produce respirator dependence, (2) produce atelectasis and recurrent infections, or (3) lead to pneumothoraces, may make pulmonary resection beneficial [120]. This should be done only if conservative measures have failed. Schneider and colleagues [120] report excellent short-term results in seven patients treated surgically for localized intractable PIE.

Congenital bronchobiliary fistula

This is a very rare condition, only 12 cases having been reported in the literature up to 1986 [86]. Only two cases have been diagnosed in the immediate neonatal period; one being found incidentally at operation for oesophageal atresia [70], the other being diagnosed at 3 days in a child who was bronchoscoped for a suspected tracheo-oesophageal fistula and was found to have an anomalous opening on the right main bronchus just beyond the carina, exuding yellow fluid; cannulation of the fistula and dye injection revealed a bronchobiliary fistula [86]. In all but one of the 12 cases on record the bronchial opening was in the right main stem bronchus, the lower communication having been to the left hepatic duct system in each case where this has been verified [86]. Apart from the two cases cited above, the age at diagnosis has ranged from 3 weeks to 6 years, following symptoms of cough productive of green or yellow sputum and repeated respiratory infections commencing within a few days of birth. Whether this anomaly arises as a result of union of an anomalous bronchial bud with an anomalous bile duct, or whether it represents a duplication of the upper gastrointestinal tract is uncertain [118]. Haight and Graves [56] performed the first successful surgical correction in 1958 and there have been seven further survivors since then [86].

Mediastinal teratoma

This tumour is a rare cause of severe respiratory distress in the newborn. Up to 1980 only five cases of extrapericardial mediastinal teratoma producing symptoms in the neonatal period could be traced, to which Rickham and Kloti added a report of the one such case treated in Liverpool [112]. This 3.7 kg infant was dyspnoeic and cyanotic from birth and had inspiratory stridor when admitted at the age of 8 h. Radiography revealed a large mass in the anterior mediastinum and left hemithorax [Figure 22.18(a,b)]. Because of deterioration in her condition a thoracotomy was performed on the following day, revealing a large multicystic anterior mediastinal mass (Figure 22.19) compressing the trachea and bronchi. This was removed successfully. Histology revealed a benign teratoma consisting of an assortment of epithelial-lined cysts, some lined by squamous epithelium and some by tall columnar mucus-secreting epithelium; in addition there were numerous glandular structures resembling pancreatic acini.

There is no doubt that in this case the mass increased in size rapidly over a period of 24 h, and similar observations have been made by others [122]. It is therefore imperative to operate immediately when the diagnosis of an anterior mediastinal mass causing symptoms has been made.

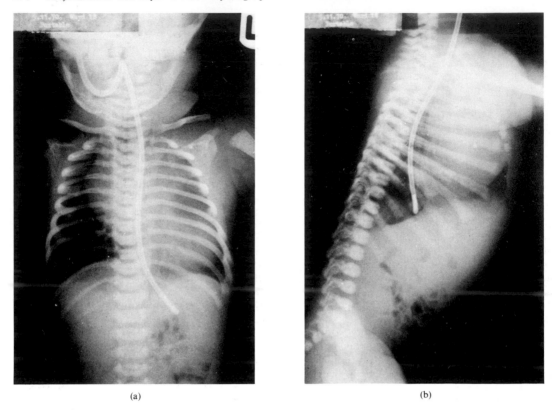

(a)   (b)

Figure 22.18 Mediastinal teratoma. (a) Large mass in left side of chest. (b) Lateral view shows the mass to be in the anterior mediastinum

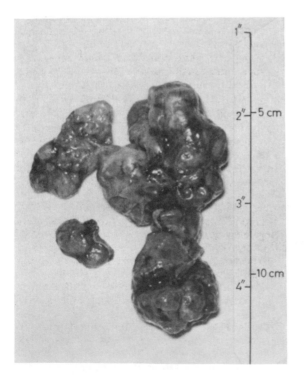

Figure 22.19 Same case as Figure 22.18. The large multicystic teratoma which was removed from the anterior mediastinum

References

1. Allen, R.P., Taylor, R.L. and Reiquam, C.W. (1966) Congenital lobar emphysema with dilated septal lymphatics. *Radiology*, **86**, 929–931
2. Andersen, E.A., Hertel, J., Pedersen, S.A. and Sørensen, H.R. (1984) Congenital chylothorax: management by ligature of the thoracic duct. *Scand. J. Thorac. Cardiovasc. Surg.*, **18**, 193–194
3. Anderson, K.D. and Chandra, R. (1976) Pneumothorax secondary to perforation of sequential bronchi by suction catheters. *J. Pediat. Surg.*, **11**, 687–693
4. Aranda, J.V., Stern, L. and Dunbar, J.S. (1972) Pneumothorax with pneumoperitoneum in a newborn infant. *Am. J. Dis. Child.*, **123**, 163–166
5. Asellius, G. (1640) *De lactibus, sive lacteis venis, quarto vasorum mesarai coruum genere, novo invento*, Leydon, Milan
6. Azizkhan, R.G., Canfield, J., Alford, B.A. and Rodgers, B.M. (1983) Pleuroperitoneal shunts in the management of neonatal chylothorax. *J. Pediat. Surg.*, **18**, 842–850
7. Bain, A.D. and Scott, J.S. (1960) Renal agenesis and severe urinary tract dysplasia: a review of 50 cases with particular reference to the associated anomalies. *Br. Med. J.*, **i**, 841–846
8. Bashour, B.N. and Balfe, J.W. (1977) Urinary tract anomalies in neonates with spontaneous pneumothorax and/or pneumomediastinum. *Pediatrics*, **59** (Suppl.), 1048–1049
9. Beau, A., Prévot, J. and Azambourg, J.P. (1969) Détresse respiratoire aiguü et kyste bronchogénique chez le nouvcau-né. *Ann. Chirurg. Infant.*, **10**, 495–503
10. Bensoussan, A.L., Braun, P. and Guttman, F.M. (1975) Bilateral spontaneous chylothorax of the newborn. *Arch. Surg.*, **110**, 1243–1245
11. Berberich, F.R., Bernstein, I.D., Ochs, H.D. and Schaller, R.T. (1975) Lymphangiomatosis with chylothorax. *J. Pediat.*, **87**, 941–943
12. Berg, T.J., Pagtakhan, R.D., Reed, M.H., Langston, C. and Chernick, V. (1975) Bronchopulmonary dysplasia and lung rupture in hyaline membrane disease. Influence of continuous distending pressure. *Pediatrics*, **55**, 51–54
13. Berlinger, N.T., Porto, D.P. and Thompson, T.R. (1987) Infantile lobar emphysema. *Ann. Otol., Rhinol. Laryngol.*, **96**, 106–111
14. Binet, J.P., Langlois, J., Belloy, A., Chollet, M., Pottemain, M. and Conso, J.F. (1972) Traitement chirurgical des emphysèmes pulmonaires malformatifs du nourrisson. *Ann. Chirurg. Infant.*, **13**, 59–64
15. Birdsell, P., Wenworth, P., Reilly, B.J. and Donohue, W.L. (1966) Congenital cystic adenomatous malformation of the lung. *Can. J. Surg.*, **2**, 350–356
16. Bliek, A.J. and Mulholland, D.J. (1971) Extralobar lung sequestration associated with fatal neonatal respiratory distress. *Thorax*, **26**, 125–130
17. Bolande, R.B., Schneider, A.F. and Boggs, J.D. (1956) Infantile lobar emphysema. *Arch. Pathol.*, **61**, 289
18. Bornhurst, R.A. and Carsky, E.W. (1964) Fetal hydrothorax. *Radiology*, **83**, 476–479
19. Brazy, J.E. and Blackmon, L.R. (1977) Hypotension and bradycardia associated with air block in the neonate. *J. Pediat.*, **90**, 796–798
20. Buntain, W.L., Isaacs, H. Jr, Payne, V.C. Jr, Lindesmith, G.G. and Rosenkratz, J.G. (1974) Lobar emphysema, cystic adenomatoid malformation, pulmonary sequestration, and bronchogenic cyst in infancy and childhood: a clinical group. *J. Pediat. Surg.*, **9**, 85–93
21. Buntain, W.L., Woolley, M.M., Mahour, G.H., Isaacs, H. and Payne, V. Jr. (1977) Pulmonary sequestration in children: a twenty-five year experience. *Surgery*, **81**, 413–420
22. Campbell, D.P. and Raffensperger, J.G. (1972) Congenital cystic disease of the lung masquerading as diaphragmatic hernia. *J. Thorac. Cardiovasc. Surg.*, **64**, 592–595
23. Campbell, P.E. (1969) Congenital lobar emphysema. Etiological studies. *Aust. Paediat. J.*, **5**, 226
24. Campbell, R.E. (1970) Intrapulmonary interstitial emphysema: a complication of hyaline membrane disease. *Am. J. Roent.*, **110**, 449–456
25. Chernick, V. and Avery, Mary E. (1963) Spontaneous alveolar rupture at birth. *Pediatrics*, **32**, 816–824
26. Chernick, V. and Reed, M.H. (1970) Pneumothorax and chylothorax in the neonatal period. *J. Pediat.*, **76**, 624–632
27. Ch'in, K.Y. and Tang, M.Y. (1949) Congenital adenomatoid malformation of one lobe of lung with general anasarca. *Arch. Pathol.*, **48**, 221–229
28. Chunn, V.D. and Geppert, L.J. (1962) Spontaneous rupture of the oesophagus in the newborn. *J. Pediat.*, **60**, 404–407
29. Cockayne, E.A. and Gladstone, R.J. (1917) A case of accessory lungs associated with hernia through a congenital defect of the diaphragm. *J. Anat.*, **52**, 64–96
30. Conway, D.J. (1951) Origin of lung cysts in childhood . *Arch. Dis. Child.*, **26**, 504–529
31. Craig, J.M., Kirkpatrick, J. and Neuhauser, E.B.D. (1956) Congenital cystic adenomatoid malformation of the lung in infants. *Am. J. Roent.*, **76**, 516–526
32. Crawford, T.J. and Cahill, J.L. (1971) The surgical treatment of pulmonary cystic disorders in infancy and childhood. *J. Pediat. Surg.*, **6**, 251–255
33. Curci, M.R. and Dibbins, A.W. (1980) Bilateral chylothorax in a newborn. *J. Pediat. Surg.*, **15**, 663–665
34. Davis, C.H. and Stevens, G.W. (1930) Value of routine radiographic examinations of the newborn based on a study of 702 consecutive babies. *Am. J. Obstet. Gynecol.*, **20**, 73–76

35. De, N.C. and Harper, J.R. (1972) Renal agenesis and pulmonary hypoplasia. *Br. Med. J.*, **3**, 696–697
36. Decancq, H.G. Jr (1965) The treatment of chylothorax in children. *Surg. Gynecol. Obstet.*, **121**, 509–512
37. Defoort, P. and Thiery, M. (1978) Antenatal diagnosis of congenital chylothorax by gray scale sonography. *J. Clin. Ultrasound*, **6**, 47–48
38. DeLuca, F.G., Wesselhoeft, C.W. Jr and Frates, R. *J. Thorac. Cardiovasc. Surg.*, **70**, 260–264
    Hendren, W.H. (1972) Pneumoperitoneum secondary
39. Demos, N.J. and Teresi, A. (1975) Congenital lung malformations: A unified concept and a case report. *J. Thorac. Cardiovasc. Surg.*, **70**, 269–264
40. De Paredes, C.G., Pierce, W.S., Johnson, D.G. and Waldhausen, J.A. (1970) Pulmonary sequestration in infants and children: A 20 year experience and review of the literature. *J. Pediat. Surg.*, **5**, 136–147
41. Depp, D.A., Atherton, S.O. and McGough, E.C. (1974) Spontaneous neonatal pleural effusion. *J. Pediat. Surg.*, **9**, 809–812
42. Donahoe, P.K., Stewart, D.R., Osmond, J.D. and Hendren, W.H. (1972) Pneumoperitoneum secondary to pulmonary air leak. *J. Pediat.*, **81**, 797–800
43. Emery, J.L. (1956) Interstitial emphysema, pneumothorax and air-block in the newborn. *Lancet*, **i**, 405–409
44. Engle, W.A., Lemons, J.A., Weber, T.R. and Cohen, M.D. (1984) Congenital lobar emphysema due to a bronchogenic cyst. *Am. J. Perinatol.*, **1**, 196–198
45. Eraklis, A.J., Griscom, N.T. and McGovern, J.B. (1969) Bronchogenic cysts of the mediastinum in infancy. *New Engl. J. Med.*, **281**, 1150–1155
46. Everhart, J.K. and Jacobs, A.H. (1939) Chylothorax. *J. Pediat.*, **15**, 558–562
47. Fagan, C.J. and Swischuk, L.E. (1972) The opaque lung in lobar emphysema. *Am. J. Roent.*, **114**, 300–304
48. Fischer, H.E., Lucido, J.L. and Lynxwiler, C.P. (1958) Lobar emphysema. *J. Am. Med. Ass.*, **166**, 340–345
49. Fischer, W., Potts, W.J. and Holinger, P.H. (1952) Lobar emphysema in infants and children. *J. Pediat.*, **41**, 403–410
50. Flye, M.W. and Izant, R.J. (1972) Extralobar pulmonary sequestration with esophageal communication and complete duplication of the colon. *Surgery*, **71**, 744–752
51. Franken, E.A. Jr and Buehl, I. (1966) Infantile lobar emphysema: Report of two cases with unusual roentgenographic manifestations. *Am. J. Roent.*, **98**, 354–357
52. Gerle, R.D., Jaretzki, A., Ashley, C.A. and Berne, A.S. (1968) Congenital bronchopulmonary – foregut malformation. *New Engl. J. Med.*, **278**, 1413–1419
53. Geubelle, F., Karlberg, P., Koch, G., Lind, J., Wallgren, G. and Wegelius, C. (1959) L'aeration du poumon chez de nouveau-né. *Biol. Neonate.*, **1**, 169

54. Greenough, A., Dixon, A.K. and Roberton, N.R.C. (1984) Pulmonary interstitial emphysema. *Arch. Dis. Child.*, **59**, 1046–1051
55. Gross, R.W. and Lewis, J.E. (1945) Defect of the anterior mediastinum. *Surg. Gynec. Obstet.*, **80**, 549–554
56. Haight, C. and Graves, W.H.: as quoted by Weitzman, J.J., Cohen, S.R., Woods, L.O. Jr and Chadwick, D.L. (1968) Congenital bronchobiliary fistula. *J. Pediat.*, **73**, 329–334
57. Hall, R.T. and Rhodes, P.G. (1975) Pneumothorax and pneumomediastinum in infants with idiopathic respiratory distress syndrome receiving continuous positive airway pressure. *Pediatrics*, **55**, 493–496
58. Haller, J.A., Gollady, E.S., Pickard, L.R., Tepas, J.J. 3rd, Shorter, N.A. and Shermeta, D.W. (1979) Surgical management of lung bud anomalies: lobar emphysema, bronchogenic cysts, cystic adenomatoid malformations, and intrapulmonary sequestration. *Ann. Thorac. Surg.*, **28**, 33–43
59. Halloran, L.G., Silverberg, S.G. and Salzberg, A.M. (1972) Congenital cystic adenomatoid malformation of the lung. *Arch. Surg.*, **104**, 715–719
60. Heald, F. and Wilder, T.S. (1949) Pneumomediastinum in the newborn infant. *J. Pediat.*, **34**, 325–330
61. Hendren, W.H. and McKee, D.M. (1966) Lobar emphysema of infancy. *J. Pediat. Surg.*, **1**, 24–39
62. Hislop, A. and Reid, L. (1970) New pathological findings in emphysema of childhood: 1. Polyalveolar lobe with emphysema. *Thorax*, **25**, 682–690
63. Holzel, A., Bennet, E. and Vaughan, B.F. (1956) Congenital lobar emphysema. *Arch. Dis. Child.*, **31**, 216–221
64. Howie, V.M. and Weed, A.S. (1957) Spontaneous pneumothorax in the first ten days of life. *J. Pediat.*, **50**, 6–15
65. Izzo, C. and Rickham, P.P. (1968) Neonatal pulmonary hamartoma. *J. Pediat. Surg.*, **3**, 77–83
66. Jaffa, A.J., Barak, S., Kaysar, N. and Peyser, M.R. (1985) Antenatal diagnosis of bilateral congenital chylothorax with pericardial effusion. *Acta Obstet. Gynecol. Scand.*, **64**, 455–456
67. Janet, H., Boegner, E. and Laquerriere, Mme (1936) Chylothorax chez un nouveau-né. *Bull. Soc. Pédiat. Paris*, **34**, 577–585
68. Jones, J.C., Almond, C.H., Snyder, H.M., Meyer, B.W. and Patrick, J.R. (1965) Lobar emphysema and congenital heart disease in infancy. *J. Thorac. Cardiovasc. Surg.*, **49**, 1–10
69. Kabelka, M. and Kolihová, E. (1971) Aspects of surgical treatment of congenital pulmonary malformations with tension behaviour in the newborn. 1. The differential diagnosis and indications for surgery. *Z. Kinderchir.*, **10**, 360
70. Kalayoğlu, M. and Oclay, I. (1976) Congenital bronchobiliary fistula associated with esophageal atresia and tracheo-oesophageal fistula. *J. Pediat. Surg.*, **11**, 463–464
71. Karlberg, P.J.E. (1958) Breathing and its control in

premature infants. In *Physiology of Prematurity*, Transactions of the Second Conference, 1957, Princeton, NJ (ed. J.T. Lanman), Josiah Macy Jr, Foundation, New York

72. Klein, Z.L. (1970) An accessory lobe of lung in a newborn. *Pediatrics*, **45**, 118–122

73. Korngold, H.W. and Baker, J.M. (1954) Nonsurgical treatment of unilobar obstructive emphysema in the newborn. *Pediatrics*, **14**, 296–304

74. Kosloske, A.M., Martin, L.W. and Schubert, W.K. (1974) Management of chylothorax in children by thoracentesis and medium-chain triglyceride feedings. *J. Pediat. Surg.*, **9**, 365–371

75. Krueger, C.S., Sherafat, M. and Reagan, L.B. (1968) Spontaneous pneumothorax in newborn infants. *Surgery*, **64**, 498–502

76. Kuhns, L.R., Bednarek, F.J., Wyman, M.L., Roloff, D.W. and Borer, R.C. (1975) Diagnosis of pneumothorax and pneumomediastinum in the neonate by transillumination. *Pediatrics*, **56**, 355–360

77. Kuruvilla, A.C., Kesler, K.R., Williams, J.W. and McGee, M.J. (1987) Congenital cystic adenomatoid malformation of the lung associated with prune belly syndrome. *J. Pediat. Surg.*, **22**, 370–371

78. Kwittken, J. and Reiner, L. (1962) Congenital cystadenomatoid malformation of the lung. *Pediatrics*, **30**, 759–768

79. Lampson, R.S. (1948) Traumatic chylothorax. *J. Thorac. Surg.*, **17**, 778–791

80. Landing, B.H. (1957) Anomalies of the respiratory tract. *Pediat. Clin. N. Am.*, **4**, 73–102

81. Leape, L.L. and Longino, L.A. (1964) Infantile lobar emphysema. *Pediatrics*, **34**, 246–255

82. Leininger, B.J., Barker, W.L. and Langston, H.T. (1970) Tension pneumoperitoneum and pneumothorax in the newborn. *Ann. Thorac. Surg.*, **9**, 359–363

83. Lewis, J.E. and Potts, W.J. (1951) Obstructive emphysema with a defect of the anterior mediastinum. *J. Thorac. Surg.*, **21**, 438–443

84. Liberman, M.M., Abraham, J.M. and France, N.E. (1969) Association between pneumomediastinum and renal anomalies. *Arch. Dis. Child.*, **44**, 471–475

85. Lincoln, J.C.R., Stark, J., Subramanian, S., Aberdeen, E., Bonham-Carter, R.E., Berry, C.L. *et al.* (1971) Congenital lobar emphysema. *Ann. Surg.*, **173**, 55–62

86. Lindahl, H. and Nyman, R. (1986) Congenital bronchobiliary fistula successfully treated at the age of three days. *J. Pediat. Surg.*, **21**, 734–735

87. Lipscomb, A.P., Thorburn, R.J., Reynolds, E.O.R., Stewart, A.L., Blackwell, R.J., Cusick, G. *et al.* (1981) Pneumothorax and cerebral haemorrhage in preterm infants. *Lancet*, **i**, 416–418

88. Lubchenco, L.O. (1959) Recognition of spontaneous pneumothorax in premature infants. *Pediatrics*, **24**, 996–1004

89. McBride, J.T., Wohl, M.E., Strieder, D.J., Jackson, A.C., Morton, J.R., Zwerdling, R.G. *et al.* (1980) Lung growth and airway function after lobectomy in infancy for congenital lobar emphysema. *J. Clin. Invest.*, **66**, 962–970

90. Macklin, C.C. (1939) Transport of air along sheaths of pulmonic blood vessels from alveoli to mediastinum. *Arch. Intern. Med.*, **64**, 913–926

91. Macklin, C.C. (1940) The impediment to circulation occasioned by pulmonic interstitial emphysema and pneumomediastinum. *J. Mich. State Med. Soc.*, **39**, 756–759

92. Mauney, F.M. Jr and Sabiston, D.C. (1970) The role of pulmonary scanning in the diagnosis of congenital lobar emphysema. *Am. Surg.*, **36**, 20–27

93. Michelson, E. (1977) Clinical spectrum of infantile lobar emphysema. *Ann. Thorac. Surg.*, **24**, 182–196

94. Miller, K.E., Edwards, K.D., Hilton, S., Collins, D., Lynch, F. and Williams, R. (1981) Acquired lobar emphysema in premature infants with bronchopulmonary dysplasia: an iatrogenic disease? *Pediat. Radiol.*, **138**, 589–592

95. Milsom, J.W., Kron, I.L., Rheuban, K.S. and Rodgers, B.M. (1985) Chylothorax: an assessment of current surgical management. *J. Thorac. Cardiovasc. Surg.*, **89**, 221–227

96. Monclair, T. and Schistad, G. (1974) Congenital pulmonary cysts versus diaphragmatic hernia: A differential diagnosis in the newborn. *J. Pediat. Surg.*, **9**, 417–418

97. Muayed, R., Azmy, A.F., Fyfe, A.H. and Cochran, W. (1986) Congenital cystic adenomatoid malformation of the lung. Potential diagnostic pitfall. *Z. Kinderchir.*, **41**, 107–108

98. Murray, G.F. (1967) Congenital lobar emphysema. *Surg. Gynec. Obstet.*, **124**, 611–624

99. Murray, G.F., Talbert, J.L. and Haller, J.A. Jr (1967) Obstructive lobar emphysema of the newborn infant. Documentation of the 'mucus plug syndrome' with successful treatment by bronchotomy. *J. Thorac. Cardiovasc. Surg.*, **53**, 886–890

100. Nelson, R.L. (1932) Congenital cystic disease of lung. *J. Pediat.*, **1**, 233–238

101. Nelson, T.Y. (1957) Tension emphysema in infants. *Arch. Dis. Child.*, **32**, 38–41

102. Ogata, E.S., Gregory, G.A., Kitterman, J.A., Phibbs, R.H. and Tooley, W.H. (1975) Pneumothorax in the respiratory distress syndrome: incidence and effect on vital signs, blood gases and pH. *Pediatrics*, **58**, 177–183

103. Pardes, J.G., Augh, Y.H., Blomquist, K., Kazam, E. and Magid, M. (1983) CT diagnosis of congenital lobar emphysema. *J. Comp. Ass. Tomogr.*, **7**, 1095–1097

104. Perlman, M., Williams, J. and Hirsch, M. (1976) Neonatal pulmonary hypoplasia after prolonged leakage of amniotic fluid. *Arch. Dis. Child.*, **51**, 349–353

105. Peterson, H.G. and Pendleton, M.E. (1955) Contrasting roentgenographic patterns of the hyaline membrane and fetal aspiration syndromes. *Am. J. Roent.*, **74**, 800–817

284

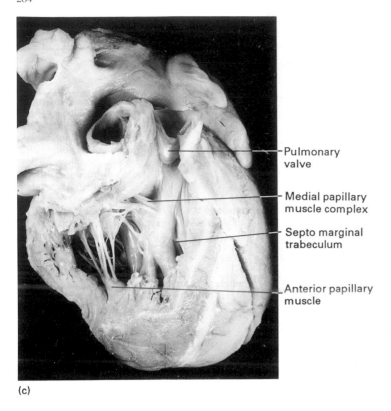

-Pulmonary
valve

- Medial papillary
muscle complex

- Septo marginal
trabeculum

Anterior papillary
muscle

(c)

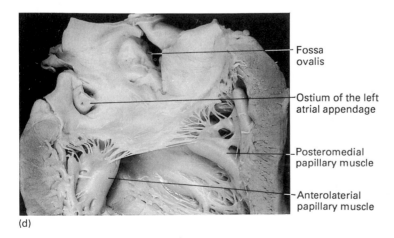

- Fossa
ovalis

-Ostium of the left
atrial appendage

Posteromedial
papillary muscle

- Anterolaterial
papillary muscle

(d)

Figure 23.1 (c) Anterior right ventricular wall excised to reveal the inlet and
outlet zones separated by the septomarginal trabeculum and the anterosuperior and septal leaflets of the tricuspid valve. (d) The left heart opened to
illustrate the posterior aspect of the mitral valve. The anterior leaflet is deeper
than the posterior leaflet.

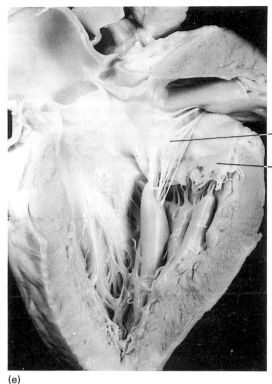

—Anterior mitral leaflet

—Posterior mitral leaflet

(e)

Figure 23.1 (e) The left ventricle opened to demonstrate the relationship of the mitral and aortic valves. Note the asymmetry of the mitral leaflets and their papillary muscles

surface of the right atrium is characterized by the fossa ovalis and the orifice of the coronary sinus. The fossa ovalis is encircled by the limbus, the superior portion of which forms the septum secundum. The floor of the fossa ovalis is formed by a fibromuscular flap valve which guards the foramen ovale. The foramen ovale is probe-patent at its superior margin in virtually all neonates, but interatrial blood flow is prevented by the valve mechanism once the left to right atrial pressure gradient is established soon after birth. However, distention of either atrium or reversal of the normal intra-atrial pressure gradient may allow shunting, a factor of considerable pathological significance. The anterior wall of the right atrium is the atrial appendage which is triangular with a broad base and a blunt apex encircling the right border of the ascending aorta.

The left atrium has a smooth walled posterior chamber and a narrow hook-shaped appendage which extends forward encircling the leftward margin of the pulmonary trunk. The posterior chamber receives the four pulmonary veins on its superior margin and is related to the coronary sinus inferiorly. The body of the left atrium is the most posterior portion of the heart, being closely related to the oesophagus posteriorly and the left and right bronchi superiorly.

Enlargement of the left atrium exerts pressure on the left bronchus and is a cause of atelectasis, particularly of the left lower lobe. Enlargement of the left atrial appendage is visible as a convexity inferior to the pulmonary conus on the left heart border. Internally the left atrium has a roof which receives the four pulmonary veins, a posterior wall, and an anterior wall which contains the ostium of the appendage and is closely related to the ascending aorta. The floor of the left atrium is formed by the mitral valve. The septal surface is oblique consisting of a smooth area overlying the fossa ovalis and a roughened flap valve anteriorly. The differ-

Table 23.3 Morphological differences between the right and left atria

	Right atrium	*Left atrium*
Appendage	Blunt with broad base	Hook shaped with narrow base
Crista terminalis	Delimits body of atrium from appendage	Absent
Fossa ovalis	Has limbus	Has flap valve
Remnants of venous valves	Present	Absent

Table 23.8 Continued

Name of syndrome	Clinical features	Cardiac lesion	Aetiological factors: chromosomal abnormalities
Ivemark	A syndrome associated with isomerism (see text)	Anomalies of venous drainage. Endocardial cushion defects. Conotruncal abnormalities	Sporadic
Kartagener	Situs inversus. Absent frontal sinus in some. Bronchiectasis. Upper and lower airway infections frequent: pansinusitis, otitis, pneumonia	Anomalies of venous return, endocardial cushions, septation and of great vessels. Dextrocardia	Autosomal recessive
Laurence-Moon-Biedl-Bardet	Mental retardation, obesity, hypo-genitalism, retinitis pigmentosa	Tetralogy of Fallot	?
Leopard Multiple lentigines	Multiple dark spots on skin present at birth. Physical and mental retardation (mild). Hypogonadism	Pulmonary stenosis. Prolonged P-R interval and QRS complex. Aortic stenosis	Autosomal dominant
18 Long arm deletion	Mental and physical retardation. Narrow or atretic auditory canal. Cleft palate. Long hands; tapering fingers. Undescended testicles	Variable	Long arm deletion of chromosome 18
Marfan	Connective tissue defect resulting in tall stature, thin limbs, hypotonia, scoliosis, narrow palate, lens subluxation and lung malformation	Dilatation or aneurysm of aorta or pulmonary artery. Aortic valve and mitral valve incompetence (50%)	Autosomal dominant
Noonan Male Turner	Physical and some mental retardation. Characteristic facies with epicanthic folds; ptosis of eyelids; low-set ears. Webbed neck. Cubitus valgus. Pectus excavatum. Small penis. Undescended testicles. Occurs in male and female	Pulmonary stenosis. Septal defect. Left ventricular obstruction or non-obstructive myopathy	Sporadic. No chromosomal abnormality
Osteogenesis imperfecta	Fragile bones, blue sclera	Weakness of the media of arteries, aneurisms, valvular incompetence	Autosomal dominant
Pseudo-Hurler Polydystrophy Mucolipidosis III	Physical and mental retardation. Similar to Hurler syndrome but milder	Aortic stenosis and incompetence	Autosomal recessive
Radial aplasia-thrombocytopenia	Absent or hypoplastic radius and sometimes other limb defects. Thrombocytopenia. Eosinophilia	Variable; 25%	Autosomal recessive
Rubella	Mental and physical retardation. Deafness, cataract, anaemia, thrombocytopenia. Hepatosplenomegaly. Obstructive jaundice. Osteolytic trabeculation in metaphyses with subperiosteal rarefaction. Interstitial pneumonia	Patent ductus. Pulmonary artery branch stenoses. Septal defect. Carditis. Lesions may cause heart failure	Rubella virus transmitted from mother. May persist in excretions of infant for months
13 Trisomy	Gross mental retardation. Microcephaly. Cleft lip and palate. Widespread skeletal abnormality. Single umbilical artery. Early death	Ventricular and atrial septal defects. Patent ductus. Other gross defects 80%	Trisomy for large part of D group (13-15) chromosome
18 Trisomy	Mental and physical retardation. Small mouth and palpebral fissures. Short sternum. Limb abnormalities. Hirsutism. Single umbilical artery. Early death	Ventricular and atrial septal defects. Patent ductus and other lesions	Extra 18 chromosome
Turner Gonadal dysgenesis	Female with short stature. Ovarian dysgenesis. Lymphoedema of hands and feet. Prominent ears. Web neck. Broad chest. Widely spaced nipples. Cubitus valgus. Horseshoe kidney. Buccal smear shows no female sex chromatin (Barr bodies)	Cardiac defect in over 20% and of these 70% have coarctation of the aorta	Sporadic. Chromosome pattern 45 XO (or mosaics XX/XO, XY/XO or part of X missing)

Table 23.8 Continued

Name of syndrome	Clinical features	Cardiac lesion	Aetiological factors: chromosomal abnormalities
VATER	'VATER' describes the main anomalies: Vertebral anomalies; vascular anomalies including VSD and single umbilical artery; anal atresia; tracheo-oesophageal fistula and atresia; radial dysplasia; polydactyly; syndactyly; renal anomaly; single umbilical artery. Physical and mental retardation (but not in all)	Ventricular septal defect and other lesions	Sporadic
Williams (see Infantile hyper-calcaemia syndrome)	Physical and mental retardation. Coarse hair. Hypoplastic nails. Hypercalcaemia occasionally found	Supravalvar aortic stenosis. Peripheral pulmonary artery stenosis. Pulmonary valve stenosis. Ventricular septal defect	Sporadic
Wolff–Parkinson–White	Paroxysmal tachycardia which may cause heart failure, ECG: short P-R interval and slurred upstroke of QRS may be found between attacks (see text)	Usually heart otherwise normal	Accessory atrio-ventricular node and conducting bundle of Kent. Sporadic

displaced pulmonary problems, e.g. pneumothorax, atelectasis, emphysema or pulmonary hypoplasia should be sought. The position of the stomach bubble may be right-sided indicating situs inversus or mid-line suggesting isomerism. The characteristic silhouettes of Fallot's tetralogy, transposition and total anomalous pulmonary venous drainage are occasionally apparent in the newborn period but more commonly appear after several months. The ratio of the transverse diameters of the heart and thorax measured on an inspiratory film gives a valuable assessment of heart size. When this ratio is above 0.6 it implies enlargement of one or more of the heart chambers. Massive enlargement usually indicates dilatation of the right atrium due to severe right heart obstruction, tricuspid regurgitation or impaired right ventricular function. The appearances of pulmonary plethora with left to right shunts may not appear for several weeks. However, the increased markings and haziness of the lung fields arising from pulmonary congestion due to anomalous pulmonary venous connection or severe left heart obstruction is often present in the first week. The reduced hilar shadows and pulmonary oligaemia of pulmonary atresia and other severe right heart obstructions may also be obvious from birth.

The electrocardiogram

The ECG changes more rapidly during the neonatal period than at any other period during childhood and interpretation is more difficult as a consequence. However, valuable information may be revealed regarding heart rhythm, enlargement of the atria, hypertrophy of the ventricles or evidence

of ischaemia. Several congenital heart lesions, e.g. tricuspid atresia and atrioventricular septal defects have a characteristic ECG pattern.

Disorders of heart rhythm occur commonly even in normal babies [43] and are usually of no consequence. Paroxysms of supraventricular tachycardia, seen often in patients with the Wolff Parkinson White syndrome, may however, be sufficiently severe to cause congestive cardiac failure. Severe bradycardia consequent upon congenital complete heart block may also result in cardiac failure.

Right atrial enlargement is indicated by a p wave greater than 3 mm in lead II. Evidence of left atrial enlargement is less common and is manifested by a biphasic p with a deep negative component in the

Table 23.9 ECG evidence of hypertrophy

Right atrial dilatation
 p wave <3 mm
Left atrial diltation
 p wave <0.07 s
Right ventricular hypertrophy
 q R in V_1
 $RV_1 > 28$ mm
 R/S $V_1 > 7.0$
 S $V_6 > 14$ mm
Upright T V_1 after 4 days
Left ventricular hypertrophy
 R $V_6 > 16$ mm
 S $V_1 > 21$ mm
 q $V_6 > 3$ mm
Combined hypertrophy
 Criteria of RVH and LVH
 R + S ub V_2 V_3 or $V_4 > 55$ mm

right chest leads. The configuration of the p wave is helpful in determining atrial situs. Normally the tallest p is in lead II (i.e. p axis +60°) whereas in situs inversus the tallest p is in lead III (p axis +120°).

Published criteria for ventricular hypertrophy in newborn are more diverse but the more helpful parameters are given in Table 23.9. Evidence of subendocardial ischaemia in the ECG is seen not infrequently in infants both with and without congenital heart abnormality who have undergone stress during the perinatal period from any cause. The changes are flattening of the T waves in many leads, mild ST segment changes and deep Q waves in leads I, QV_1 and V_6.

Two-dimensional ultrasound

In the past decade ultrasonic scanning has made a revolutionary contribution to clinical cardiology.

This technique is particularly valuable in the diagnosis and assessment of cardiovascular disorders in the newborn period, and may often avoid the need for cardiac catheterization and angiography.

An ultrasonic beam penetrates soft tissues at a constant velocity but is partially reflected at tissue interfaces. The probe containing the piezoelectric crystals not only generates the pulses of ultrasound but also detects the reflected beams. A real-time two-dimensional image is displayed on a television screen and may be recorded on videotape. The images have a high resolution and valve movements and wall motion are faithfully reproduced. Thus both intracardiac structure and myocardial function may be studied in detail. It is safe and causes little discomfort and the equipment is portable. The ultrasound beam may be directed to give sagittal, coronal, transverse or oblique views. The main echocardiographic 'windows' are along the left and right sternal borders, overlying the apex of the heart, below the left costal border near the xiphisternum and the suprasternal notch. This new technique has demanded an anatomical knowledge which allows recognition of cardiac structures in the various longitudinal, transverse and oblique sections. Some echocardiograms are shown in Figure 23.5.

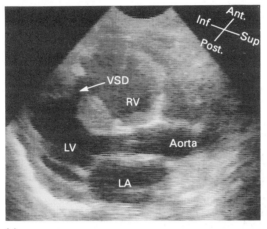

(a)

Figure 23.5 Two-dimensional echocardiograms. (a) Left parasternal long axis view of the ventricles. A large defect is present in the trabecular zone of the muscular septum. (b) Complete atrioventricular septal defect: four chamber view recorded from the apex during systole demonstrating defects above and below the posterior bridging leaflet.

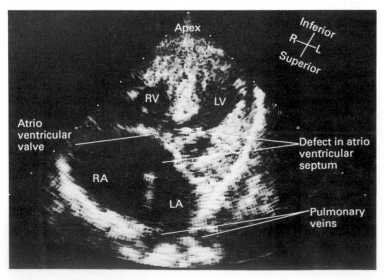

(b)

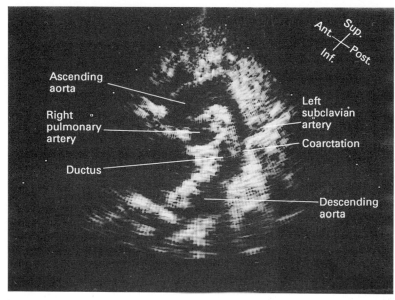

(c)

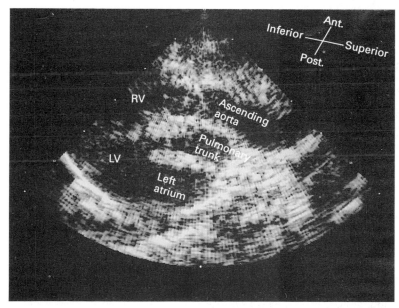

(d)

Figure 23.5 (c) Long axis view of the aorta recorded from the suprasternal notch showing hypoplasia of the isthmus and preductal coarctation. (d) Transposition of the great arteries. Unlike the normal the ascending aorta follows a parallel and anterior course to the pulmonary trunk and may be visualized in the same parasternal long axis view

Doppler ultrasound

Flow patterns within the heart and great arteries may be studied using pulsed or continuous wave ultrasound. The beam is reflected from the red blood cells and the frequency shift is proportional to the velocity of flow. Both the direction and velocity of flow along the line of the beam may be determined. Modern equipment combines two-dimensional imaging and doppler so that flow patterns at each valve and in each chamber may be systematically studied. Thus valvar regurgitation is readily detected. Estimation of the pressure gradient P at the pulmonary or aortic valves from the peak systolic velocity V (m/s), may be made from the formula $P = 4V^2$. Similarly, the systolic pressure gradient between the left and right ventricles is obtained from the velocity of flow through a ventricular septal defect.

Cardiac catheterization and angiography

Many patients presenting during the neonatal period with heart abnormalities may be diagnosed and treated without cardiac catheterization. Invasive investigation is more hazardous and more difficult during the neonatal period than at any other time because of the small size of the arteries and veins, the difficulty of manipulating rigid catheters in small heart chambers, the precarious cardiac and respiratory status and the tendency to heat loss and development of acidosis during a prolonged procedure. Two clearcut indications for cardiac catheterization in the neonatal period remain:

(1) patients requiring urgent surgery in whom echocardiography has failed to delineate the abnormalities with certainty,
(2) patients requiring interventional techniques, e.g. balloon atrial septostomy, balloon valvuloplasty or embolization of arteriovenous fistula.

These hazardous and technically difficult procedures must be undertaken by cardiologists with a detailed knowledge of congenital heart disease who have also received training in catheterization at a specialist centre. The catheterization laboratory must be equipped to undertake biplane axial angiography and facilities must be available to monitor pressure, oxygen saturation, blood gases and body temperature. The majority of catheterizations are performed under local anaesthesia but the help of a paediatric anaesthetist is essential in the presence of severe hypoxia or cardiorespiratory failure. Procedures must be undertaken in a warm environment: body temperature is maintained by a heated water blanket and heat loss further reduced by enclosing the patient in gamgee or silver foil. Blood loss in excess of 20 ml is replaced and acidosis, hypoglycaemia or hypocalcaemia carefully corrected.

Percutaneous techniques are performed but are not always successful and instruments for the dissection and cannulation of small veins and arteries must be available. In the majority of patients a catheter introduced into the femoral vein may be advanced not only to the right heart chambers and the pulmonary arteries but also through the foramen ovale to the left atrium and left ventricle. Other patients will have a ventricular septal defect allowing the catheter to pass from the right ventricle to the left ventricle and aorta. Recordings of percentage oxygen saturation and pressure are made in each catheter position. Selective angiography is carefully planned to demonstrate all of the important abnormalities. Although modern non-ionic X-ray contrasts have reduced toxicity, the volume used at each study is restricted to 6–7 ml/kg body weight and thus only two or, at the most, three angiograms may be recorded. Interventional procedures may be undertaken at the time of the diagnostic investigation providing that the patient's condition allows.

Individual defects

The variety of heart defects is almost endless but this section will concentrate on the more common defects which present during the first month. The lesions will be described in four groups according to their most common mode of presentation: they are respiratory distress, cyanosis, shock, and asymptomatic murmur.

Lesions presenting with respiratory distress

The clinical picture is one of tachypnoea, dyspnoea and feeding difficulty. Suckling may be quite impossible or the feed is not completed because of increasing fatigue and dyspnoea. Persisting hunger results in irritability, abdominal distension and regurgitation, persistent cough. Paradoxical weight gain in the presence of feeding difficulty indicates excessive fluid retention. Oedema of the face may be apparent. Systemic venous congestion results in hepatomegaly and sometimes also splenomegaly. The heart rate is persistently rapid and auscultation often reveals a gallop rhythm. A heart murmur of varying intensity may be present but in severe heart failure is commonly absent.

Various pathophysiological mechanisms are involved in the development of this syndrome. Excessive pulmonary blood flow arising from large defects in the ventricular septum or large patent ductus arteriosus result in reduced pulmonary compliance. Respiratory distress is accentuated if left ventricular failure and pulmonary congestion ensue. Obstructions to pulmonary venous return occurring in total anomalous pulmonary connection, particularly of the infradiaphragmatic variety or in mitral valve stenosis or atresia, result in severe dyspnoea. Pulmonary congestion also develops in severe aortic stenosis, in coarctation and interruption of the aorta and in a variety of disorders of the left ventricular myocardium, e.g. coronary insufficiency due to anomalous origin of the left coronary artery, endocardial fibroelastosis, cardiomyopathy, transient myocardial ischaemia due to birth asphyxia.

The defects to be described in this subgroup are listed in Table 23.6.

Ventricular septal defect (VSD)

Isolated VSD is the commonest congenital abnormality accounting for 38.3% of the cardiac patients entered in the Liverpool Registry. The majority of VSDs are haemodynamically insignificant and only 10% develop symptoms early in life. Before birth even large ventricular septal defects have little influence on the circulation because of the equalizing effect of the foramen ovale and arterial duct. During postnatal life the pathophysiology depends upon the size of the defect, the presence or absence of associated lesions and the state of the pulmonary vascular resistance. Defect size is the single most important factor in that a small defect permits insignificant shunting irrespective of other factors, whereas moderate and large defects will have a major impact on flow patterns within the heart. The association of aortic stenosis or coarctation will increase shunting at the VSD whereas right ventricular outflow obstruction will reduce, abolish or reverse the left-to-right shunt.

Large defects equalize the ventricular pressures and then the determining factor is the relative levels of vascular resistance in the pulmonary and systemic circulation. Following birth the pulmonary resistance falls progressively for several weeks allowing a proportionate increase in pulmonary flow and left-right shunt. The level of pulmonary vascular resistance attained depends on the vasometer tone of the muscularized peripheral pulmonary arteries and this varies widely. Most commonly, the pulmonary vascular resistance falls to a level somewhat above normal but which allows a pulmonary flow two or three times the systemic flow with symptoms appearing after 1–2 weeks. A small but important group retain a high pulmonary vascular resistance, have a smaller left-right shunt and no symptoms during the first months. A third group is characterized by a pulmonary vascular resistance which falls below the normal range allowing torrential pulmonary flow with shunt ratios in excess of 4:1 and the early development of severe cardiac failure.

Clinical features

The murmur of ventricular septal defect is seldom heard on the first postnatal examination but becomes audible as flow through the defect increases. The symptoms of tachypnoea, dyspnoea and feeding difficulty appear during the first few weeks. Feeds take progressively longer and are not completed resulting in periods of hunger and irritability and weight gain is poor. The development of a persistent cough indicates pulmonary congestion. The symptomatic baby will have a raised respiratory rate and subcostal indrawing. He may appear thin and anxious with a prominent praecordium. The cardiac impulse is increased sometimes with a parasternal thrill. The peripheral pulses are often somewhat collapsing in quality.

The characteristic murmur is harsh, pansystolic and maximal at the lower left sternal edge. With large defects the systolic murmur originates from turbulent flow in the main pulmonary arteries. A diastolic murmur at the apex from increased flow through the mitral valve is often heard. The systolic murmur in the important subgroup of patients with high pulmonary vascular resistance is of lower amplitude.

The electrocardiogram reveals varying patterns of hypertrophy when the defect is moderate or large but will be normal with small defects. With high pulmonary flow biventricular or left ventricular hypertrophy is usual. Right ventricular hypertrophy indicates associated pulmonary stenosis or pulmonary hypertension. The chest X-ray during the neonatal period will often be normal even in the presence of large defects, the changes of cardiomegaly and pulmonary plethora developing more commonly in the second month.

Most significant ventricular septal defects are detected by two-dimensional echocardiography providing that the septum is scanned systematically from the parasternal, subcostal and apical approaches. In the absence of an atrial septal defect the degree of dilatation of the left atrium is a useful index of pulmonary flow. Doppler echocardiography is valuable for the detection and haemodynamic assessment of ventricular septal defects. Doppler scanning of the right septal surface will usually detect anteriorly directed transeptal flow providing that the ventricular pressures are not equalized. Measurement of the velocity of the 'VSD jet' enables an estimate of right ventricular pressure to be made.

Treatment

Asymptomatic patients require careful assessment and follow-up until it is established that the defect is of trivial size or has closed spontaneously. Cardiac failure is treated initially with diuretics such as frusemide in combination with a potassium sparing agent, e.g. amiloride. Many authorities now doubt the value of digoxin in uncomplicated VSD. Systemic vasodilators such as captopril and hydralazine reduce left ventricular afterload and hence diminish the left to right shunt. Feeding by nasotracheal tube may be necessary with severe dyspnoea. Prompt and vigorous treatment of respiratory infections is imperative. Infants failing to respond to medical management and those with markedly elevated pulmonary artery pressure at 3 months of age are referred for surgery. Pulmonary artery banding is an effective palliative but many surgical teams accomplish primary closure irrespective of age or body weight with a mortality risk of 1–2%.

Prognosis

Six percent of VSDs close spontaneously in the first year and 3% per year subsequently throughout childhood [14]. Spontaneous closure is more common with small defects but occurs not infrequently with moderate and even large defects. Fifteen percent of all VSDs require surgery. Unfortunately, a significant mortality rate is still recorded with unoperated VSDs but this is mainly due to associated extracardiac anomalies.

Atrioventricular septal defects

Atrioventricular septal defects are characterized by a deficiency in the muscular portion of the atrioventricular septum together with abnormality of the atrioventricular valves.

Interatrial and interventricular communications occur in the complete type of AVSD whereas in partial AVSD there is interatrial communication only. The atrioventricular valve has five leaflets: superior and inferior bridging, anterosuperior and mural on the right and mural on the left. Separate right and left orifices are present in partial defects and a common valve orifice in the complete form of atrioventricular septal defect.

The severity of the physiological disturbance is variable and depends on the size of the atrial and ventricular defects, the degree of atrioventricular valve regurgitation and the pulmonary vascular resistance.

Clinical features

Atrioventricular septal defects, particularly in the complete form, are common in Down's syndrome. Partial AVSDs with mild regurgitation are asymptomatic in the first year and have a widely split second sound with a soft pulmonary flow murmur. With severe atrioventricular regurgitation a harsh pansystolic murmur in the lower left praecordium is heard and cardiac failure may develop. The mode of presentation and the clinical features of complete AVSD will be similar to those seen in large ventricular septal defects and the pattern will also depend on the level of the pulmonary vascular resistance.

The electrocardiogram is usually helpful in distinguishing atrioventricular septal defects from other anomalies, the main features being a superiorly orientated QRS axis and prolongation of the PR interval. Evidence of right ventricular or combined ventricular hypertrophy is usual. The radiological features are cardiomegaly and pulmonary plethora.

Cross-sectional echocardiography is especially helpful in the diagnosis and detailed assessment of atrioventricular septal defects. Apical and subcostal four chamber views demonstrate the interatrial and interventricular defects, the presence of common or separate valve orifices and will detect any significant imbalance in the size of the ventricular cavities. Pulsed doppler echocardiography will detect and provide an assessment of the severity of the valvar regurgitation.

Treatment

The medical management of congestive failure is similar to that described for ventricular septal defect. The main indication for early surgery is intractable cardiac failure. Beyond 3 months of age the spectre of pulmonary vascular disease becomes a major consideration. Corrective surgery is possible with acceptable risk even in small patients with well developed ventricles who do not have major valvar incompetence. Pulmonary artery banding has a small place in the management of atrioventricular septal defects.

Double-outlet right ventricle

Double-outlet right ventricle refers to cardiac anomalies in which both arterial trunks are connected entirely or in their greater part to the morphological right ventricle. The anatomy of these anomalies is subject to wide variation and a comprehensive classification has been provided by Wilkinson [47]. The size, site and morphology of the ventricular septal defect, which is always present, has an important influence on the clinical features and surgical management. Patients with associated pulmonary stenosis present in a similar manner to Fallot's tetralogy and are not considered in this section. The two most common variants are illustrated in Figure 23.6. Other associated anomalies are common and include coarctation of the aorta and abnormalities of the mitral valve.

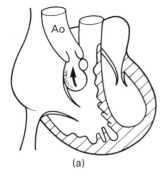 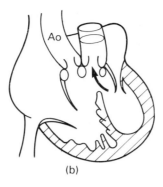

(a)   (b)

Figure 23.6 Two common variants of double-outlet right ventricle: (a) with subaortic ventricular septal defect; (b) with subpulmonary ventriculoseptal defect. The arrows indicate the direction of flow from the left ventricle

Clinical features

Evidence of cardiac failure usually appears during the first 2–4 weeks. Cyanosis may be absent or mild with subaortic ventricular septal defect but in the subpulmonary defect in which preferential streaming is from left ventricle to pulmonary artery, cyanosis is more prominent.

The physical findings resemble those of large isolated ventricular septal defect. The electrocardiogram usually reveals right ventricular hypertrophy but combined ventricular hypertrophy is not uncommon and the QRS axis is superiorly orientated in half of the patients. The chest X-ray will also be similar to that in large ventricular septal defect with cardiomegaly associated with pulmonary plethora. Cross-sectional echocardiography establishes the diagnosis with a high degree of certainty and yields valuable information regarding the positions of the arterial trunks and their relationship to the ventricular septal defect, together with details of other coexisting valvar anomalies.

Treatment

Medical treatment is given as described for large ventricular septal defect. Primary corrective surgery will yield good results in patients with subaortic ventricular septal defect, in which it is possible to insert an intraventricular tunnel connecting the left ventricle with the aorta with or without enlargement of the ventricular septal defect [26]. This approach is more difficult when the ventricular septal defect is in the subpulmonary position and alternative programmes of management are usually necessary. As the pathophysiology of this variant is more akin to transposition with ventricular septal defect, balloon atrial septostomy will improve the arterial oxygen saturation and should be performed at the initial cardiac catheterization. Corrective surgery which involves arterial switching and closure of the

ventricular septal defect will carry a high risk in the neonatal period and is best delayed to later infancy following initial pulmonary artery banding.

Double-inlet ventricle

This important group of complex defects accounts for approximately 3% of heart anomalies. Both atria empty into a large ventricular chamber which often has the morphology of a left ventricle but may also be of right ventricular or indeterminate morphology.

Hearts with double inlet left ventricle have a small right ventricle which usually connects with the aorta, the pulmonary artery arising from the main chamber. Less commonly the ventriculo arterial connections are concordant. The main chamber in double-inlet right ventricle also gives rise to both great arteries and the left ventricle is reduced to a hypoplastic pouch.

Clinical findings

The time of onset of symptoms is similar to that of large ventricular septal defect unless exacerbated by a severe associated anomaly, e.g. coarctation of the aorta or mitral stenosis. Cyanosis is mild or absent. A pulmonary systolic murmur of moderate intensity is usual unless cardiac failure is severe. Excessive flow through the mitral valve often gives rise to an apical diastolic murmur. The ECG may show either left or right hypertrophy, often with absence of the septal q in the left chest leads. Cardiomegaly, pulmonary plethora and narrowing of the vascular pedicle are the main radiological features. Echocardiography readily demonstrates the relationship of the atrioventricular valves to the main chamber, the relationship of the ventricular septal defect to the lesser chamber and the ventricular arterial connections.

Treatment

Medical treatment is similar to that for large ventricular septal defect. Banding of the pulmonary artery reduces pulmonary flow and pressure, thus relieving the symptoms of cardiac failure and preventing the development of pulmonary vascular disease. A modification of the Fontan operation may then be considered later in childhood. Some patients are suitable for 'staged septation' [16].

Transposition with large ventricular septal defect

Approximately 50% of patients with transposition have an associated VSD but many of these defects are small and of little haemodynamic significance. Ventricular septal defects in transposition may be found in the perimembranous or muscular areas of the septum, but defects extending from the inlet of the right ventricle to the left ventricular outlet are peculiar to transposition.

Clinical features

The presenting symptoms are predominantly those of cardiac failure and the onset is often earlier than simple VSD. Cyanosis is either absent or of mild degree. The auscultatory findings are a harsh systolic murmur related to the VSD and an apical diastolic murmur from excessive mitral flow. The radiological features are cardiomegaly, a narrow vascular pedicle and pulmonary plethora. The electrocardiogram is not characteristic but manifests either right ventricular or combined ventricular hypertrophy.

Treatment

The medical management is similar to that described for VSD. Of the various available operations for these high risk patients most authorities believe that arterial redirection and closure of ventricular septal defect are most likely to meet with success. Some patients with favourable features have corrective surgery without initial palliation. Frail babies with low birth weight or unfavourable anatomy undergo balloon septostomy and pulmonary artery banding and then corrective surgery in infancy or early childhood.

Persistent ductus arteriosus

The ductus is as wide as the pulmonary trunk during fetal life, but constriction occurs soon after birth so that by 1 week the majority will admit only a 2-mm probe [27]. The length and configuration of the ductus are quite variable. There is frequently widening as the ductus enters the descending aorta and

this ampulla may persist after ductal closure. The intima of the normal ductus is roughened, distinguishing it from the pulmonary trunk and the descending aorta. The ductus also differs histologically having more muscular and less elastic tissue than the great arteries. The outer layers of muscle in the media have a spiral arrangement which is important to ductal closure. Final obliteration of the ductus results from proliferation of connective tissue and ground substance in the media and intima [20].

Production of prostaglandin E_2 in the ductal wall augmented by circulating prostanoids is now thought to be important in maintaining ductal patency during fetal life [32]. Closure of the ductus is initiated by increased oxygen content in the circulating blood after the first breath [25]. Persistent ductus arteriosus is associated with birth asphyxia, birth at high altitude, congenital rubella and chromosomal anomalies and is twice as common in females.

Patency of the ductus arteriosus is an important factor in the management of premature infants and the incidence has been reported as being between 7 and 25% of all prematures [39]. The immature ductus is less responsive to oxygen and the prostaglandin relaxant mechanism is also more active in premature infants [8]. Very low birthweight premature infants requiring assisted ventilation may develop large left-to-right shunts, and the ensuing left ventricular failure prolongs the need for ventilator care.

Clinical features

Most patients who develop symptoms due to a patent ductus arteriosus during the neonatal period are born prematurely. Some will have had respiratory distress due to hyaline membrane disease and symptoms persist or increase due to the development of left ventricular failure. Others develop respiratory distress and feeding problems associated with poor weight gain during the second or third week after birth.

The characteristic appearance is a thin poorly nourished infant with increased respiratory rate and dyspnoea. The peripheral pulses are bounding and the heart rate is increased. The classic continuous murmur maximal beneath the left clavicle may be heard but more often the murmur is systolic in symptomatic patients during the neonatal period. Ventilator dependent patients with a large ductal shunt may not have an audible murmur. The chest X-ray may show cardiomegaly, enlargement of the pulmonary conus, and pulmonary plethora but may also be deceptively normal. The electrocardiogram may have increased left ventricular voltages or demonstrate combined ventricular hypertrophy. Cross-sectional echocardiography from the suprasternal approach is the most helpful investigation, often demonstrating the ductus and providing evidence of the magnitude of the shunt from the appearances of left atrial dilatation and left ventricular overactivity. The presence of intracardiac anomalies is also excluded. Doppler echocardiography demonstrates a characteristic flow pattern in the pulmonary trunk and enables an estimate of pressure difference between the systemic and pulmonary circulations.

Treatment and prognosis

Medical treatment of the premature infant with patent ductus is usually successful and only occasionally is surgical ligation necessary. Fluid restriction to 120–150 ml/kg/24 h with or without diuretic therapy will reduce pulmonary congestion and may encourage ductal closure. Digoxin may have little beneficial effect [2]. Maintenance of the haemoglobin level above 10 g/100 ml is also important. Indomethacin, a prostaglandin synthetase inhibitor has been used to close the ductus in symptomatic premature infants [19,21]. Most success is achieved when indomethacin 0.2 mg/kg is given intravenously during the first 3 weeks of life. Administration may be repeated once or twice on successive days. Hyperbilirubinaemia and impaired renal function are contraindications to indomethacin. The main side effects are transient oliguria and gastrointestinal bleeding.

Surgical ligation of the ductus may be achieved even in the smallest prematures with an operative mortality of less than 1%. Premature infants with patent arterial ducts but without symptoms are managed expectantly, spontaneous closure commonly occurring within 1–3 months.

Aneurism of the arterial duct

A diverticulum is commonly present at the aortic or pulmonary ends of the ductus following closure. Rarely the aortic diverticulum will enlarge to form an aneurism which may present as a mediastinal mass or lead to rupture, dissection, thrombosis and embolism and recurrent laryngeal or phrenic nerve palsy. Endocarditis is sometimes present. Surgical excision is life saving.

Aortopulmonary window

An error of septation of the aortopulmonary septum gives rise to a defect between the ascending aorta and the pulmonary trunk in the presence of separate semilunar valves. This rare anomaly is important because surgical correction is made before the development of intractible cardiac failure or irreversible pulmonary vascular disease. Associated anomalies include patent ductus arteriosus, ventricular septal defect, aortic interruption, Fallot's tetralogy and aortic stenosis.

Clinical features

The onset, symptoms and clinical findings are similar to those of large persistent ductus arteriosus. The murmur from flow through the defect is usually systolic rather than continuous. Cardiomegaly and pulmonary plethora are seen on X-ray and combined ventricular hypertrophy on the electrocardiogram. Echocardiography using high parasternal short axis scans will usually enable visualization of the defect.

Treatment

A short period of pre-operative medical treatment is followed by closure of the defect using heart lung bypass.

Truncus arteriosus

Failure of fusion of the infundibulotruncal endocardial cushions gives rise to a single arterial trunk which provides the systemic, the pulmonary and the coronary circulations. The arterial valve has from two to six leaflets and overrides a large ventricular septal defect. The truncal valve is often regurgitant and occasionally stenotic. The pulmonary arteries may arise separately or there may be a short common pulmonary trunk. Coarctation or interruption of the aortic arch occurs in 11–19%. Free flow of blood from the truncus to the pulmonary circulation leads to severe volume loading of the left ventricle but in addition lowers the aortic diastolic pressure thus reducing coronary perfusion. Truncal valve regurgitation if present is a further adverse factor.

Clinical features

The onset of symptoms is earlier and more severe than with larger ventricular septal defect. Cyanosis is of mild degree or absent. The peripheral pulses are collapsing and the praecordial impulse increased. The first heart sound is followed by an ejection click and a harsh ejection systolic murmur. The second heart sound is single and an early diastolic murmur at the lower left sternal edge is heard in the presence of truncal regurgitation. The chest X-ray shows cardiomegaly, with prominence of the ascending aorta and pulmonary plethora. One-third of patients have a right aortic arch. The electrocardiogram often reveals left ventricular hypertrophy and strain. Cross-sectional echocardiography enables a detailed diagnosis to be made with confidence and cardiac catheterization is seldom required during the neonatal period.

Treatment

Transient improvement may follow treatment with digoxin and diuretics but the prognosis without surgery is very poor, death occurring either in the first months from intractable failure or later in childhood from progressive pulmonary vascular disease. Most authorities favour corrective surgery at 3–6 months. This is achieved by excision of the pulmonary arteries from the truncus, interposition of a homograft valve between the right ventricle and pulmonary arteries and closure of the ventricular septal defect. Very small and ill patients in whom the risks of open heart surgery are excessive may be palliated by pulmonary artery banding.

Coarctation of the aorta

More than half of patients with coarctation of the aorta develop cardiac failure during the first month and this anomaly leads the list of causes of cardiac failure during the neonatal period. Intracardiac anomalies co-exist in 45% of patients and these include ventricular septal defect, double inlet ventricle and transposition. The neonatal mortality rate for symptomatic patients as recorded in the Liverpool Registry was 51%. Most commonly a discrete waist or shelf narrows the aortic lumen immediately proximal to or opposite to the insertion of the arterial duct. Less often the coarctation is postductal or proximal to the origin of the left subclavian artery. Tubular hypoplasia of the aortic isthmus is frequently present in association with a discrete coarctation. Extension of the ductal tissue into the wall of the aortic isthmus may increase the aortic constriction at the time of closure of the ductus.

The pathophysiology of coarctation syndrome is incompletely understood. Dilatation of the right ventricle is often present in patients diagnosed during the first few days and must develop prenatally, possibly due to constriction of the ductus. Postnatally, perfusion of the descending aorta may be dependent on right to left shunting through the ductus in severe coarctation. Subsequent constriction of the ductus will then impair renal perfusion resulting in fluid retention, pulmonary congestion and acidosis. Within the heart excessive left ventricular afterload may lead to left ventricular failure, pulmonary congestion and pulmonary hypertension. In the presence of a septal defect, left-to-right shunting within the heart is increased.

Clinical features

The onset of dyspnoea and feeding difficulty is common during the first 10 days, occasionally in the first 2 days or later in the neonatal period. Symptoms are often progressive and cardiovascular shock may develop with alarming rapidity. The physical signs are those of cardiac failure: tachypnoea, intercostal recession, hepatomegaly, tachycardia and gallop rhythm. The femoral pulses are weak or absent, the arm pulse stronger unless shock has developed. A discrepancy of more than 20 mmHg between arm and leg blood pressures is usual. Murmurs are not heard in the more ill patients.

The chest X-ray shows cardiomegaly and pulmonary congestion. The ECG usually demonstrates severe right hypertrophy associated with flattening or inversions of the T waves in the left ventricular leads. The echocardiographic features are of dilatation of the right heart chambers and a pulmonary trunk markedly wider than the ascending aorta. Careful scanning with the probe in a high upper parasternal or suprasternal position will usually reveal the coarctation. Associated intracardiac anomalies are also diagnosed. The importance of establishing a complete diagnosis echocardiographically cannot be overemphasized as angiography carries a considerable risk in these very sick patients.

Management

Treatment is directed towards the preparation for urgent operation and the requirements will vary from simple anticongestive measures to full scale resuscitation. Diuretic therapy, e.g. frusemide 1–2 mg/kg intravenously is given. If the diuresis is poor an infusion of prostaglandin E 10–50 ng/kg per min is commenced. Successful dilatation of the ductus is manifested by improvement of the femoral pulses and diuresis. Metabolic acidosis is corrected with intravenous sodium bicarbonate. Persistent hypotension and oliguria may improve with inotropic support, e.g. dopamine 5–10 μg/kg per min. Patients with pulmonary oedema or severe acidosis will require assisted ventilation. Surgical relief of the coarctation is undertaken after a brief period of medical treatment: it is usually unwise to delay more than 12–24 h as the improvement with medical management is usually transitory.

Interruption or atresia of the aortic arch

Interruption refers to an anomaly in which a segment of the aortic arch or isthmus is absent whereas in arch atresia a segment is represented by a solid cord. The obstructed or absent segment may be between the left subclavian artery and the ductus, between the left carotid artery and the left subclavian or rarely between the innominate and left carotid arteries. A ventricular septal defect of the malalignment type is nearly always present and other associated anomalies include subaortic stenosis, truncus arteriosus, aortopulmonary window and transposition. Blood flow to the descending aorta is by means of the ductus arteriosus. Aortic interruption may be associated with thymic aplasia as part of the di George syndrome.

Clinical findings and diagnosis

The presentation and physical findings are similar to coarctation but the onset is earlier and the symptoms more severe. If the duct remains widely patent the pulses may be normal, but some discrepancy is usually present, the left arm and femoral pulses being weaker. Occasionally both subclavian arteries arise from the lower segment giving rise to weakness of all the limb pulses. The echocardiogram will usually demonstrate the arch anomaly, the ductus and the associated intracardiac abnormalities.

Treatment

The medical management is similar to that for coarctation but the surgical management is more difficult and is the subject of controversy. Early reports described a staged operation with reconstruction of the aortic arch and banding of the pulmonary trunk. Recently improved results have been achieved with early primary correction using cardiopulmonary bypass.

Disorders of the myocardium

A variety of myocardial disorders may give rise to cardiorespiratory distress during the neonatal period and these are listed in Table 23.6.

Transient myocardial ischaemia

Symptoms of impaired myocardial function together with electrocardiographic changes of myocardial ischaemia are commonplace in babies suffering fetal distress or perinatal asphyxia. The clinical picture ranges from tachypnoea, to respiratory distress, to hypotensive cardiac failure and cardiogenic shock. The more severely affected may also have cerebral complications and renal failure. The normal transitional changes in the pulmonary circulation may fail resulting in residual pulmonary hypertension and right-to-left shunting at the foramen ovale and the ductus. Ventricular dilatation and papillary muscle dysfunction may be manifest by the characteristic murmurs of tricuspid or mitral regurgitation [38]. The electrocardiographic changes include flattening or inversion of the T waves and deep Q waves in leads I, II, III, AVL and V_{5-6}. If supportive therapy is successful competence of the mitral and tricuspid valves is restored and the clinical and electrocardiographic changes of myocardial ischaemia resolve.

Cardiomyopathy in infants of diabetic mothers

Babies of diabetic and prediabetic mothers are large and plump with plethoric features. Respiratory distress is common and a proportion have evidence of a transient hypertrophic cardiomyopathy. Symptoms of cardiac failure develop and a murmur due to mitral or tricuspid regurgitation may be heard. The heart is enlarged and the QRS voltages in the praecordial leads are strikingly increased.

Echocardiography reveals hypertrophy which is generalized but which particularly involves the ventricular septum. The response to treatment is good and the cardiovascular changes resolve after several weeks or months.

Primary endocardial fibroelastosis

Endocardial fibroelastosis is associated with several valvular lesions and particularly with left heart hypoplasia but this section is concerned with primary endocardial fibroelastosis occurring as an isolated disorder. The appearance is of a dense white lining to the left atrium and left ventricle. The aetiology is uncertain but some reports suggest an autosomal recessive mode of inheritance. The left ventricular diastolic volume increases and the ejection fraction is depressed. The left atrium is dilated particularly if mitral insufficiency ensues. One-third of patients, the most severely afflicted, develop symptoms within the first 3 months.

Clinical features

The onset is usually abrupt with dyspnoea, tachypnoea, cough and feeding difficulty. Sweating, pallor and peripheral cyanosis indicating low cardiac output are often present. The heart sounds are muffled with a gallop rhythm. There is usually no murmur at the time of onset but a mitral insufficiency murmur may develop. The heart is always enlarged with a cardiothoracic ratio of 60–80%. The chest X-ray may also show left atrial enlargement and left lower lobe atelectasis from secondary bronchial compression. The ECG reflects the changes of left ventricular hypertrophy and strain in the majority of patients but right ventricular hypertrophy may be seen in the neonatal period. The dilatation and disordered function of the left ventricle is immediately apparent on echocardiographic scanning. The thickened endothelium reflects unusually dense echoes. Aortography is often necessary to exclude anomalous origin of the left coronary artery from the pulmonary trunk which may produce similar clinical features.

Treatment and prognosis

Patients with respiratory distress are nursed in humidified oxygen. Intravenous frusemide, 1 mg/kg,

distinguishing feature. The second heart sound is single. A crescendo-decrescendo murmur in the upper praecordium or in the back indicates flow through a ductus arteriosus or collateral arteries and usually indicates pulmonary atresia. A harsh to-and-fro murmur at the lower left sternal edge suggests the absent pulmonary valve syndrome. The electro-cardiogram usually shows evidence of right ventricu-lar hypertrophy either with increased R/S ratio in V_1 or an upright T V_1. The chest X-ray in the neonate may not show the characteristic coeur en sabot configuration. In 25% the aortic arch and descend-ing aorta are to the right of the spine. In the presence of cyanosis the pulmonary vascular mark-ings are diminished. The haemoglobin level and haematocrit will not demonstrate the normal phy-siological decline during the first months.

Diagnosis

Echocardiography reveals the anatomy in consider-able detail. Long axial views reveal the ventricular septal defect and its relationship to the overriding aortic valve, the obstruction of the right ventricular infundibulum and the disproportion in size between the aortic and pulmonary valves. A parasternal short axis view should reveal the bifurcation of the pulmonary trunk and allow assessment of the calibre of the right and left pulmonary arteries. The presence of a ductus arteriosus or collateral arteries may also be demonstrated. Doppler echocardiogra-phy will detect a high systolic flow velocity in the pulmonary artery or a continuous flow pattern if a ductus is present.

Treatment

Many babies with Fallot's tetralogy will not require treatment during the neonatal period. Cyanotic patients, however, require detailed investigation. Maintenance of ductal patency with prostaglandin is imperative in the patient with pulmonary atresia. In most centres, babies requiring surgery during the first month are referred for palliative rather than corrective surgery and a modified Blalock–Taussig shunt is the procedure of choice. Cardiac catheter-ization and balloon dilatation of the right ventricular outflow and pulmonary valve is an alternative that has met with some success in Liverpool.

Pulmonary atresia and critical pulmonary stenosis with intact ventricular septum

Pulmonary atresia implies lack of continuity between the ventricular cavity and the pulmonary trunk. Pulmonary atresia with ventricular septal defect is included in the section on Fallot's tetralogy.

Pulmonary atresia also occurs occasionally with transposition, corrected transposition, double-inlet left ventricle, tricuspid atresia and in the complex heart defect associated with the asplenia syndrome. This section, however, is concerned with pulmonary atresia and critical pulmonary stenosis with intact ventricular septum, which is the second most fre-quent defect to present with cyanosis at birth.

Wide variation in the morphology of the right heart structures occurs in this condition. The obstruction to right ventricular outflow is an imper-forate valve in more than 80% and obstruction at the infundibulum in the remainder. The pulmonary trunk is usually patent above the valve diaphragm but is hypoplastic to varying degree. The right and left pulmonary arteries are usually well formed. The tricuspid valve is often stenotic and regurgitant with dysplastic cusps and short chordae tendineae. Less commonly Ebstein's anomaly of the tricuspid valve occurs. The right ventricular cavity ranges from the diminutive through the normal and is rarely enlarged. The right ventricular wall is usually thickened but rarely is as thin as parchment (Uhl's anomaly). The right ventricular cavity may be partially obstructed with spongy myocardium and endocardial fibroelastosis is common. In the pre-sence of severe right ventricular hypoplasia the cavity may be connected to the coronary arteries by sinusoids. The right atrium is always dilated, some-times massively so.

Haemodynamics

In the fetus with pulmonary atresia caval blood passes through the foramen ovale to the left atrium and left ventricle. The right ventricular stroke volume depends on the degree of tricuspid regurgi-tation or on the flow through sinusoids. The ductus is small as it carries only the 7% of cardiac output directed to the lungs. Following birth pulmonary blood flow is dependent on ductal patency. The left ventricle carries the additional burden of the pul-monary circulation. Myocardial oxygenation is com-promised by right-left shunting at the foramen ovale and may be further depressed in the presence of sinusoids by shunting of right ventricular blood to the coronary circulation.

Clinical features and diagnosis

The appearances immediately after birth are often normal but cyanosis and tachypnoea increase rapidly during the first day or two. Hepatomegaly, oedema and gallop rhythm also develop at an early stage. A systolic murmur of variable intensity is usually present from tricuspid regurgitation but ductal flow less commonly results in an audible continuous murmur.

The electrocardiogram demonstrates the increased left ventricular hypertrophy and strain and the tall peaked p waves of right atrial dilatation are a common feature. The QRS complexes of the right chest leads reflect the wide variation in right ventricular development but are most commonly of reduced amplitude. The cardiac shadow on X-ray is enlarged due mainly to right atrial dilatation and the lung fields are underperfused.

The echocardiogram is usually diagnostic. The subcostal view reveals the dilated right atrium and abnormal tricuspid valve, the parasternal long axis view, the atretic right ventricular outflow and its relationship to the pulmonary trunk. The dimensions of the right ventricle and tricuspid valve may be measured. Doppler echocardiography will detect tricuspid regurgitation and ductal flow.

Cardiac catheterization and angiocardiography are only necessary in the neonatal period if echocardiography fails to demonstrate the anatomy in sufficient detail to plan the management. Echocardiography may fail in some patients to distinguish between atresia and critical stenosis of the pulmonary valve, a distinction that is vital because the latter may be treated by balloon dilatation. A prostaglandin infusion is commenced prior to the procedure, to improve the oxygenation and also to improve angiographic visualization of the pulmonary arteries. Cardiac catheterization usually reveals suprasystemic right ventricular pressure. Right ventricular angiocardiography allows assessment of the right ventricular cavity, the size and incompetence of the tricuspid valve and the presence of sinusoids. The pulmonary arteries are demonstrated by left ventricular angiography.

Treatment and prognosis

Immediate resuscitation is frequently required and consists of correction of metabolic acidosis and ductal dilatation by prostaglandin infusion 10–50 ng/kg per min. Treatment with digoxin and diuretics are often necessary. The treatment of choice for patients with critical pulmonary stenosis is balloon pulmonary valvuloplasty performed at the time of initial cardiac catheterization. The surgical management of pulmonary atresia with intact ventricular septum remains controversial. Some authorities recommend early pulmonary valvotomy when the right ventricle is well developed whereas in many centres the initial operation is an aortopulmonary shunt.

In Liverpool, a three-stage surgical management has achieved encouraging results:

(1) modified Blalock shunt in the first days,
(2) patch repair of the right ventricular outflow using cardiopulmonary bypass at 3–4 months of age,
(3) closure of the atrial septal defect and Blalock shunt once right ventricular growth is adequate.

Pulmonary atresia with intact ventricular septum remains a challenging problem with high operative risks because of the severity and diversity of the anomalies of the right ventricle. Adverse factors are severe stenosis of the tricuspid valve, small right ventricular cavity and extensive sinusoid formation and these factors may preclude a successful outcome to the staged management. A modification of the Fontan operation after initial palliative shunt operation will then be the only alternative.

Tricuspid atresia

The term tricuspid atresia includes a group of malformations in which the right atrioventricular valve is absent or imperforate and thus the only pathway for systemic venous blood is through the foramen ovale or atrial septal defect to the left atrium. The incidence is approximately 1% of all congenital heart defects. Usually the floor of the right atrium has no connection with the ventricular myocardium but there are rare examples in which the right atrium is separated from a ventricular cavity by an imperforate membrane. The left ventricle and mitral valve are larger than normal while the right ventricle is hypoplastic. With concordant ventriculo-arterial connections the pulmonary artery is connected to the right ventricle which fills by way of a ventricular septal defect. A minority of patients also have transposition.

Cyanosis is always present because of the obligatory shunting from right to left atrium but the degree of hypoxia is determined by the level of pulmonary flow. With concordant ventriculo-arterial connection, pulmonary flow is usually restricted by the size of the VSD but may be supplemented by flow through the ductus. In the minority of patients with ventriculo-arterial discordance pulmonary flow and pressure are increased and pulmonary vascular disease develops at an early age.

Clinical features

Half of the patients present on the first day with cyanosis and four-fifths within the first month. The minority of patients who have increased pulmonary flow may present somewhat later with tachypnoea, dyspnoea or evidence of cardiac failure. The mean birth weight is below normal and postnatal growth also tends to be slow. The systolic murmur which is usually present is due to the VSD. The chest X-ray reflects the haemodynamics but the features are not pathognomonic. With diminished pulmonary blood flow the heart is not enlarged, and the lung fields are oligaemic. The minority with pulmonary plethora also have cardiomegaly. Tricuspid atresia is one of the few cyanotic lesions demonstrating left ventricular hypertrophy and left axis deviation.

catheterization is undesirable in the neonatal period.

Treatment and prognosis

Palliative or open heart surgery has met with little success in the first year. Critically ill patients in the neonatal period may require acid-base correction, assisted ventilation, digoxin and diuretics. Ductal patency will improve pulmonary blood flow and is achieved by a prostaglandin E infusion. Reduction of pulmonary vascular resistance and hence right ventricular pressure holds the promise of spontaneous improvement during the second and third weeks.

Transposition

The term transposition is applied to hearts in which the aorta arises mainly or completely from the morphological right ventricle and the pulmonary artery mainly or completely from the left ventricle. It is the commonest defect to present with cyanosis at birth. Associated defects are common and may have a major influence on the clinical course. The incidence of associated defects is shown in Table 23.10.

Table 23.10 The incidence of associated abnormalities in 142 cases of transposition from the Liverpool registry

	No.	*(%)*
Ventricular septal defect	36	(25.3)
Persistent ductus arteriosus	34	(23.9)
Coarctation	8	(5.6)
Ventricular septal defect and pulmonary stenosis	7	(4.9)
Tricuspid valve anomalies	6	(4.9)
Pulmonary stenosis	4	(2.8)
Total anomalous pulmonary venous return	1	(0.7)

Transposition of the great arteries has the following important implications: (1) cyanotic caval blood recirculation to the aorta; (2) pulmonary venous blood recirculation to the lungs; (3) shunting between the circulations is essential for life, must be bidirectional and the magnitude of shunting in each direction must be equal. Survival during the first few days is usually dependent on bidirectional shunting through the foramen ovale in addition to aortopulmonary shunting by way of the ductus. The few transpositions with a large atrial septal defect may and is in danger from congestive cardiac failure and

The presence of a small VSD or small ductus will have little influence on the degree of cyanosis. However, the baby with transposition and large ventricular septal defect will present with respiratory distress from torrential pulmonary blood flow

and is in danger from congestive cardiac failure and progressive pulmonary vascular disease rather than severe hypoxia.

Pulmonary valve stenosis or left ventricular outflow obstruction in addition to VSD will encourage bidirectional shunting and the degree of cyanosis then depends on the level of pulmonary blood flow.

The associated abnormalities will also have an important influence on the growth and development of the ventricular chambers. The left ventricular myocardium in simple transposition develops to a thickness which is commensurate with the left ventricular pressure whereas the right ventricle hypertrophies to enable it to support the systemic circulation. Persistence of the ductus arteriosus or the presence of a large VSD or pulmonary stenosis will prevent the underdevelopment of the left ventricular myocardium and this is a factor of major importance in determining the surgical management.

Clinical features and diagnosis

Prominent cyanosis on the first day of life is the dominant feature in 90% of transpositions. Mild degrees of cyanosis and later presentation are associated with significant ASD, VSD or PDA. An increased respiratory rate is usual and dyspnoea may develop subsequently with increase in pulmonary blood flow. The peripheral pulses are of good volume and the cardiac impulse increased. Auscultation at the initial examination usually reveals single heart sounds and the murmur if present is of low amplitude. A more obvious murmur indicates an associated VSD or pulmonary stenosis. The typical chest X-ray findings are of cardiomegaly and an 'egg-shaped' cardiac contour with increased pulmonary vascular markings, but these changes may not become apparent for several weeks. The electrocardiogram may also be normal at the time of presentation but right ventricular hypertrophy soon develops.

The diagnosis is established by two-dimensional echocardiography (Figure 23.3(d)). The ventriculo-arterial connections, the positional relationships of the semilunar valves and the associated lesions are identified. Cardiac catheterization is no longer required for initial diagnosis and angiography is avoided during the neonatal period if possible.

Treatment

The introduction of balloon atrial septostomy by Rashkind in 1964 transformed the early management of transposition [35]. The balloon catheter is introduced percutaneously into a femoral vein. The tip of the catheter is positioned in the left atrium, the balloon is inflated with dilute X-ray contrast medium and forcefully withdrawn to the right atrium rupturing the flap valve of the foramen ovale. The improvement in oxygen saturation is often striking and immediate. Patients who are severely hypoxic and acidotic may require resuscitation with intravenous sodium bicarbonate. Dilatation of the ductus arteriosus with a prostaglandin E infusion is also helpful.

The surgical management of transposition has been the subject of several controversies and treatment policies vary widely in the major centres. The atrial redirection operations of Senning and Mustard held sway until Jatene's success with the arterial redirection operation in 1975. Jatene's operation is the procedure of choice for transposition with large VSD as the results of atrial redirection and VSD closure are poor [22]. The ideal management of simple transposition is less certain. The Senning and Mustard operations are accomplished at 3–6 months

of age with low risk whereas arterial redirection must be performed in the first weeks before the left ventricular pressure declines. The operative risk is higher but this may be counterbalanced by a superior long-term prognosis. Transposition VSD with pulmonary stenosis may require staged management, the initial operation being a Blalock shunt followed at 3–4 years by a Rastelli operation, i.e. VSD closure and connection of right ventricle to pulmonary artery with a valved conduit.

Total anomalous pulmonary venous connection

The pulmonary veins form alongside the developing lung buds and have connections with the foregut veins. A venous channel grows from the developing left atrium to the pulmonary veins. With further development connections with the splanchnic plexus

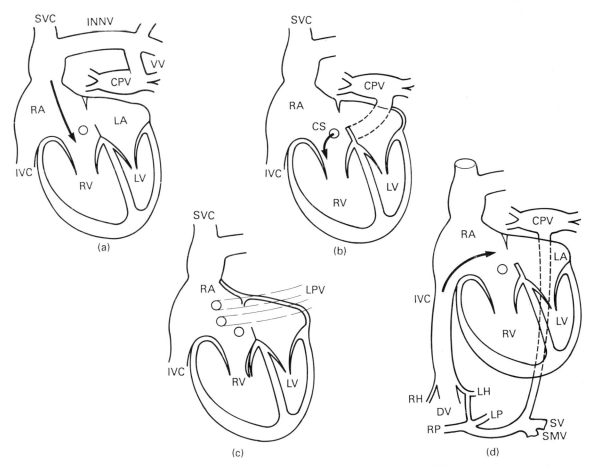

Figure 23.7 Four of the more common patterns of total anomalous pulmonary venous connection. (a) Supracardiac type with connection to the innominate vein; (b) connection to the coronary sinus; (c) cardiac type with connection to the right atrium; (d) infra-diaphragmatic type. The arrows indicate the preferential flow of pulmonary venous blood. CPV, common pulmonary vein; CS, coronary sinus; DV, ductus venosus; IVC, inferior vena cava; INNV, innominate vein; LH, left hepatic vein; LP, left portal vein; RH, right hepatic vein; RP, right portal vein; SMV, superior mesenteric vein; SV, splenic vein; SVC, superior vena cava

are lost and the common pulmonary vein is incorporated into the body of the left atrium. If the common pulmonary vein fails to develop, connections with the systemic venous system persist and enlarge.

The anastomosis may be with the anterior cardinal veins, the sinus venosus or the omphalomesenteric system and occasionally there is more than one connection. Thus the pattern and sites of anomalous pulmonary venous connection are varied and the most common are shown in Figure 23.7. Associated major cardiac malformations may co-exist especially in the presence of isomerism. The major haemodynamic factors are: the admixture of pulmonary and systemic venous blood in the caval veins or right atrium, obligatory right-to-left atrial shunt and obstruction to pulmonary venous return. The degree of cyanosis depends not only on the level of pulmonary blood flow but also the site of connection of the pulmonary veins. With infradiaphragmatic connections oxygenated blood is directed towards the foramen ovale. Severe obstruction to pulmonary venous return is always present in the infradiaphragmatic type because flow is from the descending channel and through the hepatic capillaries. Obstruction also occurs in a considerable proportion of the supracardiac types and to some extent with pulmonary venous connections to the coronary sinus.

The main determinant of pulmonary artery pressure in this condition during the neonatal period is the severity of pulmonary venous obstruction. Patients with infradiaphragmatic type always have severe pulmonary hypertension and a majority of cardiac and supracardiac types have some elevation of pulmonary artery pressure. Flow through the foramen ovale is often suboptimal resulting in reduced left ventricular stroke volume and poor development of the left ventricle.

Clinical findings

The most constant feature is tachypnoea, the onset and severity of cyanosis being variable. With severe pulmonary venous obstruction symptoms appear early and progress rapidly with failure to establish feeding, deteriorating peripheral circulation and hepatomegaly. With less severe obstruction the picture is of gradually increasing tachypnoea, dyspnoea, feeding difficulty and mild cyanosis. Increased pulmonary flow is manifested by a prominent right ventricular impulse, wide splitting of the second sound and an ejection systolic murmur in the pulmonary area. Occasionally, a continuous murmur from flow through the anomalous channel may be heard.

Investigation

Pulmonary venous obstruction leads to a characteristic ground glass appearance of the lung fields with small or normal sized heart, a picture that has some of the features that obtain in the respiratory distress syndrome. With less pulmonary venous obstruction the lung fields are plethoric and the heart size increased. The classic 'snowman' cardiac silhouette seldom appears before 3 months. The ECG shows right ventricular hypertrophy and normal or poor left ventricular activity. Two-dimensional echocardiography will usually confirm the diagnosis and reveal the detailed anatomy of the anomalous veins. Dilatation of the right atrium and right ventricle in comparison with the smaller left heart chambers is immediately apparent. Four-chamber views show no evidence of pulmonary venous connection to the left atrium and reveal a common pulmonary vein posterior to the left atrium. A suprasternal approach will often reveal the four pulmonary veins. A search is then made for an ascending or descending vein or marked dilatation of the coronary sinus. Cardiac catheterization and angiography are performed if the anatomical detail is not clear.

Treatment

Diuretic therapy may bring about transient improvement but the best results are obtained when surgery is undertaken without delay.

Lesions presenting with circulatory shock

Successful treatment of shock depends on rapid diagnosis of the underlying cause and it is important to be aware of the non-cardiac and cardiac causes. Shock at or soon after birth is usually related to intrapartum asphyxia, intracranial haemorrhage or fetal blood loss. Subsequently, sepsis with Gram-negative organisms and endotoxaemia is the most important cause. The cardiac causes are listed in Table 23.7.

The appearance is of pallor, mottling, peripheral or central cyanosis and coolness of the peripheries. The respirations are shallow or gasping with apnoeic episodes and the infant may be hypotonic and unresponsive. The pulses are weak or impalpable. The liver and spleen may be enlarged, often markedly so. Oliguria is an early feature and rapid progress to anuria is usual.

The shock syndrome may appear with alarming rapidity or develop progressively in a baby with cardiac respiratory distress or cyanosis.

Hypoplastic left heart syndrome

The designation hypoplastic left heart syndrome applies to a group of conditions in which the left ventricle is markedly reduced in size together with stenosis or atresia of the aortic and mitral valves.

This group of abnormalities ranks tenth in the incidence list and accounts for almost a quarter of the deaths due to heart abnormality occurring in the first month. The left ventricular cavity is usually slitlike with fibroelastotic changes in the endocardium. The mitral annulus is small with abnormalities of the cusps, chordae and papillary muscles. The left atrium is usually small. In the most common variant the aortic valve is atretic and the ascending aorta reduced in calibre to 2 or 3 mm. The aortic arch and its branches are more normally developed but a preductal coarctation co-exists in one-fifth of patients.

Restriction at the mitral valve results in severe pulmonary congestion. Pressure and flow in the aorta is dependent on the degree of ductal patency. Constriction of the arterial duct results in generalized systemic hypoperfusion and diverts more of the right ventricular output to the lungs thus intensifying the pulmonary congestion. Impaired coronary perfusion accelerates the right ventricular failure. Metabolic acidosis and renal impairment rapidly ensue.

Clinical features

The condition at birth is often satisfactory but the onset of tachypnoea, dyspnoea and feeding difficulty is usual within 2 or 3 days. Rapid progression to circulatory collapse soon follows. The peripheral pulses become weak or absent or the femoral pulses may be stronger than the upper limb pulses. Auscultatory findings are: a gallop rhythm, single second sound and a pulmonary ejection click. A systolic murmur if present is due to tricuspid regurgitation. Pulmonary crepitations or even evidence of haemorrhagic pulmonary oedema may be present.

The chest X-ray usually shows moderate cardiomegaly and the hazy pulmonary vascular markings of congestion. Less commonly the heart size is small and the lungs have a ground glass appearance similar to that of the respiratory distress syndrome. The electrocardiogram reflects reduced left ventricular voltages often with a qR pattern in V_1. A tall peaked p wave of right atrial enlargement is usual. The hypoplastic nature of the left ventricular structures and the ascending aorta together with dilatation of the right atrium, right ventricle and pulmonary artery is readily apparent on the two-dimensional echocardiogram.

Management and prognosis

More than 90% of patients die during the neonatal period and until recently few attempts at surgical palliation were made because of the dismal long-term prognosis. Limited success using a staged procedure has been achieved by Norwood *et al.* [31].

Initial palliation includes division of the pulmonary trunk, forming an anastomosis between the aortic arch and the proximal pulmonary trunk, a systemic artery to pulmonary anastomosis and atrial septectomy. A 'corrective' operation using a modification of the Fontan operation may then be feasible several years later. If surgery is to be considered initial treatment is with a prostaglandin infusion to maintain ductal patency.

Critical aortic valve stenosis

Less than 5% of patients with aortic valve stenosis have obstruction of such severity as to result in hypotensive heart failure. Commonly the aortic valve is thickened and dysplastic with a small eccentric orifice. The valve annulus may also be small. The left ventricular wall is hypertrophied and often exhibits endocardial fibroelastosis. The cavity may be dilated or show a varying degree of hypoplasia.

Clinical features

The onset of symptoms is usually sudden and within a few weeks of birth. The pulses are weak or impalpable. A systolic murmur of low intensity, together with a gallop rhythm, is present. The chest X-ray shows cardiomegaly and pulmonary congestion. The electrocardiogram may demonstrate flattening or inversion of the T waves but the QRS voltages are often normal. Two-dimensional echocardiography reveals the anatomy of the aortic valve and left ventricle and provides an assessment of left ventricular function. An estimate of the systolic pressure gradient at the aortic valve may be made using Doppler echocardiography.

Management

Anticongestive therapy will produce transient improvement but the prognosis without surgery is very poor. Operation using cardiopulmonary bypass offers the best prospect of survival.

Lesions presenting with an asymptomatic murmur

The detection of a heart murmur is the most common mode of presentation of heart abnormalities. Differentiation between organic and innocent murmurs during the neonatal period is more difficult than later in childhood. A brief discussion is given of abnormalities that are asymptomatic during the neonatal period followed by a note on innocent murmurs. The more common anomalies are listed in Table 23.11.

Table 23.11 Asymptomatic murmur

Ventricular septal defect
Atrial septal defect
Persistent ductus arteriosus
Pulmonary stenosis
Fallot's tetralogy
Aortic stenosis
Coarctation of the aorta

Ventricular septal defect

The murmur usually appears after the first few days and is initially quite soft and maximal at the lower left sternal edge. The murmur subsequently becomes louder and harsher and may be accompanied by a thrill. The ECG and chest X-ray are usually normal.

Atrial septal defect

The ejection systolic murmur of atrial septal defect is produced by increased pulmonary blood flow and accompanied by fixed splitting of the second sound. The murmur is soft and frequently passes undetected during the neonatal period. The chest X-ray and ECG are usually normal.

Persistent ductus arteriosus

Early in the neonatal period the murmur is systolic rather than continuous, maximal in the pulmonary area and propagated to the back. With significant ductal flow the peripheral pulses are collapsing. The ECG may show left ventricular hypertrophy but the chest X-ray is usually normal.

Pulmonary stenosis

The hallmark of pulmonary stenosis is an ejection systolic murmur preceded by an ejection click, maximal in the pulmonary area and propagated to the back. The murmur is soft and blowing in mild stenosis, harsh and accompanied by a thrill in more severe lesions. The ECG may show right ventricular hypertrophy but the chest X-ray is usually normal.

Fallot's tetralogy

More than half of neonates with Fallot's tetralogy are acyanotic and asymptomatic. The murmur which derives from the pulmonary stenosis is usually of grade 3/6 intensity, maximal in the third left interspace and propagated to the back. It is commonly mistaken for the murmur of VSD. The ECG shows right ventricular hypertrophy but the chest X-ray is often normal.

Aortic stenosis

The majority of patients with aortic stenosis go undetected during the neonatal period and it is only the more severe lesions which generate a harsh ejection systolic murmur at the left sternal edge and aortic area during the neonatal period. An ejection click is audible in valvar stenosis. The chest X-ray and ECG are often normal.

Coarctation of the aorta

Rather more than half of neonates with coarctation are asymptomatic. The systolic murmur is usually of low amplitude, ejection in type and equally well heard in the praecordium and interscapular region. The femoral pulses are weak and delayed in comparison with the right arm pulse. The ECG often reveals right rather than left ventricular hypertrophy. The chest X-ray is often normal.

Innocent murmurs

Approximately 60% of babies have transient systolic murmurs during the first days, many of which are related to turbulence at the site of the closing ductus. Diagnosis of a systolic murmur as innocent is based more on the exclusion of heart abnormality rather than the auscultatory features of the murmur. Serial examination during the first days may reveal diminishing intensity in the case of an innocent murmur whereas organic murmurs often become harsher and louder. If doubt remains after careful assessment, a chest X-ray, an electrocardiogram and perhaps an echocardiogram should be obtained and careful follow-up made until either the murmur has disappeared or its innocence has been established. Careful counselling of the parents is essential if undue anxiety is to be prevented.

Arrhythmias

Marked variations in heart rate and rhythm are common in healthy neonates. Sinus pauses, atrial and ventricular premature beats and junctional escape rhythms have been detected in a significant proportion of healthy neonates using 24-h ECG tape recording [43] and are of little importance. Occasionally, however, arrhythmia is a symptom of myocarditis or cardiomyopathy or co-exists with a congenital heart abnormality. A brief description of the more significant arrhythmias will be given.

Sinus bradycardia

Transient bradycardia occurs in association with apnoeic spells and convulsions and during the regurgitation of feeds. More persistent bradycardia is caused by profound hypoxia, hypothermia, hypothyroidism, intracranial haemorrhage and digoxin toxicity.

Supraventricular tachycardia

Paroxysmal supraventricular tachycardia is an uncommon but important cause of cardiac failure during the neonatal period. Attacks also occur before birth and cause fetal distress or hydrops foetalis. The majority have a re-entry mechanism for their tachycardia and one-quarter to one-half will show evidence of the Wolff–Parkinson–White syndrome on the interval electrocardiogram. The majority have a structurally normal heart but some have defects such as Ebstein's anomaly of the tricuspid valve. Heart rates of up to 300/min are not uncommon and symptoms of poor feeding, irritability, dyspnoea and pallor soon appear. The electrocardiogram reveals aberrant P waves, long PR interval and usually normal QRS configuration. Flattening or inversion of the T waves usually develops. Urgent treatment is required and the safest and most effective means of restoring sinus rhythm is direct current counter shock; 1–2 J/kg is usually sufficient. Digoxin is commenced because recurrent attacks are usual. Other antiarrhythmic drugs such as propranolol and flecainide may be required in addition. The longer-term prognosis is good and treatment may often be discontinued after 1 year.

Complete atrioventricular block

Failure of conduction of atrial impulses to the ventricle is usually due to a block between the atrial myocardium and the atrioventricular node. An escape rhythm with a fairly constant rate of from 45–80 beats/min persists. In some patients without structural defects heart block develops as a consequence of the transfer of anti SS-A/Ro antibodies from mothers who have lupus erythematosis [41]. A minority have associated defects such as corrected transposition.

The prognosis is determined by the heart rate and the severity of associated lesions if present. Cardiac failure is more likely to develop with heart rates below 50 beats/min and then survival is unlikely without permanent pacing. The development of reliable small implantable pacemakers and improved epicardial leads has made possible the long-term pacing of the smallest patients.

References

1. Anderson, R.H., Becker, A.E., Lucchese, F.E., Meier, M.A., Rigby, M.L. and Soto, B. (1983) Sequential segmental analysis. In *Morphology of Congenital Heart Disease. Angiocardiographic, Echocardiographic and Surgical Correlates*, Castle House, Tunbridge Wells, pp. 1–22

2. Baylen, B., Meyer, R.A., Karfhagen, J., Benzig, G. III, Bubb, M.E. and Kaplan, S. (1977) Left ventricular performance in the critically ill premature infant with patent ductus arteriosus and pulmonary disease. *Circulation*, **55**, 182–188

3. Bound, J.P. and Logan, W.F.W.E. (1977) Incidence of congenital heart disease in Blackpool 1947–1971. *Br. Heart J.*, **139**, 445–450

4. Bourne, G.L. and Benirschke, K. (1960) Absent umbilical artery. *Arch. Dis. Child.*, **35**, 534

5. Braudo, M. and Rowe, R.D. (1961) Auscultation of the heart – early neonatal period. *Am. J. Dis. Child.*, **101**, 575–586

6. Carlgren, L.E. (1969) The incidence of congenital heart disease in Gothenberg. *Proc. Ass. Eur. Cardiol.*, **5**, 208

7. Coceani, F. and Olley, P.M. (1973) The response of the ductus arteriosus to prostaglandins. *Can. J. Physiol. Pharmacol.*, **51**, 220–225

8. Coceani, F., White, E., Bodack, E. and Olley, P.M. (1979) Age dependent changes in the response of the ductus arteriosus to oxygen and Ibuprofen. *Can. J. Physiol. Pharmacol.*, **57**, 825–831

9. Craig, W.S. (1962) Admissions and readmissions from district to the special care baby unit of a maternity hospital. *Br. Med. J.*, **ii**, 1139–1144

10. de la Cruz, M.V. and Nadal-Ginard, B. (1976) Rules for the diagnosis of visceral situs, trunco-conal morphologies and ventricular inversions. *Am. Heart J.*, **84**, 19–32

11. de la Cruz, M.V., Berrazueta, J.R., Arteaga, M., Attie, F. and Soni, J. (1976) Rules for diagnosis of arterio-ventricular discordances and spatial identification of ventricle. *Br. Heart J.*, **38**, 341–354

12. Deanfield, J., Leanage, R., Stroobant, J., Crispin, A.R., Taylor, J.F.N. and Macartney, F.J. (1980) Use of high kilovoltage filtered beam radiographs for detection of bronchial situs in infants and young children. *Br. Heart J.*, **44**, 577–583

13. Dickenson, D.F., Arnold, R. and Wilkinson, J.L. (1981a) Congenital heart disease amongst 160,480 liveborn children in Liverpool 1960–1969 – implications for surgical treatment. *Br. Heart J.*, **46**, 55–62

14. Dickenson, D.F., Arnold, R. and Wilkinson, J.L. (1981b) Ventricular septal defect in children born in Liverpool 1960–1969. Evaluation of natural course and surgical implications in an unselected population. *Br. Heart J.*, **46**, 47–54

15. Dickenson, D.F., Arnold, R. and Wilkinson, J.L. (1982) Outcome of treatment for neonates referred to a supraregional cardiac centre 1976–1978. *Arch. Dis. Child.*, **57**, 328–333

16. Ebert, P.A. (1984) Staged partitioning of single ventricle. *J. Thorac. Cardiovasc. Surg.*, **88**, 908–913

17. Esscher, E. and Michaelsson, B. (1975) Cardiovascu-

lar malformations in infant deaths: 10 year clinical and epidemiological study. *Br. Heart J.*, **37**, 824

18. Fontan, F. and Boudet, E. (1971) Surgical repair of tricuspid atresia. *Thorax*, **26**, 240–248

19. Friedman, W.F., Hirschlklau, M.J., Printz, M.P., Pitlick, P.T. and Kirkpatric, S.E. (1976) Pharmacologic closure of patent ductus in premature infants. *New Engl. J. Med.*, **295**, 526–529

20. Gittenberger-de-Groot, A.C. (1977) Persistent ductus arteriosus: most probably a primary congenital malformation. *Br. Heart J.*, **39**, 610–618

21. Heymann, M.A., Rudolph, A.M. and Silverman, N.H. (1976) Closure of the ductus arteriosus in premature infants by inhibition of prostaglandin synthesis. *New Engl. J. Med.*, **295**, 530–533

22. Jatene, A.D., Fontes, V.F., Paulista, P.P. *et al.* (1976) Anatomic correction of transposition of the great vessels. *J. Thorac. Cardiovasc. Surg.*, **72**, 364–370

23. Jones, R.W.A., Bawmer, J.H., Joseph, M.C. and Shinebourne, E.A. (1976) Arterial oxygenation and response to oxygen breathing in differential diagnosis of congenital heart disease in infancy. *Arch. Dis. Child.*, **51**, 667–673

24. Kenna, A.P., Smithells, R.W. and Fielding, D.W. (1975) Congenital heart disease in Liverpool 1960–1969. *Q. J. Med.*, **173**, 17–44

25. Kennedy, J.A. and Clark, S.L. (1942) Observations on the physiological reaction of the ductus arteriosus. *Am. J. Physiol.*, **136**, 140–147

26. Kirklin, J.W., Harp, R.A. and McGoon, D.C. (1964) Surgical treatment of origin of both vessels from right ventricle, including cases of pulmonary stenosis. *J. Thorac. Cardiovasc. Surg.*, **48**, 1024–1036

27. Mitchell, S.C. (1957) The ductus arteriosus in the neonatal period. *J. Pediat.*, **51**, 12

28. Mitchell, S.K., Korones, S.B. and Berendes, H.W. (1971) Congenital heart disease in 56109 births. Incidence and neonatal history. *Circulation*, **43**, 323–332

29. Mustard, W.T., Keith, J.D., Trusler, G.A., Fowler, R. and Kidd, L. (1964) The surgical management of transposition of the great vessels. *J. Thorac. Cardiovasc. Surg.*, **48**, 953–958

30. Nora, J.J. and Nora, A.H. (1976) Recurrence risks in children having one parent with a congenital heart disease. *Circulation*, **53**, 801

31. Norwood, W.I., Lang, P. and Hansen, D.D. (1983) Physiologic repair of the aortic atresia – hypoplastic left heart syndrome. *New Engl. J. Med.*, **308**, 23–26

32. Olley, P.M. and Coceani, F. (1981) Prostaglandins and the ductus arteriosus. *Annu. Rev. Med.*, **32**, 375–385

33. Partridge, J.B., Scott, O., Deverall, P.B. and Macartney, F.J. (1975) Visualisation and measurement of the main bronchi by tomography as an objective indicator of the thoracic situs in congenital heart disease. *Circulation*, **51**, 188–196

34. Peltonen, T. and Hirvonen, L. (1963) The ductus venosus. *Acta Pediat.*, **52**, 202

35. Rashkind, W.J. and Miller, W.W. (1966) Creation of an atrial septal defect without thoracotomy. A palliative approach to complete transposition of great arteries. *J. Am. Med. Ass.*, **196**, 991–992

36. Rastelli, G.C., Wallace, R.B. and Angley, P.A. (1969) Complete repair of transposition of the great arteries with pulmonary stenosis. A review and report of a case corrected by using a new surgical technique. *Circulation*, **39**, 83–95

37. Rowe, R.D. and Cleary, T.W. (1960) Congenital cardiac malformation in the newborn period. Frequency in a childrens hospital. *Can. Med. Ass. J.*, **83**, 299–302

38. Rowe, R.D. and Hoffman, T. (1972) Transient myocardial ischaemia of the newborn infant. A form of severe cardio-respiratory distress in full term infants. *J. Pediat.*, **81**, 243–250

39. Rowe, R.D., Freedom, R.M., Mehriyi, A. and Bloom, K.R. (1981) Patent ductus arteriosus. In *The Neonate with Congenital Heart Disease*, 2nd edition, W.B. Saunders, Philadelphia, p. 273

40. Rudolph, A.M. and Heymann, M.A. (1967) The circulation of the foetus in utero: methods for studying distribution of blood flow, cardiac output and organ flow. *Circulation Res.*, **21**, 163

41. Scott, J.S., Maddison, P.S., Taylor, P.V., Esscher, E., Scott, O. and Skinner, R.P. (1983) Connective tissue disease antibodies to ribonucleoprotein and congenital heart block. *New Engl. J. Med.*, **309**, 209–212

42. Senning, A. (1959) Surgical correction of transposition of the great arteries. *Surgery*, **45**, 966–980

43. Southall, D.P., Richards, J., Mitchell, P., Brown, D.J., Johnston, P.G.B. and Shirebourne, E.A. (1980) Study of cardiac rhythm in healthy newborn infants. *Br. Heart J.*, **4**, 14–20

44. Tynan, M.J., Becker, A.E., Macartney, F.J., Quero-Juanez, M., Shinebourne, E.A. and Anderson, R.H. (1979) Study of cardiac rhythm in healthy newborn infants. *Br. Heart J.*, **43**, 14–20

45. Van Praagh, A. (1972) The segmental approach to diagnosis in congenital heart disease. *Birth Defects*, **8**, 4–23

46. Wilcox, B.R. and Anderson, R.H. (1985) *Surgical Anatomy of the Heart*, Gower Medical Publishing Ltd, London

47. Wilkinson, J.L., Wilcox, B.R. and Anderson, R.H. (1981) The anatomy of double outlet right ventricle. In *Paediatric Cardiology* (eds R.H. Anderson, F.J. Macartney, E.A. Shinebourne and N. Tynan). Vol. 5, Churchill Livingston, Edinburgh, pp. 397–407

The surgery of congenital heart defects

D.I. Hamilton

Introduction

Further developments and changes in the management of congenital heart defects have occurred since the last edition of this book. Some of these changes will be discussed here and, because a number of new approaches have been included, it has been necessary to exclude some of the material from the last edition. Reference will be made to this material where it still applies to current practice.

Approximately 1% of infants suffer from congenital heart disease and 40% of these will die before their fifth birthday [16,32]. Certain defects such as total anomalous pulmonary venous connection (TAPVC), transposition of the great arteries (TGA), and truncus arteriosus carry a high mortality (85%) during the first year of life.

Neonatal mortality increases with the severity of the defects and with multiplicity of defects, some of which may compensate each other, but which may compound the haemodynamic response and the degree of cardiac failure or cyanosis. It is clear from reviewing clinical results and postmortem material, that morbidity and mortality relate to an underestimation of the complexity and multiplicity of the heart defect(s) if this has resulted in an incomplete surgical repair. Thus, it behoves the cardiologist to give a comprehensive and detailed diagnosis (anatomical and physiological) and with the advent of two-dimensional echocardiography and doppler echocardiography this is now usually possible.

Before 1970 little corrective intracardiac surgery had been attempted in this age group [21]. Closure of the persistent ductus arteriosus (PDA), resection of coarctation of the aorta and division of an obstructive vascular ring were practised. Certain palliative procedures, such as the creation of a systemic to pulmonary artery shunt in cyanotic conditions [13,60] and banding of the main pulmonary artery [42], to restrict pulmonary blood flow, were available. Open heart surgery has been performed extensively in infants during the past 15 years and the indications for corrective surgery are increasing [36]. Primary closure of isolated ventricular septal defects (VSD) is now practised in the first 6 months of life in most centres in preference to pulmonary artery banding as a first stage. Infants suffering from interruption of the aortic arch in association with VSD and PDA present in the first weeks of life in congestive cardiac failure. Improved management, including radical surgical correction, has resulted in a higher survival rate in this group of neonates. This success also leads to an increased demand for secondary and tertiary open-heart procedures as the child grows, particularly where it has been necessary to insert man-made conduits and valves, rather than providing a more natural reconstruction with some 'growth potential'. We have found that the most successful approach to infants with pulmonary valve atresia, hypoplastic right ventricle and hypoplasia of the tricuspid valve is a three-stage policy combining early palliative treatment in the first week of life with two further open-heart procedures.

The intravenous administration of prostaglandin E_1 can be effective in maintaining patency of the ductus arteriosus in the neonate [45]. This is helpful in a variety of conditions where pulmonary blood flow is dependent on duct patency or where distal thoracic and abdominal aortic blood flow is provided via the persistent ductus (severe preductal coarctation of the aorta and arch interruption). Metabolic acidosis, hypoxia and oliguria usually respond to intravenous prostaglandin therapy and the neonate enters the operating theatre in a much improved condition generally. Infants requiring palliative systemic to pulmonary artery shunts often benefit from a short period of therapy with prostaglandin and 'emergency surgery' can often be delayed for 24–48 h.

There has been further evolution in the concept of 'systemic to pulmonary artery' shunting in recent years. This procedure was introduced by Blalock and Taussig [13] initially to treat children who had survived to an older age, in spite of cyanotic heart conditions. We have performed 98 'shunts' in children under 3 months of age during the period 1980–85. Some of these have been aimed at stimulating severely underdeveloped branch pulmonary arteries to grow, in the absence of adequate blood flow from the right ventricle or main pulmonary artery. This becomes necessary when the branch pulmonary arteries are 'disconnected' from each other. By shunting into one or both branch pulmonary arteries in the first 3 months of life, such arteries can be salvaged in preparation for reconstructive surgery at an older age. The addition of microvascular techniques into the paediatric cardiac surgeon's armamentarium has facilitated such work considerably.

Surgery without cardiopulmonary bypass for defects with increased pulmonary blood flow

Persistent ductus arteriosus (PDA)

The ductus arteriosus usually lies between the origin of the left main pulmonary artery and the inferior aspect of the aortic arch, immediately distal to the origin of the left subclavian artery. It develops from the distal portion of the left sixth aortic arch. Galen knew of its existence in the second century and it was described in detail by Leone Carceno in 1574. Monro [41] of Philadelphia suggested ligation in 1907 but this was not achieved successfully until 1938 [29]. The incidence of PDA has been assessed by Anderson [2] as 1 per 2500–5000 live births and comprises 12% of all cases with congenital heart disease [26]. Wood [62] gave a figure of 14.5% and Maude Abbott [1] quoted an incidence of 9.2%. She pointed out that the condition is more common in girls than boys.

The ductus usually closes soon after birth. Christie [19] reported that approximately 65% are still open 2 weeks after birth, 12% at 8 weeks and 1–2% at 12 months of age. Unless the ductus is large in calibre symptoms are usually mild or are absent when it occurs as an isolated defect. When it is persistent in association with other defects of the cardiovascular system, symptoms are usually present. The ductus may play a life-sustaining role in supplying blood into the pulmonary circulation (natural shunt), beyond a critical obstruction in the right side of the heart (tricuspid or pulmonary valve atresia). It is now possible to manipulate the ductus pharmacologically, maintaining its patency by the administration of prostaglandin E_1 intravenously (see below).

The ductus arteriosus forms, with the patent foramen ovale, a bypass mechanism away from the pulmonary circulation *in utero*. After birth, as the pulmonary vascular resistance falls, flow from the aorta through the PDA into the pulmonary circulation increases. It is customary to advise closure of the ductus at any age, if it is thought that the left-to-right shunt is causing congestive heart failure which is not responding to medical therapy (e.g. premature infants), and after term in all children to prevent the later development of cardiac failure, pulmonary vascular disease and hypertension, subacute bacterial endocarditis (SBE) and the late complications of calcification and aneurysm formation.

The duct is often thin walled and its structure differs from that of the walls of the aorta and pulmonary artery. Surgically, it should be handled with great respect and delicacy and it should not be incorporated in any reconstructive procedure. It is inadvisable to use the ductus in the reconstruction of coarctation of the aorta or interruption of the aortic arch, particularly in the neonatal period. Provided that the physical signs are classic, it is not necessary to perform cardiac catheterization preoperatively. The ductus can be demonstrated by echocardiography. If the signs are atypical, differentiation from aortopulmonary window (fistula) and coronary artery fistula must be made. The closure of aortopulmonary window requires cardiopulmonary bypass. When associated intracardiac defects are suspected, full investigation is recommended.

PDA in the premature infant

Following the development of special care baby units there has been an improvement in the survival of premature infants. Many of these babies suffer from respiratory distress syndrome and the ductus is usually patent because of prematurity. Intermittent positive-pressure ventilation is required but this is not always sufficient to control congestive cardiac failure adequately. These tiny infants, weighing as little as 500 g, withstand thoracotomy and ligation of the ductus remarkably well and this can be a helpful addition to their conventional medical management, and is often a turning point towards recovery. Others fail to respond and succumb to the complications of infection or respiratory disease postoperatively.

Surgical closure

It is sometimes necessary to close a PDA in infancy when the left-to-right shunt into the lungs is large. More frequently, the ductus is closed as part of a more extensive operation aimed at correcting the additional abnormalities at the same time.

Two procedures are available: ligation or division. Ligation was suggested by Blalock [10] and by Gross [29], who subsequently preferred division [28]. Conklin and Watkins [20] advised division and suture of the wall of the aorta and pulmonary artery rather than of the ductus itself. Bickford [9] reported 122 patients who had PDAs of less than 7 mm diameter ligated. Recanalization occurred in less than 1%. In 106 cases having PDAs greater than 7 mm in diameter, simple ligation was followed by recanalization in 16%. As a result of these observations we employ a particular method of ligation (see below). PDAs of more than 1 cm in diameter and those which are very short should be divided.

Surgical technique

Ligation

The chest is opened through a left thoracotomy in the third or fourth intercostal space. The mediastinal pleura is incised vertically over the thoracic aorta below the superior intercostal vein. The pleura is dissected anteriorly off the lateral aspect of the aorta and ductus and is retracted with stay sutures.

The inferior and superior aspects of the ductus are freed from surrounding areolar tissue before any attempt is made to pass an instrument around it. The recurrent laryngeal nerve is identified as it leaves the vagus nerve and loops around the medial end of the PDA. A small pouch of pericardium, usually containing fluid, extends a few millimetres along the superior aspect of the ductus. This is displaced medially using sharp or blunt dissection.

Curved forceps (Negus or Waterston) are used to isolate the ductus completely. Two ligatures of thick braided silk are then passed around it. If dissection proves difficult or when the PDA is large, tape slings are passed around the thoracic aorta above and below the level of the ductus. This precaution can be invaluable in the event of haemorrhage from torn ductal tissue. The first ligature is tied down on the aortic end of the ductus. Broad ligature material minimizes trauma to the friable wall and it can be tied more tightly than thinner material. The central portion of the ductus is transfixed and ligated with a fine suture which is passed around the duct to close its lumen and force any blood remaining in the duct centrally. Finally, the remaining ligature is tied at the medial end of the duct. The thrill which was palpable over the main pulmonary artery should now have been abolished. As the 'run off' from the systemic circulation has been closed, there should be an improvement in both systolic and diastolic elements of the blood pressure. The mediastinal pleura is sutured back over the aorta and ductal ligatures. We do not drain the chest routinely following this operation but great care is taken not to traumatize the lung on suturing the chest wall tissues. A chest X-ray is taken immediately the child arrives in the recovery ward to check that the lung is fully expanded. If this technique is adopted, it is essential that the anaesthetist keeps the lungs fully expanded throughout the closure of the intercostal muscle layer.

Division

Although hypotensive anaesthesia can be employed to facilitate the ligation of the large PDA, it is probably wiser to divide PDAs of more than 1 cm in diameter and those which are associated with pulmonary hypertension.

Side-biting occlusion clamps are placed on the walls of the aorta and pulmonary artery, and the duct is divided or resected. Sutures are passed through the wall of the aorta and pulmonary artery to close both stumps securely.

During the neonatal period ductal tissue is soft. On one occasion following the repair of a preductal coarctation of the aorta with a subclavian arterial onlay flap, the ductus was ligated at either end with strong linen thread. The infant returned to the ward with femoral pulses that were easily palpable initially. These diminished after a few hours and the child died subsequently. At postmortem examination it was apparent that the linen ligature had cut through the duct wall and a rosette of intimal tissue had invaginated into the aortic lumen, causing obstruction to blood flow. For this reason we prefer to divide the patent ductus in the neonatal period.

The results of closure of PDA in infancy are summarized in Table 24.1.

Table 24.1 Results of surgical closure of PDA in infants under 3 months of age at Royal Liverpool Children's Hospital, 1980–85

PDA closure	No.	Deaths
'Simple'	47	1
'Complex'	14	2
Ligation	57	3
Division	4	0

Postoperative complications

These include pneumothorax, haemothorax, wound infection and hoarseness of the voice, inability to

the heart by blood or clots (tamponade), inadequate ventilation, and arrhythmias. The duration of circulatory arrest or cardiopulmonary bypass also may have a profound influence on postoperative recovery [51], as can the length of the operative procedure, or acute pre-operative haemodynamic deterioration [50]. This information should accompany the patient to the postoperative recovery ward.

Facilities for postoperative care

Transfer of the patient from the operating theatre to the area of postoperative care takes place at a particularly vulnerable time and should be well-planned in advance. The distance between the two facilities should be as short as possible and without obstruction to patient movement. The receiving unit, notified of the patient's impending arrival, prepares all necessary monitoring and support equipment, while the theatre staff confirm that any requisite lifts are available and working before the patient leaves the operating room.

The amount of cardiorespiratory support and monitoring necessary during the actual transfer varies according to the patient's condition and operative procedure. In general, it is essential to have a clear indication that ventilation and cardiac output are adequate. Following an uncomplicated, closed operation, this may involve simply watching the infant breathe and observing his apical impulse or peripheral pulses, which are usually easily seen in a small baby. At the other extreme, the safe transport of a patient who has been haemodynamically unstable may require a portable monitor to display the electrocardiogram and arterial pressure trace, battery-driven infusion pumps for uninterrupted delivery of inotropes, immediate availability of a portable defibrillator, and continuous hand ventilation from an oxygen cylinder. The baby's body temperature must be maintained also, either in a heated incubator or by thermal insulation. Immediately upon arrival in the intensive care unit, the electrocardiogram and pressure monitoring lines are attached and the chest drains are unclamped to release any accumulated air or fluid. There is, not infrequently, a brief period of instability after movement of the neonate from the operating theatre, and it is important that an experienced member of the surgical team remains at the bedside until he is satisfied that the chest X-ray, haemodynamics and ventilation are acceptable.

The intensive care or high dependency unit should provide an environment for the safe and efficient nursing of small infants. Ideally, this is geographically separate from both adult cardiac patients and other non-cardiac babies, such that the staff may concentrate on management of the small and rapidly changeable patient, his parents may be given a sensitive degree of privacy and support, and the risk of cross-infection is minimized. Approximately 80–100 ft^2 of space should be available for each infant, and adjoining staff rooms are essential for accessibility of doctors, interviewing of parents, and relief of stress during nursing shifts. For intubated patients, a 1:1 nurse:patient ratio is appropriate, while extubated patients may be nursed on a 1:2 ratio. Equipment requirements include pressure, temperature and electrocardiogram monitors; doppler or sphygmomanometer blood pressure recorders; infusion pumps for delivery of 0.1–25 ml/h; incubators or overhead heaters; and apnoea monitors. Laboratory facilities should be readily available for the measurement of arterial blood gases, haemoglobin, serum potassium, glucose, calcium and sodium on a 24-h basis, with capability to carry out other routine bacteriology, haematology and biochemistry investigations as needed. A portable X-ray service is essential, and most postoperative cardiac intensive care units also have a sector scanner or doppler echocardiography machine available.

Subsystem management

Cardiovascular subsystem

Although comparatively little information is available concerning structure and function of the normal newborn human heart, it seems likely that there are important anatomical and biochemical differences which influence cardiac performance. Resting cardiac output in the newborn, based on body weight, is two to three times greater than an adult [81], emphasizing the physiological demands which are present at birth. A balanced ventricular architecture is also present at birth, and the left ventricle subsequently acquires dominance, contributing almost the entire ventricular septum [16]. However, sarcomere arrangement is random in the fetus and the ventricle of newborn lambs shows considerably more distensibility [59] and less contractility than adults [80]. Augmentation of cardiac output in the neonate is thus achieved predominantly by increasing heart rate rather than stroke volume. At the same time, cardiac muscle in the neonate probably has a greater capacity for anaerobic metabolism which makes it less susceptible to hypoxic injury.

Following cardiac surgery, an adequate cardiac output is manifest by warm, pink extremities, easily palpable foot pulses, a good urine output and a normal serum potassium level. In the neonate, these signs are virtually as reliable as direct measurement of cardiac output and predict a 90% probability of survival [50]. When cardiac output is measured by dye dilution [70] or thermodilution [60], an index of more than 2 litres/min per m^2 also correlates well with uncomplicated recovery from open heart surgery. Conversely, systemic arterial blood pressure is a poor indicator of cardiac output because an increased systemic resistance will maintain blood pressure at the expense of tissue perfusion, even in the presence of severely impaired cardiac output.

The earliest indication of low cardiac output in the neonate is often diminished production of urine followed by weakening of the peripheral pulses and augmentation of the core–toe temperature gradient. Arterial blood gases subsequently show a reduction in pO_2 and metabolic acidosis, while a low ($<28 mmHg$) systemic mixed venous pO_2 and peripheral cyanosis also reflect poor tissue perfusion. If conscious, the patient becomes restless. Hyperthermia rapidly supervenes in severe low cardiac output with rectal temperatures in excess of 40°C, and tachycardia is almost invariably present. The myocardial reserves of the neonatal heart are less well developed than at a later age, and cardiac function can deteriorate with alarming rapidity. Early recognition and swift intervention are mandatory to control this potentially lethal situation and mitigate secondary damage to other organs. In some cases, it may be necessary to start intensive treatment even before the exact cause of low cardiac output has been investigated fully.

The management of low cardiac output is facilitated by a clear appreciation of those factors which determine ventricular function. These are (1) preload, (2) afterload, (3) contractility, (4) heart rate and rhythm, and (5) synergy.

Preload

Physiologically, preload is defined as end-diastolic sarcomere length and determined by the size, shape, thickness and transmural pressure of the ventricle. Considering the different thickness and shape of the two ventricles, it is not surprising that preload may be different on the right and left sides of the heart. In clinical practice, preload is assessed by measurement of mean atrial pressure and adjusted by transfusion of blood or plasma.

Afterload

Within the intact cardiovascular system, afterload represents the impedance against which blood is ejected from the heart, or the systolic tension of the ventricle. It is approximated (in the absence of outflow obstruction) by systolic pressure in the great vessels, which in turn reflects peripheral vascular resistance. Reduction of afterload can be effected by a variety of vasodilators with a view to improving ventricular function and stroke volume.

Contractility

Although simply defined as the tension produced by a given amount of shortening in isolated muscle experiments, contractility of the intact ventricle is more difficult to translate into a clinical context. It is generally accepted to be the changes in stroke volume which are not due to changes in preload or afterload, and hence reflects the contractile state of the heart muscle itself. Those pharmacological agents which affect contractility are called inotropes. At the present time, three general groups of inotropic agents are known to increase contractility of the heart – cardiac glycosides (digoxin and its derivatives), catecholamines or adrenergic agents (adrenaline, isoprenaline, dopamine, and dobutamine) and non-adrenergic phosphodiesterase inhibitors.

Heart rate

The dependence of cardiac output upon heart rate is summarized by the equation

cardiac output = heart rate × stroke volume

The mean normal heart rate in the neonate ranges from 119 beats/min at birth to 163 beats/min at the end of the first month of life [1,64]. At low heart rates, there is a corresponding reduction in cardiac output due to the neonate's limited capacity to increase stroke volume [80]. A reduced diastolic filling time at higher rates may embarrass both cardiac output and coronary artery perfusion. Cardiac rhythm is important also, between 10% and 15% of cardiac output normally resulting from the atrial contribution in sinus rhythm.

Synergy

The way in which different areas of the ventricle contract to bring about changes in ventricular volume has been shown to influence the ejection fraction of patients with a variety of congenitally deformed hearts [31]. Although poorly defined in the neonate, this factor may become an important determinant of cardiac output in patients with complex ventricular morphology or in whom areas of damaged myocardium have paradoxical movement.

In addition to the above determinants of ventricular function, impaired cardiac output may result also from tamponade or residual intracardiac defects. Real-time and doppler echocardiography in the postoperative intensive care unit have proved to be invaluable for the investigation of such complications. An intrapericardial collection of fluid with reduced atrial filling, diagnostic of cardiac tamponade, can be demonstrated by sector scanning [84], as can residual intracardiac shunts with the aid of contrast echocardiography [97]. Estimation of ventricular function during adjustment of inotropes and ventilation may also be helpful. It is likely that the colour echo-doppler will be even more useful in this context.

Timely and skillful management of the cardiovascular subsystem is essential after both open and closed procedures in the neonate. There is, not infrequently, a period of haemodynamic instability followed by a gradual improvement in cardiac function during the next 2–3 days. Appropriate, and sometimes aggressive, treatment of low cardiac output in the early postoperative period is often rewarded with eventual survival of the baby, providing irreversible damage to other organ systems has not occurred.

Preload is first adjusted to an optimal level by transfusion of blood (if the packed cell volume is less than 35%) or plasma (when packed cell volume exceeds 35%). In the neonate, either left or right atrial pressure may be higher, and thus limiting, depending upon relative resistance in the pulmonary and systemic vascular beds and the underlying cardiac malformation. In general, a mean atrial pressure of 20 mmHg should not be exceeded because of the propensity to pulmonary oedema on the left side and ascites on the right side of the circulation. If there is uncertainty whether a higher filling pressure will benefit cardiac output, gentle pressure over the liver may be used to cause a temporary increase in venous return; if this is followed by an increase in systemic blood pressure, expansion of the patient's blood volume is usually beneficial. If the blood pressure is unchanged or, more importantly, falls, the heart is already working at a maximal filling pressure and any further distension will pass onto the descending limb of the Starling curve.

Inadequate preload

There are several causes of inadequate preload after open heart operation. The most obvious is haemorrhage, which should be readily apparent from the amount of chest drainage. In the presence of brisk bleeding, drainage should be measured and replaced every 15–30 min to avoid wide variations in filling pressure and the need for rapid transfusion. Peripheral vasodilatation in the small infant who returns from the operating theatre cold and constricted also may require a surprising amount of volume expansion. This is often equal to as much as 50% (but rarely exceeds 100%) of the patient's calculated blood volume. A corresponding rise in peripheral temperature should follow, indicating improved filling of previously collapsed vessels.

Post perfusion capillary leak

The most sinister cause of a low atrial pressure which transfusion supports only temporarily is post perfusion capillary leak [17,51]. Characteristically, the systolic arterial pressure and central venous pressure fall repeatedly, and, after a few hours, an increase in abdominal girth measurements indicates formation of ascitic fluid. Arterial oxygen saturation usually declines both as the result of a similar fluid leak into the lung and because progressive abdominal distension compromises ventilation. Diminishing urine production signifies prerenal failure which may progress to established tubular necrosis. Treatment of this complex and incompletely understood syndrome is largely empirical. There is some evidence that improving cardiac output by administration of inotropes will facilitate repair of capillary damage and attenuate loss of fluid from the intravascular space by achieving adequate tissue perfusion at a lower filling pressure. Peritoneal dialysis has been used to treat the renal complications and (theoretically) remove activated complement factors. A simple measure which has been effective in some patients is abdominal compression, either by application of a circumferencial crepe bandage or intermittent abdominal pulsation [41]. This probably works by support of the right atrial filling pressure and mechanical limitation of ascities through increasing intra-abdominal pressure. However, mechanical ventilation (particularly with a pressure ventilator), is invariably compromised and must be adjusted accordingly. Finally, as a last resort, we have successfully managed some patients who suffered a massive (5–10 times their blood volume/24 h) and continuing capillary leak by intravenous reinfusion of ascitic fluid. The advantages of this technique are accurate replacement of volume, conservation of serum proteins, freedom from plasma preserving agents and economy. However, there is a possible risk of infection, reinfusion of activated complement, and pulmonary dysfunction from protein aggregates, such that it must be used with caution at the present time.

Afterload reduction

Afterload reduction frequently benefits cardiac output in the postoperative patient by counteracting vasoconstriction, thus allowing the ventricle to eject blood with less work and lower oxygen consumption by the heart [2]. It can be used safely only if the systemic arterial blood pressure is at least normal (a systolic of about 70 mmHg in the neonate) and preferably above normal because lower levels (particularly in the presence of left ventricular hypertrophy) embarrass coronary perfusion. There is now considerable clinical experience with a variety of vasodilators (Table 25.1), and the selection for a particular patient often reflects institutional preferences as well as pharmacological advantages. The

Table 25.1 Vasodilating agents used for afterload reduction

Vasodilator	Mechanism of action	Dose/route of administration	Onset and duration of action	Advantages	Disadvantages
Phenoxy-benzamine	α-blocker arterial dilatation	1 mg/kg given i.v. over 15–30 min	Delayed onset (30–60 min) Duration 12–24 h	Ease of administration	Reflex tachycardia. Long duration. Cerebral and coronary resistance unaltered
Phentol-amine	α-blocker arterial dilatation	i.v. infusion 0.01 mg/kg per min	Immediate onset Short-lived	Possible pulmonary vasodilator	Hypotension Tachycardia
Sodium nitroprusside	Relaxation of venous and arterial smooth muscle	i.v. infusion 1–10 µg/kg per min	Immediate Short-lived	Inexpensive Rapid and accurate control	Metabolized to cyanide. Toxicity with high doses or prolonged infusion (>24 h) Sensitive to light
Nitroglycerin	Decreased venous and coronary arterial tone	i.v. infusion 0.5–3.0 µg/kg per min Topical - 5 mg patch. Released over 24 h	1–4 min onset Half-life of metabolites 2 h about	Improves coronary blood flow Non-toxic	Unpredictable delivery due to absorption on plastic or dependence on cutaneous circulation
Hydralazine	Relaxes arteriolar smooth muscles	0.5–1 mg/kg per h by i.v. infusion	Immediate onset Half-life 2–3 h	Improves renal and hepatic blood flow	Reflex tachycardia. Hepatotoxicity
Captopril	Block angiotensin II and aldosterone production	Oral - 8-hourly 0.1 mg/kg increasing to 2 mg/kg	Onset 30 min Duration 8 h	Balanced vasodilator (arterial and venous)	Excreted via kidney i.v. preparation not generally available. First dose can cause hypotension
Chlorpromazine	α-blockade Central effects Direct dilatation of blood vessels	i.v. dose 0.1–0.3 mg/kg	Onset 5–10 min: duration variable	Readily available	Tachycardia Cardiac depression Extrapyramidal side effects

simplest (but least precise) option is topical application of nitroglycerin, which will be effective in mild vasoconstriction without severe impairment of ventricular function. The intravenous infusion of nitrates allows more exact regulation of blood pressure and frequently is used in combination with inotropes and volume expansion to counteract secondary hypotension. When the need and tolerance for sustained vasodilatation have been established, phenoxybenzamine or captopril may be useful.

Arrhythmias

Although less frequent in neonates than adult cardiac patients, arrhythmias may seriously impair cardiac function because of the neonatal heart's dependence upon a comparatively fast rate. Virtually all patients have temporary ventricular pacemaker wires left at the time of open heart operation and most will also have atrial pacing wires. These are useful both in diagnosis of conduction disturbances and their treatment. Pacing wires generally remain *in situ* for 6–8 days after operation, by which time surrounding adhesions should localize any haemorrhage following their removal. They should be taken out only after the presence of a stable (preferably sinus) rhythm has been confirmed and they should be removed early in the day, so that any complications (such as bleeding) are readily identified and treated. In patients with persistent pyrexia, the ends of the pacemaker wires are sent for culture, although other signs of mediastinal infection are usually a more reliable guide to deep-seated infection.

of low birthweight twins with both members suffering from inguinal hernia in the neonatal period and ten pairs of twins each with only one member being affected by this condition.

The higher incidence of inguinal hernia on the right than on the left is related to the fact that the right testis descends at a later date than the left and hence the right processus vaginalis obliterates later than the left [22,61]. The association of undescended testis and inguinal hernia is common and 16 out of 130 neonates (12.3%) in our series have undescended testes.

Other associated congenital abnormalities seen in our series include myelomeningocele, eight (6.2%), congenital heart disease, 14 (10.8%), hypospadias, three (2.3%), solitary kidney and refluxing ureter, one (0.8%), malrotation, two (1.5%), imperforate anus, one (0.8%), talipes equino varus, one (0.8%), Rhesus incompatibility, one (0.8%) and ectopic adrenal in hernia, one (0.8%).

Although the occurrence of inguinal hernia may have been influenced genetically in some instances, perinatal factors appear to play a more important role in its aetiology. Prematurity is the most important risk factor. Harper *et al.* reported that 11 of 37 infants weighing less than 1000 g developed an inguinal hernia [23]. The cumulative risks of infants born in Liverpool in 1981 developing inguinal hernias before 6 months of age were calculated to be 0.6% for full-term boys and 0.09% for full-term girls compared with 7.0% for preterm boys (<36 weeks) and 1.0% for preterm girls (<36 weeks), representing a tenfold increase in risk in preterm infants [7]. In the same series, very low birthweight babies (<1500 g) had a 20-fold increase in risk of inguinal hernia. Similar results were obtained in other epidemiological studies [38,41,57]. It has been postulated that inguinal hernia is more likely to develop when preterm delivery, with its accompanying increase in intra-abdominal pressure, occurs prior to the obliteration of the processus vaginalis which normally proceeds after 32 weeks of gestation. It has also been suggested in one series that intrauterine growth retardation is also associated with an increase in neonatal inguinal hernia [38] although this finding has not been confirmed in the Liverpool series [41].

Increased abdominal pressure is likely to be important in precipitating an inguinal hernia even after delivery, particularly in premature babies. It has been calculated that enteral feeds given to healthy underweight infants amount to an adult equivalent for weight of more than 3 gallons a day. Definite increased abdominal pressure was present in 16 (12.3%) of our cases and the causes include necrotizing enterocolitis, eight, malrotation, two, imperforate anus, one and the presence of a ventriculoperitoneal shunt for the treatment of hydrocephalus, five.

The presence of respiratory problems and the use of mechanical respiratory support have been found not to be associated with increased prevalence of hernia but are predictive of bilateral rather than unilateral hernia. In our series, 11 babies had respiratory distress syndrome and six required ventilation.

Pathological anatomy

The processus vaginalis has the same anatomical relationship with the cord structures as the peritoneum, lying anterior to the vas deferens and spermatic vessels in the male and to the round ligament in the female. The cremasteric muscle covers the hernial sac. The inguinal canal in the neonate is short and the external inguinal ring nearly overlies the internal ring allowing herniotomy to be performed without opening the inguinal canal.

Incarceration refers to interference with the normal progression of bowel contents in that part of the bowel confined in the hernial sac. Most clinicians use the terms incarceration and irreducibility synonymously [18]. The risk of incarceration in childhood inguinal hernia is substantial (5–18%) [24] and this risk has been reported to be further increased in the first few months of life. In our series 53 (40.8%) had incarceration.

Unrelieved incarceration can lead to intestinal obstruction or gangrene secondary to strangulation. In strangulation, there is venous obstruction of the contents of the hernial sac, leading ultimately to gangrene. The term 'strangulated hernia' is used somewhat loosely by different authors; some use it to describe hernias with commencing vascular changes of the contents [10], others restrict it to hernias with gangrenous contents [56]. In most series of childhood inguinal hernia the frequency of overt gangrenous changes necessitating bowel resection is low (0–1.8%) [1,10,18,24] and in our series none had progressed so far. These figures, however, should not be misinterpreted to suggest that the risk of bowel strangulation in neonatal inguinal hernias is negligible but should rather be interpreted as a satisfactory standard of care in these centres.

An incarcerated inguinal hernia in a neonate poses a serious threat to the viability of the testis as the pressure-effect of the incarcerated hernia contents may jeopardize the precarious vascular supply of the testis causing strangulation of the testis with subsequent infarction and atrophy [4,40,49]. Friedman *et al.* found that 38.4% of male infants with incarcerated hernia in their series had potential gonadal compromise [20]. The incidence of testicular atrophy following incarceration of inguinal hernia has been reported to be between 2.3% and 15% [8,10,26,30,42]. In our series out of 53 incarcerated hernias, eight (15.1%) had reversible ischaemia and one (1.9%) had irreversible ischaemia of the testis. Subsequent atrophy of the testis was detected in two (3.8%).

The contents of the hernia usually have reduced spontaneously at operation after the baby is anaesthetized when emergency surgery is undertaken for incarcerated hernias. In our series, bowel was present in the sac in five (3.8%). Two of these patients had Richter's hernia. Richter's hernia occurs when a portion of the intestinal circumference is incarcerated in the neck of the hernia. According to previous reports, Richter's hernia is extremely rare in children [52]. As the affected segment is small, it may escape clinical detection. Evidence of intestinal obstruction may also be lacking as obliteration of the bowel lumen is incomplete. Unrecognized, the entrapped knuckle of bowel may become gangrenous.

In females, an incarcerated hernia often contains the ovary and the fallopian tube in a sliding manner. This occurred in one of our two female patients.

Splenic tissue (as a result of splenogonadal fusion) and adrenal tissue are occasionally found along the hernial sac [5,39,46,50]. We had one baby with a piece of ectopic adrenal tissue found on his spermatic cord during elective herniotomy.

Interstitial inguinal hernias are rarely described in children [35]. Festen quotes a frequency of between 1 and 2% [19]. We have no such experience.

Incidence

The exact incidence of childhood inguinal hernia is unknown but has been estimated to be 10–20 per 1000 live births [16,33,37,55]. The peak incidence is in early infancy with up to 20% presenting in the first month of life [55]. Boys are more commonly affected than girls. The reported male to female ratio of childhood inguinal hernia ranges from 4:1 [55] to 22:1 [32]. In our series of 130 neonates, 128 were boys and only two were girls. Prematurity accounted for an increasing number of babies presenting with inguinal hernias in the neonatal period in recent years (Figure 26.1). Overall, 62 babies (47.7%) were premature. Eleven babies were small for dates. The condition affected the right side

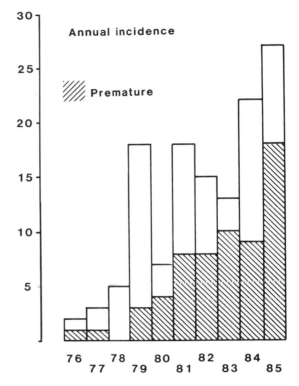

Figure 26.1 Annual incidence of neonatal inguinal hernia in Alder Hey Children's Hospital

more often than the left side but bilateral involvement was also common, particularly in premature babies, of whom more than half had bilateral hernias (Table 26.1).

The incidence of incarceration in childhood has been variously reported as being between 1.6% [22] and 18% [10] of all cases and is said to be more than 50% during the first 3 months of life [44]. In our series of 130 neonates, 53 (40.8%) presented with incarceration. We did not observe an increased incidence of incarceration in premature babies – of 62 premature babies, 17 (27.4%) developed incarceration. This should not be interpreted as suggesting a low risk of incarceration in premature babies

Table 26.1 Location of hernia

	Right n (%)	Left n (%)	Bilateral n (%)
Number of premature babies	25 (40.3)	4 (6.5)	33 (53.2)
Number of term babies	44 (64.7)	8 (11.8)	16 (23.5)
Total number of babies	69 (53.1)	12 (9.2)	49 (37.7)

as it may only be the result of early diagnosis and early treatment of hernias in premature babies in our hospital.

Clinical picture

Symptoms

The presenting feature is commonly the discovery of a groin swelling when the baby cries. When incarceration has occurred the swelling becomes irreducible and painful and the baby screams and becomes irritable. Vomiting of gastric contents is common in incarceration and is usually secondary to peritoneal irritation. When vomiting becomes bile-stained, intestinal obstruction has to be suspected. There is usually no change in bowel habit. Constipation sets in when there is complete intestinal obstruction. Passage of blood per rectum is uncommon and suggests the possibility of strangulated bowel.

Signs

On examination, a groin swelling may be evident. If the swelling has reduced, the experienced examiner will be able to find that the cord is thickened. Sometimes this sign is not definite and the diagnosis may have to depend on a reliable history. When incarceration has occurred, the groin swelling becomes obvious on inspection and it is firm and tender on palpation. The child may be dehydrated if he/she has had repeated vomiting. If intestinal obstruction is present, signs such as abdominal distension or hyperactive bowel sounds will be noticed. If there is bowel strangulation the baby will become toxic. When there is peritonitis, there will be abdominal tenderness and rebound tenderness. An important point of consideration is that in Richter's hernia, the groin swelling may not be obvious and features of intestinal obstruction may be absent.

Examination of the scrotum and testes is essential in all boys with inguinal hernia. The association of inguinal hernia with undescended testis has been mentioned in a previous section. When incarceration has occurred, this part of the examination is even more important in view of the high risk of strangulation of the testis in such circumstances. Scrotal oedema and testicular engorgement are not uncommonly observed. Absence of testis in the scrotum is sometimes noticed and suggests the impaction of an undescended or retractile testis within the hernia. Any sign of compromise of testicular circulation should lead to a greater urgency for the relief of incarceration.

Rectal bimanual examination of the internal inguinal ring has been suggested to be of value in differentiating incarcerated hernias from hydroceles and inguinal adenitis and in ascertaining whether the hernia has been completely reduced [11,13,43,52]. We do not routinely perform this procedure but we do recognize its possible usefulness in difficult clinical situations.

Radiological investigations

Plain abdominal X-ray of an infant with an incarcerated inguinal hernia may occasionally aid the diagnosis by showing air in the inguinoscrotal fold or asymmetrical folds [15].

Herniography [6,9,17,28,29,58,59], the use of contrast such as urografin injected into the peritoneal cavity to outline a hernia sac or patent processus vaginalis, is now seldom practised. Some surgeons employ this technique in situations where physical signs of a hernia are dubious. Others use it to help them to decide if contralateral groin exploration should be performed in cases of unilateral inguinal hernia. Complications are not uncommon. We do not think this investigation is of much value and we do not utilize it.

Differential diagnosis

The differentiation of an incarcerated inguinal hernia in a neonate from other conditions is achieved clinically. A tense hydrocele may mimic a hernia but will not have a history of reducibility. The swelling in a hernia usually has a more prominent inguinal component whereas that in a hydrocele has a more obvious scrotal presentation. An occasional clinical problem arises in the premature baby who develops vomiting and abdominal distension and is noticed to have an inguinoscrotal swelling. It may then be difficult to decide whether this is an incarcerated inguinal hernia causing intestinal obstruction or necrotizing enterocolitis aggravating a hydrocele. A rectal bimanual examination will be helpful if bowel is felt at the internal inguinal ring in the former and blood found per rectum in the latter. The demonstration of intramural gas in plain abdominal X-ray will also be useful in ascertaining the diagnosis of necrotizing enterocolitis.

An incarcerated inguinal hernia may also be mistaken for neonatal torsion of testis. This occurred once in our series. It must also be added that occasionally a small incarcerated hernia may be associated with torsion of testis [4]. In either event of incarcerated hernia or torsion of testis, urgent attention has to be directed to the salvage of the testis. Emergency exploration is advisable if incarceration is unrelieved or if torsion of testis is suspected.

The differentiation of an incarcerated hernia from inguinal lymphadenitis usually is not difficult.

Management

Infants with inguinal hernias should have elective herniotomy as early as possible after diagnosis because of the risk of incarceration. Premature babies pose a special clinical problem as they often have associated medical problems presenting a higher anaesthetic risk as well as suffering more frequent postoperative apnoeic episodes than term babies [31,45,53]. In a survey of paediatric surgeons Rowe and Marchilda found that 30% were reluctant to operate on premature infants with a reducible hernia [47]. We believe that although there is no urgency to operate on such babies, they should have elective herniotomy performed before they are discharged from hospital [21]. However, herniotomy in a premature baby is a difficult procedure and should be done by an experienced surgeon both to minimize operating time (and hence anaesthetic risk) and to ensure adequacy of surgery.

Reduction of incarcerated hernia

Rest, sedation and elevation of the foot end of the cot are often successful in reducing an apparently irreducible hernia. We do not recommend the time-honoured method of placing an ice-pack on the groin as its only effect is to make the infant cry, thus making reduction of the hernia even more difficult. Unless there is evidence that strangulation has progressed to a dangerous degree (as shown by the fact that the infant is in shock and the inguinal swelling is extremely tender), taxis, i.e. gentle efforts at manual reduction of the swelling, should be attempted. Constant pressure on the fundus of the hernia in the direction of the cord is successful surprisingly frequently, but this manoeuvre demands patience and persistent efforts for a reasonable length of time are often required. In the past, reports suggested that nearly 50% of incarcerated inguinal hernias required emergency herniotomy [10,18] but very few patients were actually found to have strangulation. It is our experience that taxis correctly carried out can obviate the necessity of emergency operation in the majority of cases. In our series of 53 incarcerated hernias, 40 (75.5%) were reduced in this manner. After the hernia is reduced, the infant should be kept in hospital for 24–48 h to allow the oedema in the inguinal region to subside after which herniotomy is carried out. Some authors recommend that taxis should not be attempted if symptoms have persisted for more than 8 [17] to 12 [54] h but in our experience the length of the clinical history bears no relationship to the success or failure of taxis. Each patient should be assessed clinically on an individual basis.

Pre-operative management

In infants whose hernia was reduced by taxis 1 or 2 days previously and in infants with irreducible hernias whose general condition is satisfactory, the operation can be performed without any special pre-operative therapy. The shocked, dehydrated infant who has lost quantities of water and electrolytes by prolonged vomiting must be resuscitated by naso-gastric suction and intravenous fluid therapy.

Operation

The standard operation is simple ligation of the hernial sac without opening the external ring. Repair of the posterior wall of inguinal canal is not necessary. It cannot be overemphasized that herniotomy in the neonate is a delicate procedure and should not be left in the hands of the unsupervised surgical apprentice. This is particularly the case when herniotomy is performed on a premature baby and when emergency hernitomy is carried out for incarceration, during which the sac is friable and oedematous and tissue planes are difficult to define.

The infant is placed supine on the operating table. Preparation of the operative field should include both the groin and the scrotum to allow access to the testis. A 1.5-cm incision is made along the skin crease in the groin just lateral to the pubic tubercle (Figure 26.2a). The subcutaneous fat is held up in between two pairs of forceps and incised with diathermy. The Scarpa's fascia is next incised. A pair of scissors is then introduced into the depth of the wound and the blades opened to clear the external ring and the cord of surrounding tissues (Figure 26.2b). The cord is delivered into the wound. In difficult situations one can move the testis upwards and downwards to help the identification of the cord. The cremasteric muscle on the cord is split open along its length and the hernial sac is exposed. The sac is held with a pair of forceps and first the testicular vessels and then the vas deferens which lie successively posteriorly are gently separated from the sac by blunt dissection with fine tissue forceps. Further separation of alveolar tissues around the entire circumference of the sac completes the dissection.

The sac is opened in between pairs of mosquito forceps and the contents can be inspected (Figure 26.2c). Usually the sac is empty. Even at emergency herniotomy for an incarcerated hernia, the hernia not infrequently reduces spontaneously when the infant is anaesthetized; should this occur it is extremely unlikely that bowel viability has been jeopardized. The peritoneal cavity need not be explored unless the hernial sac contains fluid which is dirty and heavily blood-stained. If bowel is present in the sac and remains incarcerated the

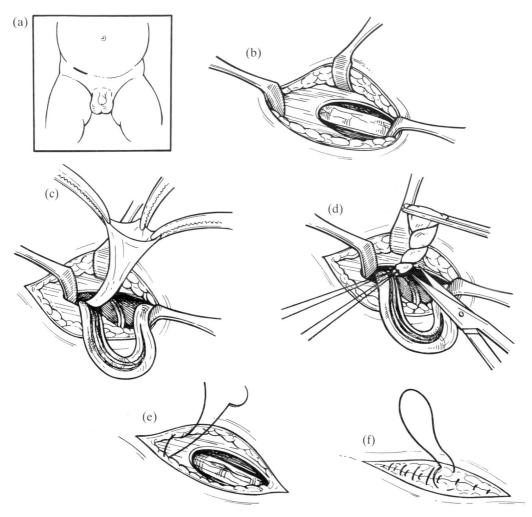

Figure 26.2 (a) Skin incision. (b) Exposure of external inguinal ring. (c) Isolation and opening of hernial sac. (d) Transfixion and ligation of hernial sac. (e) Subcutaneous stitching of superficial fascia. (f) Subcuticular stitch.

constriction ring should be released. The viability of the bowel is then assessed. If viability is doubtful, the bowel is wrapped in packs soaked with warm saline for a few minutes. A return of pinkish coloration, arterial pulsations and peristaltic activity usually occurs. Any doubtful small areas can be oversewn with interrupted seromuscular stitches. If the bowel is non-viable, resection and primary end-to-end anastomosis are carried out in the groin wound. The bowel is then returned to the peritoneal cavity. The testis has to be inspected in incarcerated hernias. If it is clearly gangrenous, orchidectomy is performed. More often, the testis is swollen and looks blue due to venous obstruction. This usually improves after the hernia is reduced. The tunica albuginea may need to be incised to relieve tension

in the testes. In our series, only one testis was obviously gangrenous and removed. Eight testes showed ischaemic changes which improved at operation and were left behind. Of these only one was discovered to have atrophied during follow-up.

Dissection of the hernial sac at the external inguinal ring may or may not have included the fundus of the sac. If the fundus has not been included, the sac is divided at the external ring after a mosquito forceps has been applied proximally. Gentle traction is applied to the proximal part of the sac which is then twisted (Figure 26.2d). The alveolar tissue, spermatic vessels and vas are swept away from the sac with a piece of gauze until the preperitoneal pad of fat is seen at the neck of the sac. The neck of the sac is then doubly transfixed

and the sac is removed. It is of paramount importance that the testis is replaced in the scrotum as it
can easily be dislocated upwards during cord dissection in a neonate. If there is an associated undescended testis, a formal orchidopexy is performed,
placing the testis in the dartos pouch. The Scarpa's
fascia and subcutaneous fat are sutured successively
with interrupted fine catgut stitches (Figure 26.2e).
The skin is closed with a continuous subcuticular
absorbable suture or with adhesive strips (Figure
26.2f).

In females, the sac should always be opened for
examination during herniotomy as the ovary and the
Fallopian tube often lie in the wall of the hernial sac
as sliding elements. In such instances, the hernial sac
can be ligated distal to the ovary and the Fallopian
tube. A purse-string stitch is then placed around the
neck of the sac externally. The proximal sac with the
ovary and the Fallopian tube are invaginated and
the purse-string stitch is tied [61]. An alternative
method is to incise the sac wall on either side of the
ovary and the Fallopian tube to create a U-shaped
flap. This flap with the ovary and the Fallopian tube
is then inverted through the internal ring into the
peritoneal cavity. The edges on either side of the
flap are reapproximated with stitches near the
internal ring, thus reconstituting a complete hernial
sac. Routine herniotomy can then be performed. In
rare instances, when the 'ovary' is not normal-
looking, the possibilities of testicular feminization
and hermaphroditism may have to be considered and
a gonadal biopsy is advisable.

The question of whether the opposite side should
be explored in cases of unilateral inguinal hernia is
a vexed one. According to a survey in 1981, the
majority of American surgeons practise routine
contralateral exploration [48]. There is a high yield
with such an approach but the debatable point is
how often will the contralateral asymptomatic
patent processus vaginalis develop into a symptomatic hernia. In our series, of 53 infants presenting with
unilateral inguinal hernia initially, 12 (12.9%) subsequently developed contralateral hernia. This incidence is slightly higher in premature babies
(19.4%). We do not feel that these figures justify
the bilateral approach in infants with unilateral
hernia. We do, however, agree with Potts [40] who
recommended that only if the hernia is on the left side
should the opposite side be explored because an
isolated left-sided hernia is much rarer than a right-
sided or a bilateral one.

Postoperative management

If the child's general condition is satisfactory,
feeding can be resumed soon after the operation.
The healthy, full-term neonate can usually be
discharged on the day of operation if herniotomy is
done electively or on the day after the operation if
emergency herniotomy is done for incarceration.
The premature baby is more prone to postoperative
attacks of apnoea and bradycardia and should
therefore be observed closely after operation for 24–
48 h in hospital. In our series, of 62 premature
babies undergoing herniotomy, seven (11.3%) had
postoperative apnoeic attacks.

Results

Results of neonatal inguinal herniotomy are generally gratifying. However, advanced incarceration of
inguinal hernia can still carry significant mortality
and morbidity and this is not uncommon in developing countries [11]. In our series of 130 neonates with
inguinal hernia, there were five deaths, four of
which were unrelated to the hernia – three died of
complications of myelomeningocele, and one died
of advanced necrotizing enterocolitis without herniotomy. The remaining death concerns a very
premature baby (26 weeks' gestation) with respiratory distress syndrome and congenital heart disease
who had respiratory problems after herniotomy. He
went on to develop heart failure on postoperative
day 5 and died on day 13 from his cardiorespiratory
problems.

Table 26.2 Complications of inguinal herniotomy in relation to gestational age

	Term infants (n)	Premature infants (n)	Total (n)
Recurrence	0	3	3
Wound infection	3	0	3
Scrotal haematoma	2	2	4
High testis	0	1	1
Atropic testis	1	1	2
Postoperative/respiratory problem	0	7	7
Total	6 (8.8%)	14 (22.6%)	20 (15.4%)

fetus in which closure of the normally formed umbilical ring has failed to take place; either of these explanations would account for the fact that the liver is very rarely eviscerated in gastroschisis and also for the low incidence of non-gastrointestinal anomalies in gastroschisis. Thomas and Atwell [119] suggest that gastroschisis is most probably the end result of intrauterine rupture of an incarcerated hernia of the cord and theorize that this could result from constriction of the intercoelomic communication by over-rapid development of the abdominal musculature. De Vries [29] takes the argument a stage further and suggests that the disruption leading to gastroschisis occurs in the paraumbilical somatopleure as a result of infarction due to disturbances in the circulation to the somatopleure at its junction with the body stalk during involution of the right umbilical vein. That the siting of the gastroschisis defect is connected with umbilical vein involution is borne out by his observation of two cases of left-sided gastroschisis in which the left rather than the right umbilical vein had involuted. Hoyme and colleagues [58] suggest that most cases of gastroschisis are the result of an intrauterine vascular accident involving the omphalomesenteric artery. More recently, however, Glick and colleagues [45] claim to have established the 'missing link' between exomphalos and gastroschisis by documenting *in utero* rupture of a small exomphalos; between 27 weeks and 34.5 weeks of gestation the ultrasound appearances changed from those of a small hernia of the cord to a typical gastroschisis. The condition of the bowel at delivery was consistent with relatively late evisceration. Even more recently Bulut and colleagues [17] have reported what they term a 'pregastroschisis', namely, a gastroschisis-like anomaly, with a sac, within which lay distal ileum with an atresia but without evidence of contact with amniotic fluid. The description suggests that this was a true sac, but unfortunately there is no histological information about it.

Several experimental models of gastroschisis have been studied. Sherman and colleagues [113] produced evisceration by creating small abdominal wall defects in fetal rabbits. Decreased intestinal length and enteritis were produced after only 4 days of exposure to amniotic fluid. Haller and colleagues [54] used a similar technique in fetal lambs and were able to study bowel that had been eviscerated for 10 to 30 days. They documented progressive damage to the neuronal plexuses. Aoki *et al.* [4] also used rabbits and made a special study of the apparent shortening of the eviscerated bowel; the high density of mesenteric vessels indicated that the bowel was 'concertinad', which accords with clinical observations [42]. Klück and colleagues [73] developed a gastroschisis model in the chick embryo and found that the characteristic picture of gastroschisis only evolved when the eviscerated bowel was exposed to urine. From a combined study undertaken in Rotterdam and Glasgow [123] which involved further chick experiments as well as clinical (including prenatal) observations it was concluded that the fibrous coating of the eviscerated bowel is a late occurrence and directly related to changes in amniotic fluid composition, and that both associated intestinal atresia and postoperative hypoperistalsis in the absence of obstruction are also late gestational events caused by ischaemia due to compression of bowel and mesentery in a small defect. Bond and colleagues [12] in San Francisco, in a clinical study which correlated prenatal sonographic findings with clinical outcome could not correlate either time of exposure to amniotic fluid or defect size to eventual clinical outcome. No doubt the rapidly amassing volume of prenatal data in these cases will continue to shed light on the pathogenesis of the condition.

Incidence

Exomphalos and gastroschisis are not common anomalies, but are considerably more common than is apparent to the surgeon, who probably sees only approximately 50% of the total number of cases [127]. This fact was established by McKeown, McMahon and Record [81] who surveyed all infants born during the years 1941–51 in Birmingham (UK). Of the 69 infants with exomphalos (representing an incidence of 1 in 3200) only 34 were live born.

During the decade 1976–85 the Liverpool Malformations Registry documented 78 cases of exomphalos and gastroschisis. Of these, 20 were aborted fetuses (five spontaneous), nine were stillborn and nine died shortly after birth without having been transferred for surgery.

The birth prevalence of exomphalos plus gastroschisis in Liverpool and environs was 1 in 2280 live and stillbirths during the period 1967–75, and 1 in 2780 during the period 1979–83. There can be little doubt that increasing numbers of terminations of pregnancy following prenatal diagnosis have had an influence on birth prevalence. Cases admitted from the area represented by these figures account for only a small proportion of the total admissions to the Liverpool Regional Neonatal Surgical Centre. Over a period of 33 years we have treated 191 cases of exomphalos and 74 cases of gastroschisis. During the 22 years reviewed in the 2nd edition of this book the figures for exomphalos and gastroschisis were 145 and 33 respectively; during the subsequent 11 years the corresponding figures were 45 and 42, a remarkable change in relative incidence. In the exomphalos cases males predominated over females in the ratio of 2:1 whereas in gastroschisis the sexes were affected equally.

Aetiology

It is obvious that exomphalos is caused by some fault in very early embryonic development, but the aetiology of the condition is unknown. Both exomphalos and gastroschisis have been produced experimentally in rodents. In a strain of mice with a genetic predisposition to exomphalos the incidence was increased tenfold by exposure of the animals to low oxygen pressure on the ninth day of gestation [62]. Abdominal wall defects have been induced in rats by folic acid deficiency [90] and by the administration of trypan blue [43], salicylates [128] and streptonigrin [129].

Exomphalos, but not gastroschisis, is a well-recognized feature of the chromosomal trisomy syndromes [74]. The 45 cases which we have treated during the period 1975–85 included two cases each of trisomy 13 (Patau's syndrome), trisomy 18 (Edward's syndrome) and trisomy 21 (Down's syndrome).

The great majority of cases of exomphalos are sporadic, but from time to time familial cases are reported and this has to be borne in mind when parents are counselled [80]. Cases have been reported in two generations of families [56,93], with a possibility of sex-linked inheritance in one family [56]. Our 1953–74 series included two brothers, each with a small exomphalos containing a Meckel's diverticulum, but no other anomalies. Familial cases of the Beckwith–Wiedemann syndrome (see page 382) are encountered more frequently. In the family included in our series of these patients [65] as well as in others [75] the pattern was that of autosomal dominant inheritance (with incomplete penitrance and variable expressivity), but two recent reports [11,14] of the syndrome affecting one of a pair of monozygotic twins suggests a multifactorial aetiology. Duplication of the short arm of chromosome 11 has been found in two unrelated cases, suggesting that the responsible gene or genes may be located on that chromosome [131].

Salinas and colleagues [102] in 1979 reported on the familial occurrence of gastroschisis in two unrelated families and could find no previous familial cases in the literature. This was followed by a report of gastroschisis and exomphalos occurring in siblings [40]. The first reported case of gastroschisis in twins (dizygotic) was possibly related to maternal alcohol consumption [104].

Additional anomalies

Anomalies associated with exomphalos

It has long been recognized that exomphalos is frequently associated with other abnormalities, indicative of a general interference with early embryonic development. Moore [86] found that they occurred in 37% of 236 collected cases. In the analysis of our 1953–74 series of 145 cases for the second edition of this book we found that the same percentage (37%) of infants had one or more additional major anomaly. Table 27.1 lists only the major anomalies found in that series; in addition there were 49 non-obstructive malrotations, 21 Meckel's diverticula (almost always associated with hernias of the cord rather than larger defects), 17 relatively minor cardiovascular anomalies, 16 undescended testes and eight penile anomalies. In addition, large numbers of minor craniofacial and limb anomalies were recorded, almost all of these being features of chromosomal trisomy and Beckwith–Wiedemann syndrome cases.

Our more recent series (1975–85) of 45 cases has been analysed in the manner suggested by Moore [86] and later by Knight and colleagues [74] into 'syndrome' and 'non-syndrome' groups. This is a more meaningful type of analysis than was applied to our earlier series, firstly because it has important prognostic significance [74] (see Table 27.2), and secondly because it allows for a distinction to be made between associated anomalies which are part of a complex syndrome (of which the exomphalos may be a comparatively minor feature) as opposed to more isolated additional anomalies. Both Moore [86] and Knight [74] included cases of Cantrell's pentalogy [19] and of cloacal exstrophy in the syndrome-related group; we have not treated any case of the former and the latter are discussed elsewhere (see Chapter 50).

The 14 'syndrome' cases listed in Table 27.2 exhibited the numerous dysmorphic features typical of the various syndromes. (The features of the Beckwith–Wiedemann syndrome are described in the next section and for excellent descriptions of the three trisomies the reader is referred to Knight and

Table 27.1 Major additional anomalies in 145 cases of exomphalos[a], 1953–74

Major cardiovascular anomalies	26
Malrotation with obstruction[b]	19
Upper urinary tract anomalies	19
Bladder exstrophy	6
Imperforate anus	6
CNS malformations (hydrocephalus, spina bifida)	4
Ileal atresia	3
Prune-belly syndrome	3
Diaphragmatic hernia	2
Duplication cysts	2
Hamartomas (biliary, anorectal)	2
Duodenal atresia	1
Sacrococcygeal teratoma	1

[a] Cases of cloacal exstrophy not included (see Chapter 50)
[b] Cases with Ladd's bands

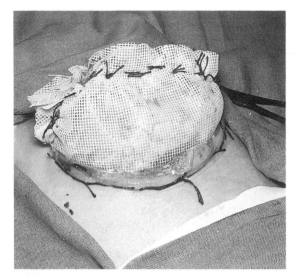

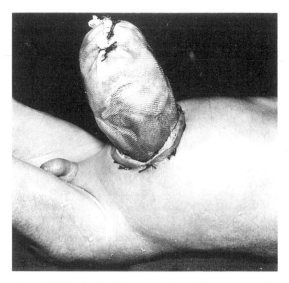

Figure 27.20 Silastic pouch. There is a large abdominal wall defect following excision of an exomphalos sac. Dacron-reinforced silastic has been sutured to the full thickness of the abdominal wall and fashioned into a pouch

Figure 27.21 Silastic 'silo'. A pouch of this type must be suspended from the roof of the incubator by an elastic band

dressing which is subsequently sprayed with povidone-iodine at frequent intervals. If the sac is an elongated one a suture placed through its apex is tied to an elastic band which is looped over a wooden spatula placed across the roof hole of the incubator (Figure 27.21). There should be no tension on the sac and the baby's position should be checked frequently and adjusted if there is any pull on the elastic band.

At intervals of 2–3 days, as judged by the ease with which the sac can be compressed, it is reduced in size, either by placing a lower row of sutures across it or by ligation if it is tubular in shape. This is best done under light anaesthesia, and full aseptic technique must be employed. Excessive 'crowding' within the sac must be avoided as this will result in its premature separation from the abdominal wall. Ideally, after the sac has been reduced in size two or three times over a period of 7–10 days it should be possible to remove it and close the abdominal wall in layers. If, however, this is not achieved and the sac separates after a week or more it will be found that the viscera are covered by a pseudomembrane which prevents evisceration. In our experience, such a membrane will usually contract and epithelialize quite rapidly if it is protected by sterile dressings and antiseptic applications, and as long as an enteric fistula does not complicate the situation.

Seashore and colleagues [109] reported that porcine skin grafts and human amniotic membrane used as biological dressings provide effective control of wound infection after premature separation of a silastic pouch. Anderl and colleagues [3] have used mesh skin autografts successfully in such cases and Hutson and Azmy [61] report favourably on the use of preserved dura and pericardium in these problem cases. It must be stressed that sepsis is always a hazard while a silastic sac remains *in situ*.

Use of synthetic fascial 'gusset'

Schuster [107] no longer uses the silastic method but, in cases where primary repair is impossible, prefers to bridge the gap between the rectus muscles with Teflon mesh over the intact sac, usually without skin closure initially. The mesh is excised in stages, the skin usually being closed at the second stage. Stone [115] uses a similar gusset but uses polypropylene fabric, excises the sac and covers the patch with mobilized skin flaps; the gusset is retained permanently.

Closure of gastroschisis defects

One of the notable achievements of paediatric surgery in the 1970s was the marked improvement in the chances of survival for infants with gastroschisis. That this was due in some measure to the introduction of the silastic techniques cannot be denied, but there have been many reports of equally good and sometimes better survival rates being achieved by the use of the conventional methods of primary full-thickness closure or skin flap closure [20,36,38].

The most important single factor which has improved survival rates is undoubtedly the widespread use of intravenous feeding in the postoperative period, but a second important factor has been the widespread adoption of the simple manoeuvre of thorough stretching of the abdominal wall during operation [66,78,96].

As stated previously, surgery should not be delayed once measures have been taken to improve the infant's general condition. The protective intestinal bag is left on until the infant is anaesthetized and lying on a warmed mattress on the operating table. Throughout the operation careful attention must be paid to keeping the exposed bowel warm. It is first gently cleaned with warmed aqueous chlorhexidine. Any loose exudate or debris is removed but no attempt should be made to remove the adherent 'peel' as this can cause excessive bleeding and even perforation. Furthermore, removal is unnecessary as the 'peel' resolves when the bowel is returned to the peritoneal cavity. Preoperative nasogastric suction and rectal irrigations will have decompressed the bowel to some extent but further improvement can usually be achieved by gently 'milking' the bowel contents upwards and downwards [121]. Enterotomies [28] for deflation of the bowel have no advantage over these methods and should not be carried out [100]. The abdominal wall defect almost always has to be enlarged before the viscera can be returned to the abdomen and this should be done by vertical incision upwards and downwards (Figure 27.22). The abdominal wall should now be thoroughly stretched, starting in the flanks and working towards the midline, between two fingers inside and the thumb outside. This manoeuvre can double the capacity of the abdomen [96] and can allow it to accommodate seemingly impossible amounts of bowel (Figure 27.23)

The intestine must be inspected from end to end for atresias and any sharp kinks should be straightened out by careful dissection. Gangrenous bowel must be resected. In cases with lesser degrees of serosal reaction primary anastomosis may be feasible and is preferable to exteriorization [78,96], but the latter may be unavoidable if the intestine is grossly thick and rigid. If there is doubt about bowel viability, especially if a large proportion of the bowel is in question a 'second look' policy is wise as the vascularity of the bowel may be much better than appearances suggest [125]. We agree with Lewis and colleagues [78] and van Hoorn and colleagues [125] that most atresias are best left alone at the initial operation and can be dealt with after 2–3 weeks of intravenous alimentation, by which time the intestine will be in a more normal state, allowing resection and anastomosis to be done with minimal risk.

Primary layered closure can be done without difficulty in the rare cases with small amounts of

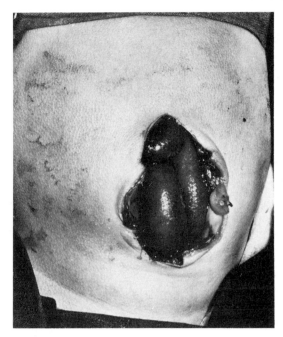

Figure 27.22 Primary closure of gastroschisis. The small abdominal wall defect has been extended by vertical incisions upwards and downwards. Thorough stretching of the abdominal wall has permitted replacement of the viscera

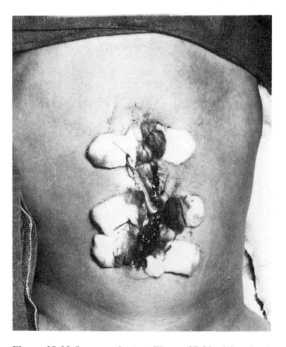

Figure 27.23 Same patient as Figure 27.22. After further stretching of the abdominal wall closure has been achieved. Horizontal mattress deep tension stitches have been tied over 'dental rolls'

prolapsed bowel and in those in which a major resection has been necessary. It can also be achieved in a surprisingly high proportion of 'full-blown' cases if abdominal wall stretching and intestinal decompression have been used to maximal effect [20,36]. It should only be done, however, if the surgeon and anaesthetist are satisfied that the infant's lung compliance and cardiac return are not being compromised. Some authors [96,119] insist that simple skin closure without undermining is the procedure of choice. Wesson and Baesl [134] describe a technique for preservation of the umbilicus.

If the viscera cannot be accommodated in the peritoneal cavity without 'crowding' the alternatives available are as for the large exomphalos. Coverage of the bowel with undermined skin flaps has a low incidence of sepsis but the large ventral hernia requires later correction. Use of a silastic sac carries the risk of sepsis and premature separation of the prosthesis, but if staged reduction of the viscera can be achieved in 7–10 days without complications the child will be left with a sound abdominal wall or, at worst, a small ventral hernia. As in the case of omphalocele, cases in which the sac separates prematurely can usually be managed conservatively by virtue of pseudomembrane formation. The use of the synthetic fascial 'gusset' is also applicable to the unclosable gastroschisis. Schuster [107] recommends the use of a lining of thin silastic sheeting between the Teflon and the bowel; both he and Stone [115] record some problems with infection.

Opinions vary about the necessity for performing a gastrostomy for decompression in cases of gastroschisis. We have not employed gastrostomy in these cases for several years and find that decompression via a nasogastric tube is perfectly adequate.

Postoperative management

After repair of a small exomphalos postoperative management is usually quite straightforward; oral intake can usually be started after 48 h of nasogastric suction and intravenous fluids.

Babies with the Beckwith–Wiedemann syndrome can present special problems. Hypoglycaemia is the main hazard. Blood glucose levels should be estimated routinely at least twice daily during the first postoperative week and immediately if the infant develops signs of hypoglycaemia. Intensive and prolonged treatment may be required in some cases [24]. Hypocalcaemia may also be encountered in BWS cases [65]. If the tongue is very large it may fall back, causing respiratory obstruction when the infant is lying supine. This complication can be prevented by nursing the child in the face-down head-down position [65]. Feeding difficulties due to the macroglossia can usually be overcome by the use of an extra-long soft teat, but occasionally tube feeding may be necessary.

Ventilatory support may be necessary postoperatively and is of particular benefit in the babies who have had a primary fascial closure and have a tense abdomen. These babies benefit greatly from a short period of elective ventilation. In any other cases, if respiratory efforts are weak when spontaneous breathing recommences at the end of the operation, the endotracheal tube should be left *in situ* and ventilatory support given; it is rarely required for more than 48 h.

In cases of gastroschisis a prolonged period of ileus can be anticipated, particularly when the bowel has been grossly thickened and matted. During this time the bowel must be kept decompressed by continuous nasogastric suction and nutrition maintained by total intravenous parenteral nutrition (see Chapter 5), which may have to be continued for several weeks. Oral feeding should never be attempted while a silastic prosthesis is *in situ*. When gastrointestinal function returns in these cases malabsorption and intestinal hurry can be very troublesome and lactose-free or predigested feeds may have to be given until normal feeds are tolerated.

Sepsis is a constant hazard while a silastic sac is *in situ*. Antibiotics are given (usually penicillin and gentamicin) and modified if necessary according to bacteriological findings. Strict aseptic technique must be used if the silastic sac has to be redressed. While a central venous line is in place for intravenous feeding the danger of septicaemia exists and frequent blood culture is advisable. Prophylactic nystatin reduces the risk of *Candida* septicaemia [42].

As mentioned earlier, serum protein levels are likely to be abnormally low at birth in babies with gastroschisis [53]. Protein losses are also heavy when a silastic sac has been applied [141]. Serum protein levels are estimated daily and plasma is infused daily in the early postoperative period.

Conservative management of exomphalos

If infection and rupture of the sac can be prevented, the skin of the anterior abdominal wall will slowly grow over it, thus forming a ventral hernia which, because of cicatrization, is usually not as large as those produced by staged operations. The method consists in repeated application of an antiseptic lotion to the sac, which after a few days forms a dry eschar. This separates after about 3 weeks, leaving a granulating surface which gradually epithelializes from the edges.

The use of mercurial antiseptics [48] should be avoided as it has been shown [34] that they can produce blood and tissue levels of mercury well above minimum toxic levels. Safe alternatives are 65% or 70% alcohol or 1% aqueous gentian violet [21]. Once a thick scab has formed, a dry antiseptic

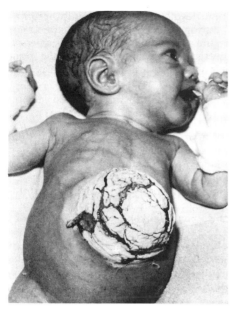

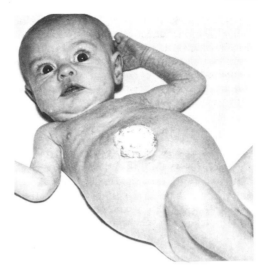

Figure 27.25 Same case as in Figure 27.24 after 7 weeks' conservative treatment

Figure 27.24 Large exomphalos treated conservatively

powder can be used (Figures 27.24 and 27.25). Systemic antibiotics should always be given. The ventral hernia usually requires repair at a later date, but occasionally it disappears completely.

The advantage of non operative management is obvious in the case of the infant who is in poor general condition, or who has anomalies that carry a very poor prognosis, for example trisomies 13 and 18. It might also be the treatment of choice in babies with other major anomalies which require more urgent surgery than the exomphalos; for example oesophageal atresia. The principal disadvantage of the method is the fact that the abdominal viscera are not inspected and hence the danger exists of underlying unrecognized anomalies [82] causing complications, notably intestinal obstruction, which may also result from adhesion formation between intestine and sac. In addition, the conservative method is time consuming. Depending on the size of the exomphalos, the infant may be in hospital for up to 5 months [37]. Despite these disadvantages and despite improvements in surgical results there are many who still regard this method as the one of choice in selected cases, notably the 'giant' sacs [21,37,47,133].

Results

In 18 series of intact exomphalos collected from the literature of 1959–69 mortality averaged 41.5% [95].

Despite advances in surgical techniques and particularly in general management, overall mortality remains around 25% [74,84,108] a fact which is largely attributable to associated severe anomalies.

In Liverpool our mortality figures for exomphalos have fallen from 40% for the period 1953–66 to 20% for the period 1975–85. As will be seen from Table 27.2 the nine deaths in the 1975–85 series included seven 'syndrome-related' cases and two 'non-syndrome' cases. The latter included a child with pulmonary hypoplasia who died without surgery and a child with oesophageal atresia and subglottic stenosis who died of tracheostomy complications. We cannot, however, afford to be complacent about our low mortality in the 'non-syndrome' group as there is little doubt that in recent years we have seen a shift in the pattern of referrals towards the less severe end of the spectrum, consequent on prenatal diagnosis and selective abortion; this probably accounts for the unusually low incidence of cardiac malformations in the 1975–85 series. Of the syndrome-related cases, the deaths of the trisomy 13 and 18 patients were not surprising but the death of three BWS patients out of seven was more remarkable; one of these was a very unusual BWS, having a huge exomphalos, low birth weight, RDS and intraventricular haemorrhage (IVH). IVH was the cause of death in another of the BWS cases whilst the third died at 16 months, cause obscure. In general the prognosis for BWS is good if they can be tided over the neonatal period, and despite the numerous anomalies they have the potential for

perforation has occurred, the anaesthetist should be asked to inject air by syringe down the nasogastric tube. The mucosa of the pyloric canal will then be seen to bulge through the incision and any perforation, however small, would be noticeable by the escape of air bubbles from it.

The pylorus is returned into the abdomen. It is usually not necessary to stop any bleeding from the cut muscle by cautery or ligation as this is mainly due to venous engorgement brought about by delivering the tumour into the wound. It will stop as soon as the pylorus is returned into the abdominal cavity.

The abdominal wound is closed in layers. For the skin, we prefer a running subcuticular suture of 4/0 catgut which eliminates the necessity of removing skin sutures later on. If an intravenous infusion has been set up it is wise to keep it going in the immediate postoperative period rather than to remove it at the end of the operation, especially in the child who has had a considerable period of starvation and whose hepatic glycogen stores are depleted to such an extent that hypoglycaemia may occur before an adequate caloric intake can be established [77,147].

Postoperative management

The baby is returned to the ward when fully conscious. He is kept lying flat on his side and a close watch is kept in case he vomits and aspirates vomitus. Oral feeding is started 4 h after operation and, when established, intravenous fluids are discontinued. The pyloric feeding regimen used in the Royal Liverpool Children's Hospital (Alder Hey) is outlined in Table 28.3

Gastric stasis probably lasts for 12 h or more after operation and some surgeons therefore advocate a late start to feeding [144], resting the stomach for 18–24 h postoperatively. The incidence of postoperative vomiting is said to be reduced by such a

Table 28.3 Pyloric regimen, Alder Hey Children's Hospital

Hours postoperatively	Amount (ml)	Feed
4	4	5% glucose water
6	4	Milk
8	8	5% glucose water
10	8	Milk
12	15	5% glucose water
14	15	Milk
16	25	5% glucose water
18	25	Milk
20	30	5% glucose water
22	30	Milk
24	45	5% glucose water
26	45	Milk

Table 28.4 Delayed pyloric feeding regimen

Hours postoperatively	Amount (ml)	Feed
18	15	5% glucose water
21	15	5% glucose water
24	30	5% glucose water
27	30	5% glucose water
30	30	½ st milk
33	45	½ st milk
36	45	F/S milk

Then increased by 15 ml each feed to the full amount for expected weight. Small vomits should be ignored. If large amounts are vomited then aspirate stomach and return to previous step in regimen

regimen and the period of hospital stay is not lengthened [103]. We have used such a feeding schedule (Table 28.4) and have found the results satisfactory but the infants seem restless and hungry and cry and swallow air more obviously on the delayed schedule than the prompt one. If all goes well on either regimen of feeding the infant can be discharged 72 h after operation, though this is a minimum time under the most favourable circumstances and in general it would be difficult to reduce the average postoperative stay to less than 4 days [112]. A short stay in hospital greatly reduces the risk of cross-infection, a risk forever present in children's wards. If there is any postoperative vomiting, feeds may have to be temporarily reduced in quantity or be omitted altogether. At times when there is a lot of gastric mucus it may be helpful to wash the stomach out with warm saline. Sitting the baby up during and between feeds often prevents vomiting in those cases where there is an associated hiatus hernia [60].

Medical treatment

The medical treatment of pyloric stenosis is based on the fact that if the infant can be kept alive, the symptoms will ultimately disappear, probably because the pyloric canal, taking part in the infant's general growth, will ultimately be wide enough to allow food to pass into the duodenum without hindrance. Medical treatment consists of dietetic methods, gastric lavage and the administration of antispasmodics.

Careful graduated feeding at 3- or even 2-hourly intervals and refeeding after the child had vomited were recommended in the beginning of this century [86,172].

Gastric lavage with warm normal saline was popularized by Kussmaul [97] in 1869. It is of especial use when there is gastritis and a lot of thick mucus in the stomach.

Atropine was recommended by von Struempel [157] in 1904 but was not found to be very effective until Swensgaard [161] introduced methylatropine nitrate which can be given in watery or alcoholic solution. Later on the drug was dispensed in the form of lamellae which are given sublingually before feeds. Scopolamine (scopolamine methylnitrate), given by mouth in doses 0.1 mg six times daily 15 min before each feed, has an even better spasmolytic effect.

The disadvantages of medical treatment are that its progress is uncertain and that the infant needs expert nursing care in hospital for a prolonged period [165].

Balloon dilatation of the pylorus

Balloon dilatation of the pyloric canal has been tried successfully at Alder Hey Children's Hospital. The balloon is inserted under gastroscopic control. Preliminary reports suggest that the technique is as effective as pyloromyotomy (P.K.H. Tam, personal communication).

Results

In the past the early mortality rate for Ramstedt's operation remained high; in the UK the overall mortality rate was estimated to be as high as 25% as late as the Second World War [138]. In recent years many large series have been published from paediatric surgical centres in Europe and North America showing a very low operative mortality [15,52,73]. Current mortality rates are well under 1%.

The myotomy heals by fibrous scarring and if seen some months later looks remarkably normal. The radiological appearances remain abnormal for long periods after Ramstedt's operation and if the obstructed pylorus is bypassed by some other procedure, the classic radiological signs persist for many years. Gastric emptying is measurably faster and duodenogastric reflux found more commonly in children after pyloromyotomy than in normal controls [168] and this may be the basis of the dyspepsia reported by Soloweijczyk in 24 out of 41 patients 15–30 years after operation [151]. There is clearly a need for detailed long-term studies to determine whether the incidence of gastritis and peptic ulceration is significantly higher. In childhood, growth and development is normal and abdominal symptoms are absent [114,159]. Berglund and Rabo [16,17] found no difference in the later mortality rate for boys operated on between 1922 and 1942 from that of the general population, though intriguingly a disproportionate number of them died violent deaths in later years – a statistic for which there is no obvious explanation.

Atwell and Levick [7], mindful of associated urinary tract problems, suggest that infants should be followed to ensure freedom from urinary infection.

References

1. Ahmed, S. (1970) Infantile pyloric stenosis associated with major anomalies of the alimentary tract. *J. Pediat. Surg.*, **5**, 660
2. Anas, P. and Miller, R.C. (1971) Pyloric duplication masquerading as hypertrophic pyloric stenosis. *J. Pediat. Surg.*, **6**, 664
3. Arey, L.B. (1966) *Developmental Anatomy*, W.B. Saunders, Philadelphia
4. Arias, I., Schoor, J.B. and Fraad, L.M. (1959) Congenital hypertrophic pyloric stenosis with jaundice. *Pediatrics*, **24**, 338–342
5. Armstrong, G. (1777) An account of the diseases most incident to children from their birth to the age of puberty etc. London
6. Atwell, J.D., Cook, P.L., Strong, L., Hyde, I. (1977) The interrelationship between vesico-ureteric reflux, trigonal abnormalities and a bifid pelvi-calyceal collecting system: a family study. *Br. J. Urol.*, **49**, 97–107
7. Atwell, J.D., Levick, P. (1981) Congenital hypertrophic pyloric stenosis and associated anomalies in the genito-urinary tract. *J. Pediat. Surg.*, **16**, 1029–1035
8. Beardsley, H. (1788) *Congenital hypertrophic stenosis of the pylorus. Cases and observations by the Medical Society of New York*. F. Meigs, New Haven
9. Belding, H.H. and Kernohan, J.W. (1953) A morphologic study of the myenteric plexus and musculature of the pylorus. *Surg. Gynec. Obstet.*, **97**, 322–334
10. Bell, M.J. (1968) Infantile pyloric stenosis: experience with 305 cases at Louisville Children's Hospital. *Surgery*, **64**, 983–989
11. Bell, M.J., Ternberg, J.L., Keating, J.P., Moedjona, S., McAlister, W. and Shackelford, G.D. (1978) Prepyloric gastric antral web: a puzzling epidemic. *J. Pediat. Surg.*, **13**, 307–314
12. Belloli, G., Locatelli, G. and Bedogni, L. (1979) The treatment of congenital pyloric atresia. *Ped. Med. Chir.*, **1**, 53–56
13. Bennett, R.J. Jr (1937) Atresia of the pylorus. *Am. J. Dig. Dis.*, **4**, 44
14. Benson, C.D. and Adelman, S. (1979) Prepyloric and pyloric obstruction. In *Pediatric Surgery*, Vol. 2, (ed. M.M. Ravitch, K.J. Welch, C.D. Benson, E. Aberdeen and J.G. Randolph) Year Book Medical Publishers, Chicago
15. Benson, C.D. and Coury, J.J. (1951) Congenital intrinsic obstruction of the stomach and duodenum in the newborn. *Arch. Surg.*, **62**, 856–866
16. Berglund, G. and Rabo, E. (1973) A long-term follow-up investigation of patients with hypertrophic pyloric stenosis – with special reference to the physical and mental development. *Acta Paediat. Scand.*, **62**, 125–129
17. Berglund, G. and Rabo, E. (1973) A long-term follow up investigation of patients with hypertrophic pyloric stenosis – with special reference to heredity

and later morbidity. *Acta Paediat. Scand.*, **62**, 130–132

18. Berman, J.K. and Ballenger, F. (1942) Prepyloric membranous obstruction. *Bull. Indiana Univ. Med. Center*, **4**, 14–16

19. Blair, P. (1717) An account of the dissection of a child. *Phil. Trans.*, **30**, 631

20. Blumhagen, J.D. (1986) The role of ultrasonography in the evaluation of vomiting in infants. *Pediat. Radiol.*, **16**, 267–270

21. Bommen, M. and Singh, M.P. (1984) Pyloric duplication in a preterm neonate. *J. Pediat. Surg.*, **19**, 158–159

22. Boyden, E.A., Cope, J.G. and Bill, A.H. (1967) Anatomy and embryology of congenital intrinsic obstruction of the duodenum. *Am. J. Surg.*, **114**, 190–202

23. Bronsther, B., Nadeau, M.R. and Abrams, M.W. (1971) Congenital pyloric atresia – a report of three cases and a review of the literature. *Surgery*, **69**, 130–136

24. Brown, R.P. and Hertzler, J.H. (1959) Congenital prepyloric gastric atresia – a report of two cases. *Am. J. Dis. Child.*, **97**, 857–862

25. Browne, D. (1951) The technique of Ramstedt's operation. *Proc. Roy. Soc. Med.*, **44**, 1057–1059

26. Burnett, H.A. and Halpert, B. (1947) Perforation of the stomach of a newborn infant with pyloric atresia. *Arch. Path.*, **44**, 318–320

27. Cantley, E. and Dent, C.T. (1903) Congenital hypertrophic pyloric stenosis and its treatment by pyloroplasty. *Med. -chir. Trans.*, **86**, 471

28. Carter, C.O. (1961) Genetic factors in pyloric stenosis. *Proc. Roy. Soc. Med.*, **54**, 453–454

29. Carter, C.O. (1976) Genetics of common single malformations. *Br. Med. Bull.*, **32**, 21–26

30. Carter, C.O. and Evans, K.A. (1969) Inheritance of congenital pyloric stenosis. *J. Med. Genet.*, **6**, 233–254

31. Casasa, J.M., Lafuente, J.M., Boix-Ochoa, J., Tornio, R., Infente, D. and Carol, J. (1977) Gastrin and gastric acidity in hypertrophic pyloric stenosis. *Ann. Chir. Infant.*, **18**, 363–369

32. Chang, C.H., Perrin, E.V. and Bove, K.E. (1983) Pyloric atresia associated with epidermolysis bullosa: special reference to pathogenesis. *Pediat. Pathol.*, **1**, 449–457

33. Chaves-Carballo, E., Harris, L.E. and Lynn, H.B. (1968) Jaundice associated with pyloric stenosis and neonatal small bowel obstructions. *Clin. Pediat.*, **7**, 198–202

34. Cochran, W.D. (1975) Infantile hypertrophic pyloric stenosis. *Arch. Dis. Child.*, **50**, 907

35. Cockaigne, E.A. and Penrose, L.S. (1934) Congenital pyloric stenosis in first cousins. *Lancet*, **i**, 898

36. Cordua, E. (1892) *Ein Fall von einem monstrosen Blindsac des Dickdarms*. Dieterich, Goetingen

37. Cremin, B.J. (1967) Neonatal prepyloric membrane. *S. Afr. med. J.*, **41**, 1076–1079

38. Cremin, B.J. and Klein, A. (1968) Infantile pyloric stenosis: a 10 year survey. *S. Afr. med. J.*, **42**, 1056–1060

39. Crooks (1828) Estomac se terminant en cul-de-sac. *Arch. Gen. Med.*, **17**, 264

40. Czeizel, A. (1972) Birthweight distribution in congenital pyloric stenosis. *Arch. Dis. Child.*, **47**, 978–980

41. Davis, D.A. and Douglas, K.R. (1961) Congenital pyloric atresia, a rare anomaly. *Ann. Surg.*, **153**, 418–422

42. Davison, G. (1946) The incidence of pyloric stenosis. *Arch Dis. Child.*, **21**, 113–114

43. De Spirito, A.J. and Guthorn, P.J. (1957) Recovery from meconium peritonitis associated with diaphragmatic obstruction of the prepyloric mucosa. *J. Pediat.*, **50**, 599–602

44. Devroede, G. and Beaudry, R. (1971) Small bowel volvulus, malabsorption and mucosal diaphragm of the pylorus. *Am. J. Dig. Dis.*, **16**, 953–958

45. Dineen, J.P. and Redo, S.F. (1963) Pyloric obstruction due to mucosal diaphragm. *Surgery*, **53**, 674–676

46. Dodge, J.A. (1970) Production of duodenal ulcer and hypertrophic pyloric stenosis by administration of pentagastrin to pregnant and newborn dogs. *Nature, Lond.*, **225**, 284–285

47. Dodge, J.A. (1973) Infantile pyloric stenosis, inheritance, psyche and soma. *Ir. J. med. Sci.*, **142**, 6–18

48. Dodge, J.A. (1974) Changing incidence of congenital pyloric stenosis. *Br. med. J.*, **1**, 640

49. Dodge, J.A. (1974) Maternal factors in infantile hypertrophic pyloric stenosis. *Arch Dis. Child.*, **49**, 825

50. Dodge, J.A. (1975) Infantile hypertrophic pyloric stenosis in Belfast. *Arch Dis. Child.*, **50**, 171–178

51. Dodge, J.A. (1975) Infantile hypertrophic pyloric stenosis. *Arch Dis. Child.*, **50**, 907

52. Donovan, E.J. (1946) Congenital hypertrophic pyloric stenosis. *Ann. Surg.*, **124**, 709–715

53. Ducharme, J.C. and Bensoussan, A.L. (1975) Pyloric atresia. *J. Pediat. Surg.*, **10**, 149–150

54. Dufour, H. and Fredet, P. (1908) La sclerose hypertrophique du pylore chez le nourisson et son traitement chirurgical. *Revue Chir.*, **27**, 208–253

55. Evans, N.J. (1982) Pyloric stenosis in preterm infants after transpyloric feeding. *Lancet*, **ii**, 665

56. Farack, U.M., Goresky, C.A., Jabbari, M. and Kinnear, D.H. (1974) Double pylorus: a hypothesis concerning its pathogenesis. *Gastroenterology*, **66**, 596–600

57. Felsher, B.F., Asch, M., Carpio, N. and Woolley, M. (1973) Unconjugated hyperbilirubinaemia in neonates with congenital gastrointestinal obstruction. *Gastroenterology*, **64**, 151–152

58. Finsen, V.R. (1979) Infantile hypertrophic pyloric stenosis – unusual familial incidence. *Arch Dis. Child.*, **54**, 720–721

59. Finny, C.E. (1908) Duodenal ulcers with perforation in an infant with hypertrophic stenosis of the pylorus. *Proc. Roy. Soc. Med.*, **2**, 67–70

60. Forshall, I. (1955) The cardio-oesophageal syndrome in childhood. *Arch Dis. Child.*, **30**, 46–54

61. Franken, E.A. and Saldino, R.M. (1969) Hypertrophic pyloric stenosis complicating esophageal atresia with tracheo-esophageal fistula. *Am. J. Surg.*, **117**, 647–649

62. Freer, E. (1924) Die angeborene pylorusstenose. In *Handbuch der Kinderkrankheiten.* Verlag Vogel, Berlin

63. Friesen, S.R., Boley, J.O. and Miller, D.R. (1956) The myenteric plexus of the pylorus. *Surgery*, **39**, 21–29

64. Garrow, E. and Hertzler, J. (1966) Hypertrophic pyloric stenosis with jaundice: a case report of one family. *J. Pediat. Surg.*, **1**, 284–287

65. Georgi, B.A., Slim, M.S. and Muffarrij, A.B. (1984) Pyloric duplication simulating pyloric stenosis. *Ann. Paediat. Surg.*, **1**, 130–133

66. Gerber, B.C. (1965) Prepyloric diaphragm, an unusual abnormality. *Arch. Surg.*, **90**, 472–480

67. Glasson, M.J., Bandrevics, V. and Cohen, D.H. (1973) Hypertrophic pyloric stenosis complicating esophageal atresia. *Surgery*, **74**, 530–535

68. Gray, S.W. and Skandalakis, J.E. (1972) *Embryology for Surgeons*, W.B. Saunders, Philadelphia

69. Grob, M. (1957) *Lehrbuch der Kinderchirurgie*, Georg Thieme, Stuttgart

70. Grochowski, J., Szafran, H., Sztefko, K., Janik, A. and Szafran, Z. (1980) Blood serum immunoreactive gastrin level in infants with hypertrophic pyloric stenosis. *J. Pediat. Surg.*, **15**, 279–282

71. Grosfeld, J.L., Boles, E.T. and Reiner, C. (1970) Duplication of the pylorus in the newborn. *J. Pediat. Surg.*, **5**, 365–369

72. Grosfeld, J.L., O'Neill, J.A. and Clatworthy, H.W. (1970) Enteric duplication in infancy and childhood. An 18 year review. *Ann. Surg.*, **172**, 83–90

73. Gross, R.E. (1953) *The Surgery of Infancy and Childhood*, W.B. Saunders, Philadelphia

74. Hambourg, M.A., Mignon, M. and Ricour, C. (1979) Serum gastrin levels in hypertrophic pyloric stenosis of infancy. *Arch. Dis. Child.*, **54**, 208–212

75. Hart Hansen, O., Kronborg, O. and Pedersen, T. (1972) The double pylorus. *Scand. J. Gastroenterol.*, **7**, 695

76. Hart Hansen, O., Pedersen, T. and Johansen, A. (1974) Double pylorus: an overlooked lesion? *Gastroenterology*, **67**, 1082

77. Henderson, B.M., Schubert, W.K., Hug, G. and Martin, L.W. (1968) Hypoglycaemia with hepatic glycogen depletion: a post-operative complication of pyloric stenosis. *J. Pediat. Surg.*, **3**, 309–316

78. Henderson, J.L., Mason Brown, J.J. and Taylor, W.C. (1952) Clinical observations on pyloric stenosis in preterm infants. *Arch. Dis. Child.*, **27**, 175–178

79. Herweg, J.C., Middlekamp, J.N., Thornton, H.K. and Reed, C.A. (1962) A search into the etiology of hypertrophic pyloric stenhosis. *J. Pediat.*, **61**, 309–310

80. Hicks, L.M., Morgan, A., Andersen, M.R. (1981) Pyloric stenosis – a report of triplet females and notes on its inheritance. *J. Pediat. Surg.*, **16**, 739–740

81. Hight, D.E., Benson, C.D., Philippat, A.I. and Hertzler, J.H. (1981) Management of mucosal perforation during pyloromyotomy for infantile pyloric stenosis. *Surgery*, **90**, 85–86

82. Hildanus, F. (1646) *Opera Omnia*. Joh. Beyerns, Frankfurt

83. Hirschsprung, H. (1888) Fälle van angeborenen Pylorusstenose, beobachtet bei Saenlingen. *Jb. Kinderheilk.*, **28**, 61

84. Holladay, L.J. (1946) A case report of congenital aplasia of the pylorus. *J. Indiana St. med. Ass.*, **39**, 350–351

85. Hyman, P.E., Clarke, D.D. and Everett, S.L. (1985) Gastric acid secretory function in pre-term infants. *J. Pediat.*, **106**, 467–471

86. Ibrahim, J. (1905) *Die angeborenen Pylorusstenose in Senglingsalter*, S. Karger, Berlin

87. Iwai, N., Nanri, M., Hashimoto, K., Kaneda, H. and Majima, S. (1984) Serum gastrin levels and lower oesophageal sphincter pressures in infants with congenital hypertrophic pyloric stenosis. *Z. Kinderchir.*, **39**, 234–236

88. Janik, J.S., Akbar, A.M. and Burrington, J.D. (1978) The role of gastrin in congenital hypertrophic pyloric stenosis. *J. Pediat. Surg.*, **13**, 151–153

89. Jona, J.Z. (1978) Electron microscopic observations in infantile hypertrophic pyloric stenosis. *J. Pediat. Surg.*, **13**, 17–20

90. Kadowaki, H., Takenchi, S. and Nakahira, M. (1981) Congenital pyloric atresia. *Am. J. Gastroenterology*, **76**, 449–452

91. Kammerer, G.T. (1969) Duplication of the stomach resembling hypertrophic pyloric stenosis. *J. Am. med. Ass.*, **207**, 2101–2102

92. Kekomaki, M. and Kuitunen, P. (1974) Simultaneous occurrence of congenital pyloric web and hiatal insufficiency in an infant. *Helv. Paediat. Acta*, **29**, 595–598

93. Kelsey, D., Stayman, J.W., McLaughlin, E.D. and Mebane, W. (1968) Massive bleeding in a newborn infant from a gastric ulcer associated with hypertrophic pyloric stenosis. *Surgery*, **64**, 979–989

94. Keramidas, D.C. (1974) Congenital pyloric atresia in siblings. *Arch. Surg.*, **108**, 123

95. Keramidas, D.C. (1974) Congenital incomplete prepyloric diaphragm in infants and children. *Surgery*, **75**, 690–694

96. Kornfield, H.J. (1962) Pyloric atresia and its repair. *Surgery*, **51**, 569–573

97. Kussmaul, A. (1869) *Ueber die Behandlung der Magenerweiterung.* H.M. Pappen und Sohn, Freiburg

98. Laron, Z. and Horne, L.M. (1957) The incidence of infantile pyloric stenosis. *Am. J. Dis. Child.*, **94**, 151–154

99. Larsen, G.L. (1966) Limitations of roentgenographic examination in the diagnosis of infantile hypertrophic pyloric stenosis. *Surgery*, **60**, 768–772

49. Lecco, T.M. (1910) Zur Morphologie des Pankreas Annulare. *Sitzungsber. Akad. Wissensch.*, **119**, 391–406

50. Lenz, W. (1963) Chemicals and malformations in man. *Proceedings of the Second International Conference on Congenital Malformations.* International Medical Congress, New York

51. Lister, J. (1986) *Complications of Paediatric Surgery*, Baillière Tindall, London, pp. 85–90

52. Lloyd, J.R. and Clatworthy, H.W. (1958) Hydramnios as an aid to the early diagnosis of congenital obstructions of the alimentary tract: A study of the maternal and fetal factors. *Pediatrics*, **21**, 903–909

53. Longo, M.F. and Lynn, H.B. (1967) Congenital duodenal obstruction. Review of 29 cases encountered in a 30 year period. *Mayo Clin. Proc.*, **42**, 423–430

54. Louw, J.H. (1952) Congenital intestinal atresia and severe stenosis in the newborn. *S. Afr. J. Clin. Sci.*, **3**, 109–129

55. Louw, J.H. (1952) Congenital duodenal stenosis and mongolism. *S. Afr. Med. J.*, **26**, 521

56. Louw, J.H. (1959) Congenital intestinal atresia and stenosis in the newborn. *Ann. Roy. Coll. Surg. Engl.*, **25**, 209–234

57. Lynn, H.B. (1962) In *Pediatric Surgery* (ed. C.D. Benson, W.T. Mustard, M.M. Ravitch, W.H. Snyder Jr. and K.J. Welch), Year Book Medical Publishers, Chicago, pp. 663–670

58. Lynn, H.B. and Espinas, E.E. (1959) Intestinal atresia. *Arch. Surg.*, **79**, 357–361

59. Mackenzie, W.C., Lang, A., Friedman, M.H.W. and Calder, J. (1960) Congenital atresia of the second part of the duodenum with associated obstruction of the biliary tract. *Surg. Gynec. Obstet.*, **110**, 755–758

60. Madden, J.L. and McCann, W.J. (1956) Congenital diaphragmatic occlusion of the duodenum, with a report of 3 cases. *Int. Abstr. Surg.*, **103**, 1–15

61. Marshall, J.M. (1953) Gastro-jejunal ulcers in children. *Arch. Surg.*, **67**, 490–492

62. Mishalany, H.G., Der Kaloustian, V.M. and Ghandour, M. (1970) Familial congenital duodenal atresia. *Pediatrics*, **46**, 629–632

63. Molenaar, J.C. and Looyen, S.G. (1974) Wind sock web of the duodenum. *Z. Kinderchir.*, **14**, 164–171

64. Mooney, D., Lewis, J.E., Connors, R.H. and Weber, T.R. (1987) *Am. J. Surg.*, **153**, 347–349

65. Morton, J.J. and Jones, T.B. (1936) Obstructions about the mesentery in infants. *Ann. Surg.*, **104**, 864–891

66. Moutsouris, Chr. (1966) The 'solid stage' and congenital intestinal atresia. *J. Pediat. Surg.*, **1**, 446–450

67. Nixon, H.H. and Tawes, R. (1970) Etiology and treatment of small intestinal atresia: Analysis of a series of 127 jejunoileal atresias and comparison with 62 duodenal atresias. *Surgery*, **69**, 41–51

68. Noblett, H.R. and Paton, C. (1970) Intrinsic duodenal obstruction associated with interposition of the pancreas. *Proc. Int. Paediat. Surg. Congr., Melbourne*, **2**, 329

69. Pierro, A., Cozzi, F., Colarossi, G., Irving, I.M., Pierce, A.M. and Lister, J. (1987) Does fetal gut obstruction cause hydramnios and growth retardation? *J. Pediat. Surg.*, **22**, 454–457

70. Raffensperger, J., Johnson, F.R. and Greengard, J. (1961) Non-mechanical conditions simulating obstructive lesions of the intestinal tract in the newborn infant. *Surgery*, **49**, 696–700

71. Raine, P.A.M. and Noblett, H.R. (1977) Duodenal atresia with biliary anomalies and unusual gas pattern. *J. Pediat. Surg.*, **12**, 763–765

72. Rangecroft, L. and Courtney, D.F. (1980) The use of transanastomotic feeding tubes in neonatal duodenal obstruction. *Z. Kinderchir.*, **29**, 268–270

73. Reid, I.S. (1973) Biliary tract abnormalities associated with duodenal atresia. *Arch. Dis. Child.*, **48**, 952–957

74. Reid, I.S. (1973) The pattern of intrinsic duodenal obstructions. *Aust. N.Z. J. Surg.*, **42**, 349–352

75. Reid, I.S. (1973) Intrinsic duodenal lesions: Clinical features. *Aust. N.Z. J. Surg.*, **43**, 158–160

76. Richardson, W.R. and Martin, L.W. (1969) Pitfalls in the surgical management of the incomplete duodenal diaphragm. *J. Pediat. Surg.*, **4**, 303–312

77. Rickham, P.P. (1954) Annular pancreas in the newborn. *Arch. Dis. Child.*, **29**, 80–83

78. Rickham, P.P. (1966) Emergency alimentary-tract surgery in the newborn. *Br. Med. J.*, **1**, 78–79

79. Rowe, M.I., Buckner, D. and Clatworthy, H.W. Jr (1968) Windsock web of the duodenum. *Am. J. Surg.*, **116**, 444–449

80. Salonen, I.S. (1978) Congenital duodenal obstruction. *Acta Paediat. Scand.* (Suppl. **272**), 1–86

81. Salonen, I.S. and Mäkinen, E. (1976) Intestinal blind pouch – and blind loop – syndrome in children operated previously for congenital duodenal obstruction. *Ann. Chir. Gynaecol.*, **65**, 38–45

82. Schnaufer, L. (1986) Duodenal atresia, stenosis and annular pancreas. In *Pediatric Surgery* (ed. K.J. Welch, J.G. Randolph, M.M. Ravitch, J.A. O'Neill, Jr. and M.I. Rowe) 4th edn, Year Book Medical Publishers Inc., Chicago, pp. 829–837

83. Stauffer, U.G. and Irving, I. (1977) Duodenal atresia – long term results. *Progr. Pediat. Surg.*, **10**, 49–60

84. Suga, M., Morita, K., Okabe, I., Azuma, Y., Munakata, K. and Ishihara, M. (1983) Congenital duodenal stenosis and ampulla of Vater. *J. Jap. Soc. Pediat. Surg.*, **19**, 919–923

85. Tan, H.L., Jones, P.G. and Auldist, A.W. (1985) Gallstones and duodenal atresia. *Ann. Acad. Med. Singapore*, **14**, 604–608

86. Tandler, J. (1902) Zur Entwicklungsgeschichte des menschlichen Duodenum in frühen Embryonalstadien. *Morphol. Jahrb.*, **29**, 187–216

87. Tchirkow, G., Highman, L.M. and Shafer, A.D. (1980) Cholelithiasis and cholecystitis in children after repair of congenital duodenal anomalies. *Arch. Surg.*, **115**, 85–86

88. Tiedemann, F. (1818) Cited by Reitano, R. (1932)

Sul pancreas anulare. *Arch. Ital. di Anat. e Istol. Pat.*, **3**, 755

89. Tieken, T. (1901) Annular pancreas. *Trans. Chicago Path. Soc.*, **4**, 180–190
90. Verga, G. (1972) Le pancréas annulaire est-il vraiment cause d'occlusion duodénale chez le nouveauné? *Ann. Chir. Infant.*, **13**, 275–276
91. Vidal, E. (1905) Quelques cas de chirurgie pancréatique. *Ass. Franç. Chir.*, **18**, 739–747
92. Waterston, D.J., Bonham Carter, R.E. and Aberdeen, E. (1962) Oesophageal atresia. Tracheo-oesophageal fistula. *Lancet*, **i**, 819–822
93. Wayne, E.R. and Burrington, J.D. (1973) Management of 97 children with duodenal obstruction. *Arch. Surg.*, **107**, 857–860
94. Weisgerber, G. and Boureau, M. (1982) Résultats immédiats et secondaires des duodéno-duodénostomies avec modelage dans le traitement des obstructions duodénales congènitales complètes du nouveau-né. *Chir. Pédiat.*, **23**, 369–372
95. Weissberg, H. (1935) Eine Pancreas annulare bei einem menschlichen Embryo von 16 mm Länge. *Anat. Anz.*, **79**, 296–301
96. Weitzman, J.J. and Brennan, L.P. (1974) An improved technique for the correction of congenital duodenal obstruction in the neonate. *J. Pediat. Surg.*, **9**, 385–388
97. Wesley, J.R. and Mahour, G.H. (1977) Congenital intrinsic duodenal obstruction. A 25 year review. *Surgery*, **82**, 716–720
98. Wilkinson, A.W., Hughes, E.A. and Stevens, L.H. (1965) Neonatal duodenal obstruction. *Br. J. Surg.*, **52**, 410–424
99. Williams, T. and Baker Meio, I. (1977) Personal communication
100. Young, D.G. and Wilkinson, A.W. (1966) Mortality in neonatal duodenal obstruction. *Lancet*, **ii**, 18–20
101. Young, D.G. and Wilkinson, A.W. (1968) Abnormalities associated with neonatal duodenal obstruction. *Surgery*, **63**, 832–836
102. Young, I.D., Kennedy, R. and Ein, S.H. (1986) Familial small bowel atresia and stenosis. *J. Pediat. Surg.*, **21**, 792–793

31

Malrotation and volvulus of the intestine

James Lister

Historical notes

The embryology of normal intestinal rotation was described during the last century by the anatomists His [17] (1880) and Mall [28] (1898). The embryological explanation of malrotations of the midgut is based on the classic work of Frazer and Robbins [9] in 1915 and Dott [6] in 1923. The first successful operation on a neonate with malrotation of the intestine was probably that reported by Higgins [16] in 1923, but the operative procedures did not become standardized until 1937 when Ladd [23] described the operative procedure which now bears his name. In the 1950s Snyder and Chaffin [34] in the USA and Grob [14,15] in Switzerland did much to clarify our understanding of this subject.

Embryology and pathology

Normal intestinal rotation

During the fourth week of intrauterine life the primitive intestine lies in the median sagittal plane. During the next 6 weeks the intestines grow at a faster rate than the coelomic cavity, and the rapidly developing liver forces them to protrude into the physiological hernia in the umbilical cord. The cranial part of the intestinal loop in the hernial sac corresponds to the jejunum and the ileum as far distal as the omphalomesenteric duct, the caudal part to the lower ileum and the colon. The gut enters the hernial sac at a point corresponding to the duodenojejunal junction and leaves it at a point corresponding to the primary colonic flexure. While the primitive intestinal loop lies in the umbilical hernia, it rotates around the axis of the superior mesenteric artery through 90 degrees in an anticlockwise direction (as seen when viewing the embryo from the front), so that the duodenojejunal junction no longer lies cranial to the primitive colonic flexure but in a transverse plane and to the right of it (Figures 31.1 and 31.2).

After the tenth week of intrauterine life the coelomic cavity has grown sufficiently to permit the intestine to return into it. The return of the intestine into the abdominal cavity is accompanied by further rotation of the intestine in an anticlockwise direction around the axis of the superior mesenteric artery. The duodenojejunal loop rotates through a further 180 degrees, i.e. it rotates through a total 270 degrees, until it comes to lie behind and to the left of the superior mesenteric artery (Figure 31.3). The caecocolic loop also rotates in an anticlockwise direction through a further 180 degrees until the caecum finally comes to lie to the right of the superior mesenteric artery with the colon crossing in front of the artery. The caecum, being the bulkiest part of the prolapsed intestine, is the last to return into the abdomen (Figure 31.3). By the end of the 11th to 12th week of intrauterine life the total rotation of the caecocolic loop through 270 degrees has been completed and the caecum has come to lie in the right hypochondrium beneath the liver. The caecum then descends slowly by differential growth during the rest of fetal life until, at birth, it has reached its final position in the right iliac fossa.

Finally, certain parts of the intestine become fixed to the posterior abdominal parietal peritoneum by forming adhesions to it. The fixation of the posterior surface of the duodenum and of the ascending colon defines the root of the mesentery, which now runs from the duodenojejunal flexure obliquely downwards and to the right to the ileocaecal junction.

These three parts of rotation – the first 90 degrees occurring while the intestine is in the umbilical hernia, the next 180 degrees as it returns to the coelomic cavity and the final 90 degrees during

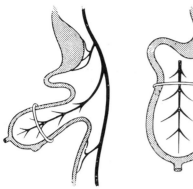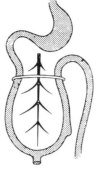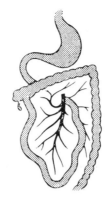

Figure 31.1–31.3 Normal rotation of fetal intestine (after Grob)

fixation – were described as Stages I, II and III by Frazer and Robbins [9] and most authors retain this staging [30]. However, it must be remembered that this is an ongoing process, Stage II being such a quick one that few embryos have been demonstrated actually showing the gut returning to the abdominal cavity [34].

It is also important to emphasize that the rotation of the midgut loop is not the rotation of the postarterial loop around the pre-arterial one, but the rotation of both loops around the superior mesenteric artery; Snyder and Chaffin [34] point out that the duodenojejunal flexure has swung beneath the artery long before the second stage of rotation of the caecocolic loop, and they suggest that arrest in the movement of the duodenojejunal segment may set the stage for arrest of the caecocolic segment. The practical significance is that surgical procedures should be directed as much to the duodenojejunal loop as to the caecocolic one.

Intestinal malrotation

Considering how complicated the process of rotation is in the normal fetus, it is not surprising that many things may go wrong and that the gut may take up a considerable number of abnormal positions.

Complete non-rotation

Complete non-rotation, i.e. the absence of any fetal rotation is rarely seen, though Kantor [18] reported it as an incidental finding in 0.2% of contrast studies of the gastrointestinal tract. The patient has a common longitudinal mesentery serving small and large bowel and running vertically downwards in the midline of the abdominal wall. Our experience of this condition, like others [6,14], has been when it is associated with exomphalos, gastroschisis and posterolateral diaphragmatic hernias [30].

Incomplete rotation (non-rotation)

This usually means that no further rotation has occurred after the initial anticlockwise rotation of the primitive intestinal loop through 90 degrees. In these cases the duodenum and small intestine remain on the right side of the superior mesenteric artery, and the caecum and colon remain on the left side (Figure 31.4). The condition is frequently

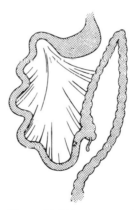

Figure 31.4 Non-rotation (after Grob)

further complicated by the formation of congenital adhesions between various coils of bowel and the parietal peritoneum. There were two such cases in our series.

Malrotation

'Malrotation' is a term which embraces a number of different types of abnormal rotation. In the commonest variety of this anomaly rotation occurs through 180 degrees; the duodenum comes to lie behind the superior mesenteric artery or fails to cross the midline and lies wholly to the right of the artery. The caecum does not reach its normal

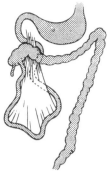

Figure 31.5 Incomplete rotation. Malrotation Type 1 (after Grob)

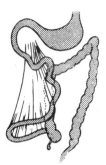

Figure 31.6 Malrotation Type 2 (after Grob)

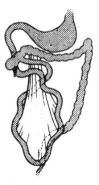

Figure 31.7 Malrotation Type 3 (after Grob)

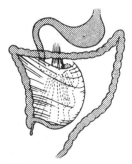

Figure 31.8 Malrotation with mesocolic hernia (after Grob)

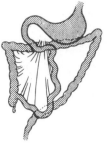

Figure 31.9 Complete clockwise rotation through 180 degrees (after Grob)

position, but comes to lie anterior to the duodenum, and abnormal adhesions form, running from the caecum across the duodenum to the parietal peritoneum in the right hypochondrium (Figure 13.5). These adhesions, which are often called Ladd's bands, tend to obstruct the second part of the duodenum.

In the less common and more complicated types of malrotation there is first a normal rotation through 90 degrees in the anticlockwise direction, followed by an abnormal rotation in a clockwise direction through 90 or 180 degrees. In all types of malrotation the duodenum comes to lie in front of the superior mesenteric artery. The proximal colon either comes to lie behind the mesentery of the small intestine (Figure 31.6) or ascends from behind the mesentery towards the right in front of the duodenum (Figure 31.7). Occasionally the mesocolon may envelope the whole of the small intestine in the shape of a hernial sac, thus forming a mesocolic hernia, as happened in one of our cases (Figure 31.8).

If the clockwise rotation is completed through a full 180 degrees, the transverse colon comes to lie behind the superior mesenteric vessels, and the caecum and ascending colon lie in the right side of the abdomen in the normal position (Figure 31.9).

Situs inversus

This may be associated with various degrees of malrotation. In one of our cases there was situs inversus of liver, spleen and foregut, whilst the hindgut was in the normal position. In another there was a total situs inversus with malrotation.

Miscellaneous

Miscellaneous types of malrotation which do not quite fit into the systems outlined above are also occasionally seen. The duodenum and colon may be in the normal position, but the duodenum may be spirally twisted on itself, as happened in one of our cases. Others are described in the literature [25].

In two more of the cases in this series the duodenum lay in front of the superior mesenteric vessels, but was crossed anteriorly by the portal vein, which obstructed it.

In most cases of non-rotation and malrotation the root of the mesentery has only a very narrow attachment to the posterior abdominal wall instead of the normal long oblique attachment. When the whole of the small intestine is suspended from a mesentery with a narrow attachment to the posterior abdominal wall around the origin of the superior mesenteric vessels, there is considerable danger that the small intestine will twist around the axis of the mesenteric vessels, thus causing a volvulus, as occurred in 48 (44%) of our neonatal cases.

There are many additional varieties of obstruction caused by failures in rotation and fixation, including duodenojejunal obstruction by kinks and bands which may occur even in the presence of complete rotation [26,35].

Incidence

The condition is not common and only half of the cases present with symptoms during the neonatal period [15]. During 32 years, 1954–85, 108 infants were admitted to the Liverpool Neonatal Surgical Centre with symptoms due to malrotation of the intestine. There were 69 boys and 39 girls. It is generally stated that boys are affected about twice as often as girls [17,36]. Cases of malrotation associated with exomphalos (see Chapter 27) are not included amongst these 108 cases, nor are infants who had an intrinsic duodenal obstruction as well as malrotation (see Chapter 30).

Clinical picture

Family history

Reference to abnormal family histories of infants born with malrotation was not found in the literature. It is therefore surprising that in 22 of the 108 in this series there was an abnormal family history. Ten mothers had had previous abortions, six had had stillbirths and in ten cases siblings were known to have been born with other severe malformations.

Pregnancy history

No reference to abnormal pregnancy histories of the mothers of infants with malrotation has been made in the literature. In this series there were 15 mothers who gave an abnormal pregnancy history: five suffered from toxaemia, five from hydramnios and one each from hypertension, hyperemesis, threatened abortion, diabetes and epilepsy.

Associated malformations

The very common association of exomphalos and gastroschisis with malrotation has already been referred to: these cases are not included in the series nor are cases of diaphragmatic hernia and malfixation. Of the other associated severe malformations, by far the commonest is duodenal atresia or stenosis [12,20]. Fifty-three such cases occurred during the period of review: they are discussed in Chapter 30. In Gross's large series of 156 cases of malrotation in infancy and childhood [15] five were found to have pyloric stenosis and two of our infants suffered from this condition.

We also saw two cases each with gastro-oesophageal reflux, meconium ileus, jejunal atresia and anorectal anomalies as well as one each with oesophageal atresia, myelomeningocele, hydro-nephrosis and prune-belly syndrome. One child had a patent ductus arteriosus and short bowel. One very important group were the seven neonates with Hirschsprung's disease who had malrotation: one of these developed intestinal obstruction due to an incomplete volvulus which was at first considered to be due to his Hirschsprung's disease: the possibility of this association has been reported by others and must always be considered [8].

Presenting symptoms and signs

In every one of the cases in this series vomiting was the presenting symptom tending to start on the third to fifth day of life. The vomiting is usually due to duodenal obstruction. It is said that occasionally the vomitus may not be bile-stained, but all the infants in this series vomited yellow or greenish material. Projectile vomiting, indicating a high duodenal obstruction was observed in 16 infants. Blood stained vomitus is rarely seen but suggests bowel strangulation.

As the obstruction in malrotation is usually only partial [11], meconium stools, and later on milk stools, are usually passed; two children were constipated and three had loose stools. If intestinal strangulation due to volvulus develops, some blood may be passed per rectum, as was the case in 12 of the infants in this series.

Abdominal distension was not a constant feature. At first it may only be noticed in the epigastrium; later on, especially in infants with volvulus, distension will become generalized. Extreme distension was noticed in only four cases in this series, including three with a gangrenous volvulus and one with a perforation of the stomach. Tenderness may be elicited on abdominal palpation: this, like blood stained vomit or the passage of blood per rectum, is ominous, suggesting infarction of the strangulated bowel.

Dehydration secondary to vomiting will develop rapidly and was gross in 20% of our neonates. In a

5-day-old infant the weight had dropped by 550 g since birth.

Pyrexia and sometimes hyperpyrexia can occur with dehydration or in association with gangrenous gut. It indicates a bad prognosis and was present in 14 infants in this series.

Jaundice is less commonly noticed, and also has a bad prognosis, as it may be associated with gangrenous intestine. We observed 14 such infants. Surprisingly, the infants do not seem to suffer from any abdominal pain [21].

Differential diagnosis

Clinically it is often impossible to differentiate the condition from other types of high incomplete intestinal obstruction. It is characteristic of neonates with malrotation that the obstruction, being incomplete, is associated with mild symptoms and signs, and the medical attendant may, therefore, not take the condition very seriously at first. Strangulation and gangrene of the intestine may, however, develop very rapidly. Some infants with gangrenous intestine remain in remarkably good general condition for a number of hours until they suddenly collapse and become very shocked and ill.

Radiological investigation

In many cases a straight abdominal radiographic picture in the upright position will reveal evidence of partial obstruction by outlining a distended stomach and proximal duodenum with little or no air in the rest of the intestine (Figure 31.10): this evidence in a child who has had intermittent vomiting of bile is often all that is required. On rare occasions the straight X-ray may be more specific (Figure 31.11). However, a child who has been vomiting may expel all the air from his stomach and duodenum and then the straight abdominal X-ray will give inadequate information; the great danger of accepting such a film as normal and delaying operation in a child who has potentially strangulated bowel has led to a demand for contrast studies, especially in a child who has been vomiting bile. Contrast medium can be given by mouth and may demonstrate dilated stomach and duodenum (Figures 31.12 and 31.13), a duodenojejunal flexure to the right of midline, jejunal loops to the left and even occasionally may show the twisting intestine distal to the partially obstructed duodenum.

It should be emphasized that modern non-ionic contrast-media should be used (see Chapter 8). Not only is there a risk of aspiration of barium in a vomiting baby, but also, as in one of our early cases, inspissated barium can result in colonic perforation, even after a successful operation for malrotation.

Air is a very satisfactory contrast medium and 20–30 ml injected through a nasogastric tube which is

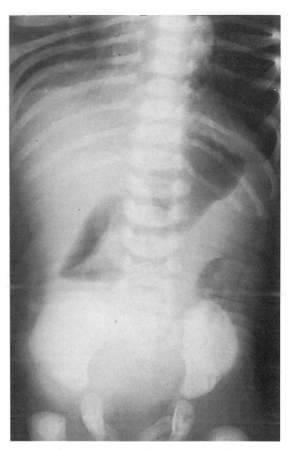

Figure 31.10 Malrotation of the intestine. Stomach and duodenum are distended with air. There is little air in the rest of the abdomen, mainly on the left side

then clamped off, will usually reveal the duodenal obstruction when a radiograph is taken in the upright position (Figure 31.14). Some radiologists [1,2] suggest that a prone film is of great value in demonstrating pooled air in the duodenum. Intramural air seen in the straight X-ray is ominous evidence of infarction. The presence of free intraperitoneal air indicates perforation, but in general the straight X-ray will demonstrate obstruction but not give evidence of the vascular state of the small intestine; supine or prone films occasionally show thickened oedematous jejunal walls [1].

Theoretically a contrast enema should be of value [38] in revealing a malplaced caecum; however, it may be difficult to localize the caecum because it can be obscured by flooding of the small bowel with barium and, indeed, the redundant pelvic colon in the neonate may mislead the radiologist into believing he has filled the colon

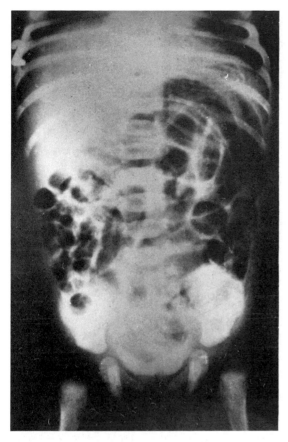

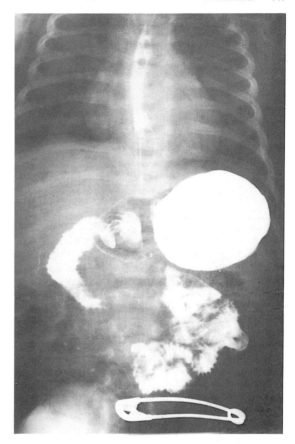

Figure 31.11 Straight X-ray of abdomen, showing dilated small bowel on the left and undilated small bowel enclosed in mesocolic hernial sac (cf. Figure 31.8) (X-ray courtesy of Dr Claudio de Souza Leite, Rio de Janeiro)

Figure 31.12 Barium meal in a case of malrotation of midgut with obstruction of the distal duodenum

when the barium reaches the hepatic flexure, or even the upper sigmoid colon [1]. Furthermore, Kiesewetter and Smith [19] found that 5% of their midgut malrotations had a normally sited colon and certainly the mobile caecum frequently lies in the right iliac fossa. Air injected into the colon through a rectal tube may again serve as a very effective contrast medium (Figure 31.15) and avoids some of the problems of barium.

In a review of 32 cases of malrotation Simpson, Leonidas and Krasna [32] attempted to correlate plain film patterns with underlying pathology; they were unable to draw firm conclusions and believed barium studies essential for specific diagnosis, preferring upper gastrointestinal studies as being a more direct approach to demonstrate the obstruction.

In our earlier series of 83 cases, seven were admitted having had a diagnostic barium meal in the referring hospital. Of the remaining 76 patients, one was moribund on admission and was not investigated and 75 had straight X-rays in the erect position

which were considered sufficiently diagnostic in all but 13. Of the 13 patients in whom the first radiological examination was equivocal, three were diagnosed at repeat straight X-ray, and five each at barium meal or barium enema. None of the 25 cases admitted during the decade 1976–85 had had contrast studies before admission.

Ultrasound has been used to demonstrate abnormality of rotation of the midgut loop by showing an abnormal relationship of the superior mesenteric vein to the superior mesenteric artery [10]. This is a non-invasive investigation and useful as confirmatory evidence and may in the future be used more frequently.

Treatment

Operation is always indicated, but it must be admitted that one infant in this series, in whom the diagnosis was confirmed by a barium meal, stopped

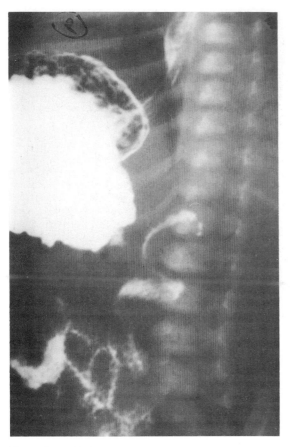

Figure 31.13 Barium swallow in a case of malrotation of midgut with volvulus. The oblique view shows the dilated stomach and the spiral twists of the small intestine

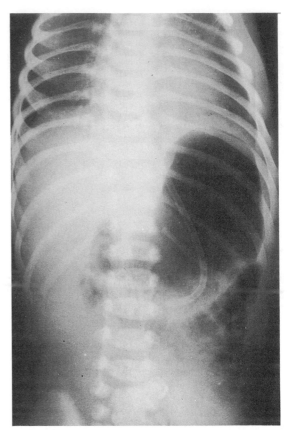

Figure 31.14 Malrotation of midgut. Twenty ml air has been injected into the stomach. The stomach and distended proximal duodenum are outlined. There is very little air in the rest of the intestine

vomiting without surgical intervention and showed no further abnormal symptoms. There is, however, little doubt that in such a case, where a volvulus has probably untwisted itself, it is very likely that symptoms will recur.

Pre-operative management

In dehydrated infants the water and electrolyte balance must be restored by intravenous therapy and in all infants the stomach must be continuously aspirated via a nasogastric tube.

Operation

The abdomen is opened through the standard supraumbilical transverse incision (see Chapter 6). All the intestines are now withdrawn from the abdominal cavity and covered with warm moist packs (Figure 31.16). It is of the utmost importance to eviscerate all the intestines as otherwise it will be

impossible for the surgeon to recognize the type of malformation present. If a volvulus is present, it is usually in a clockwise direction; it must now be untwisted. Twists of two, three or even more complete circles are not uncommon. Once the gut has been untwisted the cyanosis usually disappears and the pink colour of the intestine returns.

In the common type of malrotation where rotation is incomplete (see Figure 31.5) the caecum will be found in the right hypochondrium, fixed by adhesions passing across the second and third parts of the duodenum to the lateral abdominal wall. Ladd's procedure, i.e. division of the adhesions, mobilizing the caecum and placing it in the left side of the abdomen, has now to be carried out (Figure 31.17). The duodenum has then to be inspected carefully and freed from any adhesions causing kinks. When this has been done the duodenum will be seen coursing down the right side of the abdomen.

In cases of inverse rotation in which the transverse colon lies behind the mesenteric vessels, it is often possible to place the colon in front of the mesenteric vessels by rotating the whole of the gut through 360 degrees in an anticlockwise direction. At the same time it is often possible to displace the duodenum to the right and thus avoid any further compression of this segment of intestine.

If the small intestine is inside a mesocolic hernial sac, the sac must not be resected because it contains the colonic vessels in its wall. The intestine should be pulled out of the sac, which should then be fixed to the posterior abdominal wall.

Whatever the type of malrotation encountered, it is of the utmost importance that all adhesions between intestinal loops and between the intestine and the parietal peritoneum be meticulously and completely divided until the whole length of the intestine from the first part of the duodenum to the sigmoid colon can be demonstrated to be free from adhesions and kinks. This often needs time-consuming careful dissection, but once this has been completed it is most unlikely that the infant will have subsequent episodes of intestinal obstruction or volvulus [31]. In three cases in this series it was

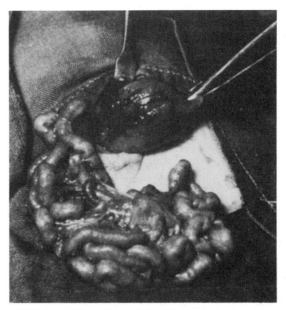

Figure 31.16 The whole of the small intestine has been withdrawn from the abdomen. The stomach is seen protruding through the left side of the transverse incision. The volvulated small intestine is suspended from two loops, the most proximal segment of jejunum and most distal segment of ileum, respectively

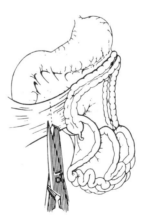

Figure 31.17 Division of Ladd's band

necessary to perform a relaparotomy because of recurrent volvulus; in all of them it was found that the original adhesions had not been divided completely.

If the operation is carried out carefully and completely, additional fixation of the colon to the left side of the abdomen [20] or stabilization of the colonic mesentery [3] in order to prevent recurrence of volvulus and obstruction is not necessary and may do more harm than good.

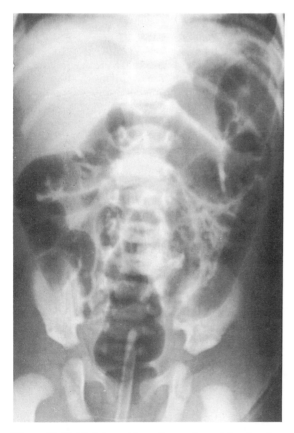

Figure 31.15 Air injected into the newborn infant's colon outlines the whole colon on radiography

Many authorities advise that if the infant's general condition is satisfactory at the end of the operation, appendicectomy should be performed, as subsequent inflammation of an appendix lying in the left hypochondrium may give rise to bizarre symptoms and difficulty in diagnosis [38]. Appendicectomy was carried out in 12 cases in this series, but should never be attempted if the caecum is cyanosed or oedematous, as leakage from the appendix stump may lead to disaster. Invagination of the appendix without its removal is recommended by some; it certainly avoids contamination but, again, should not be done in the presence of inflammatory changes in the caecum. Before the abdomen is closed, care must be taken to make sure that there is no coexisting intrinsic obstruction of the duodenum. If air is injected into the stomach and massaged through the duodenum under direct vision, any obstruction can usually be easily observed. It is therefore not often necessary to pass a catheter from the stomach along the duodenum, as advised by a number of authors [27], and since this procedure is both cumbersome and traumatic, it is best avoided if possible.

Postoperative management

Details of routine postoperative management are described in Chapter 5. Duodenal dilatation and vascular changes in the volvulated small intestine may cause prolonged postoperative ileus, and continuous gastric suction and intravenous therapy may have to be continued for periods of 48 h or more.

Results

There is hardly any other neonatal condition in which the results obtained by surgical treatment in various centres differ so much. This is partly explained by the fact that most authors have published series of all their cases of malrotation, including neonates and older children. It must also be remembered that malrotation is often associated with other serious abdominal conditions such as exomphalos, intrinsic duodenal obstruction, diaphragmatic hernia, etc. The published results differ markedly, depending on the types of cases which are included.

The operative mortality rate for cases of malrotation in infants and older children has dropped spectacularly during the last 40 years. In 1922 the mortality rate was still more than 99% [5]. Today one might expect that the mortality rate for an operative procedure not entailing resection and anastomosis of intestine (i.e. malrotation without gangrenous volvulus) would be negligible. Unfortunately this is not the case. In our series of 108 cases there were 21 deaths: six were moribund on admission, one of them having no operation: these were all very small babies; all had gangrenous bowel and one had Down's Syndrome and severe heart disease. Three more had gut resected for gangrene and died, one from septicaemia and two following further operations for recurrent obstruction due to adhesions. There were six very small prematures with additional problems such as neonatal hepatitis, kernicterus. *E. coli* meningitis, severe congenital heart defect and pyelonephritis. Four full-term babies, however, had deaths which should have been avoidable: one had sepsis due to leakage from an anastomosis which had been made in the presence of peritonitis when an enterostomy would have been preferable, and three died of bronchopneumonia associated probably with vomiting and inhalation, one being a late death at 5 weeks when there was a recurrence of the volvulus. During the 10 years from 1976 to 1985, however, only two of 25 babies died, one with gangrene of the entire midgut and one of renal insufficiency related to his prunebelly syndrome.

Volvulus without malrotation

During the same period of 33 years from 1953 to 1985 when 83 cases of volvulus associated with malrotations were seen, there were 19 cases of volvulus without malrotation. This is the primary postnatal volvulus of the small intestine described by Pellerin and Bertin [29] which occurs mainly in normal, healthy full-term babies and carries a high mortality. Our cases were equally distributed between males (ten) and females (nine) and there was no significant maternal history nor abnormalities of pregnancy.

Anatomy and pathology

In only one case did the volvulus occur around a band. In the remainder there was no clear evidence of the aetiology of the twist. One child had a gangrenous cyst of the left ovary, one had bilateral undescended testes and one had pulmonary stenosis.

Clinical picture

All our patients except one had a history of intermittent bile-stained vomiting from birth. In four the vomiting had been severe enough to result in evidence of dehydration. Abdominal distension was present in ten, and in four there was bleeding per rectum.

These children tended to present rather earlier than children with malrotation and volvulus; nine were admitted in the first 24 h of life and another four on the second or third day; only six were over 1 week old when admitted.

Treatment

Of the 19 cases, 15 required resection for gangrenous bowel, the remaining three having the volvulus untwisted. One, with extensive gangrene, was moribund on admission and died before operation.

Results

In spite of the very rapid progression to gangrene of the twisted bowel in this condition and the poor prognosis attached to it by others [29], there were only four deaths in our series: one attributable to associated congenital heart disease, one to a respiratory infection in a child who was found at autopsy to have pulmonary fibroelastosis, one who died from a short gut having had a massive resection, and the one who died without operation.

One child had a wound disruption and another had a recurrent obstruction due to adhesions, but all children were trouble-free when discharged from follow-up 1–3 years after operation.

Extensive bowel resection

It was in the group of children with volvulus without malrotation that our only late death occurred, due to an inadequate length of bowel remaining after resection for infarction. Neonates with vascular obstruction of the gut due to volvulus of any type are particularly suitable for a 'second look' procedure; at the first laparotomy frankly gangrenous bowel is excised and a double-barrelled enterostomy made leaving the bowel of doubtful viability in the abdomen. The tendency at this stage should be to err on the side of under-resection rather than over-resection. After 12–24 h the abdomen is opened again, and a decision made as to how much further resection, if any, is required; a new double enterostomy or an anastomosis can then be made.

The use of hyperbaric oxygen in the period between the two operations was shown to improve survival rates in experimental animals [33]; it was not clear whether this improvement was due to reduction in clostridial infection [4] or to bowel decompression [37]. Experimentally, there is some evidence that infarction can be reduced by the infusion of low molecular weight dextran [24]. Krasna and his colleagues [22] treated two patients with low molecular weight dextran in the intervening period, undoing the midgut volvulus at the first operation but resecting no bowel; one case required no resection and the other was found to have viable 17 cm of jejunum and 6 cm of ileum, an amount just sufficient to support life (see Chapter 32).

References

1. Berdon, W.F., Baker, D.H. and Leonidas, J. (1968) Advantages of prone positioning in gastrointestinal and genitourinary roentgenologic studies in infants and children. *Am. J. Roent.*, **103**, 444–455
2. Berdon, W.F., Baker, D.H., Bull, S. and Santulli, T.V. (1970) Midgut malrotation and volvulus; which films are most helpful? *Radiology*, **96**, 375–384
3. Bill, A.H. and Grauman, D. (1966) Rationale and technic for stabilization of the mesentery in cases of non-rotation of the midgut. *J. Pediat. Surg.*, **1**, 127–136
4. Brummelkamp, W.H., Hoogendijk, J.L. and Boerema, I. (1961) Treatment of anaerobic infections by drenching the tissue with oxygen under high pressure. *Surgery*, **49**, 299–302
5. Davis, D.L. and Poynter, C.W.M. (1922) Congenital occlusions of the intestines. *Surg. Gynec. Obstet.*, **34**, 35–41
6. Dott, N.M. (1923) Anomalies of intestinal rotation. *Br. J. Surg.*, **11**, 251–286
7. Dott, N.M. (1927) Volvulus neonatorum. *Br. Med. J.*, **1**, 230–231
8. Filston, H.C. and Kirks, D.R. (1981) Malrotation the ubiquitous anomaly. *J. Pediat. Surg.*, **16**, 614–620
9. Frazer, J.E. and Robbins, R.H. (1915) On facts concerned in causing rotation of the intestine in man. *J. Anat. Physiol.*, **50**, 75–110
10. Gaines, P.A., Saunders, A.J.S. and Drake, D. (1987) Midgut malrotation diagnosed by ultrasound. *Clin. Radiol.*, **38**, 51–53
11. Gardner, C.E. and Hart, D. (1934) Anomalies of intestinal rotation as a cause of intestinal obstruction. *Arch Surg.*, **29**, 942–981
12. Glover, D.M. and Barry, F.M. (1949) Intestinal obstruction in the newborn. *Ann. Surg.*, **130**, 480–511
13. Grob, M. (1953) *Uber Lagenabnormalien des Magendarmtrackies Infolge Storungen der foetalen Darmdrehung*, Beno Schwabe, Basle
14. Grob, M. (1957) *Lehrbuch der Kinderchirurgie*, Georg Thieme Verlag, Stuttgart
15. Gross, R.E. (1953) *Surgery of Infancy and Childhood*, W.B. Saunders, Philadelphia
16. Higgins, T.T. (1923) A case of intestinal obstruction in a newborn infant. *Br. J. Surg.*, **11**, 382–384
17. His, W. (1980) *Anatomie menschlicher Embryome*, F.C.N. Vogel, Leipzig
18. Kantor, J.L. (1934) Anomalies of the colon: their roentgen diagnosis and clinical significance. Resumé of ten years study. *Radiology*, **23**, 651–662
19. Kiesewetter, W.B. and Smith, J.W. (1958) Malrotation of the midgut in infancy and childhood. *Arch. Surg.*, **77**, 483–491
20. Knutrud, O. and Eek, S. (1960) Combined intrinsic duodenal obstruction and malrotation. *Acta Chir. Scand.*, **119**, 506–517
21. Koop, C.E. (1953) Intestinal obstruction in the neonatal period. *Adv. Pediat.*, **6**, 63
22. Krasna, I.H., Fox, H.A., Schneider, K.M. and

Becker, J.M. (1973) Low molecular weight dextran in the treatment of necrotising enterocolitis and midgut volvulus in infants. *J. Pediat. Surg.*, **8**, 615–622

23. Ladd, W.E. (1937) Congenital duodenal obstruction. *Surgery*, **1**, 878–885

24. Lepley, D., Man, J. and Ellison, E.H. (1962) Superior mesenteric venous occlusion: a study using low molecular weight dextran to prevent infarction. *J. Surg. Res.*, **2**, 403

25. Lewis, J.E. (1966) Partial duodenal obstruction with incomplete duodenal rotation. *J. Pediat. Surg.*, **1**, 47–53

26. McIntosh, R. and Donovan, E.J. (1939) Disturbances of rotation of intestinal tract: clinical picture based on observations in 20 cases. *Am. J. Dis. Child.*, **57**, 116–166

27. Madden, J.L. and McCann, W.J. (1955) Symposium on critical emergencies. *Surg. Clins N. Am.*, **35**, 441–450

28. Mall, F.P. (1898) Development of the human intestine and its position in the adult. *Johns Hopkins Hosp. Bull. Balt.*, **9**, 197–208

29. Pellerin, D. and Bertin, P. (1972) Volvulus primitif postnatal du grele. *Ann. Chir. infant.*, **13**, 83–94

30. Rees, J.R. and Redo,S.F. (1968) Anomalies of intestinal rotation and fixation. *Am. J. Surg.*, **116**, 834–841

31. Schultz, L.R., Lasher, E.P. and Bill, A.H. (1961) Abnormalities of rotation of the bowel. *Am. J. Surg.*, **101**, 128–133

32. Simpson, A.J., Leonidas, J.C. and Krasna, I.H. (1972) Roentgen diagnosis of midgut malrotation: value of upper gastro-intestinal radiographic study. *J. Pediat. Surg.*, **7**, 243–252

33. Smith, B., Okamoto, E., Leal, E. and Clatworthy, H.W. (1968) Hyperbaric oxygen in the treatment of volvulus of the midgut. *J. Pediat. Surg.*, **3**, 32–35

34. Snyder, W.H. and Chaffin, L. (1954) Embryology and pathology of the intestinal tract. *Ann. Surg.*, **140**, 368–380

35. Soper, R.T. and Selke, A.C. (1970) Congenital extrinsic obstruction of the duodenojejunal junction. *J. Pediat. Surg.*, **5**, 437–443

36. Stewart, D.R., Colodny, A.L. and Dagget, W.C. (1976) Malrotation of the bowel in infants and children: a 15 year review. *Surgery*, **79**, 716–720

37. Stewart, J.S.S., Keddie, N.C., Middleton, M.D., Hopkinson, W.I. and Williams, K.G. (1964) Gut decompression with hyperbaric oxygen. *Lancet*, **i**, 699

38. Swenson, O. (1958) *Pediatric Surgery*, Appleton Century Crofts, New York

32

Intestinal atresia and stenosis, excluding the duodenum

James Lister

Historical notes

The first case of small intestinal atresia recorded in the literature was that of Goeller [43] who, in 1683, described the autopsy findings in a stillborn female child with atresia of the terminal ileum. Eleven years before this Binninger [7] had recorded the postmortem findings of a 36-h old infant with atresia of the colon. The third case of atresia reported in the literature was perhaps the most astonishing. Horch [55], in 1696, described a girl who, despite constant vomiting, survived for 22 days and was found at autopsy to have atresia of the lower ileum with a gap between the proximal and distal segments of intestine. Bland Sutton [10] in 1889, was the first to diagnose an ileal atresia in a living neonate and to attempt to treat it by operation. He performed an ileostomy, but the child died a few hours later. Fockens [38] in 1911 reported the first successful operation for intestinal atresia; his patient was still alive and well over 40 years later [125]. According to Kreuter [65], Nelaton in 1855 was the first to attempt operative treatment of a colonic atresia by performing a colostomy; the child died. It was not until 1922 that Gaub [42] succeeded in keeping alive a boy with atresia of the sigmoid colon, by performing a colostomy proximal to the atresia. The first successful resection and anastomosis of a colonic atresia was reported by Potts as recently as 1947 [91].

Pathological anatomy

Bland Sutton [10] classified atresia of the bowel as of three types. In Type 1 there is continuity of the bowel wall, the lumen being blocked by one or more septa (Figure 32.1a). In Type 2 the two blind ends of the gut are connected by a fibrous cord of varying length; the mesentery is either intact or shows a V-shaped defect between the two blind segments [67] (Figure 32.1b). In Type 3 the two intestinal segments are separated by a gap. This type is frequently associated with a V-shaped gap in the mesentery (Figure 32.1c). In stenosis there is either a narrowing of the segment of the intestine or the two intestinal segments are separated by a septum with a small, usually central, opening. Multiple atretic segments, producing an appearance resembling a string of sausages [44], are not uncommon (Figures 32.1d and 32.2).

In some cases of intestinal atresia the intestine is found to be arranged in a spiral around a central mesenteric vessel, the mesentery running like a spiral staircase from the central vessel to the intestine (Figure 32.3). This abnormality has been named the 'apple-peel syndrome' by Santulli and Blanc [107], 'Christmas tree deformity' by Weitzman and Vanderhoof [126] and 'maypole atresia' by Nixon and Tawes [88]. In these cases the spiral formation of the distal small bowel is due to an associated deficiency of its mesentery [133], the branches of the superior mesenteric artery to jejunum and ileum are absent and the vascular stalk around which the distal ileum forms its spiral represents a somewhat precarious retrograde flow from the middle colic artery through the terminal part of the superior mesenteric artery [59]. This particular type of atresia seems to form a separate group: familial incidence has been reported [11,83] but it has also been reported on two occasions in one member of a pair of identical twins [80,132], suggesting that the condition is not always inherited.

Martin and Zerella [80] proposed a modification of Bland Sutton's classification, combining his Type (b) and (c) into Type II, reserving multiple atresia

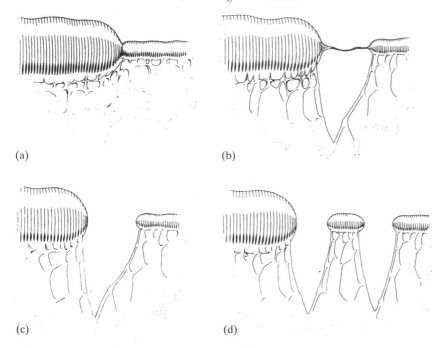

(a)   (b)

(c)   (d)

Figure 32.1 Types of intestinal atresia and stenosis

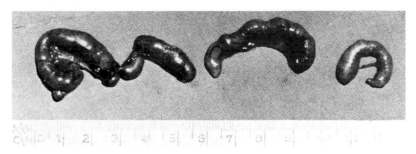

Figure 32.2 Multiple atretic intestinal segments excised at operation

(Bland Sutton type (d)) for Type III and adding Type IV for the 'apple-peel' deformity. They pointed out that in their Type I, the membrane or diaphragm atresia, there was no shortening of bowel length or associated anomalies whilst in Type II, where there was discontinuity of bowel the gut might be short and associated anomalies might be seen. In their Types III (multiple atresias) and IV (apple-peel) short bowel was common but associated anomalies were not seen.

Whatever the type of the atresia, the pathological changes caused by the intestinal obstruction are always the same. The intestine proximal to the obstruction becomes enormously dilated and hypertrophied [21] except in the upper jejunum, where the muscle layers may be thinned and deficient [114]. The mucosa of the distended proximal bowel tends to be flattened whilst in the narrow bowel distal to the obstruction there appears to be villous hyperplasia. The dilatation is maximal just proximal to the atresia and here the diameter of the gut may be several times that found in an adult. The intestinal distension interferes with the venous return from the bowel so that the dilated segment is often cyanosed and necrotic areas are not uncommon. At operation peristaltic movements can be

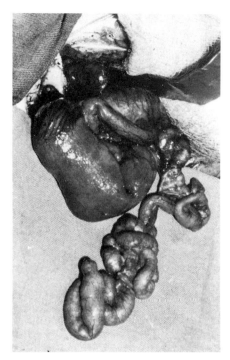

Figure 32.3 Atretic intestine arranged in a spiral around a central vessel

observed in the proximal dilated gut but, as Nixon [86] has pointed out, these contractions are ineffective in moving along the intestinal contents.

The diameter of the distal intestine is minute, and the gut is often no thicker than a pipe-cleaner. In cases of stenosis the distal intestine contains meconium and air. With atresia, the distal intestine may be empty but more often than not contains greyish mucus or some meconium.

Embryology

Many theories have, from time to time, been put forward to explain the causation of intestinal atresia. For many years the most convincing explanation [45] was a presumption of a failure of recanalization following a stage in development when the intestinal lumen was obliterated. Tandler [117] described the development of the duodenum during the second month of gestation; in embryos of 8.5 mm and 14.5 mm there was such proliferation of the epithelium that the lumen was plugged; this was followed by an increase in the diameter of the surrounding mesoderm, formation of vacuoles in the epithelium and the coalescence of these vacuoles around the 20-mm stage to re-form the lumen. Forssner [41] confirmed these findings in 1907 though Schridde

[110] denied them in 1908. Johnson [60] in 1910 described vacuolization in the oesophagus, duodenum and possibly the ileocaecal region. Lynn and Espinas [77] found epithelial proliferation and/or vacuolization to be present in the duodenum in every embryo they studied between 5 and 8 weeks, though complete occlusion was only seen in one-third of them; they also showed occlusion of the ileum in some cases. Moutsouris [84] found no obliteration of the lumen in the small bowel. We have found apparent complete occlusion in the duodenum (see Chapter 30) but reconstructions show this appearance to be due to the serpentine course of the lumen.

There is considerable doubt therefore that any atresias or stenoses below the level of the duodenum can be regarded as malformations occurring during the critical first 8 weeks of development; rather they are deformities resulting from intra-abdominal pathological catastrophes occurring at a much later period after the organs have been formed. It has long been known that the intestine distal to an atresia may contain bile-stained meconium [68], indicating that the lumen must have been complete after the 11th week of intrauterine life when bile is first secreted – and long after the stage of epithelial proliferation. Furthermore, the meconium in the bowel distal to an atresia may contain squamous epithelial cells and lanugo [86] and Keith [61] states that swallowing commences only after the third month.

Bland Sutton [10] suggested that ileal atresias might be associated with excessive resorption of the vitelline duct; but this also would need to be a very early malformation. However, a careful search will frequently reveal evidence of an intrauterine accident resulting in atresia or stenosis. Of our 172 cases of atresia and stenosis, 71 showed evidence of accidents to the bowel after its formation.

Meconium peritonitis causing adhesions, strangulation and vascular damage to the intestine is frequently associated with intestinal atresia [40]; there was evidence of meconium peritonitis in 36 of our 172 cases. Nixon found evidence of meconium peritonitis in 10 of 33 cases in his first series [86] and 61 of 127 in his second series [87] when he included macroscopic or microscopic findings. Meconium peritonitis could be secondary to bowel infarction and not a primary aetiological factor (see Chapter 35).

Volvulus of a part of the small intestine resulting in the twisting off of a segment of gut may cause atresia [40,76,86,112]; we had 43 such cases in our series. The review by de Lorimier, Fonkalsrud and Hays [28] showed evidence of intrauterine bowel infarction in 42% of 449 patients but this must include some cases where the volvulus affects the grossly distended atretic loop, heavy with packed meconium hanging free in the abdominal cavity [65] as happened in four of our cases, and also other causes of bowel infarction mentioned below.

In 1873, Ahlfeld [1] pointed out that a persistent omphalomesenteric duct may cause atresia by its continuous pull on the intestine. Atresia due to pulling or nipping off of a loop of intestine within the sac of an exomphalos or hernia was described by Nixon [86], who also described six cases of segmental volvulus where the lesion was attached to the posterior aspect of the umbilicus [88]; in our series there were three ileal atresias associated with exomphalos and two with gastroschisis.

Intrauterine intussusception as a cause of intestinal atresia was mentioned by Chiari [18] in 1888 and there have been numerous reports in the literature [14,44,76,86]. Todani, Tabuchi and Tanaka [121] analysing 24 cases of atresia with intussusception in Japan, suggest this is a very late intrauterine catastrophe. We have seen a striking example of this condition (Figure 32.4).

The so-called vascular theory, which postulated that failure of the blood supply to the gut may cause intestinal atresia, was first evolved over a century ago [58,109]. In 1952, Forshall, Hall and Rickham [40] pointed out that the V-shaped defect in the mesentery frequently found in intestinal atresias suggested an obliteration of the mesenteric blood vessels as a cause of the atresia. Such a gap was present in 18 of our cases. Louw [71], studying cases of intestinal atresia in the Hospital for Sick Children, Great Ormond Street, and noticing that there was frequently an associated vascular insufficiency, had the brilliant idea of producing intestinal atresia in fetal puppies by interrupting their mesenteric blood supply. Experimental work has also shown that an intraluminal diaphragm can be caused by tying a ligature round the intestine of a fetal puppy [76]. Atresia of the colon can be produced by similar means in puppies [73]. It has also been shown [23] that perforation of fetal rabbit intestine may result in healing without trace, stenosis or residual atresia. Koga and his associates [63] have studied the

pathological process following vascular insults to the small intestine of puppies *in utero* and shown that when all the blood supply to a 2 cm length of small bowel is ligated at 45–55 days' gestation a stenosis measuring less than 2 cm could be found up to 7 days after the ligation and at 11 days this portion was an atretic cord. A possible clinical example of such an insult was reported by Foglia and his colleagues [39]. Detailed studies of lamb models of atresia have shown histological and histochemical changes consistent with vascular insult [47].

Two types of atresia are of particular interest in relation to aetiology because of their familial incidence. The jejunoileal atresia with absent dorsal mesentery and an 'apple-peel' deformity [31,107] has an obvious vascular deficiency, but has also been shown to have a familial incidence [11,83,104,132] – suggesting an autosomal recessive condition. The frequent association with abnormalities of rotation of the midgut loop suggests a possible inherited tendency to atresia of the small bowel with a superimposed environmental factor. Multiple atresias of both small and large bowel with an intact mesentery and no evidence of vascular insufficiency have also been described in families; Mishalany and Der Kaloustian [82] described two siblings in the Lebanon who had multiple diaphragms, and Guttman *et al.* [46] reported five patients from three related French-Canadian families with multiple atresias from stomach to rectum; Martin, Leonidas and Amoury [79] reported two siblings born in Missouri with similar multiple atresias whose mother came from the same area in Quebec as Guttman's families. Further cases were described by Daneman *et al.* [25], Teja *et al.* [119] and Arnal-Monreal *et al.* [2]. Rittenhouse and his colleagues [106], in describing a single similar case, suggested that since the septa were both transverse and longitudinal and had their own muscularis mucosae they were unlikely to be the result of epithelial plugging but were possibly due to an intrauterine ulcerative process. Rickham and Karplus [104], in reporting single jejunoileal

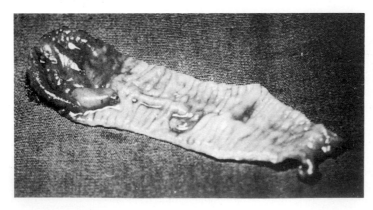

Figure 32.4 Distal blind segment in a case of intestinal atresia. The segment is opened up and shows an intussusception at the apex

atresias occurring in two aunts and two nephews who were siblings, postulated a modified dominant inheritance whereas in Mishalany's [82] and Guttman's [46] families it seemed that an autosomal recessive gene mode of inheritance was present – as in the 'apple-peel' syndrome.

Prem Puri and his colleagues [94] reviewed 59 neonates with intestinal atresia: 19 (32%) were found to have multiple atresias: seven of these occurred in three families, whilst 12 were non-hereditary. In all the hereditary cases and in six of the non-hereditary cases, microscopic examination of the bowel distal to the atresia showed multiple lumina, each with its own mucosa and submucosa, but all sharing a common muscular coat; some of the lumina showed inflammatory changes but these were believed to be the result of the obstruction not its cause: there was no evidence of bile pigment, lanugo or squares in these lumina. They concluded that all cases of hereditary multiple intestinal atresias are a consequence of a malformative process of the gastrointestinal tract rather than an ischaemic process occurring at a later stage of development: some support for this conclusion is provided by the fact that patients with hereditary multiple atresias tend to have more associated congenital anomalies than those with non-hereditary atresias.

Incidence

Estimates of the incidence of intestinal atresia vary enormously; early estimates at around 1 per 20 000 live births [124] were too low because many cases born at home were missed [33,37]. More recent estimates in the UK [36,71], the USA [17,50] and Germany [125] suggest an incidence of 3000 between 1 per 1500 and 1 per 300. In a review of 24 centres, a WHO report [22] showed an overall incidence of 0.09 per 1000 total births, but this figure included duodenal stenoses and atresias except those associated with Down's syndrome. In the first edition of this book, the 143 children with intestinal atresia in the Alder Hey series collected over 12 years represented an incidence of 1 per 5000 live births, which compares with the 1 per 9000 obtained from the WHO figures including duodenal atresia with Down's syndrome. The WHO figures ranged from 0.05 per 1000 births in Belfast to 0.76 in the Queen Victoria Hospital in Melbourne, or approximately 1 in 20 000 to 1 in 1300. Undoubtedly there are regional variations.

In our series, over 33 years, of 172 intestinal atresias and stenoses below the duodenum there were 58 involving jejunum, 72 ileum, seven colon and 35 multiple. There were 95 girls and 79 boys. The associated abnormalities found are listed in

Table 32.1 Associated major malformations and pre-operative complications in 172 intestinal atresias below the duodenum

Meconium peritonitis	32
Volvulus	30
Intestinal rotational anomalies	18
Perforation of bowel	18
Exomphalos	6
Skeletal anomalies	3
Major heart defects	3
Down's syndrome	2
Myelomeningocele	2
Gastro-oesophageal reflux	2
Hamartomatous cyst jejunum	2
Anorectal anomaly	2
Coarctation of aorta	1
Biliary atresia	1
Ectopia vesical	1
Oesophageal atresia	1
Cleft palate	1
Duplication cyst jejunum	1

Table 32.1. The presence of two cases of Down's syndrome is of some interest – one of them was found to have a duodenal membrane with a narrow orifice at 6 months of age. Our figures are similar to those found in the review compiled by the Surgical Section of the American Academy of Pediatrics [28], and those of Nixon and Tawes [88] and others [26,34,51].

Clinical picture

Maternal history

The maternal history again differs from that found in duodenal atresias. Of 93 cases with an accurate record of the length of pregnancy, only 16 were delivered under 36 weeks, and of a total of 120 with a maternal history available, 32 had hydramnios; one of these with a history of hydramnios also had oesophageal atresia, and of the remainder, 25 had obstruction in the jejunum and only four had ileal atresias. Hydramnios in the mother has long been recognized as a possible indication of alimentary tract obstruction in the fetus [118] and attention is drawn to it from time to time [30,70,85], indeed, polyhydramnios in the mother should be regarded as a positive indication for detailed ultrasound examination of the fetus to allow prenatal diagnosis of alimentary tract obstructions. Threatened abortion, toxaemia of pregnancy, jaundice in the first trimester, severe anaemia, antepartum haemorrhage and glycosuria were examples of complications of pregnancy found in 20 women.

Presenting symptoms and signs

Vomiting

Bile-stained vomiting is the most common presenting symptom of intestinal atresia. Its significance and differential diagnostic importance have been discussed in Chapter 31. In general, the higher the obstruction, the earlier and the more forceful is the vomiting. In low intestinal obstruction the onset of vomiting may be delayed for 24 h or even more and it is never forceful or profuse. Of 58 cases of jejunal atresia, 44 vomited during the first day and in only 14 was vomiting first observed on the second or third day after birth. Of the 72 infants with ileal atresia, only 36 started vomiting during the first 24 h and five never vomited at all. Of the seven babies with colonic atresia, three vomited from birth, one had one slight vomit and three none at all. Bile-stained vomiting does not necessarily mean that the infant is suffering from intestinal obstruction but nevertheless demands its exclusion [24].

Abdominal distension

This is frequently observed; the higher the site of the obstruction, the less marked is the distension. In more than half of the jejunal atresia cases in this series no abdominal distension was noted and in the others it was slight or moderate. Distension was absent in only nine of the 72 ileal atresia cases, in three it was moderate and in all the others it was gross. In low intestinal obstruction the distension is generalized and may be extreme, as the newborn infant's relatively poor abdominal muscles allow enormous ballooning of the abdominal wall (Figure 32.5). The abdominal skin is often tightly stretched and shiny, and large veins can be seen coursing over the abdomen in the subcutaneous tissues. It has been said that these dilated veins are a sign of peritonitis, but this is not invariably the case.

Abdominal distension present at birth is indicative of meconium peritonitis or meconium ileus [88].

Severe abdominal distension is a dangerous condition in newborn infants. Neonatal breathing is practically entirely diaphragmatic in nature and any interference with diaphragmatic contractions markedly reduces pulmonary excursion [95].

Visible peristalsis

This is an inconstant sign. It was noticed in less than a fifth of our cases and it may be observed in a perfectly normal premature infant with a thin abdominal wall.

Constipation

Constipation is often not absolute even in atresia. Only 30 of the 58 jejunal and 36 of the 72 ileal atresias had no bowel action at all.

Normal meconium was passed by 20 jejunal and six ileal atresia cases, and after rectal examination a further four infants passed meconium. In the remaining cases grey plugs of mucus were passed per rectum, except in one child with gangrenous bowel who passed a melaena stool. None of the children with colonic atresia passed any stools.

Diagnostic difficulties

Two conditions may easily be mistaken for intrinsic intestinal obstruction. Hirschsprung's disease may give a very similar clinical picture to low ileal or

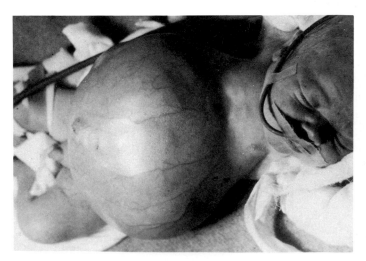

Figure 32.5 Gross abdominal distension in a newborn infant

colonic atresia [116]. In neonates with Hirsch-sprung's disease the forceful expulsion of flatus and some meconium on removing the examining finger from the rectum with subsequent deflation of the baby's lower intestine, often gives the clue. Differential diagnosis is further discussed in Chapter 37.

Similarly, meconium ileus may be mistaken for an intrinsic intestinal obstruction and is discussed in Chapter 36; a family history and the fact that the child is distended at birth may point to the diagnosis.

Intestinal stenoses are often difficult to diagnose as their symptoms and signs may be very variable. There was bile-stained vomiting in all our 17 cases, but this may be delayed for several weeks after birth. Abdominal distension tended to vary, and in all cases meconium and, later on, milk stools were passed. We have experienced great difficulty in the diagnosis of three cases with low ileal stenosis, who originally presented with bile-stained vomiting and abdominal distension which subsided without treatment. Subsequently they had further attacks of quickly subsiding intestinal obstruction. Straight radiography, barium follow-through and barium enema examination, and rectal biopsies were all perfectly normal. These children failed to thrive and gain weight, and extensive studies to identify an absorption anomaly were carried out without anything abnormal being discovered. All three finally obstructed completely and at laparotomy the presence of an ileal stenosis was found.

Clinical examination

This is often not very informative. It is rare to palpate a mass or discover tenderness on abdominal examination; in only seven of our cases was a mass palpated. On auscultation, increased high-pitched intestinal noises may occasionally be heard. Rectal examination should never be omitted except in very low birthweight babies. The little finger only should be used and great care should be taken not to injure the infant's delicate anal mucosa. The presence and nature of meconium, the presence of flatus, may all give a lead to the diagnosis. Limited experience in rectal examination of small infants may lead to the mistake of diagnosing a high rectal obstruction when the rectum is perfectly normal. It is often forgotten that in a small infant the rectosigmoid junction can be easily reached by the examining finger and that the acute angle between the rectum and sigmoid colon may give one the illusion of having come up against an obstruction.

Radiography

A radiographic picture of the infant's abdomen in the upright position confirms the diagnosis in the vast majority of cases. Newborn infants swallow air continually; this reaches the intestine within 1 h and the anus sometimes as early as 3 h [123] and certainly within 12 h after birth [16,131]. There should be fluid levels, and by studying the number, size and site of these fluid levels, as well as the absence or presence of air in the intestine distal to the obstruction, it is usually possible not only to diagnose a complete or incomplete obstruction, but also to define the anatomical level of the obstruction (Figure 32.6). Plain radiography may fail to differentiate between atresia and stenosis of the lower ileum or colon and such conditions as Hirsch-sprung's disease and the meconium plug syndrome [5]. A barium meal has little place in the diagnostic armamentarium and its dangers have already been refered to (Chapter 31). X-rays after a contrast meal should be reserved for complicated cases of incomplete obstruction such as malrotations (see Chapter 31) and intestinal stenoses, and instead of barium one of the new non-ionic contrasts should be used (see Chapter 8). Contrast enema, however, may be of value in intraluminal or functional obstruction (see Chapters 29, 36 and 37); in colonic atresia, contrast studies after colostomy may give detailed information of the lesion (Figure 32.7). When studying the plain radiograph of the abdomen of an infant with an intestinal atresia, the inexperienced may be tempted to make a diagnosis of incomplete obstruction by observing some air bubbles in the distal colon; these are usually due to air which has been introduced into the colon during a rectal examination.

Examination of the meconium

As indicated in the discussion of the pathogenesis of the condition, examination of the meconium is of no practical value and therefore we do not recommend it.

Treatment

Pre-operative treatment

In obstruction of the lower small intestine, symptoms may take some time to develop, and it is not surprising that admission to hospital of some of the children with intestinal atresia distal to the duodenum may occasionally be delayed. This explains the frequent occurrence of such fatal complications as severe bacterial peritonitis or gangrene of the intestine (see Table 32.1). Only 51 of our 172 cases were admitted when under 24 h old, and 27 were more than 4 days old on admission. Most of the latter suffered from intestinal stenosis, but our oldest case was a premature infant with jejunal

460

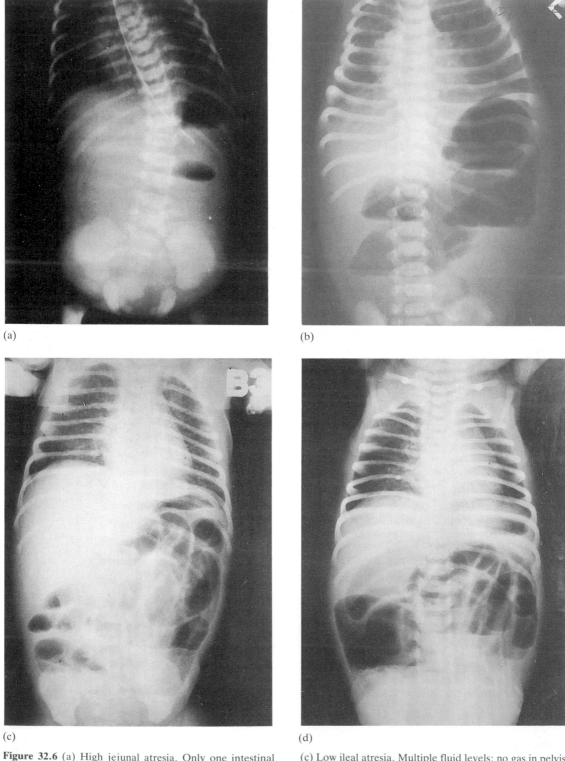

(a)

(b)

(c)

(d)

Figure 32.6 (a) High jejunal atresia. Only one intestinal fluid level; no gas in lower abdomen. (b) Atresia of mid-jejunum. Large fluid levels but relatively few in number.

(c) Low ileal atresia. Multiple fluid levels; no gas in pelvis. (d) Colonic atresia. Multiple fluid levels; one very large fluid level in the region of the caecum; no gas in pelvis

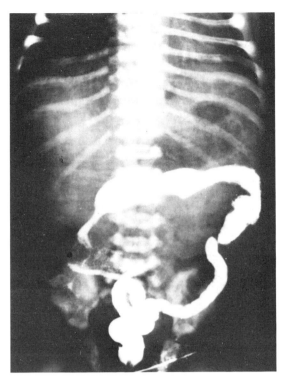

Figure 32.7 Colonic atresia demonstrated after colostomy with the colon filled from below per rectum and from above per colostomy

atresia, who was 13 days old on admission and had not had any intravenous therapy.

Because of their age on admission and the consequent fluid and electrolyte loss prior to admission, many of these infants suffer from dehydration and disturbances of their blood chemistry, and will need intravenous resuscitation prior to operation. In addition, their abdominal distension has to be relieved by suction. Fortunately, it is possible to deflate the abdomen of the newborn infant completely by continuous, low negative pressure gastric suction and we have not found any need to employ infants' intestinal tubes for this purpose.

The danger of infarction of bowel, however, is always present and operation must not be delayed more than an hour or two: abdominal deflation and intravenous resuscitation must therefore be achieved as quickly as possible.

Operation

General operative management and anaesthesia are discussed in the appropriate chapters.

It is our practice in all cases with obstruction of the intestine below the duodenum to open the abdomen through a transverse incision placed just above the umbilicus in the centre of the epigastrium (Figure 32.8a). Initially, this muscle-cutting incision should not be longer than 6–7.5 cm. A longer incision is frequently not necessary and, in addition, is time consuming to close. Should it be found that the initial incision is too short for adequate exposure, it is a small matter to enlarge it.

In all cases of neonatal intestinal obstruction an excess of intraperitoneal fluid will be encountered on opening the peritoneum and a specimen of this fluid should always be collected and sent for bacterial culture. The fluid is usually clear and yellow in colour but in cases with intestinal strangulation the fluid may be blood-stained.

It is usually best to deliver the dilated as well as the collapsed loops of the intestine into the wound and to wrap them immediately into packs moistened with warm saline. Because of the frequent association of intestinal atresia with meconium peritonitis, difficulty may be experienced in delivering the intestinal loops just proximal to the obstruction and it may be necessary to divide numerous and often vascular adhesions and bands before it is possible to deliver the terminal atretic segment into the wound.

Prior to 1922 the operative mortality for intestinal atresia was 95–100% [27] and in 1952 it was still 80% even in wellknown paediatric surgical centres [71].

This high mortality was in part due to difficulties with the actual anastomotic technique, but mainly due to the prolonged ileus and failure of the anastomosis to work during the postoperative period. It was shown by Nixon [86] that the main reason for these bad results was the fact that the enormously dilated segment of the intestine proximal to the atresia was unable to perform effective peristaltic movements. In addition, the excessive distension of this segment of intestine often interferes with the blood supply and hence the vitality of the gut, and allows bacteria to traverse the intestinal wall, causing peritonitis [52]. Furthermore, because of the marked inequality of the intestinal segments proximal and distal to the obstruction, there is a considerable danger that the distal loop of intestine will kink after an anastomosis has been performed [98].

It should be remembered that Louw's experimental work showed that the blood supply of the proximal end of the distal bowel as well as of the distal end of the proximal bowel could be deficient and the functional efficiency of that bowel may be questionable [74]. Doolin *et al.* [32] in experimental work on lamb fetuses showed that myoelectric activity in the micro-bowel immediately distal to the atresia was considerably reduced thus contributing to the postoperative functional obstruction. It is,

authors [8,87] have found that a one-layer anasto-mosis is associated with an increased frequency of intestinal leaks and have, therefore, reverted to a two-layer anastomosis.

It is advisable to perform the anastomosis with the aid of intestinal clamps, and here we have found the use of bulldog clamps most satisfactory (Figure 32.11). We have not found that the 'aseptic' anasto-mosis advocated by Swenson [115] has marked advantages. It is difficult to perform and the lumen of the anastomosed gut tends to become narrowed.

Despite the resection of considerable lengths of the intestine proximal to the obstruction, the remaining proximal gut will still be distended with air and intestinal contents and should be decom-pressed. Aspiration of the gut either with a needle and syringe or with aid of a special aspirator is not very effective, and decompressing the intestine by passing a long metal suction tube along its lumen [44] is very traumatizing to the neonatal intestinal mucosa. We have found that decompressing the intestine by passing a size 12 F Foley's catheter along its lumen is most effective and causes little trauma (Figure 32.12).

After the anastomosis is completed, it should be tested by removing the bulldog clamps and allowing intestinal gas to distend the intestine, watching for the telltale escape of air bubbles (Figure 32.13). The gap in the mesentery is then closed by grasping the free margins with pairs of curved mosquito forceps and tying a ligature around them (Figure 32.8e). Nixon and Tawes again pointed out [88] that, because of the unequal length of the margins of the mesenteric gap, simple approximation of the mar-gins may cause kinking; they therefore advised that a tuck should be taken in the edge of the proximal mesentery to prevent it. The survey of the Surgical Section of the American Academy of Pediatrics [28] did not show any advantage in decompressing types of anastomosis over 'end-to-back' anastomosis pro-vided there was adequate excision of proximal dilated bowel and this excision seemed particularly important in jejunal atresias where the mortality is somewhat higher. However, when the atresia is complicated by perforation and bacterial peritonitis, or if vascular integrity is in doubt because there has been a volvulus of the dilated proximal blind loop, a primary anastomosis is especially hazardous and liable to leak; some sort of venting enterostomy should be made (Figure 32.14). Gross [45], after many years' experience, recommended a Mikulicz double-barrelled enterostomy; Santulli [101] devised a proximal enterostomy with a side-to-end anastomosis to the distal intestine; the Bishop–Koop [9] distal enterostomy, the proximal bowel being anastomosed to it end to side – first designed

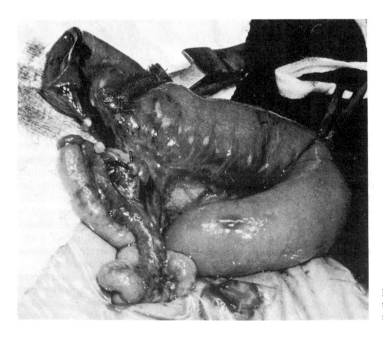

Figure 32.11 The proximal and distal intes-tinal segments just prior to the commence-ment of an end-to-back anastomosis

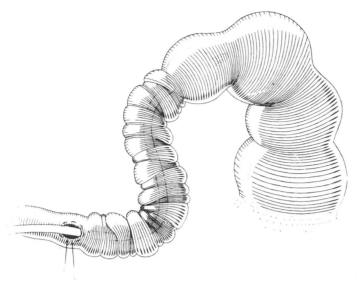

Figure 32.12 Decompressing the distended intestine with the aid of a Foley's catheter

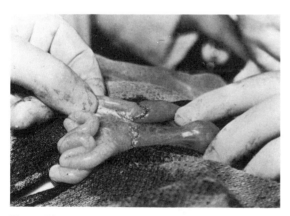

Figure 32.13 Testing the end-to-back anastomosis at the completion of operation

for the treatment of meconium ileus – can also be applied to the intestinal atresia situation.

Halsband and Rehbein [48] used a double tube technique – a wide-bore tube and a finer one, both introduced into the bowel proximal to the anastomosis, the former to drain the distended loop and the latter to irrigate the distal bowel. We have found the Bishop–Koop technique to be the most satisfactory: it has the advantage of being an effective enterostomy without the disadvantage of excessive fluid loss when the bowel begins to function.

Stenosis, as distinct from atresia, accounted for less than 5% of our series: in one case a longitudinal incision through the stenosed area was closed transversely, but a limited resection and end-to-end anastomosis is more satisfactory.

One of the patients with colonic atresia died of his multiple anomalies before operation; the others were all managed with primary colostomies. This staging of correction was recommended by Boles, Vassy and Ralston in 1976 [12] though other authors [74] have recommended excision and end-to-end anastomosis. In a review of 19 cases of colonic atresia Powell and Raffensperger [93] concluded that resection and ileo-transverse colostomy was the treatment of choice for atresias proximal to the splenic flexure, but for atresias distal to the splenic flexure colostomy a staged procedure was indicated.

Multiple atresias present special problems in management. They formed just over 20% of our cases, a figure which compares with the majority of other reported series [48,75,108,115], though it is much higher than found in de Lorimier's review of 65 centres [28]. Resection of the dilated proximal segment together with portions of bowel between the multiple atresias and one anastomosis is the treatment of choice, provided an adequate amount of small bowel is left (see below). Multiple anastomoses and/or enterostomies carry a high mortality [35]. When the length of bowel involved is extensive and the number of atresias is excessive, diaphragms have been successfully perforated with a size 17 F gum elastic bougie passed along the whole length of the small intestine [35]. Late follow-up of two cases on whom this procedure had been carried out 8 and

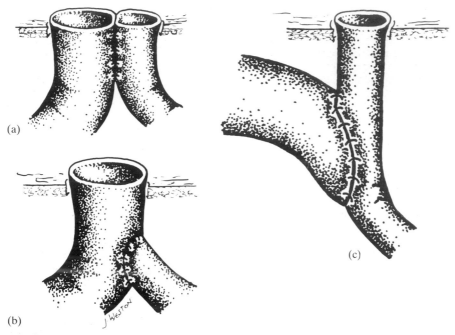

Figure 32.14 (a) Gross 'double-barrelled' enterostomy [45]. (b) 'Proximal chimney' enterostomy [108]. (c) 'Distal chimney' enterostomy [9]

9 years previously showed no evidence of any residual septum.

Postoperative treatment

Details of general postoperative management are discussed in Chapter 5 but certain special points apply to atresias of the small intestine. In spite of extensive resection of the dilated proximal small bowel, postoperative ileus may be prolonged and continuous intestinal decompression by nasogastric suction and intravenous therapy will be necessary for a period of at least 24–48 h and often more; the higher the atresia, the longer this period of ileus is likely to be. Decompression by a gastrostomy tube [54,81] has been recommended and in the high jejunal atresia a Silastic catheter can be passed in alongside the gastrostomy tube and threaded into the jejunum through the anastomosis in order to start feedings early whilst decompression of the stomach continues; where there is no gastrostomy, such a Silastic tube can also be passed through nose and oesophagus during operation and threaded through the anastomosis in a similar fashion. Improvements in parenteral feeding have undoubtedly reduced the urgency of commencing either oral or tube feeding (see Chapter 5). When the gastric aspirations are reduced in both quantity

and bile content sufficiently to commence oral feeding this must be started with very small quantities and increased very slowly in order to avoid vomiting and the dangers of aspiration.

Lactose intolerance is common following intestinal procedures in the newborn and malabsorption and diarrhoea are quite frequent problems even when relatively minor lengths of small bowel have been resected, especially if the ileocaecal valve has been included in the resection. It should be remembered that an unknown amount of small bowel may have been lost as a result of the pathological catastrophe which caused the atresia, for example in multiple atresias or the 'apple-peel' deformity. Problems can often be avoided by starting the babies on a formula containing medium chain triglycerides and casein hydrolysate (Pregestamil) (see Chapter 5); where even this formula is not tolerated total parenteral nutrition is indicated.

Results

Prior to 1950 very few infants survived operations for intestinal stenosis and atresia [111]; even in Ladd's and Gross's expert hands, only nine out of 52 infants operated on in the Boston Children's Hospital prior to 1951 survived [69]. Results in the

1950s and 1960s improved but the overall mortality rate remained between 20 and 30% even in the best hands [28,49,88,127]. In the 1970s and 1980s however, partly as a result of the introduction of total parenteral nutrition further improvements could be expected. So-called 'unavoidable' deaths associated with gross prematurity and multiple other severe anomalies will always occur and, as the case material will differ from hospital to hospital, comparisons are often very difficult. There should be virtually no mortality in the uncomplicated case of intestinal atresia below the level of the duodenum. We have had no deaths in this group of cases in the Liverpool Neonatal Surgical Centre. We have seen that severe associated abnormalities are less common in jejuno-ileal than in duodenal atresia and it is therefore not surprising that deaths due to associated anomalies are not frequent; only three of our infants died because of an associated anomaly. Rescorla and Grosfeld reported an 87% survival rate in 52 cases of jejunoileal atresia and 100% survival in colonic atresias [100].

In the Liverpool series the mortality rate was nearly 30% in 75 cases from 1954 to 1967; it fell to 25% in 58 cases from 1968 to 1975 and in the 10 years from 1976 to 1985 there were five deaths in 39 cases, a mortality rate of 12.8%. One of these deaths was the result of associated anomalies including severe congenital heart disease; three had massive resections being left with small intestine measured at 35 cm, 30 cm and 24.5 cm and survived on total parenteral nutrition for 1, 4 and 5 months. The last death was from septicaemia within 12 h of operation and 36 h from birth, in a child where there had been intrauterine perforation of the gut and premature rupture of the membranes.

Morbidity also in recent years has improved due to better control of already existing infection, improved surgical techniques and a reduction of the number of anastomotic leaks. Parenteral nutrition allows long-term management of postoperative ileus, both that due to abnormal gut motility and that due to early adhesions. Second laparotomies are consequently undertaken less frequently. In our experience late obstruction due to postoperative adhesions is very rare though Wilkins and Spitz found a total incidence of adhesive obstructions in five out of 74 small bowel atresias [128].

Many of the earlier complications could have been avoided by earlier diagnosis; of the first 75 cases in our series less than one-third were admitted during the first day of life and one-quarter did not arrive until they were more than 4 days old. Even from 1968 to 1975, of 58 cases only 21 (63%) were admitted under 24 h of age, 15 (26%) from 24–48 h and a similar number from 48–96 h, the remaining seven children (12%) being over 4 days old when admitted.

From 1976 to 1985, in spite of the increasing influence of ultrasound in antenatal diagnosis and the known early onset of vomiting, out of the 39 jejunoileal atresias the majority were admitted at 24 to 48 h of age: five jejunal and two ileal atresias were admitted during the first 24 h but two jejunal and four ileal atresias were not admitted until the third day and seven jejunal and one ileal atresia were over 4 days old on admission. Some paediatricians, obstetricians and midwives are still slow to recognize the significance of vomiting though they always recognize abdominal distension very quickly. The seriousness of green vomiting cannot be over-emphasized.

Long segment bowel resection

Another cause of high mortality is the loss of extensive lengths of small bowel. Apart from any bowel lost by resection because of its severe dilatation, the total length of remaining small intestine measured accurately in autopsy material together with the length of resected bowel frequently amounts to much less than the average length of normal small intestine in the newborn. Willis Potts himself in 1955 [92] doubted whether a newborn infant could survive the loss of more than 15% of his small intestine.

In 1967 Rickham [102] defined extensive small bowel resection as an excision leaving not more than 75 cm of small bowel; this amounts to a 70% resection of the average neonatal small bowel of 250 cm, though the normal length varies considerably [99] and measuring methods are of variable accuracy [103].

Pilling and Cresson [90] reported the first successful extensive resection in 1957, Wilkinson, Hughes and Toms [129] reported one successful case in 1963 and by 1965 Kuffer *et al.* [67] could find six successful cases in the literature. However, seven survivors out of 17 cases were reported from Liverpool in 1968 [103] and nine patients surviving from 10–18 years were reported in 1977 [105]; one of these survivors had a measured length of 26 cm jejunum anastomosed to ascending colon at his neonatal operation.

Parenteral nutrition

All these children with massive resection require long-term intravenous alimentation, defined as a period exceeding 4 weeks when at least 50% of the necessary calories are supplied intravenously (see Chapter 5). There is no doubt that improved results in these children are attributable to their support by intravenous feeding over a period of weeks or even months during which, by a combination of growth and adaptation which is not fully understood, they compensate for their original short bowel [62].

Oral feeding must be started very slowly, usually some 2–4 weeks after operation; the first feeds given are very small amounts of hypo-osmolar glucose solution (1%) gradually increased to normal osmolarity and to larger quantities. Next electrolyte and amino acid mixtures may be introduced and then elemental feeds (Nutri 2000 (Nutricia) [113], Flexical (Mead Johnson), Vivonex (Eaton). All these substances are started in low concentrations to prevent diarrhoea. It may be 3–6 months, or even 12 months when very little small intestine has been left, before a normal diet can be introduced, starting with low fat, low disaccharide feeds [48,53].

If distal ileum has been removed, vitamin B_{12} must be given [13,20]. Cholestyramines and a low fat diet with medium chain triglycerides may also be necessary in children whose terminal ileum has been resected and who may develop steatorrhoea because of failure to absorb bile salts. Cellulose or pectin may slow the intestinal transit time but response to these substances is variable.

Should diarrhoea occur during the period of increasing feeding a return to intravenous alimentation is necessary.

The prognosis depends on many factors; loss of jejunum is better tolerated than loss of ileum, and loss of the ileocaecal valve adds problems though two long-term survivors had right hemicolectomies in addition to their small bowel resections. Perhaps the most remarkable fact is that eight of the nine long-term survivors [105] had no clinical evidence of absorption difficulties at all after the age of 20 months. The only one who had a poor end result was a child whose mother would not bring him back to the hospital for follow-up, who had severe constant diarrhoea, and who apparently has a permanently deficient fat absorption.

The capacity for improvement of absorptive ability has clearly altered the limits for subtotal resection and there is a difference in whether the remaining bowel is jejunum or ileum; however, 20 cm of residual small bowel seems to be the lowest possible limit.

A variety of operative procedures have been devised for slowing transit time and increasing absorptive surfaces: these are not discussed since they are not indicated during the first 3 months of life.

Congenital segmental dilatation of intestine

Like 'a snake that swallowed the bait' is a graphic description of a segmental dilatation of the transverse colon found at autopsy on a 9-day-old infant [19], which portrays well the essential feature of this condition, i.e. localized dilatation of a single well-defined segment of intestine with more or less abrupt transition to normal bowel both proximally and distally.

Although this is not an atretic lesion it is included in this chapter because we consider that the embryogenesis of some, if not all, of these lesions may bear a relationship to the embryogenesis of some cases of intestinal atresia.

Incidence

Although we were able to review only 15 cases of segmental dilatation in 1977 [57] and several cases have been subsequently reported [4,19,64,122], we will only discuss the ten cases which were diagnosed and treated in the neonatal period, since it is not possible in cases presenting at a later age to be sure that the lesion was of congenital origin.

Pathology

All our four cases presented in the neonatal period and involved the ileum [15]. Others have been reported involving jejunum [3,57] and colon [3,19]. The feature common to all is the presence of a single 'blow-out', sometimes of gross proportions (Figure 32.15a,b) of a segment of intestine, without any evidence of intrinsic obstruction or of deficient innervation and with bowel of normal or near-normal calibre above and below. With one possible exception [57], the ileal cases have been situated at the 'Meckel's site' but in none of these cases did the blown-out segment of bowel resemble a diverticulum. Two of these ileal segmental dilatations [78,97] were contained in an exomphalos sac, and the features of Rehbein's case [97] strongly suggested that the dilatation had arisen as a result of chronic obstruction of the afferent and efferent limbs of the loop of ileum which was contained in the exomphalos sac, a type of insult to the developing intestine which in a more severe form would result in atresia. In the other case of an ileal segmental dilatation contained in an exomphalos sac [78], a very unusual type [130] of heteroplastic nodule (consisting of squamous epithelium, gastric mucosa, pancreatic tissue and lung tissue) was present in the wall of the dilated segment, suggesting a very early insult to the developing bowel. One of our own cases of ileal segmental dilatation [57] contained a very similar nodule of heteroplastic tissue, and in the case reported by Aterman and Abaci [3] areas of heteroplastic oesophageal and gastric mucosa were present in terminal ileum and caecum, which formed part of the dilated segment. The presence of such tissues in the ileum or caecum is a very rare finding [130] and suggests that these particular cases constitute a pathological entity. The remainder of the wall of the dilated segments has been unremarkable except for some vascular dilatation and thinning out of the muscle layers. Normal ganglionation has been seen in all cases.

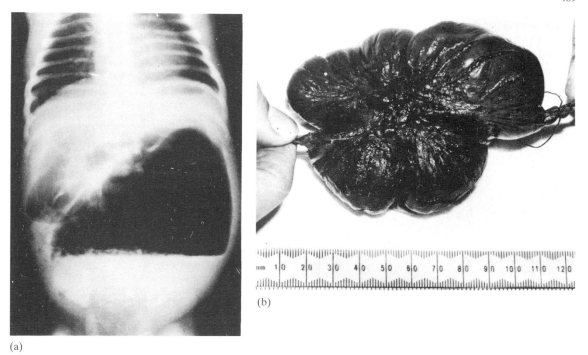

(a)

(b)

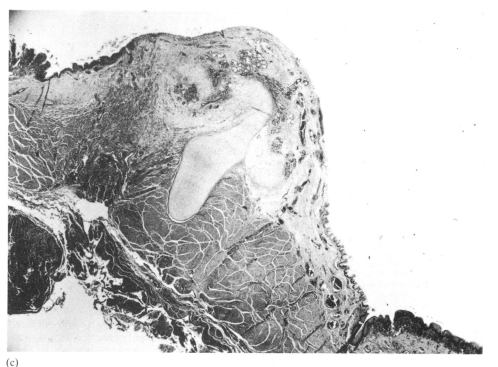

(c)

Figure 32.15 (a) Case of ileal segmental dilatation. Plain erect abdominal radiograph taken at 36 h of age, showing a grossly dilated viscus with an air/fluid level. (b) Same case as (a). Resected segment of ileum viewed from the mesenteric aspect, showing saccular dilatation and abrupt transition to narrow calibre bowel at each end. (c) Same case as (a) and (b). Section through a nodule of heteroplastic tissue on the mesenteric border of the dilated segment (haematoxylin and eosin, ×9.2). It is composed of cartilage and striated muscle. The epithelium at its base is squamous stratified, with pseudo-stratified towards the summit

Clinical picture

Of the neonatal cases which have been reported, four presented on the day of birth for treatment of other malformation (two cases of exomphalos [78,97], one case of myelomeningocele [130], one case of bladder exstrophy and covered anus, and one case of low imperforate anus). With the exception of Rehbein's patient [97], who had the dilated segment of ileum removed at the time of exomphalos repair, these infants developed signs of intestinal obstruction after admission. Infants without major external malformation were all admitted with symptoms and signs of intestinal obstruction, including abdominal distension, in the early neonatal period. The typical radiological finding was of a large, sometimes enormous (Figure 32.15a), loop of bowel distended with gas, with or without a fluid level. In three cases [3,57,122] (one ileocolic and two ileal) the dilated loop filled during the course of two ileal) the dilated loop filled during the course of a barium enema examination.

Treatment

Treatment is by resection and end-to-end anastomosis and results are good. All our four cases survived without problems. One reported case with a short gut syndrome (35 cm small intestine remaining after resection) also survived [4].

Comment

The probability of an obstructive cause in the two cases of segmental dilatation associated with exomphalos raised the possibility of a similar mechanism being involved in the pathogenesis of the other cases in which, at the time of surgery, there was no apparent extrinsic (or intrinsic) obstructive lesion. A temporary obstructive insult at an early stage of development (e.g. by vitelline vessels which subsequently involute) is a possible explanation.

References

1. Ahlfeld, F. (1880) *Die Missbildungen des Menschen*, F.W. Grunow, Leipzig
2. Arnal-Monreal, F., Pombo, F. and Capdevila-Puerta, A. (1983) Multiple hereditary gastrointestinal atresias: study of a family. *Acta Pediat. Scand.*, **72**, 773–777
3. Aterman, K. and Abaci, F. (1967) Heterotropic gastric and oesophageal tissue in the colon. *Am. J. Dis. Child.*, **113**, 552–559
4. Babut, J.M., Bracq, H., Ricour, C., Thomas, M., Boureau, M., Weisgerber, G., Soulie, J. and Braun, P. (1977) Les dilatations segmentaires congénitales de l'intestin. *Ann. Chir. infant.*, **18**, 11
5. Benson, C.D. (1955) Resection and primary anastomosis of the jejunum and ileum in the newborn. *Ann. Surg.*, **142**, 478–485
6. Benson, C.D., Lloyd, J.R. and Smith, D.J. (1960) Resection and primary anastomosis in the management of stenosis and atresia of the jejunum and ileum. *Pediatrics*, **26**, 265–272
7. Binninger, J.N. (1673) *Observationum et curationum medicinalium, centuriae quinque*, Montbelgard Hippianis
8. Bishop, H.C. (1976) Small bowel obstructions in the newborn. *Surg. Clins N. Am.*, **56**, 329–348
9. Bishop, H.C. and Koop, C.E. (1957) Management of meconium ileus; resection, Roux-en-Y anastomosis and ileostomy irrigation with pancreatic enzymes. *Ann. Surg.*, **145**, 410–414
10. Sutton, J. (1889) Imperforate ileum. *Am. J. Med. Sci.*, **98**, 457–462
11. Blyth, H. and Dickson, J.A.S. (1969) Apple peel syndrome. *J. Med. Genet.*, **6**, 275–277
12. Boles, E.T., Vassy, L.E. and Ralston, M. (1976) Atresia of the colon. *J. Pediat. Surg.*, **11**, 69–75
13. Booth, C.C. and Mollin, D.C. (1959) The site of absorption of vitamin B_{12} in man. *Lancet*, **i**, 18–21
14. Braun, H. (1902) Ueber den Angeborenen Verschluss des Duenndarms. *Bruns' Beitr. klin. Chir.*, **43**, 993
15. Brown, A. and Carty, H. (1984) Segmental dilatation of the ileum. *Br. J. Radiol.*, **57**, 371–374
16. Brown, J.J.M. (1957) Small intestinal obstruction in the newly born. *Ann. R. Coll. Surg. Engl.*, **20**, 280–297
17. Chester, S.T. and Robinson, W.T. (1957) Congenital atresia of the transverse colon. *Ann. Surg.*, **146**, 824–829
18. Chiari, H. (1888) Ueber eine intrauterine entstandene und von Darmatresie gefolgten Intussusception des Ileums. *Prag. med. Wschr.*, **13**, 399
19. Chiba, T. and Kokubo, T. (1976) Congenital segmental dilatation of the colon. *Arch. Jpn. Chir.*, **45**, 45–47
20. Clark, A.C. and Booth, C.C. (1960) Deficiency of vitamin B_{12} after extensive resection of the distal small intestine in an infant. *Arch. Dis. Child.*, **35**, 595–599
21. Cloutier, R. (1975) Intestinal smooth muscle response to chronic obstruction: possible applications in jejuno-ileal atresia. *J. Pediat. Surg.*, **10**, 3–8
22. Congenital Malformations (1966) *Bull. Wld Hlth Org.*, **34**, Supplement
23. Courtois, B. (1950) Les origines foetales des occlusions congenitales du grêle dites par atresie. *J. Chir., Paris*, **78**, 405
24. Craig, W.S. (1961) Vomiting in the early days of life. *Arch Dis. Child.*, **36**, 451–459
25. Daneman, A. and Martin, D.J. (1979) A syndrome of multiple atresias with intraluminal calcifications. *Pediat. Radiol.*, **8**, 227–231
26. Daudet, M., Chappuis, J.P. and Marion, J. (1972)

Expérience d'un service de chirurgie pédiatrique en matière d'occlusions neonatales. Commentaires à propos de 150 cas observés en 15 ans: analyse des progrés réalisés. *Ann. Chir. infant.*, **13**, 291–311

27. Davis, D.L. and Poynter, C.W.M. (1922) Congenital occlusion of the intestine. *Surg Gynec. Obstet.*, **34**, 35–41
28. De Lorimier, A.A., Fonkalsrud, E.W. and Hays, D.M. (1969) Congenital atresia and stenosis of the jejunum and ileum. *Surgery*, **65**, 819–877
29. De Lorimier, A.A. and Harrison, M.R. (1983) Intestinal plication in the treatment of atresia. *J. Pediat. Surg.*, **18**, 734–737
30. De Young, V.R. (1958) Hydramnios as a signal to the physician responsible for newborn infants. *J. Pediat.*, **53**, 277–284
31. Dickson, J.A.S. (1970) Apple peel small bowel: an uncommon variant of duodenal and jejunal atresia. *J. Pediat. Surg.*, **5**, 595–600
32. Doolin, E.J., Ormsbee, H.S. and Hill, J.L. (1987) Motility abnormality in intestinal atresia. *J. Pediat. Surg.*, **22**, 320–324
33. Dublin, L.I. (1947) Large reduction in hazards of maternity and infancy. *Bull. Metrop. Life Insur.*, **28**, 4
34. Dykstra, G., Sieber, W. and Kiesewetter, W.B. (1968) Intestinal atresia. *Arch. Surg.*, **97**, 175–182
35. El Shafie, M. and Rickham, P.P. (1970) Multiple intestinal atresias. *J. Pediat. Surg.*, **5**, 655–659
36. Feggetter, S. (1955) Congenital intestinal atresia. *Br. J. Surg.*, **42**, 378–388
37. Fishbein, M. (1949) American Academy of Pediatrics Report. *J. Am. Med. Ass.*, **139**, 1002
38. Fockens, P. (1911) Ein operativer Fall von kongenitaler Duenndarmatresie. *Zentbl. Chir.*, **38**, 532
39. Foglia, R.P., Jobst, S., Fonkalsrud, E.W. and Ament, M.F. (1983) An unusual variant of a jejunoileal atresia. *J. Pediat. Surg.*, **18**, 182–184
40. Forshall, I., Hall, E.G. and Rickham, P.P. (1952) Meconium peritonitis. *Br. J. Surg.*, **40**, 31–40
41. Forssner, H. (1907) Die angeborenan Darmund Oesophagusatresien. *Anat. Hette., Wiesbaden*, **34**, 1–163
42. Gaub, O.C. (1922) Congenital stenosis and atresia of the intestinal tract above the rectum. *Trans. Am. Surg. Ass.*, **40**, 582–640
43. Goeller, G.C. (1683) *Abortus humani monstrosi*, Norimb. Hist. Anatom. Misc. Acad. Nat. Curios
44. Grob, M. (1957) *Lehrbuch der Kinderchirurgie*. Georg Thieme Verlag, Stuttgart
45. Gross, R.E. (1953) *The Surgery of Infancy and Childhood*, W.B. Saunders, Philadelphia
46. Guttman, F.M., Braun, P., Garance, P.H., Blanchard, H., Collin, P.P., Dallaire, L., Desjardins, J.G. and Perreault, G. (1973) Multiple atresias and a new syndrome of hereditary multiple atresias involving the gastro-intestinal tract from stomach to rectum. *J. Pediat. Surg.*, **8**, 633–640
47. Haller, J.A., Tepas, J.J., Pickard, L.R. and Shermeta, D.W. (1983) Intestinal atresia: current concepts of pathogenesis, pathophysiology and operative management. *Am. Surg.*, **49**, 385–391
48. Halsband, H. and Rehbein, F. (1969) Atresien des jejunum und ileum. *Z. Kinderchir.*, **3**, 441
49. Handelsman, J.C., Abrams, S. and Corry, R.J. (1963) Improvement of therapy for congenital jejuno-ileal atresia. *Surg. Gynec. Obstet.*, **117**, 691–702
50. Hardin, C.A. and Friesen, S.R. (1960) Congenital atresia of the colon. *Arch. Surg.*, **80**, 616–619
51. Hays, D.M. (1969) Intestinal atresia and stenosis. *Curr. Probl. Surg.* Year Book Medical Publishers, Chicago
52. Heinrich, G. and Holle, F. (1956) Zur Diagnostik und Behandlung der Dünn und Dickdarmatresie beim Neugeborenen. *Dt. med. J.*, **7**, 69–72
53. Hofmann, A.F. and Poley, J.R. (1969) Cholestyramine treatment of diarrhoea associated with ileal resection. *New Engl. J. Med.*, **281**, 397–402
54. Holder, T.M. and Gross, R.E. (1960) Temporary gastrostomy in pediatric. *Surgery Pediatrics*, **26**, 36–41
55. Horch, C. (1696) *De Puella cum coalitu intestini ilei nata et per vaginti duos dei vivente.* Misc. Acad. Nat. Curios, Frankof
56. Howard, E.R. and Othersen, H.B. (1973) Proximal jejunoplasty in the treatment of jejunal atresia. *J. Pediat. Surg.*, **8**, 685–690
57. Irving, I.M. and Lister, J. (1977) Segmental dilatation of the ileum. *J. Pediat. Surg.*, **12**, 103–112
58. Jaboulay (1901) Cited by Webb, C.H. and Wagensteen, O.H. (1931) Congenital intestinal atresia. *Am. J. Dis. Child.*, **41**, 262–284
59. Jimenez, F.A. and Reiner, L. (1961) Arteriographic findings in congenital anomalies of the mesentery and intestines. *Surg. Gynec. Obstet.*, **113**, 346–352
60. Johnston, F.P. (1910) The development of the stomach and small intestine in the human embryo. *Am. J. Anat.*, **10**, 521
61. Keith, A. (1948) *Human Embryology and Morphology*, Edward Arnold, London
62. Kim, S.H. and Rickham, P.P. (1972) Parenteral lipids and amino acids in surgical neonates. *Z. Kinderchir.*, **11**, 277
63. Koga, Y., Hayashinda, Y., Ikeda, K., Inskuchi, K. and Hashimoto, N. (1975) Intestinal atresia in fetal dogs produced by localised ligation of mesenteric vessels. *J. Pediat. Surg.*, **10**, 949–953
64. Komi, N. and Kohyama, Y. (1974) Congenital segmental dilatation of the jejunum. *J. Pediat. Surg.*, **9**, 409–410
65. Kreuter, E. (1905) *Die Angeborenen Verengungen und Verschluesse des Darmkanals im Lichte der Entwicklungs-geschichte*, Habil. Schr. Erlangen
66. Kroop, H. and Thomas, C.G. (1972) An experimental model for neonatal intestinal atresia. *Am. Surg.*, **38**, 676–680
67. Kuffer, F., Fiolet, B., Oetliker, O. and Bettex, M.

(1965) Darmfunktionsproben nach subtotaler Danm resektion bei einem Säugling. *Helv. Paediat. Acta*, **20**, 19–26

68. Kuliga, P. (1960) Zur Genese der Kongenitalen Duenndarmatresien. *Beitr. path. Anat.*, **33**, 169

69. Ladd, W.E. and Gross, R.E. (1941) *Abdominal Surgery in Infancy and Childhood*, W.B. Saunders, Philadelphia

70. Lloyd, J.R. and Clatworthy, H.W. Jr (1958) Hydramnios as an aid to the early diagnosis of congenital obstruction of the alimentary tract. A study of the maternal and fetal factors. *Pediatrics*, **21**, 903–909

71. Louw, J.H. (1952) Congenital atresia and severe stenosis in the newborn. *S. Afr. J. clin. Sci.*, **3**, 109

72. Louw, J.H. (1959) Congenital intestinal atresia and stenosis in the newborn. *Ann. R. Coll. Surg. Engl.*, **35**, 209–234

73. Louw, J.H. (1964) Investigation into the etiology of congenital atresia of the colon. *Dis. Colon Rectum*, **7**, 471–478

74. Louw, J.H. (1966) Congenital atresia and stenosis of the small intestine. *S. Afr. J. Surg.*, **4**, 57

75. Louw, J.H. (1966) Jejuno-ileal atresia and stenosis. *J. Pediat. Surg.*, **1**, 8–23

76. Louw, J.H. and Barnard, C.N. (1955) Congenital atresia. *Lancet*, **ii**, 1065–1067

77. Lynn, H.B. and Espinas, E.E. (1959) Intestinal atresia. *Arch. Surg.*, **79**, 357–361

78. Marsden, H.B. and Gilchrist, W. (1963) Pulmonary heteroplasia in the terminal ileum. *J. Path. Bact.*, **86**, 532–534

79. Martin, C.E., Leonidas, J.C. and Amoury, R.A. (1976) Multiple gastro-intestinal atresias with intraluminal calcifications and cystic dilatation of bile ducts. *Pediatrics*, **57**, 268–271

80. Martin, L.W. and Zerella, J.T. (1976) Jejunoileal atresia: a proposed classification. *J. Pediat. Surg.*, **11**, 399–403

81. Meeker, I.A. and Snyder, W.A. (1962) Gastrostomy for the newborn surgical patient. *Arch. Dis. Child.*, **37**, 159–166

82. Mishalany, H.G. and Der Kaloustian, V.M. (1971) Familial multiple level intestinal atresias: report of two siblings. *J. Pediat.*, **79**, 124–125

83. Mishalany, H.G. and Najjar, F. (1968) Familial jejunal atresia: three cases in one family. *J. Pediat.*, **73**, 753–755

84. Montsouris, C. (1966) The 'solid stage' and congenital intestinal atresia. *J. Pediat. Surg.*, **1**, 446–450

85. Moya, F., Apgar, V., James, L.S. and Berrien, C. (1960) Hydramnios and congenital anomalies. *J. Am. Med. Ass.*, **173**, 1552–1556

86. Nixon, H.H. (1955) Intestinal obstruction in the newborn. *Arch. Dis. Childh.*, **30**, 13–22

87. Nixon, H.H. (1965) Podiumgespraech ueber Darmatresien und Stenosen. *Z. Kinderchir.*, **2**, 126

88. Nixon, H.H. and Tawes, R. (1971) Etiology and treatment of small intestinal atresia. Analysis of a series of 127 jejunoileal atresias and comparison with 62 duodenal atresias. *Surgery*, **69**, 41–51

89. Phelan, J.T., Lemmer, K.E. and McDonaugh, K.B. (1959) Jejunoileal atresia and stenosis. *Surgery*, **46**, 430–436

90. Pilling, G.P. and Cresson, S.C. (1957) Massive resection of the small intestine in the neonatal period. *Pediatrics*, **19**, 940–948

91. Potts, W.J. (1947) Congenital atresia of intestine and colon. *Surg. Gynec. Obstet.*, **85**, 14–19

92. Potts, W.J. (1955) Pediatric surgery. *J. Am. Med. Ass.*, **157**, 627–630

93. Powell, R.W. and Raffensperger, J.G. (1982) Congenital colonic atresia. *J. Pediat. Surg.*, **17**, 166–170

94. Puri, P. and Fujimoto, T. (1988) New observations on the pathogenesis of multiple intestinal atresias. *J. Pediat. Surg.*, **23**, 221–225

95. Rees, G.J. (1957) Neonatal anaesthesia. *Br. J. Clin. Pract.*, **11**, 822–823

96. Rehbein, F. (1959) Die Akuten Chirurgischen Baucherkrankungen beim Neugeborenen. *Langenbecks Arch. klin. Chir.*, **292**, 402

97. Rehbein, F. (1976) *Kinderchirurgische Operationen*, Hipokrates Verlag, Stuttgart

98. Rehbein, F. and Halsband, H. (1968) A double-tube technic for the treatment of meconium ileus and small bowel atresia. *J. Pediat. Surg.*, **3**, 723–726

99. Reiquam, C.W., Allen, R.P. and Akers, D.R. (1965) Normal and abnormal small bowel lengths. *Am. J. Dis. Child.*, **109**, 447–451

100. Rescorla, F.J. and Grosfeld, J.L. (1985) Intestinal atresia and stenosis. Analysis of survival in 120 cases. Surgery, **98**, 668–676

101. Rickham, P.P. (1957) Intestinal obstruction in the neonatal period. *Br. J. clin. Pract.*, **11**, 833–841

102. Rickham, P.P. (1967) Massive small intestinal resection in newborn infants. *Ann. R. Coll. Surg. Engl.*, **41**, 480–492

103. Rickham, P.P. (1968) Ansgedehute Dirnndarmresettionen beim Neugeborenen. *Z. Kinderchir.*, **5**, 2

104. Rickham, P.P. and Karplus, M. (1971) Familial and hereditary intestinal atresia. *Helv. Paediat. Acta*, **26**, 561–564

105. Rickham, P.P., Irving, I.M. and Shmerling, D.H. (1977) Long term results following extensive small intestinal resection in the neonatal period. *Progr. Pediat. Surg.*, **10**, 65–75

106. Rittenhouse, E.A., Beckwith, J.B., Chappell, J.S. and Bill, A.H. (1972) Multiple septa of the small bowel: description of an unusual case, with review of the literature and consideration of etiology. *Surgery*, **71**, 371–374

107. Santulli, T.V. and Blanc, W.A. (1961) Congenital atresia of the intestine: pathogenesis and treatment. *Ann. Surg.*, **154**, 939–948

108. Santulli, T.V., Chen, C. and Schullinger, J.N. (1970) Management of congenital atresia of the intestine. *Am. J. Surg.*, **119**, 542–547

109. Schnueppel, O. (1864) Fall von vielfacher Atresien des Duenndarms. *Arch. Heilk.*, **5**, 83

110. Schridde, H. (1908) Ueber die Epithelproliferationen in der embryonalen menschlichen speiserolire. *Virchow's Arch. Path. Anat.*, **191**, 178–192

111. Snyder, W.H., Voskamp, J.R. and Chaffin, L. (1950) Congenital atresia of the ileum. *West. J. Surg.*, **58**, 638–642

112. Spriggs, N.I. (1910) Some cases of congenital intestinal obstruction. *Lancet*, **i**, 94–98

113. Stauffer, V.G., Shmerling, D.H. and Danger, P. (1973) *Parenteral Nutrition in Paediatric Surgery*, Nutricia Symposium. H.E. Steinfert Kroese BV, Leiden

114. Suruga, K., Tsunoda, A., Fukuda, A. and Masatake, Y. (1966) Some problems of congenital intestinal atresia. *Z. Kinderchir.*, **3**, 29

115. Swenson, O. (1954) End to end aseptic intestinal anastomosis in infants and children. *Surgery*, **36**, 192–197

116. Swenson, O. and Davidson, F. (1960) Similarities of mechanical intestinal obstruction and aganglionic megacolon in the newborn infant. *New Engl. J. Med.*, **262**, 64–67

117. Tandler, J. (1902) Zur Entwickelung des menschlichen Duodenums in fruehen Embryonalstadium. *Morph. Jb.*, **29**, 187

118. Taussig, F.J. (1927) The amniotic fluid and its qualitative variability. *Am. J. Obstet. Gynec.*, **14**, 505–517

119. Teja, K., Schnatterly, P. and Shaw, A. (1981) Multiple intestinal atresias: pathology and pathogenesis. *J. Pediat. Surg.*, **16**, 194–199

120. Thomas, C.G. (1969) Jejunoplasty for the correction of jejunal atresia. *Surg. Gynec. Obstet.*, **129**, 545–546

121. Todani, T., Tabuchi, K. and Tanaka, S. (1975) Intestinal atresia due to intrauterine intussusception: analysis of 24 cases in Japan. *J. Pediat. Surg.*, **10**, 445–451

122. Wallon, P., Mitrofanoff, P. and Borde, J. (1975) Une forme rare d'occlusion neo-natale par dilatation segmentaire du grêle. *Annls Chir. infant.*, **16**, 181

123. Wash, M.G. and Mack, A. (1948) Radiographic appearance of the gastro-intestinal tract during the first day of life. *J. Pediat.*, **32**, 479

124. Webb, C.H. and Wagensteen, O.H. (1931) Congenital intestinal atresia. *Am. J. Dis. Child.*, **41**, 262–284

125. Weisschedel, E. (1953) Über angeborene Atresien und Stenosen des Dünndarmes. *Arch. klin. Chir.*, **276**, 764–766

126. Weitzman, J.J. and Vanderhoof, R.S. (1966) Jejunal atresia with agenesis of the dorsal mesentery. *Am. J. Surg.*, **111**, 443–449

127. White, J.J., Esterly, J.R., Tecklenberg, P. and Haller, J.A. (1972) Effect of changing concepts upon the diagnosis and management of intestinal atresia. *Am. Surg.*, **38**, 34–41

128. Wilkins, B.M., and Spitz, L. (1986) Incidence of postoperative adhesion obstruction following neonatal laparotomy. *Br. J. Surg.*, **73**, 762–764

129. Wilkinson, A.W., Hughes, E.A. and Toms, D.A. (1963) Massive resection of the small intestine in infancy. *Br. J. Surg.*, **50**, 715–730

130. Willis, R.A. (1968) Some unusual developmental heterotopias. *Br. Med. J.*, **3**, 267–272

131. Wolff, H.G. (1963) Klinik und Roentgenologie der Bildungsfehler des Magendarmtraktes beim Neugeborenen. *Wien. klin. Wschr.*, **69**, 592

132. Zerella, J.T. (1976) Jejunal atresia with absent mesentery and a helical ileum. *Surgery*, **80**, 550–553

133. Zwiren, G.T., Andrews, H.G. and Ahmann, P. (1972) Jejunal atresia with agenesis of the dorsal mesentery ('apple peel small bowel'). *J. Pediat. Surg.*, **7**, 414–419

33

Duplications of the alimentary tract

James Lister

Historical notes

Calder [13] in 1733 was the first to report an intestinal duplication, but following this observation there does not appear to have been any further mention of the condition in the literature until the beginning of this century. Terrier and Lecene [60] in 1904 described a duplication cyst of the ileocaecal region, and Budde [12] in 1912 published the first report of an intrathoracic duplication, arising from the stomach and passing upwards through the diaphragm. In 1937 Ladd [40] introduced the term 'duplication of the alimentary tract' for these malformations. The studies of Ladd and Gross [41] clarified the pathological anatomy of the various types of duplication.

Pathological anatomy

Duplications of the alimentary tract may be spherical or tubular structures and can occur anywhere in the alimentary tract from the tongue [29,45] to the anus. They have three characteristics.

(1) They are firmly attached to at least one point of the alimentary tract [19].
(2) They have a well developed coat of smooth muscle.
(3) The epithelial lining of the duplication always resembles some part of the alimentary tract [30].

In the chest, duplications of the alimentary tract appear as cysts in the posterior mediastinum. They may occur in isolation or there may be additional duplications beneath the diaphragm. Of our own series of 48 neonatal cases of alimentary tract duplication, 12 had intrathoracic cysts. Of these,

seven were solitary cysts in the posterior mediastinum, three had a separate cystic or tubular duplication of the intestine as well and two were communicating thoracoabdominal duplications: in one of the last the cyst extended along the concave aspect of the second and first parts of the duodenum and the greater curvature of the stomach, passed through the oesophageal hiatus, ascended through the posterior mediastinum along the right side of the oesophagus and ended in the neck, its upper end being attached to the anteroinferior margin of the fourth cervical vertebra [22] (Figure 33.1). In the other the subdiaphragmatic communication was

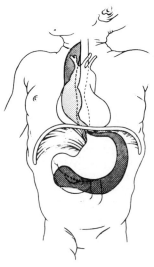

Figure 33.1 Showing position of thoracoabdominal duplication

with the jejunum. These thoracoabdominal duplications are uncommon [31]. In 1965 Hartl [32] could find only 13 reported cases in the literature. Only one of these was diagnosed during the neonatal period [24]. Only five have been seen in Liverpool in 33 years; three presented during the neonatal period, two in respiratory distress and the other with a volvulus related to the abdominal part of the duplication.

Thoracic duplications are frequently associated with other anomalies: foregut malformations are not unexpected [9,33]. Two of our cases had agenesis of one lung and two others had oesophageal atresia. Less predictably, another had an exomphalos and myelomeningocele.

Duplications of the stomach [14,26] are uncommon: Abrami and Dennison [1] found 38 in the English language literature up to 1961 but in recent years more cases have been reported [3,25,27,46,51,52]. Complete duplication extending from lower oesophagus to duodenum has only been reported on three occasions [25]; many of the smaller cysts have pancreatic tissue in their walls [23,46] and may be so closely related to the tail of the pancreas that some authors have suggested they are, in fact, pancreatic duplications [46]. Duplication cysts at the pyloric end of the stomach [2,27,37,51] tend to be quite small but present in the neonatal period with pyloric obstruction; the only gastric duplication in our series was one such as this.

As in the stomach, duodenal cysts rarely communicate with the gut [42]; the only one in our series was attached to the concave border of the duodenum lying posteriorly, but so large as almost to replace the distal half of the second and the third part of the duodenum. Two cases of cystic duplication of the duodenum associated with apparent double gall bladder have been described [4,64]; in one of them the situation was compared to the pancreatic bladder of a cat – an aberrant growth of the left ventral pancreas [64].

More commonly, abdominal duplications are attached to the jejunum, ileum or ileocaecal region [4], as was the case in 22 of our neonatal cases, three of whom also had mediastinal cysts. They may occur as globular cysts which either project into the lumen of the gut or are closely attached along the mesenteric border of the intestine, or they may be tubular in type. The larger cysts in the mesentery not infrequently cause torsion and volvulus of the intestine [35,58,65], as happened in three of our cases. Small intraluminal cysts usually occur near the ileocaecal region and may be the cause of an intussusception, as was the case in two of our infants.

Tubular duplications are less common than the spherical cysts [18]. They often reach great length and frequently have a gastric mucosal lining or may contain pancreatic glandular tissue in their walls.

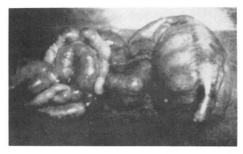

Figure 33.2 This duplication was 60 cm long and communicated proximally with the lumen of the ileum. The distal, blind end was grossly dilated

They are thus prone to develop peptic ulcers which may perforate [56], as was the case in two of our four infants with tubular duplications of the small intestine. Such duplications usually communicate with the lumen of the intestine at one end only and run along the mesenteric border of the gut. If the communication is situated proximally, the distal blind end of the duplication tube tends to dilate, and may at times reach enormous proportions (Figure 33.2).

Two infants in this series had a mesenteric cyst lined by intestinal mucosa, but not attached to the gut. Such cysts, with neither a close attachment to the alimentary tract nor a muscular wall, should not, strictly speaking, be included amongst duplications of the alimentary tract; however, they do have a lining of intestinal epithelium and are often associated with spinal malformations which suggest that their origin may be similar to the tubular duplications. These are the least common of intestinal duplications. One of our cases had a myelomeningocele, and the cyst was found at postmortem examination. In addition to myelomeningocele, exomphalos, malrotation and atresias are found with mid-gut duplications. Paddock and Aaronsen [50] reported two children with the polysplenia syndrome who had intestinal duplications and recommended that this syndrome should be excluded in children with duplications.

Duplication of the colon and rectum is less common than that of the small bowel [53]. Cysts of similar pathology to those associated with the small bowel are occasionally encountered in the proximal colon; our series includes four such cases, all intramural cysts of the caecal wall, not exceeding 3 cm in diameter yet all causing obstruction either by occlusion or by forming the head of an intussusception. Cystic duplications of the rectum also occur, usually lying behind the rectum and tending to obstruct the rectal lumen by their bulk [29]. One cyst of this type was encountered in our series, attached to the wall of a prolapsed, exstrophic rectum in an infant with exstrophy of the cloaca [36].

A second case of rectal duplication presented as a tubular mass which projected from the vulva and was adherent at its base to both the vagina and the rectum. In a third child a rectal cyst lay posterior to a narrow, anteriorly-placed anus. In all three cases, the cyst wall had two muscle layers and the lining was of well formed rectal mucosa.

A distinct variety of colonic duplication is that in which there is actual doubling of part or all of the colon. This type of malformation may be associated with spina bifida, partial or complete doubling of the lumbar and sacral spine, and duplication of the genitourinary tract [4,5,55]. There are five such cases in our series. Two of the infants had doubling of the appendix and caecum, with additional malformations in one case including exstrophy of the cloaca, bilateral double ureters, double vagina and spina bifida, and in the other a high rectal atresia with a deficient, double sacrum and a grossly shortened colon opening into the bladder (Figure 33.3). Two others had cloacal exstrophy with doubling of the whole length of a rudimentary colon

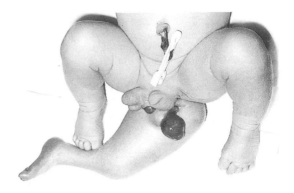

Figure 33.5 Duplication of colon, hypospadias, bifid scrotum. This prolapsed mucosa on the right communicated with bowel and discharged meconium; that on the left was a cyst

(Figure 33.4). The last child had an accessory lower limb (Figure 33.5), hypospadias and a bifid scrotum in addition to complete duplication of the distal colon.

Embryology

When discussing the possible embryological factors involved in the formation of duplications of the alimentary tract, one must distinguish between duplications which may result from localized faults in development and those which, in addition, affect the spinal cord, vertebrae, etc. [19].

At one time localized duplications were thought to be due to exceptional overgrowth of intestinal diverticula, which according to some authors [11,38,43] can frequently be seen budding out from the intestine of human as well as animal embryos. Bremer [11] thought that most of the spherical duplication cysts could be explained by this theory. He had difficulty, however, in explaining the occurrence of long tubular structures, but advanced a theory concerning their origin based on Tandler's [59] demonstration of the 'solid state' in the development of the intestine of the embryo (see Chapter 32) and of the later appearance, between the cells filling the lumen of the primitive gut, of vacuoles which finally coalesced to form the lumen of the intestine. Bremer suggested that in rare cases vacuoles could coalesce to form two lumina instead of one. However, obliteration of the intestinal lumen has not been shown to occur below the level of the duodenum in human development, and even if it did this theory could not explain those cases where the tubular duplication diverges well away from the normal bowel as it passes between the leaves of the mesentery.

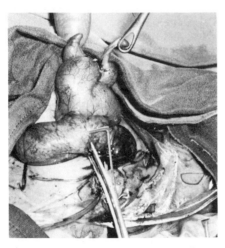

Figure 33.3 Double caecum and appendix opening into the bladder

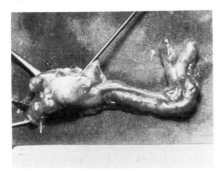

Figure 33.4 Doubling of the whole length of the rudimentary colon in a case of cloacal exstrophy

As early as 1943, Saunders [57] noticed that thoracic duplications, whether isolated or passing through the diaphragm to connect up with part of the intestine, are frequently associated with malformations of the cervical and upper thoracic vertebrae. Occasionally these duplications are attached to one of the vertebral bodies or are connected by a channel with the spinal canal [20,46]. Indeed, in 1923 Bell related anterior spina bifida to persistence of the neurenteric canal [6].

These findings gave rise to the so-called notochordal theory (Figure 33.6). Fallon, Gordon and Lendrum [20] suggested that the notochordal plate, lying originally between the ectodermic amniotic vesicle and the entodermic yolk sac, is not as usual pinched off the entoderm by ingrowth of mesodermal cells from each side, but that abnormal adhesions persist between the notochord and the roof of the developing gut. These abnormal adhesions may result in a column of entodermal cells being pulled posteriorly and cranially during the period when ectodermal and mesodermal growth exceeds that of the entoderm; such a column of cells might result in a tubular thoracic or thoracoabdominal duplication, or if only one part of it develops a lumen it may result in a cystic duplication. It will also result in

adhesion of some duplications to the vertebral column and, in some cases, abnormalities of vertebral bodies. If the adhesions occur between ectoderm and entoderm at an earlier stage this would result in a splitting of the advancing notochord with more severe interference with the development of vertebral bodies. Bentley and Smith [7] suggest a split notochord as the primary defect, herniation of the yolk sac between the two halves resulting in the subsequent duplication of the gut. It has been suggested that the notochordal theory can explain the formation of posterior mediastinal cysts but not those intra-abdominal intestinal duplications which are not associated with spinal malformations [57]. However, one does not invariably find an associated spinal abnormality even with mediastinal duplications; four of the 12 cases in this series with mediastinal duplications had no demonstrable spinal abnormality. Nor is it true that subdiaphragmatic intestinal duplications proximal to the colon are never associated with spinal malformation; a marked spinal malformation of multiple wedged or hemivertebrae was present in two of the isolated infradiaphragmatic duplications of the small intestine in our series.

Finally, it must be added that in the rare cases of duplication of the entire hindgut often associated with spina bifida and duplication of the genital and lower urinary tracts, we may be dealing with examples of caudal twinning [47,55] similar to the much rarer examples of abortive cephalic twinning which have also been described [1].

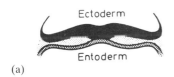

(a)

(b)

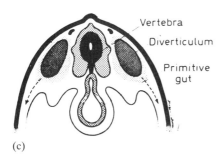

(c)

Figure 33.6 Notochordal theory of the causation of alimentary duplications (after McLetchie). (a) Adhesion between entoderm and ectoderm. (b) Duplication of notochord. (c) Formation of intestinal duplication with malformation of vertebra

Incidence

Duplications of the alimentary tract are rare. By far the biggest series, one of 67 cases, was published by Gross [29]. It is sometimes forgotten that the collection of this number of cases took nearly 30 years and that, because of their published work [41] on this subject, patients were sent to Ladd and Gross from all over the world. Even in their large series only 20 cases presented with symptoms in the neonatal period. All the other published series are smaller. In a symposium on duplications of the alimentary tract held in Paris in 1965, the combined efforts of all French paediatric surgeons could only collect 48 cases since 1949 [17], 14 of whom were seen during the neonatal period. Grosfeld, Boles and Reiner [27] reported 23 patients, in 15 of whom the lesions were collected over an 18-year period. Hocking and Young [34] reported 53 patients treated over 30 years in Glasgow but did not give an age breakdown. The 48 neonatal cases in our series represent 80% of all the children with enteric duplications seen during the last 31 years [44].

Clinical picture

Thoracic duplications

The main presenting symptom in the neonatal period is respiratory distress, brought about by the bulk of the cyst compressing the lung. As the cyst is lined with mucus-secreting epithelium, the accumulating fluid inside the cyst gradually increases in volume. In six of the 11 thoracic duplication cysts in this series, respiratory distress was the presenting symptom. In three cases it was noticed immediately after birth, in two it developed within the first week of life, and in one case during the second week. It must be added that three of these six babies had additional malformations which contributed to their respiratory distress: oesophageal atresia and agenesis of the right lung in one, and agenesis of the left lung and micrognathia in another, oesophageal atresia on its own in the last. In five cases the duplication cyst was an incidental finding: two were admitted with a thoracic myelomeningocele and three with abdominal symptoms secondary to complications of associated abdominal duplications.

As the mucosal lining of these cysts is often gastric in type, autodigestion and ulceration into the oesophagus or bronchus with repeated haematemeses or haemoptyses are common complications in older children, but are less commonly observed in neonates. If the cyst is of sufficient size it may give rise to physical signs such as dullness to percussion and diminished or absent air entry, as was noticed in two of our cases. Shifting of the mediastinum may also be observed.

Duplication of the stomach

Complete duplication of the stomach is rare and will present with abdominal distension, with or without vomiting, and a palpable mass. Small cysts may be asymptomatic, as was our case, who had oesophageal atresia, the cyst being found incidentally when a gastrostomy was being made. However, pyloric cysts are very likely to masquerade as pyloric stenosis [2,27,37,46,52,60] with projectile vomiting of gastric content. Small cysts at other levels in the stomach may present with complications such as perforation and peritonitis or haematemesis and melaena, though this is unlikely to occur in the neonatal period.

Duplication of the duodenum

These contain intestinal mucosa and do not usually communicate with the gut. If they are of sufficient size they may obstruct the duodenum, as happened in our cases, again mimicking pyloric stenosis.

Duplication of the small intestine

As stated above, small submucosal cysts only give rise to symptoms if they become the starting point of an intussusception, as happened in one of our cases.

If the cyst is large the bowel may be stretched tightly across it, causing intestinal obstruction; five of our cases with large cysts were obstructed in this way and in addition the cyst was large enough to be palpated in the abdomen (Figure 33.7). Two further

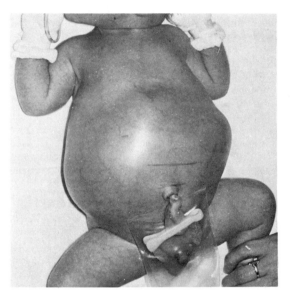

Figure 33.7 High intestinal duplication cyst, visibly distending the abdomen

children with tubular duplications presented in the same way; in these cases where the duplication only communicates with the intestine at its proximal end, the duplication can become enormously distended [54].

A cyst may cause a volvulus of the intestine [35], as occurred in two infants in our series. In one of these the volvulus had occurred before birth, resulting in a secondary intestinal atresia. Another gangrenous volvulus resulted from a tubular duplication.

One enormous tense cyst, measuring 15 cm in length and lying in the mesentery of the terminal ileum, produced partial duodenal obstruction by its weight dragging on the mesentery.

There were two perforations, one at the proximal end and one at the distal end in tubular duplications; we did not see perforation from peptic ulceration in any other lesions. The five tubular duplications, therefore, had the highest rate of serious complications: two perforations and one gangrenous volvulus, the remaining two presenting with obstruction due to gross distension of the duplication; their lengths ranged from 16 to 60 cm but this did not seem to be related to the severity of their symptoms.

Duplications of the colon and rectum

Cysts of the proximal colon, if they are of sufficient size, will cause obstruction by stretching the colon across their outer border: an associated malrotation combined with a cystic duplication of the colon has been reported as causing intermittent obstruction [39]. Three infants in our series with a caecal cyst developed intestinal obstruction in the first few days of life. In one a small palpable mass could be felt in the right iliac fossa; in another the cyst formed the apex of an intussusception and this could be felt in the right iliac fossa, confirming the diagnosis suggested by the passage of blood and mucus. In the third case the obstruction was produced by a very small intramural cyst which could not be palpated pre-operatively: one small cyst in the caecum produced bloody diarrhoea without any intussusception.

The three rectal duplications presented as visible or palpable swellings in relation to the anus, as described above. There is rarely trouble in recognizing them [15,16]; none of ours communicated with the rectum as is reported to occur in 20%.

Cases of complete duplication of the colon do not usually present with symptoms in the neonatal period unless there is duplication of the anus or an abnormal orifice in addition to a normal anus [41]. Four of our five cases of colonic doubling were discovered at operation for associated malformations: the fifth was discovered on examination of a child with an accessory lower limb.

Radiological findings

Two of our more recent duplications were diagnosed at antenatal ultrasound. This incidental finding will become more frequent. In thoracic duplications the anteroposterior radiograph may show a rounded mediastinal shadow, usually on the right, displacing the heart to the opposite side; the presence of vertebral abnormalities will be very suggestive of a duplication cyst (Figure 33.8).

The lateral radiogram of the chest will show that the tumour is in the posterior mediastinum with the trachea displaced forwards (Figure 33.9).

An abdominal duplication may show up as a dense mass displacing the intestine. Occasionally, if it communicates with the intestine, a large cyst with a fluid level may be observed. If these duplications give rise to complications such as intestinal obstruction or perforation, the typical radiographic picture

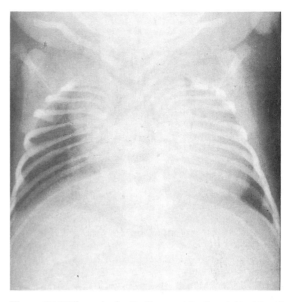

Figure 33.8 Thoracic duplication cyst in the right side of the thorax displacing the heart to the left. The vertebral abnormalities are very noticeable

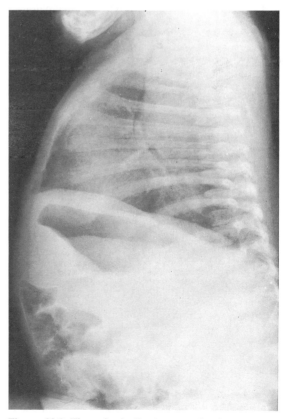

Figure 33.9 Thoracic duplication cyst in the posterior mediastinum displacing the trachea forwards

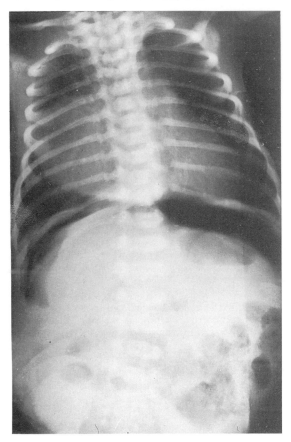

Figure 33.10 Thoracic duplication cyst on the right side and pneumoperitoneum secondary to perforated abdominal duplication

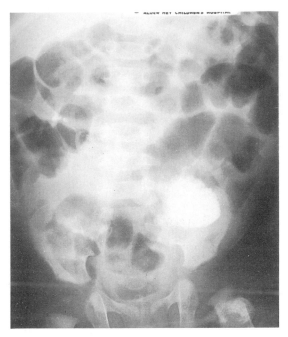

Figure 33.11 Abdominal radiograph 24 h after a barium meal showing residual barium pooling in a duplication communicating with the intestine

of the complication will be observed. Occasionally the radiological recognition of an associated thoracic duplication may indicate the diagnosis (Figure 33.10).

A barium meal is usually not very informative. If the duplication communicates with the lumen of the bowel, some barium may remain in the duplication long after all the barium has passed from the intestine (Figure 33.11). Two of our caecal duplications were demonstrated by barium enema.

Treatment

Surgical excision of the duplication is the most desirable method of treatment. This should be carried out as soon as possible because of the danger of serious complications such as obstruction, haemorrhage, perforation, etc., which may occur at any time. If the infant presents with one of these complications, an emergency operation has to be performed.

Thoracic duplications

These are best removed by a transpleural approach through a major thoracotomy (see Chapter 6). Dissection of these cysts is often comparatively easy, but some cysts are very adherent to the oesophagus and share a common muscular coat with it. These adherent cysts are best dealt with by dissection down to the neck of the cyst, which is attached to the oesophagus. The neck is clamped and the cyst is removed. The remaining mucosal lining of the cyst is then meticulously peeled off the oesophagus [10]. If the oesophagus is opened during this procedure it must be closed carefully. The thoracotomy is then closed, leaving an intercostal drain leading to the site of the operation. In those rare cases where there has been ulceration in the neonatal period with haemoptysis or haematemesis a formal excision of the cyst is practically impossible due to inflammation and scarring. Lobectomy may be indicated. Complete excision of the lining of the cyst is, however, essential, with appropriate drainage.

Thoracoabdominal duplications

These often need extensive staged operations [21]. It may be necessary to excise first the symptom-causing part, e.g. the abdominal segment if the child has presented with intestinal obstruction or the thoracic part if he presented with dyspnoea. If, however, there is no acute abdominal presentation, the thoracic portion is dealt with first. Through a mid-posterolateral thoracotomy the duplication is freed transpleurally. At the upper extremity there may be some difficulty due to local adhesions and deep attachment to bone, especially if there is an abnormal vertebral body; this extension must be freed with gouge or chisel, since infection of a residual communication could result in meningitis. The duplication is then followed downwards, where it lies free in the mediastinum to the point where it passes through the diaphragm; at that point it is pulled up as far as possible into the chest and divided between ligatures. The upper part of the duplication is then removed and the chest closed, with underwater drainage. If the general condition of the infant permits, the remaining abdominal segment is removed by an appropriate procedure; if necessary, the second stage can be postponed for a few days or even weeks. However, if the abdominal procedure had to be the first stage because of

complications, the thoracic procedure should not be delayed for more than a day or two because bleeding into the thoracic part, or even the collection of undrained secretions, may result in the development of a very large cystic lesion causing respiratory embarrassment.

Abdominal duplications

Gastric duplications

Partial gastrectomy has been performed in older children for duplications and in neonates for other reasons. However, the blood supply of the stomach coming from both ventral and dorsal borders makes possible a different approach from that applied to intestinal duplications where a common blood supply is shared by normal bowel and duplication. Excision of the duplication cyst may be performed (Figure 33.12), stripping the residual mucosal lining

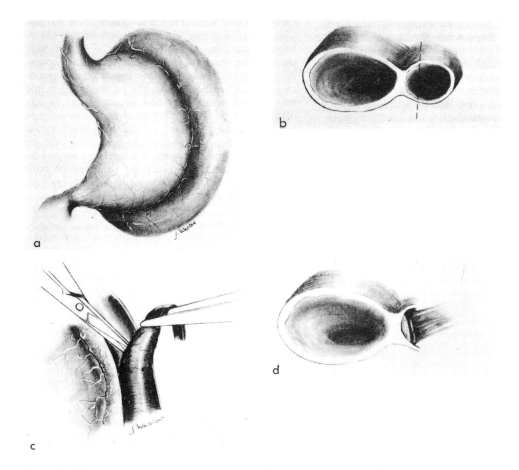

Figure 33.12 In large gastric duplications the bulk of the cyst may be excised (b) and the residual mucosa stripped (c and d) (after Lister [58])

38. Keibel, F. (1905) Zur Embryologie des Menschen der Affen und der Halbaffan. *Anat. Anz., 27* (Suppl.), 39–50

39. Kufaas, T. and Lindman, C.R. (1983) Cystic duplication of the colon combined with non-rotation anomaly initiating pyloric stenosis. *Acta Paediat. Scand., 72,* 467–468

40. Ladd, W.E. (1937) Duplications of the alimentary tract. *Sth. Med. J., 30,* 363–371

41. Ladd, W.E. and Gross, R.E. (1940) Surgical treatment of duplications of the alimentary tract. *Surg. Gynec. Obstet., 70,* 295–307

42. Leenders, E.L., Osman, M.Z. and Sukarochana, K. (1970) Treatment of duodenal duplication with international review. *Am. Surg., 36,* 368–371

43. Lewis, F.T. and Thyng, F.W. (1907) The regular occurrence of intestinal diverticula in embryos of the pig, rabbit and man. *Am. J. Anat., 7,* 505–519

44. Lister, J. and Vaos, G. (1988) Duplications of the alimentary tract. In *Operative Surgery,* 4th edn, *Pediatric Surgery,* (ed. H. Nixon and L. Spitz), Butterworths, London

45. Lister, J. and Zachary, R.B. (1968) Cystic duplication in the tongue. *J. Pediat. Surg., 3,* 491–493

46. McLetchie, N.G.B., Purvies, J.K. and Saunders, R.C. (1954) The genesis of gastric and certain intestinal diverticula and enterogenous cysts. *Surg. Gynec. Obstet., 99,* 135–141

47. McPherson, A.G., Trapnell, J.E. and Airth, G.R. (1969) Duplication of the colon. *Br. J. Surg., 56,* 138

48. Norris, R.W., Brereton, R.J., Wright, V.M. and Cudmore, R.E. (1986) A new surgical approach to duplications of the intestine. *J. Pediat. Surg., 21,* 167–170

49. Orr, M.M. and Edwards, A.J. (1975) Neoplastic change in duplications of the alimentary tract. *Br. J. Surg., 62,* 269–274

50. Paddock, R.J. and Arensman, R.M. (1982) Polysplenia syndrome: spectrum of gastrointestinal congenital anomalies. *J. Pediat. Surg., 17,* 563–566

51. Parker, B.C., Guthrie, J., France, N.E. and Attwell, J.D. (1972) Gastric duplications in infancy. *J. Pediat. Surg., 7,* 294–298

52. Ramsay, G.S. (1957) Enterogenous cyst of the stomach simulating hypertrophic pyloric stenosis. *Br. J. Surg., 44,* 632–633

53. Ravitch, M.M. (1953) Hindgut duplication. *Ann. Surg., 137,* 588–601

54. Ravitch, M.M. (1969) Duplications of the alimentary canal. In *Paediatric Surgery* (ed. W.T. Mustard, M.M. Ravitch, W.H. Snyder, K.J. Welch and C.D. Benson), Year Book Medical Publishers, Chicago

55. Ravitch, M.M. and Scott, W.W. (1953) Duplication of the entire colon, bladder and urethra. *Surgery, 34,* 843

56. Rios-Dalenz, J.C., Kress, J.W. and Montgomery, C.G. (1965) Duplication of small intestine with perforated ulcer in ectopic gastric mucosa. *Arch. Surg., 91,* 863–866

57. Saunders, R.L. (1943) Combined anterior and posterior spina bifida in a living neonatal human female. *Anat. Rec., 87,* 255–275

58. Stur, O., Zangl, A. and Zweymuller, I. (1964) Ileumduplikatur mit Volvulus bei einem Neugeborenen. *Wien. Mschr. Kinderheilk., 112,* 277–281

59. Tandler, J. (1902) Zur Entwicklung des menschlichen Duodenums im fruhen Embryonalstadium. *Morph. Jb., 29,* 187

60. Terrier, F. and Lecène, P. (1904) Un nouveau cas de kyste juxta-intestinal. *Revue Chir., 74,* 161–174

61. Torma, M.J. (1974) Of double stomachs. *Arch. Surg., 109,* 555–557

62. White, J.J. and Morgan, W.W. (1970) Improved operative technique for gastric duplication. *Surgery, 67,* 522–526

63. Wrenn, E.L. (1962) Tubular duplication of the small intestine. *Surgery, 52,* 494–498

64. Wrenn, E.L. and Favara, B.E. (1971) Duodenal duplication (or pancreatic bladder) presenting as a double gall bladder. *Surgery, 69,* 858–862

65. Yanagisawa, F. (1969) Doppelbildungen des Darmes. *Chirurg., 30,* 109

34

Neonatal necrotizing enterocolitis

James Lister and P. K. H. Tam

In the past two decades, necrotizing enterocolitis has become the most common neonatal abdominal condition requiring emergency surgery and has also emerged as the leading cause of mortality in surgical neonates. Improvement in the outcome of infants with necrotizing enterocolitis, most of whom are very low birthweight babies, requires close cooperation between paediatric surgeons and neonatologists to ensure early detection, timely intervention and appropriate aftercare of the condition.

Historical notes

The clinical and pathological features of necrotizing enterocolitis in the newborn were described in 1891 [38] but for 60 years or more the diffuse picture of the disease was interpreted as multiple conditions. The term 'necrotizing colitis' was used by Cruze and Snyder [24] in 1961 but it was Waldhausen, Herendeen and King [130] who first clearly described the disease in 1963.

The following year, Berdon and his colleagues [10] noted an increase in the incidence of the disease in a comprehensive report from The Babies Hospital, New York, and 3 years later surgical experience in the condition was reviewed from that same hospital [129]. An increase in the incidence of the condition was widely reported in the 1970s in the developed countries [15,27,28,68,81,82,99,125,131] and a similar trend has become evident in the developing countries more recently [65,106].

Incidence

The increasing emphasis on intensive neonatal care and a consequent increase in the number of surviving very low birthweight babies who are especially

liable to the development of necrotizing enterocolitis is the most important explanation for the increase in the incidence of the condition since the 1960s. There is also an increased recognition of the condition and some reports claim that up to 4–5% of all premature infants in special care centres and 25% of infants weighing less than 1200 g were affected by the condition [7,11]; a recent American study suggested that 8% of deaths in the first week of life and 15% of deaths after 1 week of life in infants below 1500 g resulted from necrotizing enterocolitis [134]. The actual incidence of necrotizing enterocolitis is in fact difficult to assess as diagnostic criteria are not always fulfilled in mild

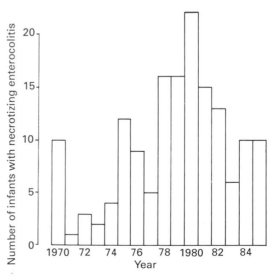

Figure 34.1 Incidence of necrotizing enterocolitis treated in Royal Liverpool Children's Hospital, Alder Hey

485

cases and calculation is further complicated by occasional outbreaks of clusters of cases in different centres [2]. The number of cases of neonatal necrotizing enterocolitis treated in Royal Liverpool Children's Hospital, Alder Hey, between 1970 and 1985 is shown in Figure 34.1. The rise in incidence culminating in a peak in the late 1970s and early 1980s reflects the increase in the number of 'at risk' infants surviving to develop this condition; the levelling off of the incidence in subsequent years may be explained partly by the neonatologists' heightened awareness of the condition resulting in early and often successful medical therapy of the infants in special care baby units and partly by more stringent indications for surgery in recent years.

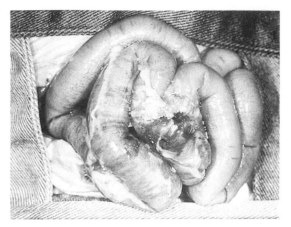

Figure 34.2 Necrotizing enterocolitis with areas of bowel gangrene and sealed off perforation

Pathological findings

Necrotizing enterocolitis can affect any part of the alimentary tract from stomach to rectum though the duodenum and rectum are rarely affected and never on their own. Of 154 cases seen in Alder Hey Children's Hospital in 1970–1985, the site of involvement was recorded in 111 cases (Table 34.1); the site was unknown in 43 cases which did not come to surgery or autopsy. Lesions ranged from extensive disease to localized involvement but even when localized one or more segments of bowel may be affected. The most commonly involved parts of the bowel were caecum and terminal ileum.

On gross examination, the bowel is dilated and friable and may be frankly necrotic with haemorrhagic areas adjoining necrotic ones; the bowel wall is thinned out and may consist of serous coat only with milk or bowel contents visible through the attenuated bowel wall. The serosa is often covered by fibrinous exudate. Air bubbles may be seen in the bowel wall, though less often than in X-rays. The mucosa shows ulceration and sloughing. Perforations may be present in necrotic areas leaving large gaps in the bowel wall, usually on the antimesenteric

side (Figure 34.2). The neighbouring bowel, viscera and omentum are sometimes successful in sealing off perforations resulting in a walled off cavity containing meconium or faeces. The peritoneal fluid becomes faeculent if there is free perforation; in other instances the fluid is bloodstained or turbid.

Histological changes range from early coagulation necrosis of the mucosa, through superficial mucosal ulceration and submucosal haemorrhage to transmural necrosis with hyaline eosinophilia and loss of nuclear detail in muscle cells and finally ends in complete gangrene of the bowel [107]; intramural gas is often seen microscopically when its gross appearance has not been detected (Figure 34.3). There is often vascular engorgement and thrombi may be seen in small mesenteric vessels and submucosal vessels [121]. Myenteric plexus ganglion cells are normal though it has been suggested that acquired aganglionic megacolon may be a late complication of the condition [126]. Healing is by rapid epithelialization [57] but fibrosis may also lead to scarring and stricture formation.

Table 34.1 Site of necrotizing enterocolitis in 111 cases in 1970–85

Localized involvement		75
Caecum and terminal ileum	30	
Distal colon	17	
Proximal colon	9	
Ileum	15	
Jejunum	2	
Stomach	2	
Extensive involvement		36
All large bowel	15	
All small bowel	8	
Small and large bowel	11	
Stomach, small and large bowel	2	

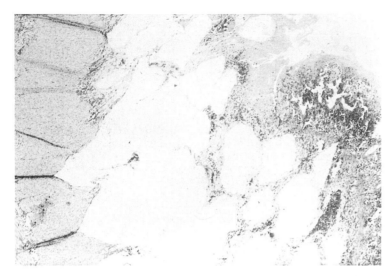

Figure 34.3 Histological changes in necrotizing enterocolitis, showing mucosal inflammation, air pockets in submucosa and transmural necrosis of muscle

Pathogenesis

Many theories of causation of the condition have been advanced, most of them valid, suggesting that the disease is a common final stage of a variety of insults in susceptible patients. Sick, premature infants are particularly at risk. The commonest situation is a multifactorial event, starting with the breakdown of the protective mucosal barrier of the intestine which then allows bacteria in the lumen to invade the intestinal wall causing intramural damage and eventual necrosis; factors such as the presence of protein substrate may facilitate bacterial growth [64,105]. The pathogenetic factors are additive in effect but in some instances, a single cause, if it is very strong, may be enough to initiate the development of necrotizing enterocolitis.

The risk for necrotizing enterocolitis is inversely related to birth weight [11,123,134]. Low birthweight itself is are associated with a number of medical problems which are themselves predisposing factors for necrotizing enterocolitis; however, there is recent experimental evidence to show that under identical conditions of hypoxia and hyperviscosity low birthweight piglets develop more frequent and more severe lesions of necrotizing enterocolitis than normal birthweight piglets, suggesting that low birth weight is itself a factor of relevance [112]. More than two-thirds of our patients weighed less than 2.5 kg at birth.

Mucosal injury is most often the result of intestinal ischaemia. Lloyd [84] argued that the hypoxia to which a premature baby was particularly prone could result in redistribution of blood flow away from the intestinal mucosa – the dive reflex of the seal [53] – and experimental work on piglets supports this theory [128]. In another experiment, the effects of the two components of asphyxia, namely hypoxia and acidosis were investigated and it was found that hypoxia played a more significant role than acidosis in causing intestinal ischaemia as well as reducing oxygen consumption especially in the terminal ileum, the commonest site of pathology [58]. In animal studies, mucosal injury may result not only from intestinal ischaemia itself but also from reperfusion during which oxygen-derived free radicals are released; to what extent this mechanism works in necrotizing enterocolitis in humans is unknown but further research is worthwhile as scavengers of oxygen-derived free radicals are available and may theoretically be helpful in reducing further intestinal damage [40]. A clinical study using Doppler ultrasound to investigate fetal and maternal circulations suggested that in some instances the hypoxic episodes are antenatal: for infants less than 2000 g birth weight, necrotizing enterocolitis occurred in seven of 26 infants with abnormal fetal Doppler patterns and none of 20 infants with normal fetal Doppler patterns [43]. Hypothermia may induce intestinal ischaemia: 94% of neonatal piglets with core-body temperature lowered 4°C for 4.5 h developed lesions ranging from superficial mucosal necrosis to transmural infarct in the small intestine [109]. Hyperviscosity may also contribute: there is experimental evidence in dogs [75] as well as clinical data [44] to support the thesis that polycythemia can cause necrotizing enterocolitis. Umbilical vein catheters for exchange transfusions have also been incriminated as interfering with portal system haemodynamics [22,127]. Corkery and his colleagues suggested that retrograde embolism or thrombosis could explain the occurrence of necrotizing enterocolitis after exchange transfusion [22], since catheters rarely reached the inferior vena cava but lay in the left branch of the portal vein; Sommerschild [115] indicated that the diameter of the portal vein in the newborn is 2–3 mm and umbilical catheters used are usually 2–2.5 mm in diameter so that great pressure variations could occur during exchange transfusion; Denes *et al.* [28] believed that an umbilical vein catheter, like an umbilical artery catheter, merely provided a portal of entry for infection; but again Touloukian, Kadar and Spencer demonstrated experimentally that mucosal necrosis could be produced [127]. Polyvinyl chloride catheters have also been cited [102] as the source of leached toxic products of unknown variety. Recent studies, however, have failed to detect difference in the frequencies of exchange transfusions or umbilical artery catheterization between normal infants and infants who develop necrotizing enterocolitis [37,61,119,124,135].

Primary mucosal lesions have been produced by hyperosmolar feeds in goats [26] and this mechanism has been implicated in the pathogenesis of necrotizing enterocolitis. This is supported by the clinical observation that premature infants fed on hyperosmolar elemental formula had a higher incidence of necrotizing enterocolitis (88%) than those fed on milk formula (25%). The presence of protein substrate to facilitate bacterial invasion has also been considered to be an important element in the pathogenesis of the condition [5,31,107]. In a series of 54 cases of necrotizing enterocolitis and 98 controls, Frantz found that all the patients with necrotizing enterocolitis but only 63% of the controls were receiving standard formula feeds on the day of the onset of the disease [37]. As a result of works on rats it was thought that breast milk, had a protective action against the development of necrotizing enterocolitis and macrophages present in fresh breast milk, but not in frozen breast milk were responsible [94]. Eyal [34], however, found that for infants with birth weight less than 1500 g a change of policy from expressed breast milk feeding to avoidance of enteral feeding for the first 2–3 weeks of life resulted in a reduction of incidence of necrotizing enterocolitis from 18% to 3% and therefore suggested initial parenteral feeding for all at risk infants. Unfed babies are, however, not free from the risk of necrotizing enterocolitis and Marchildon reported that in a series of 139 infants with this condition, 14 had not been fed [85]. La Gamma and Ostertag [93], in a retrospective review followed by a prospective study, found that dilute early enteral feeding did not affect the incidence of necrotizing enterocolitis. Whatever relevance enteral feeding has in the pathogenesis of necrotizing enterocolitis there is little doubt that it is subsidiary to the presence of bacteria: Musemeche [89] showed that necrosis developed in 75% of ischaemic bowel segments of conventionally colonized rats but none in germ-free rats whether they were fed or unfed.

The infectious aetiology of necrotizing enterocolitis is supported by experimental studies as well as clinical data. De Lemos [26] found that to produce necrotizing enterocolitis in goats, colonization of the gut with gas-forming bacteria was necessary. Musemeche [89] compared the effects of ischaemia, bacteria and substrate on the pathogenesis of intestinal necrosis in rats and concluded that the presence of bacteria was the most crucial factor. Lawrence [73] advanced the hypothesis that the environment of the neonatal intensive care unit delayed normal bacterial colonization of infants allowing growth of one or a few species of bacteria to become dominant; immature gut, especially the lower ileum, which took up macromolecules intact may therefore absorb toxic products from the growing bacteria, causing mucosal damage and initiating necrotizing enterocolitis. Clustered epidemics have been reported repeatedly [2]; based on the isolation of bacteria and the detection of their toxins in faeces, the following organisms have been implicated: *Escherichia coli* [15,25,117], *Klebsiella* [50,99], *Pseudomonas* [49,130], *Enterobacter cloacae* [96], *Salmonella [118], Clostridium difficile* [45], *Clostridium butyricum* [52,120] and *Clostridium perfringens* [62,66], which is the organism related to several diseases resembling necrotizing enterocolitis – Darmbrand [136], Pig-bel [74], and Enteritis necroticans in China and Sri Lanka [3]. Viruses which have been implicated in epidemics include rotavirus [103] and coronavirus [14,104].

A defective immunity has also been postulated to be contributory [72,133]. Bell [8] found that serum IgA in 11 neonates with necrotizing enterocolitis was significantly higher than in 11 matched controls. Dykes [30] studied eight infants with necrotizing enterocolitis, six infected controls and seven controls and found a higher IgA in infants with necrotizing enterocolitis but the difference did not reach statistical significance – it was not clear if the small size of patient population was the reason; other parameters of humoral and cellular immunity were similar in the three groups.

Several drugs have also been suspected to predispose infants to the risk of necrotizing enterocolitis. In a retrospective review of 418 infants of birth weight of less than 1500 g, the incidence of necrotizing enterocolitis was 13.4% for those who had received vitamin E for prophylaxis against sequelae of retrolental fibroplasia compared with 5.8% for controls and it was thought that hyperosmolality of the currently available vitamin E preparation was responsible [35]. Johnson and co-workers [56] confirmed this finding in a prospective double-blind clinical trial: the incidence of necrotizing enterocolitis in vitamin E treated patients was 11.9% compared with 6.5% in controls; they, however, offered the alternative explanation that this was due to vitamin E-related decrease in oxygen-dependent intracellular killing ability resulting in a decreased resistance to infection. Workers in Kentucky noticed that necrotizing enterocolitis developed in 13 of 82 infants treated with indomethacin for patent ductus closure [91]; they pursued this finding with a study in dogs and showed that gastrointestinal mucosal blood flow was significantly reduced by indomethacin treatment [91]. Clinical studies [101] have suggested that the use of xanthines, a family of drugs commonly used for the treatment of neonates with apnoeic episodes, is associated with a higher incidence of necrotizing enterocolitis in treated infants; experimentally, it has also been shown that the survival of dogs challenged with an ischaemic bowel insult is adversely affected by xanthine treatment [42].

Term infants and, rarely, older infants [114] can also develop necrotizing enterocolitis, particularly when they have congenital heart disease or have had surgical procedures for other conditions. It is believed that reduced cardiac output in infants with congenital heart disease may lead to intestinal ischaemia initiating necrotizing enterocolitis [63,79,95,113]; in our series 6% of patients had major congenital heart problems. Necrotizing enterocolitis occurring after operations was probably first described in adults by Tanner in 1968 [122] and Germain in 1973 [39]. In 1976, Kleinman reported necrotizing enterocolitis as a complication of major heart surgery in three babies [63]. Amoury observed eight cases of non-cardiac postoperative necrotizing enterocolitis in 10 years, the commonest primary conditions being gastroschisis and gastrointestinal atresias [1]; Mollitt described 11 similar cases seen over a period of 5 years [88]. In the period 1970–85, of our 154 cases of necrotizing enterocolitis, 31 (20.1%) followed operations for a wide variety of conditions: myelomeningocele 13, diaphragmatic hernia five, oesophageal atresia four, exomphalos/gastroschisis four, small bowel atresia three, anorectal anomaly two. It is interesting to note that many of these conditions were non-abdominal and had not previously been reported to be associated with the postoperative abdominal complication of necrotizing enterocolitis. Most of these babies (21/31) were term infants with no identifiable perinatal stress factors apart from the operation; the likely explanation is that major operation results in compromised mesenteric blood flow during critical periods, initiating the development of necrotizing enterocolitis.

Clinical picture

The key to the improved results now being obtained in this condition lies in early recognition of the non-specific signs of the disease and a careful supervision of the infant at risk. Any infant under 1500 g and any infant with the pathogenetic factors outlined in the previous section should be considered at risk. The commonest findings in our series were babies who became lethargic, refused feeds, developed abdominal distension and began to vomit; gross rectal bleeding was noticed in 25% and occult rectal bleeding could be detected in another 50%; there might be oliguria. The distended abdomen was usually soft initially but would become guarded and tender as the disease progressed; loops of bowel became visible and palpable and occasionally crepitus could be felt. In the presence of bowel adhesions or abscess formation, an abdominal mass could be felt; with the onset of peritonitis, the abdominal wall could become erythematous and oedematous and with the development of disseminated intravascular coagulation, petechiae could become visible. Laboratory findings were non-specific and in general indicated sepsis: white blood cell count was often elevated or decreased, differential counts showing a shift to immature forms; there might be mild anaemia, thrombocytopenia and often metabolic acidosis.

Positive diagnosis depends on operative or autopsy findings or radiological evidence of pneumatosis intestinalis in a baby with the non-specific clinical picture.

Radiological findings

The hallmark of neonatal necrotizing enterocolitis is the characteristic X-ray picture showing intramural gas (Figure 34.4) – pneumatosis intestinalis. This is often best seen in the lateral view with the baby lying supine and the X-ray beam directed from one flank to the opposite flank. It is commonly an early rather than late finding and there are cases which have been described as a mild form of the disease where intramural gas is present and a little blood may be passed per rectum but the child is never ill [51,77]. Pneumatosis intestinalis has also been shown following pneumomediastinum [76] and we have had an experience, like Robinson, Grossman and Bromley [101], where a neonate with short-lived intestinal obstruction possibly due to a meconium plug showed intramural gas which disappeared in less than 24 h.

Free intraperitoneal air is virtually pathognomonic of intestinal perforation: on rare occasions it may be a sequel of pneumomediastinum (see Chapter 20). However, in necrotizing enterocolitis perforation is not always accompanied by pneumoperitoneum.

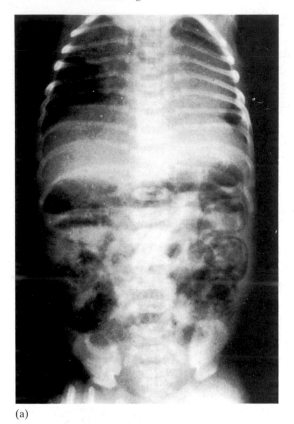
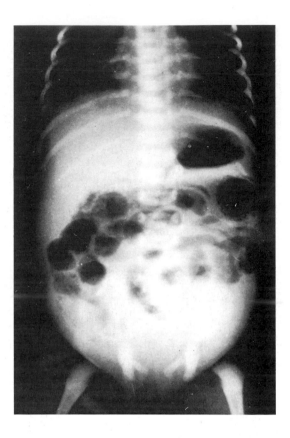

(a)

Figure 34.4 X-rays showing intramural gas. (a) Linear streaks of air in the bowel in both flanks. (b) Marked circumferential collection of air in the left upper quadrant

The disappearance of intramural air in response to treatment may be taken as a sign of improvement but it has been pointed out [78] that if there is no accompanying clinical improvement then there may still have been a perforation even though free intraperitoneal air has not been shown; the radiological finding of a gasless abdomen and increased intraperitoneal fluid may give the clue to such an indolent perforation.

A common but non-specific finding is the presence of distended loops of bowel with gas-fluid levels. However, the presence of a persistent loop of distended bowel in serial X-rays [80] is an important radiological sign suggestive of infarcted bowel (Figure 34.5).

The presence of portal vein gas (Figure 34.6) is believed to be an ominous sign suggestive of advanced disease [18]; there is some evidence that it may even be contributory to the development of septicaemia [41].

Barium enema is not necessary and may be dangerous since the friable bowel may easily be perforated. Cohen [20] reported that in cases where plain X-rays were unsatisfactory, additional information could be obtained with contrast meal studies using metrizamide, a non-ionic isotonic water-soluble compound. Schwartzentruber [111] evaluated the use of iohexol as a radiographic contrast in rats and suggested it could be useful in diagnosing bowel ischaemia but this was disputed by Erpicum and Davies on clinical grounds [33]. We do not recommend the use of contrast studies in the acute phase of necrotizing enterocolitis.

Staging

There are several classifications of necrotizing enterocolitis but the most widely adopted one is that introduced by Bell *et al.* [6] (Table 34.2).

Treatment

The importance of early recognition of the disease cannot be overemphasized and hopefully this will lead to an increase in the number of infants treated successfully by conservative measures. The surgeon should be involved with patient management before

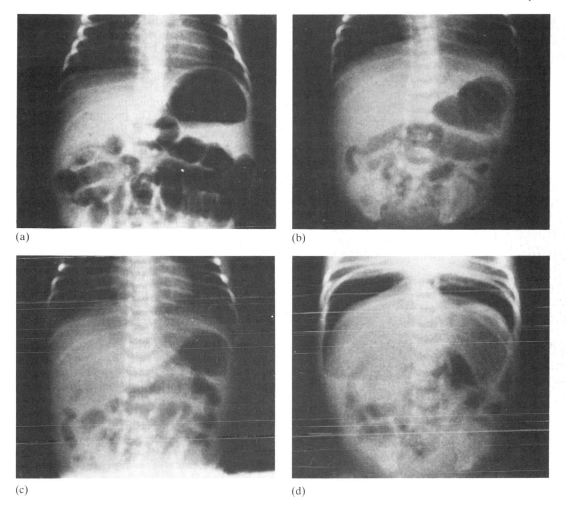

(a)

(b)

(c)

(d)

Figure 34.5 Sequential X-rays in neonatal enterocolitis. (a) Non specific distension: fixed loop in right upper quadrant apparent on day 2 (b) and persisting unchanged after 12 h (c). (d) Free air after perforation 6 h later: the loop is still unchanged and was found at operation to be infarcted terminal ileum

the disease is too advanced to allow optimal timing of any possible interventional procedure.

Initial treatment of necrotizing enterocolitis is aggressive and non-operative: oral feeding is withdrawn and nasogastric suction instituted. A venous catheter is inserted, first for the correction of fluid, electrolyte and acid-base balance, then for any necessary blood volume expanders and then for total parenteral alimentation. After blood and stool cultures are taken intravenous antibiotics are given: our first-line drugs are an aminoglycoside plus ampicillin, or cephalosporin, plus metronidazole until culture information is available; some authors prefer more powerful combinations such as cefatoxime and vancomycin [108].

The use of enteral aminoglycosides advocated by Bell *et al.* [6] remains controversial [46,59,61]; we have not used this technique. The use of low molecular weight dextran has also been recommended to reduce the tendency to intravascular coagulation and improve the perfusion of the affected gut [70]; we do not have experience of this either. The child should not be allowed to become hypoxic [59].

It is important to have regular monitoring of blood pressure and urine output, frequent clinical assessment and serial abdominal X-rays, blood cell counts, platelet counts and blood gas determinations. Blood should be cross-matched if transfusion is necessary or operation is imminent. Acidosis

né traité médicalement. *Ann. Chir. Infant.*, **7**, 261–264

88. Peiser, A. (1908) Die fötale Peritonitis. *Bruns' Beitr. Klin. Chir.*, **60**, 168–196

89. Pendergrass, E.P. and Booth, R.E. (1964) Report on a case of ruptured stomach in an infant 3 days old. *Am. J. Roent.*, **56**, 590

90. Porter, L. and Weeks, A. (1915) Megacolon and microcolon. *Am. J. Dis. Child.*, **9**, 263–299

91. Priebe, C.J., Mangahas, T. and Garrett, R. (1974) Neonatal gastric perforation not caused by congenital muscular defects. *Arch. Path.*, **98**, 422–425

92. Purcell, W.R. (1962) Perforation of the stomach in a newborn infant. *Am. J. Dis. Child.*, **103**, 66–71

93. Qvigstad, I. (1950) Spontaneous perforation of colon of newborn. *Nord. Med.*, **43**, 504–505

94. Ramos, J.F. (1950) Fetal meconium peritonitis with intra-abdominal hernia. *J. Natn. Med. Ass.*, **42**, 105–108

95. Reid, W.D. and Shannon, M.P. (1973) Necrotizing enterocolitis; a medical approach to treatment. *Can. Med. Ass. J.*, **108**, 573–576

96. Rickham, P.P. (1955) Peritonitis in the neonatal period. *Arch. Dis. Child.*, **30**, 23–31

97. Robarts, F.H. (1968) Neonatal perforation of the stomach. *Z. Kinderchir.*, **5**, 62

98. Rosser, S.B., Clark, C.H. and Elechi, E.N. (1982) Spontaneous neonatal gastric perforation. *J. Pediat. Surg.*, **17**, 390–394

99. Rosza, S. and Gross, R.J. (1953) Intrauterine perforation of Meckel's diverticulum. *Am. J. Roent.*, **69**, 944–947

100. Rubovits, W.H., Taft, E. and Neuwelt, O. (1938) The pathological properties of meconium. *Am. J. Obstet. Gynec.*, **36**, 501–505

101. Rudnew, W. (1915) Ueber die spontanen Darmperforationen bei Foeten und Neugeborenen. Inaugural Dissertation, Basle

102. Russell, T.H. (1940) Spontaneous rupture of the intestine in the newborn. *Trans. New Engl. Surg. Soc.*, **22**, 286–294

103. Shalev, J., Frankel, Avidgad, I. *et al.* (1982) Spontaneous intestinal perforation *in utero*: ultrasonic diagnostic criteria. *Am. J. Obstet. Gynaecol.*, **144**, 855–857

104. Schaupp, W., Clausen, E.G. and Ferrier, P.K. (1960) Appendicitis during the first month of life. *Surgery*, **48**, 805–811

105. Shaker, I.J., Schaefer, J.A., James, A.E. and White, J.J. (1973) Aerophagia: a mechanism for spontaneous rupture of the stomach of the newborn. *Am. Surg.*, **39**, 619–623

106. Shaw, A., Blanc, W.A., Santulli, T.V. and Kaiser, G. (1965) Spontaneous rupture of the stomach in the newborn. *Surgery*, **58**, 561–571

107. Siebold, E.A. (1825) Darmperforation in Neugeborenen. *J. Geburtsh. Frauenzimmer. Kinderkr.*, **5**, 3

108. Simpson, J.W. (1838) Notices of cases of peritonitis in the foetus *in utero*. *Edinb. Med. Surg. J.*, **15**, 390

109. Smith, A.L. and Macmahon, R.A. (1969) Perforated appendix implicating rhesus immunization in a newborn infant. *Med. J. Aust.*, **2**, 602–603

110. Snyder, W.H. and Chaffin, L. (1952) Appendicitis during the first two years of life: report on 21 cases and review of 447 cases from the literature. *Arch. Surg.*, **64**, 549–560

111. Soper, R.T. and Opitz, J.M. (1962) Neonatal pneumoperitoneum and Hirschsprung's disease. *Surgery*, **51**, 527–533

112. Speck, C.R., Moore, T.C. and Stout, F.E. (1962) Antenatal roentgen diagnosis of meconium peritonitis. *Am. J. Roent.*, **88**, 566–570

113. Sturzenegger, E. (1927) Ein Fall von mekonium Peritonitis. *Beitr. Path. Anat.*, **78**, 85–108

114. Sury, K. von (1912) Die spontane Darmruptur beim Neugeborenen. *Vjschr. gerichtl. Med.*, **43**, 91–95

115. Thelander, H.E. (1939) Perforation of gastrointestinal tract of newborn infant. *Am. J. Dis. Child.*, **58**, 371–393

116. Tibboel, D., van der Kamp, A.W.M. and Molenaar, J.C. (1981) The effect of experimentally induced intestinal perforation at an early developmental stage. *J. Pediat. Surg.*, **16**, 1017–1020

117. Tibboel, D., van der Kamp, A.W.M. and Molenaar, J.C. (1982) An experimental study of the effect of an intestinal perforation at various developmental stages. *Z. Kinderchir.*, **37**, 62–66

118. Tibboel, D. and Molenaar, J.C. (1984) Meconium peritonitis – a retrospective, prognostic analysis of 69 patients. *Z. Kinderchir.*, **39**, 25–28

119. Tucker, A.S., Soine, L. and Izant, R.J. (1975) Gastro-intestinal perforations in infancy. *Am. J. Roent.*, **123**, 755–763

120. Ungari, C. and Valiani, A. (1952) Perforated Meckel's diverticulum. *Clin. Ostet. Ginec.*, **54**, 147

121. Vargas, L.L., Levin, S.M. and Santulli, T.V. (1955) Rupture of the stomach in the newborn infant. *Surg. Gynec. Obstet.*, **101**, 417–424

122. Wagner, E.A., Jones, D.V., Koch, C.A. and Smith, D.I. (1952) Polyethylene tube feeding in premature infants. *J. Pediat.*, **41**, 79–83

123. Walstad, P.M. and Conklin, W.S. (1961) Rupture of the normal stomach after therapeutic oxygen administration. *New Engl. J. Med.*, **264**, 1201–1202

124. Wolfson, J.J. and Engel, R.R. (1969) Anticipating meconium peritonitis from metaphyseal bands. *Radiology*, **92**, 1055–1060

125. Young, D.G. (1965) Spontaneous rupture of the rectum. *Proc. Roy. Soc. Med.*, **58**, 615

126. Zerella, J.T. and McCullough, J.Y. (1981) Pneumoperitoneum in infants without gastrointestinal perforation. *Surgery*, **89**, 163–167

127. Zillner, E. (1884) Ruptura flexurae sigmoidis neonati inter partum. *Virchows Arch. Path. Anat.*, **96**, 307

36

Intraluminal intestinal obstruction

R. C. M. Cook

The commonest cause of neonatal intraluminal intestinal obstruction is cystic fibrosis, but there are a number of rare and, as yet, incompletely understood causes of intestinal obstruction in the newborn period which will be discussed at the end of this chapter.

Meconium ileus

Historical notes

In 1905 Karl Landsteiner [32] described the association of neonatal intestinal obstruction, due to inspissated meconium, with pancreatic disease. About 40 years later Anderson [1] and Farber [18,19] clarified our knowledge of the disease in a series of now classic papers. They emphasized that the disease was widespread and affected the mucus-secreting glands in many parts of the body – the lungs, pancreas and gastrointestinal tract. Glanzmann [21] suggested in 1946 that the inspissated meconium might be due to abnormal mucus production from the intestine, and in 1963 Thomaidis and Arey [54] pointed out that pancreatic causes would seem to play only a secondary role in the pathogenesis of meconium ileus. In 1953 Di Sant' Agnese et al. [11] drew attention to the fact that the disease also affected the function of the sweat glands, a discovery which had an important bearing on diagnosis. Prior to 1944 the surgery for meconium ileus was associated with virtually 100% mortality. In that year Hiatt and Wilson [24] reported the first surgical successes in four out of eight patients, describing their method of removing the abnormal meconium.

Incidence

Cystic fibrosis is the commonest lethal inherited disorder in Caucasian populations [30,40,52,58,59].

Mass screening of newborn infants suggests that the true incidence may be as high as 1 in 1800 [48], or even 1 in 1500 [59], 1 in 2000 is the accepted figure in the UK [34,48,57,58]. Ten percent of patients with cystic fibrosis were said to present at birth with meconium ileus [36], but now with more accurate diagnosis of milder cases later in childhood the proportion may fall. Although probably occurring less frequently than in Caucasians, the disease is seen in other races though the incidence in them is uncertain.

Pathological anatomy and physiology

The manifestations of cystic fibrosis are diverse and found in many different systems. The underlying biochemical abnormality – presumably of a single protein – has not been identified although membrane transport abnormalities have been found [41]. It is epithelial cells which show obvious defects particularly in their secretions and a special sensitivity to infection. This latter, often lethal, feature of the disease is not associated with demonstrable defects in immune function [35]. It is the abnormal exocrine secretions that lead to the common surgical manifestations, abnormal mucus leading to sticky meconium in the neonate and inspissated faecal masses in the older child.

Pancreas

In the pancreas the secretions are viscid and obstruct the ductules, leading to dilatation and disruption of the acini, and leaking enzymes cause local fibrosis. Ultimately only the islets of Langerhans may remain, embedded in fibrofatty tissue. In older children mild diabetes occurs [13].

Small intestine

The failure of pancreatic exocrine secretion causes abnormalities in the composition of duodenal fluid [12] and of meconium [6] in the lower small intestine, which becomes inspissated and putty-like with a high protein content due to the absence of proteolytic enzymes [33] (Figure 36.1). Additionally, absence of mucus leaves the intestinal lining unlubricated.

The distal small intestine is usually contracted, containing beads of greyish hard meconium. More proximally, the ileum and jejunum become hypertrophied and may be enormously dilated and filled with greenish-black tenacious material. The serosal surface of the dilated proximal small bowel may look inflamed, and the circulation may be impaired and the gut cyanosed (Figure 36.2).

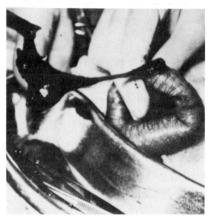

Figure 36.1 An enterostomy has been performed. The tenacity of the abnormal meconium is well shown

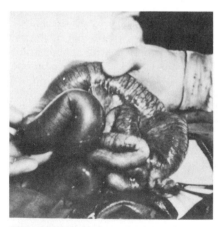

Figure 36.2 Typical appearance at laparotomy. Grossly dilated lower ileum with a poor blood supply, filled with sticky meconium

It is not surprising that gangrene and perforation of the gut, atresia, volvulus and meconium peritonitis are common complications [27,34,56]. Of 164 cases in a series at the Boston Children's Hospital Medical Centre [15], 45% presented with complications. Of 40 recent cases seen at the Regional Neonatal Surgical Unit in Liverpool, 20 had peritonitis, perforation, volvulus or atresia.

Sweat glands

Sweat glands are also involved, and defective reabsorption of sodium and chloride ions leads to high levels (>60 mg/Eq) in the sweat. This provides the basis of the standard diagnostic test [11].

Reproductive system

The reproductive system is involved, with a very high incidence of sterility in the male due to absence or atrophy of the epididymis, vas deferens or seminal vesicles. Fertility is also reduced in the female, possibly because of abnormal cervical mucus [8].

Lungs

The lungs are structurally normal at birth, but are very susceptible to infection. This susceptibility is enhanced by the secretion of abnormally viscid mucus. Interference with lung drainage and airway obstruction occurs because of this abnormal mucus, and further narrowing of the air passages is caused by hypertrophied mucous glands. Atelectasis and pneumonia may occur in the neonatal period and early death is more likely to be due to respiratory causes than to abdominal complications in the infant with meconium ileus.

Liver and bile ducts

Excess mucus blocks the fine intrahepatic ducts which dilate and proliferate. Portal fibrosis occurs, usually progresses slowly and may lead to portal hypertension in older patients.

Aetiology

Cystic fibrosis has an autosomal recessive inheritance pattern, the recurrence risk in an affected family being 1 in 4, and the sex incidence is usually said to be equal, although in the last 10 years we have seen a preponderance of female infants with meconium ileus (26:14). The manifestations of the disease are variable even in the same family. The site of the abnormal gene has been identified [30,58,59] as being on chromosome 7, but neither detection of carriers nor antenatal diagnosis of homozygotes can be carried out reliably at the present time.

Associated malformations

Apart from intestinal atresia, due to the condition itself, other malformations are rare [25] although an earlier review [9] of Liverpool cases showed several children with anomalous rotation of the gut. This, too, could be explicable in terms of the abnormal loading of the bowel in fetal life.

Clinical features

Very early intestinal obstruction and perforation may lead to intrauterine death. As stated earlier, some 10% of liveborn infants with cystic fibrosis have intestinal obstruction. The picture is of low intestinal obstruction with bile-stained vomiting and gross abdominal distension (Figure 36.3). It is usually stated that vomiting starts on the first day of life, but this is not always the case. Vomiting may be a late feature, and not occur at all before other manifestations have led to the diagnosis. In a series from the Children's Hospital in Pittsburgh [27], only 34 of 46 patients presented with vomiting. Abdominal distension, however, seems to be a common and early feature. It is often extreme, and may be present at birth. Distended loops of intestine are often visible on inspection, and palpation reveals that the intestine is filled with putty-like material that indents on pressure. In addition, strings of bead-like pellets may be felt in the right iliac fossa. Visible peristalsis is commonly observed.

Usually no meconium has been passed, but some infants are reported to have passed a little; occasionally, the meconium has appeared to be normal, or it may have been described as a greyish plug of mucus. Rectal examination usually reveals an empty rectum, or may precipitate the passage of some abnormal meconium.

The infant is usually of good birth weight, and the obstetric history is mostly unremarkable.

Special investigations

Radiography

Although the radiographic picture of the abdomen is not as specifically diagnostic as in some other types of intestinal obstruction, it is often possible to make the correct diagnosis from this examination. Gross distension of the intestine is frequently present, especially in the upper abdomen, but fluid levels are scanty and may be absent altogether [27]. Gross [22] pointed out, many years ago, the useful fact that the distended loops of bowel often vary greatly in size from one part of the abdomen to another (Figure 36.4).

Neuhauser first described [37] a mottled or coarsely granular appearance on abdominal radiographs (Figure 36.4). This is due to air bubbles which have been forced into the sticky meconium by peristaltic waves. Unfortunately, this sign is not always present [27,46] and is not specific for meconium ileus as it may be seen in other cases of intestinal obstruction in the newborn. Only 24 of 46 patients described from Pittsburgh [27] and only seven of 34 in a series from Zurich and Innsbruck [46] showed Neuhauser's sign.

Where prenatal perforation has occurred, calcification will take place in the peritoneum and be visible on plain radiographs (Figure 36.5).

A contrast enema used to be recommended as a routine to clarify the diagnosis before surgery [53]. It is doubtful if this is always necessary for diagnostic purposes, but it has taken on a new importance as a therapeutic measure in uncomplicated cases (see below, under 'Treatment').

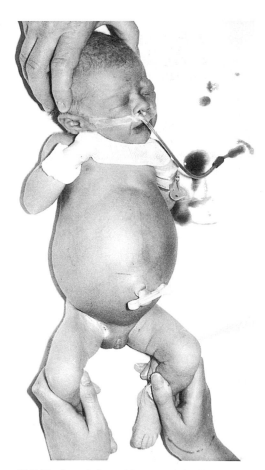

Figure 36.3 Newborn infant with gross abdominal distension due to meconium ileus

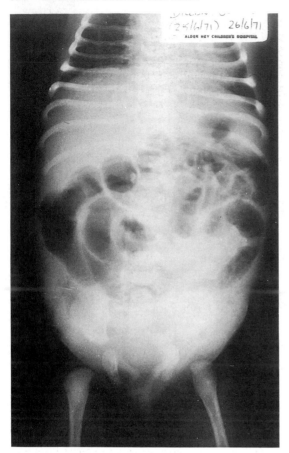

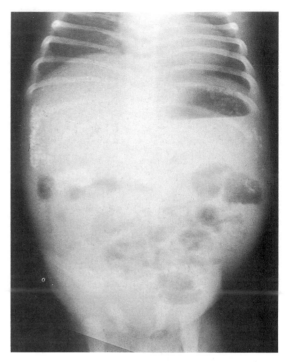

Figure 36.5 Abdominal radiograph of infant showing gross distension (due to ascites) some air in jejunum and calcification in both upper quadrants due to prenatal perforation

Figure 36.4 Abdominal radiograph of infant with meconium ileus, showing distended intestinal loops of varying size and coarsely granular masses in upper abdomen. Fluid levels are not present

Laboratory investigations

If meconium has been passed, the proteolytic activity can be measured in it. However, the absence or the presence of trypsin in the meconium is not specific enough to refute or make the diagnosis and the test has therefore been abandoned in most centres.

In meconium ileus the protein content of the meconium is abnormally high [45,47]. Schutt and Isles [47] found a 70% protein content in meconium of infants with meconium ileus compared with 9% in normal controls. The abnormally high protein (albumin) content can be recognized by a simple test using the Boehringer–Mannheim test strip. This uses tetrabromophenylphthalein as an indicator changing to a blue colour when the protein content of meconium is greater than 20 mg/g dry weight. It was initially hoped that this might provide a screening test for cystic fibrosis, but it will miss the 15–20% of infants with cystic fibrosis who do not have pancreatic insufficiency at birth. The cost of universal screening to identify cases using this and sweat tests has been estimated [35] at £10 000 for each case discovered!

The sweat test and serum trypsin levels

The fact that children with cystic fibrosis have a high concentration of sodium chloride in their sweat became the basis for the standard test for the condition [20]. Pilocarpine iontophoresis is used to ensure the collection of an adequate volume of sweat. This is not easy in small infants and at least 200 mg of sweat must be collected to obtain reliable and consistent results.

Serum immunoreactive trypsin levels are raised in neonates with cystic fibrosis, and the level can be estimated on a dried blood spot [28,29]. We have found the results consistently accurate.

Conservative treatment

The severity of obstruction varies from case to case. It has long been recognized [5] that some can be

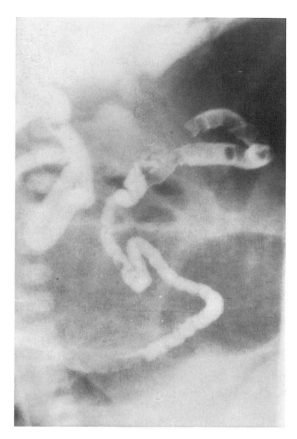

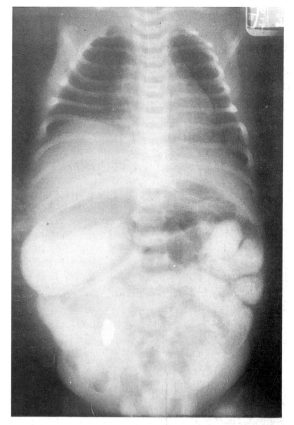

Figure 36.6 Radiograph taken during a Gastrografin enema. Contrast demonstrates the small unused colon and radiolucent areas are shown in the small intestine where the Gastrografin has seeped around pellets of meconium

Figure 36.7 Radiograph taken later than Figure 36.6. Gastrografin has reached dilated small intestine, i.e. it has penetrated the portion obstructed by hard pellets of meconium

relieved by enemas, and that surgery may be avoided. This method was popularized by Noblett [39] in 1968, since in the technique she described, the progress and success of treatment is viewed radiologically (Figures 36.6 and 7). Gastrografin is a 76% aqueous solution of sodium methyl glucamine diatrizoate together with a wetting agent. It has a high osmolarity (1900 mOsm/l) compared with plasma (300 mOsm/l) and therefore draws fluid into the lumen of the bowel, thereby loosening the obstructing material. It is an attractive technique [57], since if successful, anaesthesia, with its risk of precipitating pulmonary complications, is avoided. It can, of course, only be successful in those infants with uncomplicated intraluminal obstruction, and these complications may not be recognized on the initial plain abdominal films. Our current policy is to attempt to clear the obstruction with Gastrografin in infants with presumptive meconium ileus unless there are definite signs of complications such as free peritoneal air or calcification.

Technique

Because of its high osmolarity, Gastrografin can produce a marked fluid shift into the lumen of the bowel [23], and a reliable intravenous infusion must therefore be running during and after the enema. The Gastrografin is warmed and is injected into the rectum through a soft plain catheter using a 20 or 30 ml syringe under fluoroscopic control. Excessive pressure cannot be produced with a plain catheter which will slip out if too much force is being used to inject the contrast medium. Colonic perforations have been described [57] when using a Foley catheter as originally recommended [39]. The solution is injected in small volumes and time allowed between injections for the fluid to spread along the micro-colon (Figure 36.6). The procedure is stopped when the contrast medium reaches dilated ileum (Figure 36.7), if there is any suggestion of leakage out of the gut into the peritoneal cavity, if the infant's condition deteriorates, or after 45 min. If the infant is well, but the dilated ileum not reached the child should be returned to the ward, managed conservatively again, and a further Gastrografin enema considered 8 h or more later. When a Gastrografin enema is planned in such an infant, an operating theatre should be available in case perforation occurs or is discovered.

Operative treatment

Operation is, of course, the only method of treatment when complications such as meconium peritonitis, perforation or atresia are present. The abdomen is opened through a transverse upper abdominal incision. The appearance of the bowel is characteristic. The enormously dilated proximal intestine filled with putty-like material, the congestion of the veins over the intestinal wall, the cyanosed appearance of the gut and the narrow distal intestine containing pellets of firm meconium are all typical features of meconium ileus and the diagnosis is rarely in doubt (Figures 36.1 and 2).

A number of operative procedures have been recommended in the literature. Hiatt's and Wilson's original success was achieved by introducing a catheter through an enterotomy in the distended small bowel in order to wash out the sticky meconium with saline. It was sometimes found that multiple enterotomies were needed and the gut was often handled excessively and further damaged. The method fell out of favour, but has found a place again [38] for patients with uncomplicated meconium ileus in whom Gastrografin has not relieved the obstruction. Careful use of a Fogarty catheter may clear the obstructing meconium without the need for more than one enterotomy, and without damage to the bowel [38].

Intestinal resection has to be performed when the bowel is grossly dilated and its viability dubious, and long lengths of intestine may need to be removed. Following resection, Swenson recommended primary anastomosis, but a high incidence of anastomotic leakage led to the safer method of doing a Mikulicz type of resection and a double barrelled ileostomy [22]. Further surgery is, of course, necessary later to close the stoma.

All of these operative procedures necessitate a considerable amount of handling of the gut, causing trauma to intestine of doubtful viability, and it is not surprising that the operative mortality was high.

The Bishop–Koop [5] Roux-en-Y ileostomy avoids this excessive handling. In cases not requiring resection, the ileum is transected at the point of its maximum distension. The end of the proximal segment is then anastomosed to the side of the distal segment, leaving a free limb of distal ileum of about 4 cm in length. This open segment of ileum is brought out of the abdomen as an end ileostomy

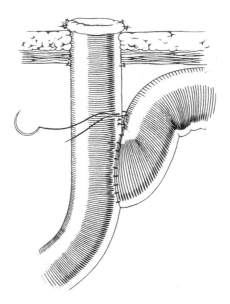

Figure 36.8 Roux-en-Y ileostomy

(Figure 36.8). In Liverpool it has been customary to vary the method slightly from that described by Bishop and Koop by hitching the proximal segment up onto the distal spout with a couple of Lembert sutures in such a way that the proximal segment enters the distal one obliquely away from the ileostomy stoma (Figure 36.8). This is designed to direct the stream of intestinal contents away from the stoma, but more importantly, when a catheter is passed through the stoma to wash out the distal segment there is no danger of the catheter going through the anastomotic stoma into the proximal segment. Such a stoma can also be made in those infants in whom resection has to be done because of very gross distension, doubtful viability of the bowel, gangrene or atresia.

When a Bishop–Koop ileostomy has been made, washouts can begin 24–36 h postoperatively, using warm normal saline rectally and via the stoma. Only 5–10 ml of fluid should be used initially through the ileostomy, but with twice or thrice daily repetition the volume can be steadily increased. Acetyl cysteine solution, or diluted Gastrografin may be used if desired, but simple saline washouts will work almost as quickly.

A wide range of procedures are therefore available for the infant who requires a laparotomy, and the most suitable procedure must be decided at operation. A short procedure with avoidance of excess handling of the 'sick' intestine is usually the best and safest, but if a stoma cannot be avoided, it must be remembered that a further operative intervention will often be necessary to close it.

After all such operative procedures, and after non-operative relief of obstruction with a Gastrografin enema, the infant is kept on continuous nasogastric aspiration and intravenous fluid replacement. Oral feeding may have to be delayed for some days after extensive surgery, and unless oral milk feeds are likely to be started early, intravenous feeding is begun. Intensive treatment of the chest is also started immediately, rather than awaiting obvious pulmonary complications. The infant is nursed in a humid atmosphere, regular physiotherapy is given, and antibiotics are used, specifically for the chest, as well as any needed to cover the intestinal surgery.

Results

The survival rate of children with meconium ileus and cystic fibrosis is not encouraging. In the early years of the Regional Neonatal Centre in Liverpool, only 64% of such infants were alive at 1 week and 46% at 4 weeks. In recent years more than 90% were alive after 1 week and 76% at 4 weeks [9]. The long-term survival remains poor, but has shown a distinct improvement – with a better quality of life. In the most recent decade analysed, 20 infants presented with simple meconium ileus. Gastrografin enemas were given to nine and four of these were successfully relieved of their obstruction. Sixteen infants were operated on – all surviving the procedure, but two died early from respiratory complications. Of 20 cases with complications, all survived the operative procedures but four died from abdominal complications and three more from respiratory disease. The infant who presents with meconium ileus does not necessarily have a poor prognosis with respect to respiratory infections later in childhood [36].

The meconium plug syndrome

Low intestinal obstruction caused by a plug of sticky meconium in the rectum or lower colon has been recognized for many years [4] and was more fully described by Clatworthy *et al.* in 1956 [7].

Aetiology

Temporary failure to pass meconium could theoretically be due either to inhibition of colonic peristalsis or to abnormal consistency of the meconium. It has been suggested [17] that colonic immaturity might allow an unusual amount of water to be reabsorbed from the meconium in late fetal life to make it harder. These infants seem to have perfectly normal colorectal function as soon as the plug has been removed, and we have found no evidence of neuronal dysplasia in this group of patients. Ellis and Clatworthy described [16] 21 cases with no abnormality in the pregnancy, but it is noteworthy that of 23 cases treated here between 1975 and 1985 nine were born by Caesarean section and four had forceps-assisted deliveries. Fibrocystic disease and Hirschsprung's disease were excluded in all our cases [55].

Clinical picture

All the infants presented with the picture of low intestinal obstruction. No meconium had been passed spontaneously. Vomiting occurred in 18 of our 23 cases, and it was bile stained in at least 12 of them. Gross abdominal distension was noted in most – especially those that had progressed to bile-stained vomiting. Visible peristalsis was another common feature and firm masses in the colon were sometimes palpable. Rectal examination demonstrated a normal anal canal and usually an empty rectum. The plug was actually palpated rectally in some. Rectal examination stimulated the passage of the plug (Figure 36.9) and the rest of the meconium in some infants.

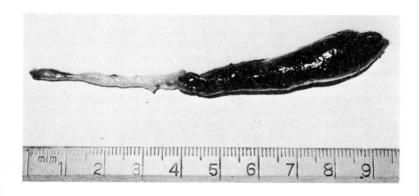

Figure 36.9 A meconium plug, nearly 10-cm long, consisting of greyish sticky mucus in its lower half and sticky meconium in its upper half

Special investigations

Radiography

Plain radiography of the abdomen shows gaseous intestinal distension, but fluid levels are uncommon. A barium enema may well reveal a normal rectum and colon while the plug shows up [16] as a translucent area low in the colon or in the rectum. We have left the choice of contrast medium to our radiologists, who often recommend changing to Gastrografin if a plug is demonstrated. This usually is very effective in stimulating emptying of the bowel but gives slightly less clear pictures.

Laboratory investigations

We have not looked for trypsin in the meconium in recent years, but note that it was invariably present when looked for in past years. Serum trypsin has been measured in many of these infants and has always been found to be normal. The sweat test is normal. We have made it a rule to do a rectal biopsy before allowing 'meconium plug' to be the discharge diagnosis. Ganglion cells were demonstrated in all instances, except one which is described below.

Treatment

In 11 cases where the meconium plug was not passed after a rectal examination, a rectal washout was effective. We consider that this should be done as a contrast enema under X-ray control to prove the diagnosis and to rule out other pathology. Even in cases with gross abdominal distension, the abdomen deflates very rapidly and oral feeding can begin within a few hours.

It will be clear from the description so far that we regard this as a diagnosis made by exclusion of other pathology. We recognize that meconium plugs may be found in other conditions and therefore fibrocystic disease and Hirschsprung's disease must always be excluded. One infant seen during this period was initially labelled as having a meconium plug. He was allowed home after a suction rectal biopsy had been taken but before the result had been seen. He was doing well and on review a few weeks later appeared to be quite normal and the fact that no ganglion cells had been seen in the biopsy was assumed to have been a technical fault – too shallow a biopsy. At 8 weeks of age he was referred back with abdominal distension and constipation and failure to thrive. Further biopsies and a barium enema confirmed that the rectum was aganglionic. He has done well after a Duhamel procedure.

Meconium obstruction in the absence of cystic fibrosis

Most large series of cases of meconium ileus contain a small proportion who do not have cystic fibrosis. The precise mechanism of obstruction in these infants remains uncertain, and it may even be doubted that they represent a specific disease or form a homogeneous group [43].

Historical notes

Isolated cases of meconium obstruction, in the absence of cystic fibrosis, and presumed to be secondary to stenosis of the pancreatic duct, were reported in 1926 and 1931. In 1957, Rickham described [42] an infant with meconium obstruction and intraluminal calcification, who showed no evidence of either cystic fibrosis or Hirschsprung's disease (Figure 36.10). The child repeatedly re-obstructed because of inspissation of the meconium. In 1969, Auburn *et al.* reported [2] a case in which partial aplasia of the pancreas resulted in abnormal meconium.

Incidence

Meconium ileus in the absence of cystic fibrosis is generally thought to be rare but is perhaps being recognized more frequently because of better survival rates and more thorough investigation. We have found ten cases over a recent 11-year period. There were 40 cases of meconium ileus associated with cystic fibrosis in the same years. All ten infants in this recent series were male.

Aetiology

The aetiology of this condition is still not clear, and, as suggested above, there is probably more than one clinical entity included under this heading [43]. Auburn's case [2] had pancreatic insufficiency due to aplasia of the dorsal anlage of the pancreas, and had multiple other anomalies. Pancreatic duct stenosis [26,31] may similarly cause insufficiency of the pancreatic exocrine secretions. The consistency of the meconium in premature infants may well be different from that in the full-term infant, but we can find no data relating to this, and although it has been implicated in 'functional' obstruction in preterm infants [50], immaturity of the neuromuscular mechanisms of the colon and rectum would seem to be a more likely explanation. Three of our infants were premature or small for dates. The histories of the pregnancies and the family histories of our patients were unremarkable but a familial form has been described [14]. Absorption studies carried out on the survivors of an earlier Liverpool series did show some abnormalities but the children were apparently normal [42,43].

Clinical picture

The presenting features were identical to children with meconium ileus who were later discovered to have cystic fibrosis. Abdominal distension and vomiting – usually bile-stained – occurred mostly in the first 24 h of life, but occasionally were delayed for several days. Rectal examination revealed an empty rectum and did not stimulate the passage of meconium. A number of cases are reported in which meconium is passed normally at first but who later develop small bowel obstruction due to retained viscid meconium [44,60].

Special investigations

Radiography

As in meconium ileus with cystic fibrosis, dilated loops of bowel with few fluid levels, the bubbly appearance of the meconium and, sometimes, calcification or even free air, make the diagnosis clear (Figure 36.10).

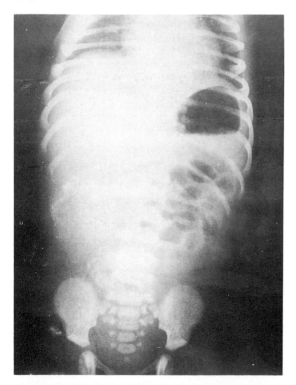

Figure 36.10 Radiograph of an infant suffering from intestinal obstruction due to meconium ileus in the absence of mucoviscidosis. Faint calcified masses can be observed on the right side of the abdomen: these were due to intraluminal calcification of meconium

Laboratory investigations

Laboratory investigations to exclude cystic fibrosis are essential after relief of the intestinal obstruction.

Treatment

As with meconium ileus associated with cystic fibrosis, a contrast enema may be indicated not only to clarify the diagnosis but also for therapeutic purposes.

Gastrografin is the medium of choice [49], and cured six out of our ten cases. Four children required laparotomy and two of these had obstruction complicated by perforation and meconium peritonitis. The surgical techniques employed are the same as for those who are later found to have cystic fibrosis, and the immediate postoperative regimen should assume that there is associated lung disease until cystic fibrosis has been ruled out.

Results

There were no deaths among the recent cases, and their course after surgery, or after Gastrografin enema clearance, was uneventful. Cystic fibrosis was ruled out in all, and suction rectal biopsy is now routine in Liverpool in such children to exclude Hirschsprung's disease or colonic neuronal dysplasia.

Milk curd obstruction

We first described this as a new disease in 1969 [10], reporting eight cases. A further 11 cases occurred in Liverpool in the next 8 years and were analysed in the second edition of this book [51]. In the ensuing 10 years we have seen a further five cases. These children were all quite normal after birth with respect to their intestinal motility. They passed normal meconium, changing to milk stools and then developed signs of low small intestinal obstruction. The obstruction was due to a hard dry mass of milk curd in the lower ileum, usually a few centimetres from the ileocaecal valve, and extending proximally for a variable distance – in some cases up to the duodenojejunal junction [43]. This syndrome seems to occur only in those infants on an artificial milk formula as opposed to breast milk [43].

Aetiology

The cause of the obstruction is not clearly understood. Only one of our most recent cases was born at full term. The others were born at between 27 and 37 weeks of gestation, and their early behaviour was unremarkable. Symptoms and signs of intestinal obstruction developed at ages ranging between 7 days and 7 weeks. The most premature infant was well until 7 weeks (gestational age was then 34 weeks) and then he quite suddenly obstructed, and perforated. Necrotizing enterocolitis was a possible cause, but the perforation was in mid ileum at the proximal end of an inspissated mass of hard curds. One of the other premature infants developed necrotizing enterocolitis after sugery to relieve his milk curd obstruction. He had a cardiac defect in addition, but had not been in heart failure, nor had he been specifically ill or hypoxic before he obstructed. It is well recognized that premature infants may have difficulty evacuating sticky faeces from the rectum and lower colon, but the picture is entirely different from the infant with small bowel curd obstruction.

Some children in our earlier series had been septicaemic and the bowel obstruction may have been precipitated by a paralytic ileus. We found [10], in some of our original patients, slight transient absorption defects for sugars and amino acids, but this was not confirmed in other reports [3]. The cause of the obstruction is undoubtedly related to artificial feeds, though additional factors must be involved otherwise the condition would be encountered much more frequently.

Clinical picture

Symptoms and signs are typical of any low small bowel obstruction. The onset is usually between a few days and a few weeks of age. Berman and Ross reported a case presenting at 6 weeks, and one of ours, as described above, occurred at 7 weeks. All have bile-stained vomiting, and abdominal distension is common. Sometimes, especially in very low birthweight infants, the solid loops of ileum can be perforated. Perforation, if it occurs, will lead to a grossly distended tender abdomen in a shocked infant. Dehydration will develop quickly in all these infants if the diagnosis and treatment are delayed.

Special investigations

An erect plain abdominal X-ray will show typical signs of low small intestinal obstruction. In some instances the picture is similar to that in meconium ileus, with grossly distended loops, Neuhauser's sign and the absence of fluid levels (Figure 36.11). A contrast enema may help to confirm the diagnosis, and again, may be therapeutic. Later absorption studies and rectal biopsies may be indicated.

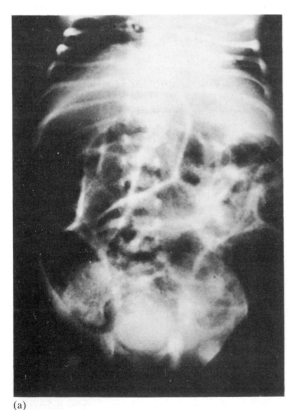

(a)

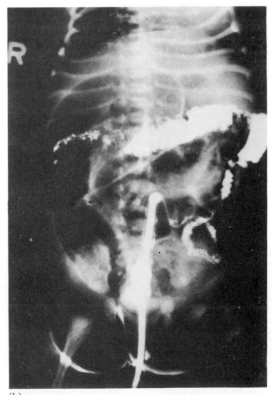

(b)

Figure 36.11 (a) Typical radiograph of a 7-day-old child with milk curd obstruction. Note the distended small bowel, absent fluid levels and Neuhauser's sign.

(b) Gastrografin enema in same patient as in (a). Normal colon. The enema was twice returned clear

Treatment

As with other intraluminal obstructions, if they are not complicated by perforations or ischaemic damage, non-operative treatment may relieve the obstruction. Gastrografin is the generally accepted agent, but to be effective it has to reflux proximal to the ileocaecal valve. It was effective in three of our recent cases. Of the others, one was perforated on admission and required an urgent laparotomy. The other was not relieved by an enema and at laparotomy was found to have an extensive obstruction with curds packing most of the ileum. At surgery, it may be possible to massage the obstructing curds into the colon without opening the bowel. In more severe cases, or where there is perforation, or bowel of dubious viability, resection is indicated. In these circumstances the construction of a Bishop–Koop ileostomy is safer than a primary anastomosis.

Results

Deaths in earlier reported series were related to metabolic and septic complications of bowel resection. Only one death occurred in the latest five infants – a small premature infant with a cardiac anomaly who became septicaemic after surgical resection of obstructed bowel and developed widespread necrotizing enterocolitis.

The survivors are growing normally and although not tested in detail, have no sign of absorption problems.

References

1. Andersen, D.H. (1938) Cystic fibrosis of the pancreas and its relation to celiac disease. *Am. J. Dis. Child.*, **56**, 344–399
2. Auburn, R., Feldman, S.A., Gadacz, T.R. and Rowe, M.I. (1969) Meconium ileus secondary to partial aplasia of the pancreas: report of a case. *Surgery*, **65**, 689–693
3. Berman, E.J. and Ross, C. (1972) Milk curd obstruction in a 6 week old infant. *J. Pediat. Surg.*, **7**, 342
4. Berti, R. (1898) Rectal blockage with fibrino epithelial plug in a newborn. *Arch. Kinderheilk.*, **24**, 463
5. Bishop, H.C. and Koop, C.E. (1957) Management of meconium ileus. *Ann. Surg.*, **145**, 410–414
6. Buchanan, D.J. and Rapoport, S. (1952) Chemical comparison of normal meconium and meconium from a patient with meconium ileus. *Pediatrics*, **9**, 304–309
7. Clatworthy, H.W. Jr, Howard, W.H.R. and Lloyd, J.R. (1956) The meconium plug syndrome. *Surgery*, **39**, 131–142
8. Cohen, L.F., Di Sant'Agnese, P.A. and Friedlander, J. (1980) Cystic fibrosis and pregnancy. *Lancet*, **ii**, 842–844
9. Cook, R.C.M., El-Gohari, M.A. and Bernard, M.

(1985) Meconium ileus: 22 years review. Presented at the European Association of Paediatric Surgeons Congress, Graz, 1985
10. Cook, R.C.M. and Rickham, P.P. (1969) Neonatal intestinal obstruction due to milk curds. *J. Pediat. Surg.*, **4**, 599–605
11. Di Sant'Agnese, P.A., Darling, R.C. and Perera, G.A. (1953) Sweat electrolyte disturbances associated with childhood pancreatic disease. *Am. J. Med.*, **15**, 777–784
12. Di Sant'Agnese, P.A., Dische, Z. and Danilezenko, A. (1957) Physicochemical differences of mucoproteins in duodenal fluid of patients with cystic fibrosis of pancreas and controls. *Pediatrics*, **19**, 252–260
13. Di Sant'Agnese, P.A. and Talamo, R.C. (1967) Pathogenesis and physiopathology of cystic fibrosis of the pancreas. *New Engl. J. Med.*, **277**, 1287–1294
14. Dolan, J. and Touloukian, R. (1974) Familial meconium ileus not associated with cystic fibrosis. *J. Pediat. Surg.*, **9**, 821–824
15. Donnison, A.B., Schwachman, H. and Gross, R.E. (1966) A review of 164 children with meconium ileus seen at the Children's Hospital Medical Center, Boston. *Pediatrics*, **37**, 833–850
16. Ellis, D.G. and Clatworthy, H.W. Jr (1966) The meconium plug syndrome revisited. *J. Pediat. Surg.*, **1**, 54–61
17. Emery, J.L. (1957) Abnormalities in meconium of the foetus and newborn. *Arch. Dis. Child.*, **32**, 17–21
18. Farber, S.J. (1944) The relation of pancreatic achylia to meconium ileus. *J. Pediat.*, **24**, 387–392
19. Farber, S.J. (1944) Pancreatic function and disease in early life. *Arch. Path.*, **37**, 238–250
20. Gibson, L.E. and Cooke, R.E. (1959) A test for the concentrations of electrolytes in sweat in cystic fibrosis of the pancreas utilizing pilocarpine by iontophorosis. *Pediatrics*, **23**, 545–549
21. Glanzmann, E. (1946) Dysporia enterobronchopancreatica congenita familiaris. *Ann. Pediat.*, **166**, 289–313
22. Gross, R.E. (1953) *The Surgery of Infancy and Childhood*. W.B. Saunders, Philadelphia
23. Harris, P.D., Neuhauser, E.B.D. and Garth, R. (1964) The osmotic effect of water soluble media on circulating plasma volume. *Am. J. Roent.*, **91**, 694–698
24. Hiatt, R.B. and Wilson, P.E. (1948) Celiac syndrome therapy of meconium ileus. *Surg. Gynec. Obstet.*, **87**, 317–327
25. Holsclaw, D.S., Eckstein, H.B. and Nixon, H.H. (1965) Meconium ileus. *Am. J. Dis. Child.*, **109**, 101–113
26. Hurwitt, E.S. and Arnheim, E.E. (1942) Meconium ileus associated with stenosis of the pancreatic ducts. *Am. J. Dis. Child.*, **64**, 443–454
27. Kalayoglu, M., Sieber, W.K., Rodnan, J.B. and Kieswetter, W.B. (1971) Meconium ileus: a critical review of treatment and eventual prognosis. *J. Pediat. Surg.*, **6**, 290–300
28. Kenny, D., Cook, A. and Tempany, E. (1978)

Activity of serum amylase in cystic fibrosis. *Clin. Chem. Acta,* **89**, 429–433

29. King, D.N. *et al.* (1979) Serum trypsin assay for dried blood specimen as screening procedure for early detection of cystic fibrosis. *Lancet,* **ii**, 1217–1218

30. Knowlton, R.G., Cohen-Haguenauer, O., Van Cong, N., Frezal, J., Brown, V.A., Barker, D., *et al* (1985) A polymorphic DNA marker linked to cystic fibrosis is located on chromosome 7. *Nature,* **318**, 380–382

31. Kornblith, B.A. and Otani, S. (1929) Meconium ileus with congenital stenosis of the main pancreatic ducts. *Am. J. Path.,* **5**, 249–262

32. Landsteiner, K. (1905) Darmverschluss durch eingedicktes Meconium-Pankreatitis. *Zentbl. allg. Path. path. Anat.,* **16**, 903–907

33. Lebenthal, E. and Baswell, D. (1983) The pancreas in cystic fibrosis. In *Textbook of Cystic Fibrosis.* ed. J.D. Lloyd-Still. J. Wright, Bristol

34. Leonidas, J.C., Berdon, W.E., Baker, D.H. and Santulli, T.V. (1970) Meconium ileus and its complications. *Am. J. Roent.,* **108**, 598–609

35. McCrae, W.M. Cystic fibrosis: Mucoviscidosis. In *Textbook of Paediatrics,* (eds J.O. Forfar and G.C. Arneill), Churchill Livingstone, Edinburgh, pp. 511–518

36. McPartlin, J.F., Dickson, J.A.S. and Swain, V.A. (1972) Meconium ileus. Immediate and long term survival. *Arch. Dis. Child.,* **47**, 207–210

37. Neuhauser, E.B.D. (1946) Roentgen changes associated with pancreatic insufficiency in early life. *Radiology,* **46**, 319–328

38. Nguyen, L.T., Youssef, S., Guttman, F.M., Laberge, J-M., Albert, D. and Doody, D. (1986) Meconium ileus: Is a stoma necessary? *J. Pediat. Surg.,* **21**, 766–768

39. Noblett, H.R. (1969) Treatment of uncomplicated meconium ileus by Gastrografin enema: a preliminary report. *J. Pediat. Surg.,* **4**, 190–197

40. Prosser, R., Owen, H., Bull, F., Parry, B., Smerkinich, J., Goodwin, H.A. *et al.* (1974) Screening for cystic fibrosis by examination of meconium. *Arch. Dis. Child.,* **49**, 597–601

41. Quinton, P.M. and Bijman, J. (1983) Higher bioelectrical potentials due to decreased chloride absorption in the sweat-glands of patients with cystic fibrosis. *New Engl. J. Med.,* **308**, 1185–1189

42. Rickham, P.P. (1957) Intraluminal intestinal calcification in the newborn. *Arch. Dis. Child.,* **32**, 31–34

43. Rickham, P.P. (1971) Intraluminal intestinal obstruction. *Prog. Pediat. Surg.,* **2**, 73–82

44. Rickham, P.P. and Boeckman, C.R. (1965) Neonatal meconium obstruction in the absence of mucoviscidosis. *Am. J. Surg.,* **109**, 173–177

45. Schachter, H. and Dixon, G.H. (1965) A comparative study of the proteins in normal meconium and in meconium from meconium ileus patients. *Can. J. Biochem.,* **43**, 381–397

46. Schennach, W., Menardi, G. and Stauffer, U.G. (1976) Zur Prognose des Mekoniumileus. *Z. Kinderchir.,* **18**, 161

47. Schutt, W.H. and Isles, T.E. (1968) Protein in meconium from meconium ileus. *Arch. Dis. Child.,* **43**, 178–181

48. Shwachman, H., Pyles, C.V. and Gross, R.E. (1956) Meconium ileus. *Am. J. Dis. Child.,* **91**, 223–244

49. Shigemoto, H., Endo, S., Isomoto, T., Sano, K. and Tagughi, K. (1978) Neonatal meconium obstruction in the ileum without mucoviscidosis. *J. Pediat. Surg.,* **13**, 475–479

50. Sieber, W.K. and Girdani, B.R. (1963) Functional intestinal obstruction in newborn infants with morphologically normal gastrointestinal tracts. *Surgery,* **53**, 357–361

51. Stauffer, U.G. and Rickham, P.P. (1978) Intraluminal intestinal obstruction. In *Neonatal Surgery,* 2nd Edition (eds P.P. Rickham, J. Lister and I.M. Irving), Butterworths, London, Chapter 34

52. Stephan, U., Busch, E.W., Kollberg, H. and Hellsing, K. (1975) Cystic fibrosis detection by means of a test strip. *Pediatrics,* **55**, 35–38

53. Swenson, O. (1958) *Pediatric Surgery,* Appleton Century Crofts, New York

54. Thomaidis, T.S. and Arey, J.B. (1963) Intestinal lesions in cystic fibrosis of pancreas. *J. Pediat.,* **63**, 444–453

55. Van Leeuwen, G., Riley, W.C., Glenn, B.A. and Woodruff, C. (1967) Meconium plug syndrome with aganglionosis. *Pediatrics,* **40**, 665–666

56. Wagget, J., Bishop, H.C. and Koop, C.E. (1970) Experience with Gastrografin enema in the treatment of meconium ileus. *J. Pediat. Surg.,* **5**, 649–654

57. Wagget, J., Johnson, D.G., Borns, P. and Bishop, H.C. (1970) The nonoperative treatment of meconium ileus by Gastrografin enema. *J. Pediat.,* **77**, 407–411

58. Wainwright, B.J., Scambler, P.J., Schmidtke, J., Watson, E.A., Law, H-Y., Farrell, M. *et al.* (1985) Location of cystic fibrosis locus to human chromosome 7cen-q22. *Nature,* **318**, 384–385

59. White, R., Woodward, S., Leppert, M., O'Connell, P., Hoff, M., Herbst, J. *et al.* (1985) A closely linked genetic marker for cystic fibrosis. *Nature,* **318**, 382–384

60. Zachary, R.B. (1957) Meconium and faecal plugs in the newborn. *Arch. Dis. Child.,* **32**, 22–24

37

Hirschsprung's disease

James Lister and P. K. H. Tam

Hirschsprung described a condition which he called sluggishness of the stool in the newborn. Although there was confusion about the aetiology of the disease for many years, the clinical picture is now well recognized. The majority (70–80%) of cases of Hirschsprung's disease are diagnosed in the neonatal period. This chapter will deal with problems of diagnosis and management of this condition in the neonatal period only. Definitive surgical procedures for Hirschsprung's disease are normally performed in older infants and will not be discussed here. Statistics in this chapter are based on an analysis of 172 neonates treated in the Royal Liverpool Children's Hospital, Alder Hey, between 1953 and 1985 with a special emphasis on the 52 recent patients managed in 1976–85. Occasional reference to interesting cases outside this series will be made for illustrative purposes.

Historical notes

In 1886, the great Danish paediatrician, Hirschsprung, gave a lecture to the Berlin Paediatric Society describing the clinical and autopsy findings in two infants whom he had treated from birth until 7 and 11 months when they died of constipation associated with dilatation and hypertrophy of the colon. Hirschsprung [78] was not the first to describe this condition; there had been previous case reports [88,93], but he was the first to recognize the fact that a congenital malformation might be the cause of the disease which later was named after him. The aetiology of the condition remained in doubt and Hirschsprung's disease was often mistaken for acquired megacolon. This is surprising, because as early as 1901 Tittel [170] reported degeneration of the cells of Auerbach's and Meissner's plexuses in

the apparently normal colon distal to the dilated segment. Similar observations were made by Hawkins [74] in 1907, Dalla Valla [37] in 1924 and Cameron [25] in 1928. Robertson and Kernohan [140], and Tiffin et al. [169] published papers prior to 1940, both of which expressed the belief that the cause of Hirschsprung's disease was the absence of peristaltic activity in the aganglionic segment of distal bowel. In 1946 Ehrenpreis [46] published a detailed review of the disease. His monograph contained a classic description of Hirschsprung's disease in the neonatal period. Finally, Swenson and Bill [156] in 1948 showed conclusively that the dilatation of the proximal colon in Hirschsprung's disease was secondary to absence of peristaltic movement in the distal narrow segment, and based their curative operation of rectosigmoidectomy on these findings. During the same year Zuelzer and Wilson [189], and Whitehouse and Kernohan [184] published histological studies showing that the disease was due to congenital aganglionosis of the distal segment of the large intestine and these findings were confirmed by the subsequent observation of Bodian et al. [15], Swenson et al. [157] and Hiatt [77].

Pathology

The basic pathology in Hirschsprung's disease is a congenital absence of intramural ganglia affecting the most distal parts of the rectum and extending proximally for a varying distance. The aganglionic segment is non-propulsive and fails to relax resulting in functional intestinal obstruction. Proximal to the aganglionic segment is a transitional zone of hypoganglionosis and more proximally the normal ganglionic bowel typically gives the appearance of 'megacolon' because of chronic distal obstruction. Tapering at the transitional zone is usually gradual although it can be either abrupt or even absent. In the majority of cases aganglionosis involves the rectum and lower sigmoid. In our series of 172 neonates the length of the aganglionic segment was recorded in 166: rectum or rectosigmoid 110 (66.3%), above sigmoid 56 (33.7%). The ultrashort segment disease reported in older children [9,43,120,143] was described in only one of our neonatal cases. Total colonic involvement (Zeulzer Wilson syndrome) [30,189] occurred in 19 (11.4%) of which two extended to mid-jejunum. Total absence of enteric innervation has been described and 21 cases have been recorded in the English literature [27,39,144]. Outside our present series, we saw one such fatal case in 1987. 'Skip-lesions' or zonal aganglionosis has also been described [151,188] but its existence is not accepted by all workers [154] as the idea is not easily explained by traditional concepts of the pathogenesis of Hirschsprung's disease. In 1987 we encountered a case of zonal involvement in which aganglionosis affected three segments: (1) rectum to descending colon, (2) distal half of ascending colon, (3) appendix; the intervening large bowel and terminal ileum were normally ganglionated.

Apart from aganglionosis, other pathological features in Hirschsprung's disease are now being increasingly identified. This improved knowledge of the abnormalities of the enteric nervous system was only made possible by the major advances in our understanding of the normal control system of intestinal motility and defaecation resulting from studies with histochemistry, immunohistochemistry and other new techniques. It is agreed that the intrinsic enteric nerve plexus (intramural ganglia and their nerve fibres) regulates normal intestinal peristalsis and the extrinsic nerves modulate the intestinal response. However, the traditional concept of inhibitory postganglionic adrenergic fibres passing from the sympathetic chain to muscle and preganglionic parasympathetic fibres from sacral outflow relaying at the intramural ganglia to continue as cholinergic excitatory fibres has now been replaced by a far more complex explanation [60,84]. The most important change is the realization that a substantial proportion of enteric nerves are non-cholinergic and non-adrenergic, their neurotransmitter being neither acetylcholine nor adrenaline. Initially, the term 'purinergic' nerves was used [24] and adenosine triphosphate (ATP) was implicated as the neurotransmitter. Serotonin (5-hydroxytryptamine) was then also shown to be present in some non-cholinergic, non-adrenergic nerves [64]. Subsequently, a large number of peptides have been identified in enteric nerves. The better known neuropeptides include substance P [137], vasoactive intestinal peptide [145], enkephalin [106], somatostatin [69], bombesin [40], cholecystokinin [99],

calcitonin gene-related peptide [34], galanin [165], neuropeptide Y [53]; novel neuropeptides are still being discovered. These 'peptidergic nerves' have undoubted roles in regulating intestinal motility; some have inhibitory actions, others have excitatory functions.

In Hirschsprung's disease, conventional histological examination of the affected bowel shows a total absence of ganglion cells in both Auerbach's and Meissner's plexus [184]; in areas normally occupied by a delicate neural matrix there is an increase in the number and size of nerve bundles and trunks [89,119,183]. A transitional zone of hypoganglionosis of variable length exists between the aganglionic and ganglionic segments and the junction tends to be more caudally located on the antimesenteric side [66].

Histochemical studies reveal that the hypertrophied nerve trunks have intense acetylcholinesterase (AChE) activity. In addition there is an abnormal proliferation of AChE-positive nerve fibres in the muscularis mucosae and lamina propria in the aganglionic bowel [62] (Figure 37.1). This histochemical feature is consistently observed in Hirschsprung's disease and has been usefully applied for diagnostic purposes [98,119]. The exact nature of these abnormal nerves remains uncertain as acetylcholinesterase can be present in all types of nerves. In long segment disease the proliferation of nerve fibres does not extend beyond the splenic flexure.

Studies of adrenergic innervation with fluorescent histochemical techniques show that the normal pericellular network of adrenergic nerves around ganglia is absent in the aganglionic segment. In the muscle layers a variable distribution of adrenergic nerves is present [7,61,62]. In the submucosa the pattern is less clear: Touloukian *et al.* [171] reported an increase of adrenergic fibres whereas Tuto [172] found an absence of these nerves.

Ultrastructural studies reveal that the non-myelinated axons (adrenergic and cholinergic) within the muscle layers of the aganglionic bowel have synaptic contacts with the muscle cells, suggesting that these nerves are functional [6,83]. The hypertrophied nerve trunks typically found in Hirschsprung's disease contain myelinated axons.

Immunohistochemical studies with general neuronal markers are now available and they allow more sensitive and specific detection of neuronal abnormalities in affected bowel segments. Using such techniques we studied resected bowel specimens from patients with Hirschsprung's disease and demonstrated intense activity of neuron-specific enolase (NSE) in the hypertrophied nerve trunks [162,163] (Figure 37.2). Other workers have used antibodies against neurofilament and other proteins and their products, and ganglion cell components [70,71,94,147,159] for immunohistochemical stud-

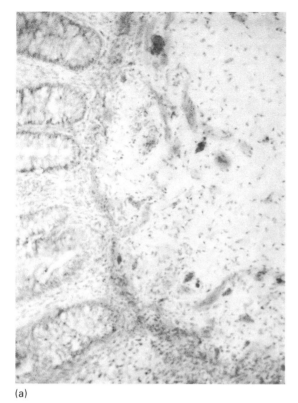

(a)

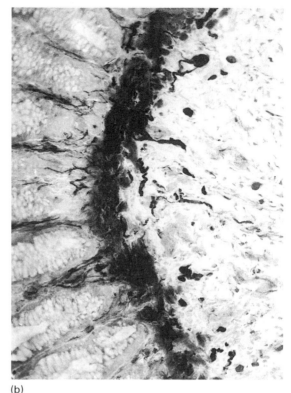

(b)

Figure 37.1 Histochemical examination of rectal biopsies for acetylcholinesterase (AChE) activity (×250), (a) Normal – minimal AChE positive nerve fibres, presence of ganglia in submucosa.

(b) Hirschsprung's disease – marked proliferation of AChE nerve fibres in lamina propria and muscularis mucosae, hypertrophical nerve bundles in submucosa, absence of ganglia

ies. Although these methods of investigation are at present used mainly for research purposes, their applications may become more widespread in future. In particular they could prove useful in areas of diagnostic difficulties for pathological variants of Hirschsprung's disease.

As early as 1952, Ehrenpreis and Pernow [49] using bioassays showed that the biologically active peptide which they termed substance P was reduced in the aganglionic bowel in Hirschsprung's disease. Advances in immunohistochemistry and radioimmunoassay subsequently identified substance P as one of the many neuropeptides involved in enteric innervation. Using these sensitive techniques, we have confirmed the findings of Ehrenpreis' study [160,161]. As substance P is now known to have an excitatory action on bowel muscle, it is likely that reduced substance P in the aganglionic bowel contributes to the lack of propulsive activity of the affected segment in Hirschsprung's disease. Other neuropeptides have now also been studied: vasoactive intestinal peptide [12,173] met-encephalin,

gastrin-releasing peptide (GRP) [100] galanin, somatostatin, calcitonin gene-related peptide [71,101] were found to be reduced in the aganglionic segment; only neuropeptide Y was shown to be increased in the aganglionic segment [71]. The exact physiological role of many neuropeptides has yet to be worked out but some are undoubtedly involved in the non-cholinergic and non-adrenergic inhibitory system. Apart from neuropeptides, serotonin (5-hydroxytryptamine) is also considered to belong to this inhibitory system; in the aganglionic segment serotonin contents were found to be reduced [141].

Pathophysiology

Previous workers have suggested that the abnormal state of contraction of the aganglionic segment is due to denervated smooth muscle being abnormally sensitive to stimuli [28,48,113,129]. Recent studies do not support this simple explanation and various other mechanisms have been postulated. Cholinergic hyperactivity may play a role: an increase in

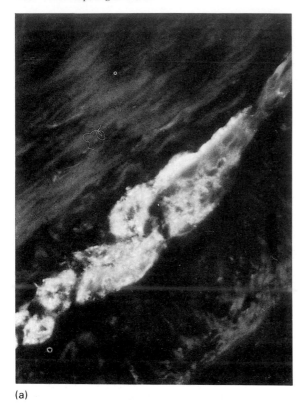

(a)

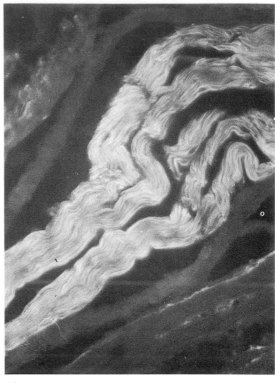

(b)

Figure 37.2 Immunohistochemical examination with antibody against neuron-specific enolase (NSE) (×400). (a) Normal – mesenteric ganglia,

(b) Hirschsprung's disease – ganglia replaced by thick nerve bundles

acetylcholine content has been demonstrated in the aganglionic bowel [86] and this may reflect an excessive stimulatory input [62,72,89]. Most workers believe that the cholinergic nervous system in the aganglionic bowel is functional (see above) but to add confusion to existing controversies on this subject some workers have provided electrophysiological evidence to suggest otherwise [174].

Abnormalities of the adrenergic innervation have also been implicated: adrenergic innervation is normally inhibitory to bowel muscle and despite increased noradrenaline content in the aganglionic bowel [171] the adrenergic nerves in the aganglionic bowel appear to be functionally defective and are incapable of the normal response of inducing muscle relaxation [125]. More recently attention has been focused on the role of the non-adrenergic and noncholinergic inhibitory system: electric field stimulation of normal bowel muscle induces relaxation preceding contraction and this relaxation is believed to be mediated by the non-adrenergic inhibitory fibres as the response is unaffected by adrenergic blockers; electric field stimulation of aganglionic

muscle however does not produce the initial relaxation response and inhibitory junction potentials are also absent [130]. This and other evidence of abnormalities of peptidergic and serotoninergic nerves described in previous paragraphs strongly suggest that defects in the non-adrenergic inhibitory system are important in the pathophysiology of Hirschsprung's disease.

Hirschsprung's related disorders

It is also important to realize that the mere presence of ganglion cells is not sufficient proof that intestinal innervation is normal [180]. It has long been recognized that some patients with clinical and radiological features identical to those of Hirschsprung's disease do not have the histological abnormality of aganglionosis and the term pseudo-Hirschsprung's disease was introduced [47]. We now know that this represents a heterogeneous group of pathological conditions some of which have remained   unquantified   even   today

[48,80,123,126,138]. The best known example is neuronal intestinal dysplasia which was first described in 1971 [118]. The affected bowel segment shows hyperplasia of the submucous and myenteric plexus, giant ganglia formation, ectopic ganglia location within the lamina propria, mild to moderate increase in acetylcholinesterase activity and reduced adrenergic activity [148]. Neuronal intestinal dysplasia can occur either in isolation or in association with Hirschsprung's disease affecting bowel proximal to the aganglionic segment [136]. The abnormalities have to be specifically looked for and may be missed if histochemical examinations are not performed on biopsy specimens. In some patients not all the characteristic histological features are present. In 1987 we encountered two neonates with neuronal intestinal dysplasia requiring surgery in this hospital; in the same year we treated ten neonates with classic Hirschsprung's disease. Other known causes of Hirschsprung-like disease include hypoganglionosis, immaturity of ganglia and hypogenesis. Hypoganglionosis is characterized by a reduction in the number of ganglion cells and nerve fibres in the intramural plexus (number of ganglion cells per unit length of intestine less than one-tenth normal, surface area of plexus per unit area less than one-fifth normal) [8,119]. Immaturity of ganglia is characterized by the histological abnormality of small monopolar ganglion cells [123] and is believed to be an important cause of functional bowel obstruction in newborns [104]. The prevalence of this clinical condition is increasing in neonatal centres where more and more premature babies are being kept alive by modern intensive care measures. Hypogenesis is a rare condition consisting of both hypoganglionosis and immaturity of ganglia [123].

In yet other patients with Hirschsprung-like presentation, no histological abnormality can be detected; it is possible that identification of the neuropathology in some of them will require more sophisticated studies including those for the non-adrenergic, non-cholinergic nerves.

Complications

The commonest complication of Hirschsprung's disease is enterocolitis; this potentially lethal condition occurred in 37 out of 172 neonates. The pathological changes in this condition resemble those in necrotizing enterocolitis in other neonates (see Chapter 34). The pathogenesis of enterocolitis in Hirschsprung's disease remains obscure. Distal obstruction resulting in stasis and bacterial overgrowth in proximal bowel is one possible explanation. A hypersensitivity reaction to bacterial antigen has also been postulated [10]. *Clostridium difficile* has been isolated in some patients with enterocolitis in one study and an aetiologic role has been implied [168]. Abnormalities of secretory functions and local immune responses of colon were observed in a study of enterocolitis in the mouse model of Hirschsprung's disease [59] but it is unclear as to whether the changes were the cause or effect of enterocolitis. An impairment of the cellular and humoral immunity has also been demonstrated in a small study involving five patients with Hirschsprung's disease complicated by enterocolitis [185]. Confirmation of the role of defective immunological defence in the aetiology of Hirschsprung's enterocolitis awaits larger studies. Eleven of our 37 patients with enterocolitis died, though in two of them death was attributable to severe congenital heart disease. The incidence of enterocolitis has not diminished – in the period 1975–85, 14 of 52 neonates with Hirschsprung's disease had enterocolitis; the mortality due to enterocolitis, however, has been reduced – only two of 14 patients died, one of them from congenital heart disease. Complications following operations are more likely to develop in patients who had enterocolitis – of 37 patients three had anastomotic leaks, two had major wound infection and one had septicaemia from colostomy necrosis. Extensive destruction of the bowel mucosa may occur during the episode of enterocolitis and survivors may encounter absorption problems. Residual mucosal changes such as polypoid mucosa, persistent granulation tissue and extensive lymphoid hyperplasia are often found in resected bowel following recovery from enterocolitis and this may explain why enterocolitis occasionally recurs in patients already treated surgically.

Another serious complication of Hirschsprung's disease is bowel perforation. This occurred in eight of our 172 cases; five were less than 4 days of age, and three were 15, 16 and 28 days old respectively when perforation was discovered. Perforation is more likely to occur in the presence of enterocolitis; only two of our eight patients did not have enterocolitis. Perforation in the absence of enterocolitis appears to be directly related to increased intraluminal pressure from distal obstruction and is more likely to occur in the bowel proximal to or at the site of the transitional zone in cases of short or intermediate lengths of aganglionosis [124]; neonatal perforation of the appendix may be caused by Hirschsprung's disease and the true diagnosis may be missed if this possibility is not considered [117]. In infants with total colonic aganglionosis, however, perforation is more often situated in the aganglionic bowel.

Aetiology and embryology

It is generally accepted that intramural ganglia originate from neural crest cells and their full development involves cell migration, distribution, differentiation and maturation; congenital aganglionosis results from abnormalities somewhere along this developmental pathway. However, the details of neither the normal embryology nor the abnormal development in Hirschsprung's disease and its newly recognized related disorders have been fully worked out. In the 1940s and 1950s, Yntema and Hammond [187] did a series of ablation experiments on chick embryos and suggested that enteric nerve cells originated solely from the neural crest at the vagal level and migrated down the gut to populate its whole extent. The histological study of human embryos by Okamoto and Ueda [128], using silver stain, seemed to confirm this view; their findings indicated that neuroblasts probably entered the oesophagus via the vagal trunks between the fifth and sixth week of gestation and migrated caudally within the muscle layers to populate the entire alimentary tract by the 12th week of gestation. The submucous plexus was formed by neuroblasts from the myenteric plexus distributing themselves across the bowel wall. They postulated that congenital aganglionosis resulted from a cessation of the craniocaudal migration of neuroblasts along the alimentary tract at various stages before the 12th week of gestation; the earlier the cessation the longer the segment of aganglionosis. Webster studied mice with congenital aganglionosis using histochemical techniques for non-specific esterase and found that neural crest cell migration was slower than normal; he concluded that aganglionosis of the rectum was due to the neural cell migration being out of phase with the longitudinal growth of bowel [181].

Although this simple and attractive hypothesis is widely accepted by paediatric surgeons there are plenty of studies to suggest otherwise. Several early workers proposed a dual origin of enteric ganglia from both vagal and trunk levels [175]; this hypothesis has been revived recently by Le Douarin [103] who performed a series of experiments on the quail–chick chimeric system and found that although the main source of enteric neurons came from the vagal neural crest, some postumbilical enteric nerve cells arose from lumbosacral neural crest. Gershon using an isotope cell labelling technique found not only a dual origin of enteric nerve cells in chick gut but also a dual gradient of differentiation and maturation of nerve cells proceeding from both ends towards mid gut. Furthermore, he was able to show that primitive nerve cells were already present in the gut before they were morphological recognizable [65]. The possibility of species variation exists but in a series of histological and immunohistochemical studies on human embryos and fetuses in this hospital we have also demonstrated the presence of a dual gradient of differentiation and maturation of enteric ganglia in humans during the ninth to 21st week of gestation [21,160]. These and other evidence have

led to an alternative hypothesis which proposes that Hirschsprung's disease and its related disorders result from abnormalities of gut microenvironment at critical stages of nerve cell development. An attractive feature of the new microenvironment theory is that unlike the old theory of arrest of neural crest cell migration it can also explain the occurrence of the increasingly recognized Hirschsprung's related disorders: different abnormalities of microenvironmental factors can result either in nerve cells not developing (Hirschsprung's disease) or developing abnormally (Hirschsprung's related disorders, e.g. neuronal intestinal dysplasia). Experimental data showing that the extracellular matrix regulates enteric neuronal development are abundant; Kumagata [96] found that cholineacetyltransferase activity of rat fetal colon culture is enhanced by the addition of fibronectin, a constituent of extracellular matrix and inhibited by the addition of antibody to fibronectin. Structural abnormalities of the bowel wall of aganglionic mice have also been identified and these include smooth muscle cell hypertrophy and overproduction of basal laminal material [167]. Co-culture experiments revealed that neural crest cells from aganglionic mice could colonize normal gut; distal gut from aganglionic mice however would not permit normal crest cells from normal mice to colonize but would promote axon growth [132]. Another important factor for enteric nerve development is the vascular supply [44]. If Urokon is injected into the inferior colic artery of the dog, the myenteric plexus is destroyed and aganglionosis results [113]. Similar results may be observed when the ganglion cells have been destroyed by *Trypanosoma cruzi* in Chagas' disease [52,95] or by accidental injuries to the arterial supply of the colon at operation [47]. The presence of abnormal arteries in Hirschsprung's disease was reported in 1966 [108]; hamartomatous changes and obliterative endarteritis were noticed in the transitional zone in three of ten patients with Hirschsprung's disease. The possibility that aganglionosis results from intrauterine intestinal ischaemia received further support from a recent histological study which detected adventitial fibromuscular dysplasia in the transitional zone of bowel specimens in 30% of patients with Hirschsprung's disease [158]. A viral aetiology for Hirschsprung's disease has also been suspected and the co-existence of intrauterine cytomegalovirus infection in Hirschsprung's disease has been reported [76].

Genetic factors play a part in the aetiology of Hirschsprung's disease. There is a definite familial incidence [13,55,56,75,105]: multifactorial inheritance is considered to be the most likely mode of inheritance although in some families, autosomal recessive inheritance is a possibility [29,63]. Three-generation transmission of Hirschsprung's disease has been reported [107]. In our series ten families had more than one member affected. In six families more than one sibling was affected; of these, two were extended kindreds with, respectively, seven and four first-degree relatives (sibs/parents/maternal cousin) affected by Hirschsprung's disease. In three other families, a cousin or an aunt was affected and in one family the father was affected.

Recurrence risk in sibs depends on the proband sex and the length of aganglionosis. For short segment index patients, the risk to brothers is about 1 in 20, and to sisters about 1 in 100; for long segment index patients the risk is about 1 in 10 irrespective of sex. Recurrence risk in children is established to be 2% for short segment patients; the risk is higher for the children of long segment patients but exact figures are not available. There is less likelihood of concordance for the length of aganglionic segment in parent and child than in sibs, i.e. a long segment parent with a short segment child and a short segment parent with a long segment child are not infrequent. In case of parent-child disease, the mother is more often involved than the father.

There is a significant association between Hirschsprung's disease and Down's syndrome [14,50,63,68,131] and this was found in 12 of our 172 patients (7%), eight of whom had congenital heart disease. Table 37.1 shows other associated anomalies. The commonest associated gastrointestinal conditions were anomalies not uncommonly seen in the general population, for example, malrotation and Meckel's diverticulum. We have not seen associated anorectal anomalies [80,177] or intestinal atresias [87]. Associated myelomeningocele [122] and congenital deafness [114] were each seen once in our series and as both conditions can result from abnormal development of the neural crest, their association with Hirschsprung's disease may have aetiological implications. The occasional association of Hirschsprung's disease with neuroblastoma, reported elsewhere [87] but not encountered in this series, has led to the concept of neurocrystopathy [16].

There were 22 mothers who had previous abortions and six mothers who had previous stillbirths. Two mothers had diabetes, an association which has been reported [22]; one mother had thyrotoxicosis and smoked heavily; one mother had ulcerative colitis and was treated with salazopyrine during pregnancy. Most mothers (60%) were aged between 20 and 30 years; 30% were between 30 and 40 years; 8% were below 20 years and only 2% were above 40 years.

Very little is known about the aetiology of Hirschsprung's related disorders and this deserves further study.

Incidence

The incidence of Hirschsprung's disease is probably about 1:5000 births [154]; higher figures (1:1000 births) [23] as well as lower figures (1:20000–1:30000 births) [15] have been reported. There is a male preponderance but this becomes less marked in long segment disease and in familial cases [80]. In the past 10 years our overall male to female ratio was 1.9:1; for short segment disease, males were three times more commonly affected than females and for long segment disease the sex distribution was equal. A racial distribution with Caucasian more commonly affected than negroes has been reported [41,51]; this series consists mainly of Caucasians.

Clinical picture

Hirschsprung's disease differs from many other alimentary tract abnormalities in that patients are usually of normal birth weight [79,105]. Premature babies are, however, not exempt from this condition – in our series 12 of the 172 (7%) weighed less than 2.5 kg at birth.

The functional intestinal obstruction in Hirschsprung's disease can be acute, recurrent or chronic. Although presentation and diagnosis may be delayed, symptoms can usually be traced to the immediate newborn period. Nowadays, because of increased clinical awareness and better diagnostic measures, an increasing proportion of patients with Hirschsprung's disease is diagnosed and treated in the neonatal period. A case report of prenatal sonographic diagnosis of Hirschsprung's disease has also been described [179] but as intestinal obstruction is functional in character and low in level,

Table 37.1 Associated anomalies in 172 neonates with Hirschsprung's disease

Down's syndrome		12
Cardiac malformation		13 (8 Down's)
GI anomalies		11
Malrotation	(5)	
Non-rotation	(1)	
Meckel's diverticulum	(4)	
Congenital short bowel	(1)	
Urological anomalies		3
Hypospadias	(2)	
Vesico-ureteric reflux	(1)	
Skeletal anomalies		3
Talipes equinovarus	(1)	
Congenital dislocation of hip	(1)	
Pes cavus	(1)	
Diaphragmatic hernia		1
Myelomeningocele (cervical)		1
Congenital profound deafness		1
Total		45

prenatal detection is unlikely to do more than raise a suspicion: the diagnosis in any event can only be confirmed postnatally. In our experience of 172 cases, 93 had symptoms and signs during the first day of life and another 61 during the first 6 days, most of these between 24 and 48 h of age; only 15 patients developed symptoms and signs between 7 days and 4 weeks. Only neonatal cases are considered here, but it is noteworthy that no patient with long segment or total colonic disease presented at Alder Hey Children's Hospital outside the neonatal period.

Vomiting

Vomiting was one of the commonest symptoms: it was recorded to have occurred at some time in 152 patients (88.4%); of these, 44 had vomiting as the sole presenting symptom. Vomiting was nearly always bile-stained; it had already progressed to faeculent vomiting in seven cases and there was haematemesis in two cases.

Reluctance to feed

Reluctance to feed, being a rather negative symptom, is not often mentioned in Hirschsprung's disease; nevertheless, it was the sole presenting symptom in four of our cases and was mentioned as an early feature in 14 more.

Passage of meconium

Some abnormality in the passage of meconium is a characteristic feature of Hirschsprung's disease and this was observed in 85% of cases. Most often there was a delay in the passage of meconium for more than 24 h after birth; in other instances only a small amount of viscid meconium was passed. In 13 cases meconium was said to have been passed normally and the child subsequently became constipated but in 13 cases bowel action was said to be entirely normal.

Abdominal distension

As a result of swallowed air, abdominal distension will be seen in most cases. Occasionally the newborn baby may present with acute, severe abdominal distension, resulting in diagnostic difficulties and even to an exploratory laparotomy. Abdominal distension will also be aggravated acutely when the disease is complicated by enterocolitis or bowel perforation. In the majority of cases however abdominal distension develops gradually and is not often obvious until after the third day of life. In the early part of this series (1954–75), abdominal distension was described amongst the presenting signs in only 34.2%; in 1976–85 it was recorded in

94.2% of cases, in half of them being described as mild. Distended loops of bowel were visible in many cases; in some, peristalsis could be seen and in one case a right iliac fossa mass was palpable. The distended abdomen was seldom tender unless complications had occurred. Abdominal distension was absent in three cases; two of these had rectosigmoid aganglionosis and one, interestingly, had near-total intestinal aganglionosis.

Rectal examination

In Hirschsprung's disease the rectum is often found to be empty and the anus described as tight. Explosive passage of flatus and meconium or faeces following rectal examination is a useful sign in pointing to the diagnosis. In 27 of our cases, the abdomen deflated visibly after rectal examination and in another 27 deflation occurred after rectal washout. However, repeated rectal examination or rectal washouts should not be carried out until after a diagnostic contrast enema has been performed since they may mask the situation by passively distending the aganglionic segment.

Enterocolitis

Of 37 cases complicated by enterocolitis. 24 were clinically obvious; of these, 12 became acutely sick, showing signs of septicaemia. The abdomen became tensely distended, vomiting became profuse and this was accompanied by frequent passage of foul-smelling flatus and loose stool. In the remaining 12 milder cases the only change observed initially was the onset of diarrhoea.

Special investigations

Radiology

A straight anteroposterior X-ray of the abdomen should be carried out in every case. The picture may be completely normal in infants who have deflated themselves, or may show multiple fluid levels indistinguishable from low intestinal obstruction due to other causes. Most commonly, multiple loops of distended bowel are shown with only an occasional fluid level (Figure 37.3). In newborn infants differentiation between dilated small and large intestine on plain radiography is difficult. There is an absence of rectal gas shadow, but this radiological finding is also not uncommonly present in normal infants. Only very occasionally is it possible by plain radiography to visualize the dilated proximal colon and the typical cone of Hirschsprung's disease narrowing towards the non-distended distal gut (Figure 37.4). In some instances the plain film will also show the colon to be loaded with meconium.

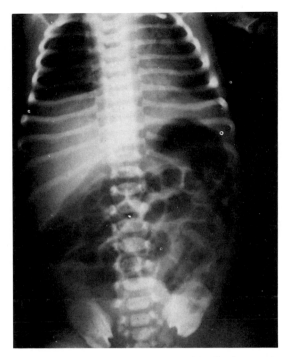

Figure 37.3 Radiograph of neonate with Hirschsprung's disease, showing gaseous distension of bowel with an occasional fluid level

Intramural gas may be seen in cases complicated by enterocolitis and pneumoperitoneum may be found in those with perforations.

Contrast enema studies are of considerable importance in the diagnosis of Hirschsprung's disease in the neonatal period [142,166]. In our series of 172 patients, a contrast enema was performed in 125 and a positive diagnosis of Hirschsprung's disease was made in 89 (71.2%); with the availability of experienced paediatric radiologists the diagnostic accuracy has improved to 76.9% in the recent decade. Barium was the most commonly used contrast medium; however, in 13 patients, because of the initial clinical suspicion of meconium plug syndrome, Gastrografin enemas were performed instead and in five (38.5%) the diagnosis was missed. We feel that Gastrografin enemas are less reliable than barium enemas in the diagnosis of Hirschsprung's disease and unless the Gastrografin enema has positively diagnosed Hirschsprung's disease a repeat enema study using barium is warranted some time later.

The demonstration of a transitional zone is the most useful radiological sign for the diagnosis of Hirschsprung's disease; this was present in 63.0% of the barium enema studies (Figure 37.5). Fluoroscopic screening is often helpful and the feature of abnormal or absent peristalsis of the distal bowel is sometimes the only clue to diagnosis [36,82]. The irregular contractions in rectum sometimes give a saw-toothed appearance especially on the anterior

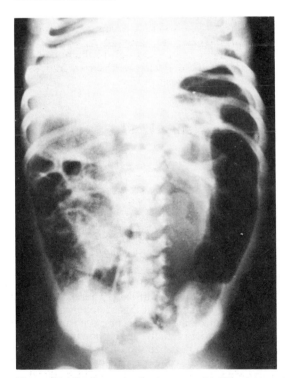

Figure 37.4 Radiograph of a neonate with Hirschsprung's disease. The grossly distended sigmoid colon narrows markedly towards its middle

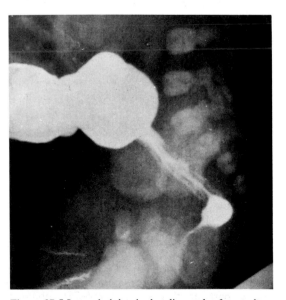

Figure 37.5 Lateral abdominal radiograph of a newborn infant with Hirschsprung's disease. The dilated sigmoid colon and narrow rectum are shown

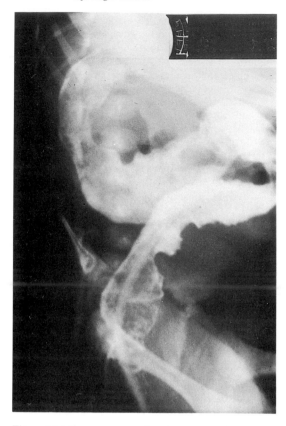

Figure 37.6 Barium enema showing saw-toothed appearance on anterior rectal wall

rectal wall (Figure 37.6). On rare occasions, mucosal ulceration may be demonstrated in cases complicated by enterocolitis (Figure 37.7); however barium enema is usually not recommended if enterocolitis is suspected on clinical grounds or plain radiography. The use of a 24-h film to show retained barium proximal to the aganglionic segment is of considerable importance [36] and this was the only abnormal radiological sign noticed in 11.1% of the barium enema studies (Figure 37.8); in one of our cases the diagnosis of total colonic aganglionosis was confirmed radiologically by the recognition of retained barium seen on IVP films 2 weeks after a barium enema (Figure 37.9). Of the 125 contrast studies, in at least 24 Hirschsprung's disease was wrongly excluded; of these one had total enteric aganglionosis, six had total colonic aganglionosis and three had long segment aganglionosis. In addition, the transitional zone seen radiologically does not always correspond to the zone found at surgery; this discrepancy was noticed in 16.7% of our recent cases, half of which proved to have total

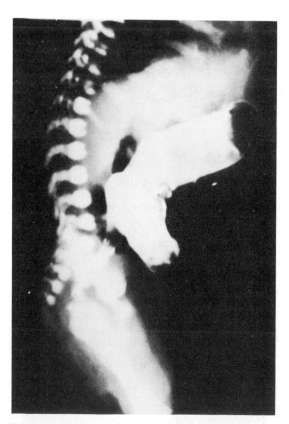

Figure 37.8 Lateral radiograph of newborn infant's abdomen 24 h after a barium enema. Some barium has been retained in the colon and the narrow rectum is clearly outlined

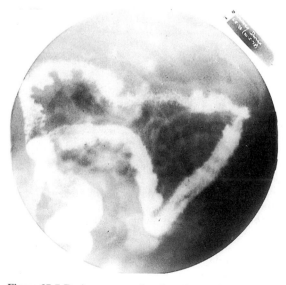

Figure 37.7 Barium enema showing ulcerated colonic mucosa in enterocolitis complicating Hirschsprung's disease

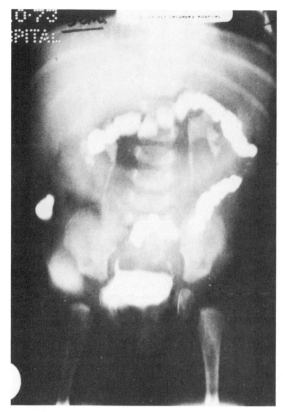

Figure 37.9 Retained contrast medium in colon noted in IVP film taken 2 weeks after barium enema in a case of Hirschsprung's disease

colonic aganglionosis at operation instead of the shorter segment involvement suggested radiologically. Contrast enema results must therefore be considered carefully in relation to the clinical picture, other investigations as well as operative and pathological findings.

Anorectal manometry

Anorectal manometry studies [102,149,150,164] have shown abnormal patterns in Hirschsprung's disease with failure of relaxation of the internal anal sphincter in response to rectal distension, and in some centres this has been used as a diagnostic technique. Howard and Nixon [85] concluded that a normal reflex response could be expected after the 40th gestational week though they would not rely on the test completely until after the second week of life. Holschneider *et al.* [81], in longitudinal studies found the internal sphincteric relaxation reflex present in only 11% of children in the first 2 days, 50% after the third day and in all normal babies

after the 12th day. Recently, the introduction of microtransducers has allowed more accurate pressure measurements in small babies and Tamate *et al.* [164] have shown that in fact prematurity and postnatal age do not influence the normal rectosphincteric reflex; hence with modern instruments, the size and age of the baby are no longer limiting factors for the use of anorectal manometry. In expert hands, this technique is reasonably accurate. Boston and Scott [18], laying emphasis on inhibition of rhythmicity rather than a drop in intraluminal anal pressure, made a correct diagnosis in 24 out of 27 neonates. Loening-Bauke *et al.* [111] used three successive falls of >5 mmHg of the anal tone associated with the inhibition of anal rhythmicity as the criteria for the presence of rectosphincteric reflex to exclude Hirschsprung's disease and reported a 75% sensitivity and 95% specificity of the technique in 25 neonates with intestinal obstruction. Anorectal electromyography is a related technique: in Hirschsprung's disease there is a reduction of spikes in the rectum and an absence of propagation of spikes from the anal canal to the rectum; initial results of its use are said to be encouraging [186]. Reports of complications of anorectal manometry are rare. However, considerable expertise is required for its proper use and interpretation, and at present the procedure is still not widely practised in the neonate.

Rectal biopsy

Definitive diagnosis of Hirschsprung's disease and its related disorders is made by histological and/or histochemical examination of the innervation pattern in biopsy specimens obtained from the rectum. Even in those cases where a laparotomy is indicated on clinical and radiological grounds rectal biopsy is preferable to an extramucosal biopsy specimen taken from the colon as aganglionosis need not necessarily extend to colon. Based on the findings of a histological study on ten neonates, Aldridge and Campbell [1] recommended that rectal biopsy should be taken at 2 cm above the anal valves (pectinate line) as a length of hypoganglionosis ranging from 0.3–1.7 cm existed in normal infants. Venugopal *et al.* [178] suggested that biopsies taken at a level of 1–1.5 cm from the pectinate line should be adequate and would avoid missing cases of ultrashort segment aganglionosis. A clue to the pathologist that the biopsy has been performed at the normally hypoganglionic level is the demonstration of stratified squamous epithelium or intermediate stratified columnar epithelium in the specimen and such findings should suggest that a repeat biopsy at a higher level is necessary.

In early days, full thickness rectal biopsy was the standard method of obtaining tissue samples for histological diagnosis. A total of 72 rectal biopsies

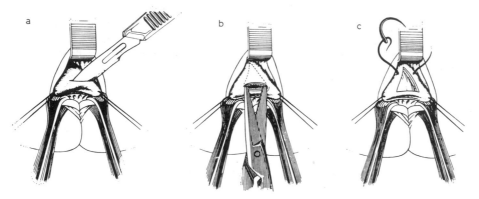

Figure 37.10 Rectal biopsy: (a) exposure of rectal mucosa and incision; (b) excision of strip of rectal wall; (c) suture of rectal wall defect

in the neonatal period were taken in this series without complication using a modification of the technique of Fisher *et al*. [54] (Figure 37.10). Under general anaesthesia the patient is placed in the lithotomy position and the anus is dilated with Hegar's dilators. The anal and lower rectal mucosa are cleaned with chlorhexidine gluconate solution (Hibitane) and a gauze swab soaked in this solution is inserted into the rectum above the operation site. The posterior wall of the anal canal is then everted by applying an Allis' tissue forceps on each side. A holding stitch on a fully curved needle is then inserted posterolaterally on each side through all the layers of the rectum at the level of the internal sphincter. Traction on these stitches will completely evert the anal canal and the posterior wall of the rectum can now be visualized by inserting a 1-cm wide malleable copper retractor into the anus and retracting the anterior wall forwards. The posterior rectal wall is now grasped with a fine-toothed dissecting forceps and a 5-mm wide and 1–1.5-cm long strip of the full thickness of the rectal wall is excised with scissors. The defect is then closed by placing interrupted 4/0 silk sutures on a 16-mm fully curved intestinal needle through all the layers of the rectal wall. The gauze pack is then removed. A stitch should be placed through the proximal end of the specimen to facilitate orientation by the pathologist. If a specimen of sufficient size is taken, following the technique outlined above, it should not be difficult to make a definite histological diagnosis by noting the absence of ganglion cells and hypertrophy of the nerve fibres in a case of Hirschsprung's disease. There have been no major complications following rectal biopsies in neonates in this series.

Full thickness rectal biopsy has the disadvantages of requiring general anaesthesia and making subsequent definitive pull-through operation more difficult. The realization that if ganglion cells are found in the superficial submucous plexus they will also be present in the myenteric plexus at the same level has led to an increasing use of superficial rectal biopsies for diagnosis. The advent of acetylcholinesterase histochemical examination means that instead of looking for the negative feature of 'absence of ganglion cells' in the submucosa by multiple serial sections, the diagnosis of Hirschsprung's disease can be made on the positive finding of increased acetylcholinesterase activity in the lamina propria and muscularis mucosae in relatively smaller specimens [3,5,26,33,97,98,121]. Specimens can be obtained either by punch biopsy using a Chevalier Jackson vocal cord biopsy forceps [133,178] or by rectal suction biopsy [127] which we prefer and have adopted as a standard procedure in recent years. No anaesthesia is required. The suction biopsy tube is passed into the infant's rectum with the cylindrical knife in the closed position. The side aperture of the biopsy capsule should face the posterior rectal wall and be positioned 1–2 cm above the pectinate line. The aperture is then opened and pressed firmly against the posterior rectal wall. Negative pressure is applied through a suction pump apparatus and maintained at 30–50 cmHg for 5 s; the suction pressure should be judiciously lowered when biopsy is attempted in small, premature infants.

The knife is closed rapidly and suction is discontinued. The biopsy specimen should be removed gently with a needle and immediately sent to the pathology laboratory in the fresh state. Complications of suction rectal biopsy are rare [139]; we only had occasional cases of transient haemorrhage but no perforations. It is desirable to have concurrent haematoxylin and eosin staining as well as acetylcholinesterase staining of the suction rectal specimen as the two examinations can be complememtary [32]. In the past 10 years, we have routinely stained our suction rectal biopsy specimens for acetylcholinesterase using Lake's modification [98] of the method of Karnovsky and Roots [90]. It is essential to have the fresh specimen snap-frozen without dehydration; this is achieved by mounting the sample in an inert medium, tissue-tak during freezing. Staining of cryostat sections can be completed in 2 h. In Hirschsprung's disease, there is proliferation of acetylcholinesterase-positive nerve fibres in the lamina propria and muscularis mucosae; if sufficient submucosa is included, thickened nerve trunks will be demonstrated (see section on Pathology).

In neuronal intestinal dysplasia, there are hyperplastic ganglia in addition to the feature of mild to moderate increase of acetylcholinesterase activity. In our experience acetylcholinesterase studies are extremely accurate when they are positive. However, occasionally false-negative acetylcholinesterase results are observed in newborns. In the past, we had several neonates who showed a normal acetylcholinesterase pattern in the rectal biopsies in the first few days of life but subsequently developed the typical Hirschsprung's disease pattern in repeat biopsies at 3–4 weeks of age. This has also been the experience of other workers [38]. Another possible error of acetylcholinesterase staining of rectal suction biopsy is the occasional false negative reports in patients with total colonic aganglionosis [97,176], for whom diagnosis may still require a full thickness biopsy. Interpretation of biopsy results demands an experienced pathologist and the use of a quantitative biochemical assay of acetylcholinesterase activity has been suggested as a simple procedure less subject to observer error [17,19], but its accuracy has been questioned [182]. Simultaneous estimation of butyrylcholinesterase activity is said to enhance diagnostic accuracy [31] but the smallness of suction rectal biopsy samples in neonates remains a technical problem for biochemical assays. High serum cholinesterase and erythrocyte acetylcholinesterase levels have also been demonstrated in patients with Hirschsprung's disease by some workers [152] but we have been unable to reproduce these results in our patients [4].

In recent years immunohistochemistry has been advocated as a new diagnostic aid (see section on Pathology). A high level of expertise is required for these investigations.

Differential diagnosis

Although Hirschsprung's disease presents as a result of intestinal obstruction in the newborn, the obstruction is not complete and therefore the differential diagnosis must include other incomplete obstructions due to intraluminal blockage of the bowel or functional disorders. Complete mechanical intestinal obstruction with air/fluid levels shown on straight X-rays of the abdomen in the erect position, such as in atresias of the small bowel, will not cause confusion, but the rather non-specific picture of clinical obstruction with erect straight X-rays showing distended loops of bowel without fluid levels presents a more difficult diagnostic problem.

Lower ileal and colonic atresia

Complete atresia of ileum or colon will present as a low intestinal obstruction but straight X-ray will show no gas in the pelvis. Incomplete obstruction by a septal or stenotic atresia of the lower ileum may present a more confusing picture; such cases tend to present after the first 6 or 7 days of life and are usually less urgent than a complete obstruction so that a barium enema may be carried out to confirm the diagnosis.

Meconium plug

Delay in the passage of meconium, with eventual passage of a meconium plug, may occur in Hirschsprung's disease [67,135] and lead to a wrong assumption of 'meconium plug syndrome': this syndrome can only validly be diagnosed after exclusion of several organic conditions (see Chapters 29 and 36). In the meconium plug syndrome the child will behave normally after passage of the plug; in Hirschsprung's disease the symptoms and signs of intestinal obstruction will recur, usually immediately, but possibly after a considerable interval. In our series 13 infants were recorded as passing meconium plugs; five of them were discharged with this diagnosis and two of these in the early part of the series died. The danger of the child being discharged with undiagnosed Hirschsprung's disease makes exclusion imperative in all cases of meconium plug syndrome, preferably by rectal biopsy.

Meconium ileus

Classically in meconium ileus due to fibrocystic disease the abdominal distension is present at birth, thus appearing earlier than in Hirschsprung's disease; plain X-rays may be diagnostic of meconium ileus. The differentiation between this condition and Hirschsprung's disease may, however, be difficult and even in the early days of life barium enema may not be diagnostic.

Malrotation

Intestinal malrotation may present a similar clinical and radiological picture of incomplete obstruction, identified by an abnormal position of caecum and ascending colon on barium enema.

Medical conditions and prematurity

Medical conditions including sepsis, hypothyroidism and hypoglycaemia may result in impaired intestinal motility. Plain films of the abdomen are likely to show gas throughout the bowel and extending well down into the pelvis; contrast enema, if done, may reveal colonic inertia and no transitional zone; diagnosis is achieved by appropriate medical tests. Increasing numbers of premature babies now survive and they often have some degree of colonic inertia; bowel motility usually improves with supportive treatment but on some occasions enterostomy is required to relieve persistent functional obstruction of distal gut; for differentiation of immature gut from Hirschsprung's disease rectal biopsy is required. Similarly in infants who have necrotizing enterocolitis without apparent predisposing causes such as perinatal stress, rectal biopsy is the only certain way to exclude Hirschsprung's enterocolitis.

Hirschsprung's-related disorders

Conditions including neuronal intestinal dysplasia, hypoganglionosis, hypogenesis, chronic intestinal pseudo-obstruction, etc., can present with clinical and radiological features identical to those in Hirschsprung's disease and histological/histochemical investigations are necessary for differentiation.

Diagnostic difficulties

The early diagnosis of Hirschsprung's disease remains difficult. The clinical diagnosis is of intestinal obstruction. Relief of the obstruction after rectal examination raises the suspicion of Hirschsprung's disease and so does relief by rectal or colonic irrigation; but particularly in the latter case, the relief may remove the possibility of radiological diagnosis. Exploratory laparotomy is notoriously unreliable in the neonatal period since there may be no macroscopic differentiation between ganglionic and aganglionic bowel. In particular, total colonic aganglionosis remains a diagnostic challenge because of atypical clinical, radiological and even histochemical features.

There were diagnostic difficulties in 34 (19.8%) of our cases. In 20 of them the wrong diagnosis was made: meconium plug 18, meconium ileus three, necrotizing enterocolitis three, malrotation one, jejunal atresia one, gastro-oesophageal reflux one, sepsis two (urinary infection one, umbilical sepsis one), vomiting and melaena with no diagnosis one. In the remaining 14 patients there was a delay in diagnosis as neonatal intestinal obstruction was relieved by washouts. The seriousness of wrong/delayed diagnosis is shown in the fact that ten of the 34 patients died: meconium ileus two, meconium plug two, gastro-oesophageal reflux one and delayed diagnosis five; of these ten deaths only one occurred after 1967. Errors and delay in diagnosis can only be avoided by increased clinical awareness and reliance upon rectal biopsy for diagnosis.

Although histological diagnosis is most easily made from rectal biopsy, the difficulty in recognizing the proximal limit of the aganglionic segment at laparotomy may still demand serial extramucosal biopsies along the colon, working proximally from the rectosigmoid, with examination of frozen sections. In the past, we had at least four cases of wrong siting of the level of enterostomy when frozen sections were not available and repeat operations were subsequently required.

Technique of extramucosal biopsy

The selected segment of colon is delivered into the wound (Figure 37.11), the biopsy site through one of the taenia coli is selected and, using a small scalpel, a strip of the wall of the colon of at least 5-mm width and 1.5-cm length is carefully dissected off the colonic mucosa (Figure 37.12). The muscular

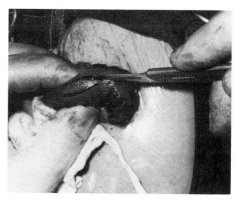

Figure 37.11 Extramucosal biopsy. The selected segment of colon is delivered through the laparotomy incision and a strip of colonic wall is outlined by incising through the serosa and muscularis

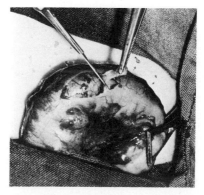

Figure 37.12 Extramucosal biopsy. The strip of serosa and muscularis is dissected off the colonic mucosa

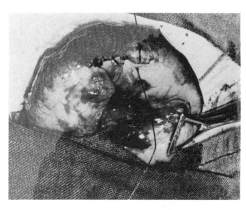

Figure 37.13 Extramucosal biopsy. Closure of the defects in the colonic muscularis and serosa

and serosal layers of the colon are then approximated using 4/0 interrupted silk sutures (Figure 37.13) of easily identifiable colour in order to facilitate recognition of the site of the biopsy at subsequent laparotomy.

Treatment

Hirschsprung's disease in the neonatal period is unpredictable in its course; in some cases the initial obstructive episode is relieved either spontaneously or by simple measures and does not recur for many weeks; in others daily washouts are necessary for a considerable period of time. But although in either of these situations conservative treatment seems reasonable [46,79,146], in both a further obstructive episode may occur without warning and the risk of enterocolitis is always present. Ehrenpreis [48] reports remarkably successful results with conservative management preceding a one-stage definitive procedure but these results have seldom been achieved outside Scandinavia [58,79,134,153].

Recurrent obstruction and necrotizing enterocolitis are potentially lethal hazards in the infant and newborn, especially if he/she is at home [11,48,105]. Rectal and colonic washouts are therefore to be regarded as short-term measures in the neonate. Bowring and Kern [20] favoured washouts to relieve the obstruction before colostomy but two of their patients, though successfully relieved of their obstruction, died of enterocolitis before colostomy; and Lividatis [110] from Sweden reported two cases of Hirschsprung's disease with enterocolitis treated by emergency colostomy after failure of conservative management.

Conservative treatment

Non-operative treatment consists of daily washouts with normal saline at 35°C. Water is not used on account of the danger of water intoxication.

A soft, well-greased rubber Jaques catheter (size 12F) should be passed per rectum and very gently manipulated up the colon, special care being taken when passing the rectosigmoid junction, which is the site where there is the greatest risk of perforation [79]. The washout is given from a funnel connected by tube to the catheter. The funnel should never be raised more than 60–70 cm above the baby. Under no circumstances should the fluid be injected under pressure as the danger of rupturing the gut is considerable. If rectal irrigation does not relieve the patient of sufficient flatus and faeces it has to be repeated. Frequent rectal washouts tend to make the infant's anus and perianal region sore and increase the risk of perforation.

Operative treatment
Pull-through procedure

Our early attempts at a primary pull-through procedure were discouraging; of four patients who had a Swenson type procedure [155] shortly after birth, two died. One collapsed 36 h after operation: permission for autopsy was refused. Another died of peritonitis resulting from an anastomosis leak. Yet another child who had a Swenson procedure during the neonatal period after a preliminary colostomy, died from faecal peritonitis resulting from a small bowel perforation. These deaths occurred more than 28 years ago and improved techniques and management would no doubt result in improved results [42,48]. Nevertheless, we are convinced that a colostomy for 6–12 months is a small price to pay for the reduced risk and simpler anatomical exposure of a delayed pull-through procedure.

Martin [116] recommends early pull-through procedure in total colonic aganglionosis if the child is in reasonable condition: like Duhamel, he brings ileum down behind the rectum but in addition, in stages, he divides the septum between ileum and aganglionic rectum and later extends this joint lumen as far as the splenic flexure, removing ascending and transverse colon. With this technique he had eight survivals out of nine cases, and follow-up from 8 months to 12 years showed satisfactory results in all but one who had recurrent diarrhoea.

Myectomy

Ultra-short segment cases suitable for rectal myectomy rarely present in the neonatal period [2]. Our single case remains constipated at 4 years.

Enterostomy

We have no doubt that colostomy is the method of choice in the treatment of neonatal Hirschsprung's disease and that this procedure should be carried out with the minimum of delay. Between 1953 and 1975 enterostomy was carried out in 109 of 120 patients, 92 in the neonatal period, four during the first admission, ten because diagnosis had been delayed and three after a failed period of conservative management. Of those who did not have a primary colostomy of ileostomy, four had a pull-through in the neonatal period with the poor results reported above, two were managed medically for 4 and 8 months respectively before a pull-through procedure and one had a myectomy in the neonatal period; three died before operation and one at laparotomy, and all these four deaths could be attributed to delay in operative treatment. Between 1976 and 1985 all 52 patients had primary enterostomy performed.

Table 37.2 Age on admission

	1953–64	1964–75	1976–85
0–24 h	2	1	4
25–48 h	14	15	25
49–96 h	24	19	12
5– 7 days	7	12	0
8–28 days	13	13	11
Total	60	60	52

Table 37.3 Age at first operation

	1953–64	1964–75	1976–85
0–7 days	10	19	29
8–28 days	32	34	24
Total	42	53	52

Tables 37.2 and 37.3 show the important changes in the age on admission and the age at first operation which contributed to the improvement of results of treatment in the last decade of our series: compared with infants during 1952–75 those during 1976–85 were admitted to hospital earlier and had their first operation at a much earlier stage. Enterostomy undoubtedly gives some protection against the ravages of enterocolitis – of 52 patients treated between 1976 and 1985 only one developed enterocolitis after enterostomy.

Pre-operative management

Once the diagnosis of Hirschsprung's disease is made, early enterostomy is indicated. Before operation, dehydration and electrolyte imbalance should first be corrected. Patients with enterocolitis can easily go into septicaemic shock and they must be treated vigorously; management should include blood and stool cultures, intensive monitoring, nasogastric decompression, intravenous fluid replacement and intravenous fluid therapy followed by prompt enterostomy. Operations should be carried out when a pathologist is available to report on frozen sections.

Operation

The level of the colostomy demands some thought; for the majority of cases, when the aganglionic bowel reaches as far proximally as mid sigmoid, a right-sided transverse colostomy provides safe decompression and leaves enough normal bowel distally to allow the pull-through procedure to be carried out without disturbing the colostomy, thus protecting the anastomosis at that stage. If, however, the aganglionic segment extends further proximally then there may not be enough bowel distally for a pull-through to be done without mobilizing the colostomy; this not only removes the existing safety valve, but is also likely to lead to the sacrificing of all the colon distal to the colostomy, since the marginal artery at the colostomy will have become thrombosed and the blood supply to that colon will be severely compromised once it has been mobilized sufficiently to perform a pull-through procedure. It is in such cases that we agree with Swenson [155] and recommend that the colostomy should be made at the most distal part of normally innervated bowel, thus allowing the colostomy to be brought down to the anus at the definitive procedure and making full use of the normal colon until that time.

It is desirable to have the proposed site of colostomy marked on the abdominal wall by the stomatherapist before operation. The colostomy can either be an end-colostomy or loop-colostomy depending on the surgeon's preference; both are satisfactory when properly performed. The end-colostomy will first be described; the description refers to a sigmoid colostomy but may be modified to adapt to any level of bowel. Under general anaesthesia, laparotomy is performed via a supra-umbilical transverse incision, this allows an adequate laparotomy and leaves the lower abdomen clear for approach for the definitive procedure. After the peritoneum is opened the sigmoid colon is identified and drawn out of the abdomen. The proposed level of colostomy should be chosen just above the transition zone and an extramucosal biopsy is taken and examined by frozen section for adequacy of ganglia. An opening is then made in the mesocolon; bowel clamps are applied and the colon transected. The distal end can be closed with continuous 3/0 silk/vicryl sutures and returned to the peritoneal cavity as in the Hartman's procedure thus eliminating the problem of prolapse of mucous fistula which is a common colostomy complication [109]. As the child's sigmoid colon can be redundant and twisted it is important to follow the course of the rectosigmoid into the pelvis to ensure that the correct bowel end is closed. The proximal bowel end is then brought out through a cruciate incision at the colostomy site marked before surgery. A 'nipple' type colostomy is created with interrupted 4/0 silk/vicryl sutures through the edge of the bowel, the seromuscular layer of the colon 1–2 cm proximal to the bowel end and the skin. In recent years, we have found the linear stapler instrument to be a useful adjunct in performing colostomy. Instead of using bowel clamps, the stapler is applied across the colon and 'fired' (Figures 37.14 and 37.15). The stapled distal end is returned to the peritoneal cavity; the stapled proximal end is brought out through a separate cruciate incision. The abdominal wound is closed and a dressing is applied to the main wound. The colostomy is then opened by trimming away the stapled bowel end; a 'nipple'-type colostomy is fashioned as usual. With the use of the stapler the operation is expedited, blood loss is minimized and faecal spillage is avoided.

The alternative to end-colostomy is loop colostomy (Figure 37.16–37.19). A W-shaped skin incision with its axis running obliquely downwards and inwards is made in the left iliac fossa mid-way between the umbilicus and anterior iliac spine. The limbs of the 'W' should be equal and about 2.5 cm long. Two small triangles of skin are completed by

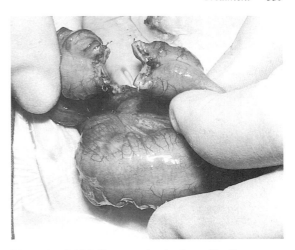

Figure 37.15 GIA linear stapler has been 'fired'

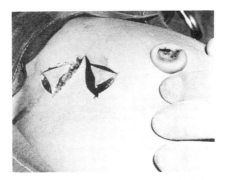

Figure 37.16 Colostomy. The central V-shaped skin flap is raised

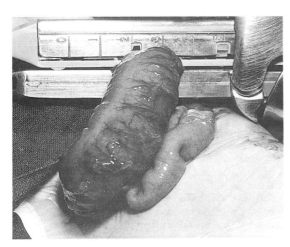

Figure 37.14 GIA linear stapler is applied across the circumference of colon

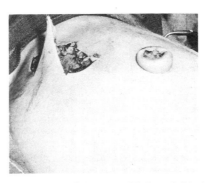

Figure 37.17 Colostomy. W-shaped skin incision in left iliac fossa. The two small triangles of skin are subsequently removed

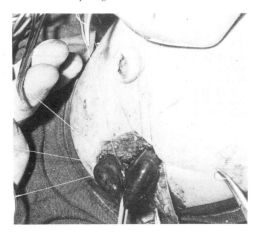

Figure 37.18 Colostomy. The selected loop of sigmoid colon is pulled out of the abdomen and an opening is made in the mesosigmoid. The peritoneum is now stitched to the circumference of the sigmoid loop.

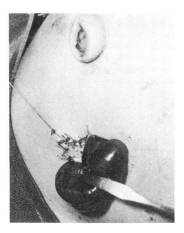

Figure 37.19 The V-shaped flap of skin has been drawn through the gap in the mesosigmoid and sewn to the opposite skin margin

joining the outer limbs of the 'W' with the apex of the central inverted 'V'. The two triangles of skin are excised and the central V-shaped flap is reflected. The external oblique aponeurosis is then split in the direction of its fibres and the underlying internal oblique and transversus abdominis muscles are cut with diathermy in the same direction as the external oblique. The peritoneum is opened and the loop of sigmoid colon is drawn out of the abdomen. An extramucosal biopsy is now taken (see above) and examined by frozen section. An opening is then made in the mesosigmoid and the parietal peritoneum is stitched to the circumference of the loop

using interrupted 4/0 silk sutures, care being taken not to perforate the bowel [35]. The abdominal muscles are then loosely approximated through the rent in a mesosigmoid using 4/0 chromic catgut. The V-shaped flap of the abdominal skin is pulled through the gap in the mesosigmoid and sutured with nylon sutures to the opposite skin margin, thus forming a skin bridge behind the sigmoid loop. At the end of the operation the colostomy is opened with the diathermy knife, and 4/0 silk/vicryl sutures are applied to approximate the colon to skin edges. This operation has now been used for many years without the problems which have previously been associated with colostomies in neonates [112,115].

Postoperative management

Nasogastric drainage and intravenous infusion are continued until postoperative ileus has disappeared. These children are often slow in establishing a normal colostomy action, the motions tending to be rather 'gritty'; many of the children are rather slow to feed. Careful attention is required to protect the abdominal skin and the use of a suitable barrier cream and colostomy bags is indicated. Most mothers soon learn how to manage the child and can look after him/her at home until the definitive procedure is carried out.

Results

Mortality in neonatal Hirschsprung's disease was high in early series with figures varying from 8 to 70% [45,48,57,81,92]. Recent reports give much lower mortality figures, varying from 0–7% [73,91,154]. Table 37.4 shows our mortality rates.

Table 37.4 Mortality (1953–85)

	1953–75	1976–85
Total number of patients	120	52
Related mortality	28 (23.3%)	2 (3.8%)
Unrelated mortality	9 (7.5%)	2 (3.8%)
Total mortality	37 (30.8%)	4 (7.7%)

Between 1953 and 1975 of our 120 patients 12 died in the neonatal period and 25 died after the neonatal period. Of 12 neonatal deaths, two occurred before colostomy, seven after colostomy and three after a definitive procedure. Of the two who died without operation one had septicaemia and one had enterocolitis. Of those who had a colostomy or ileostomy, one was misdiagnosed as fibrocystic disease and one died of congenital heart disease, three had severe enterocolitis at the time of operation, one had a perforation of the caecum before operation and one had postoperative peritonitis with no evidence of a source of leakage. The three who died following a definitive procedure have already been discussed; two had peritonitis and one probably had Gram-negative bacteraemic shock. Of 25 deaths after the neonatal period, two occurred before colostomy, 17 after colostomy (eight from unrelated causes) and six following a definitive procedure. Between 1976 and 1985, of 52 patients, two died in the neonatal period and two died after the neonatal period. Of two neonates, one died from septicaemia and enterocolitis because of delay in referral to our hospital and one died of congenital heart disease. Of two deaths after the neonatal period, one died of septicaemia and one died of aspiration pneumonia. There were no deaths in our series after 1979.

Morbidity in neonatal Hirschsprung's disease remains considerable. Between 1976 and 1985 of 52 patients, 12 (23.1%) had serious complications; four had a colostomy made in aganglionic bowel because of lack of frozen sections at operation, three had wound dehiscence requiring re-suturing, two had bowel perforation from enemas (saline one, barium one), one had postoperative peritonitis, one had bowel adhesions requiring laparotomy and one had colostomy necrosis requiring revision of colostomy. There were also nine other minor complications: five had wound infection, two had colostomy prolapse, one had colostomy narrowing and one had bleeding from suction rectal biopsy which stopped spontaneously.

These figures emphasize that there should be no complacency in the management of neonatal Hirschsprung's disease; vigilance should be exercised to ensure that an early diagnosis is made and early primary enterostomy in the ganglionic segment is performed.

References

1. Aldridge, R.T. and Campbell, P.E. (1968) Ganglion cell distribution in the normal rectum and anal canal. *J. Pediat. Surg.*, **3**, 475–490
2. Alexander, J.L. and Aston, S.J. (1974) A technique for posterior myectomy and internal sphincterotomy in short segment Hirschsprung's disease. *J. Pediat. Surg.*, **9**, 169–170
3. Andrassy, R.J., Isaacs, H. and Weitzman, J.J. (1981) Rectal suction biopsy for the diagnosis of Hirschsprung's disease. *Ann. Surg.*, **193**, 419–424
4. Bamforth, F.J., Kim, I., Isherwood, D.M. and Lister, J. (1985) Erythrocyte acetylcholinesterase in Hirschsprung's disease. *J. Clin. Pathol.*, **38**, 237–238
5. Barr, L.C., Booth, J., Filipe, H.I. and Lawson, J.O.N. (1985) Clinical evaluation of the histochemical diagnosis of Hirschsprung's disease. *Gut*, **26**, 393–399
6. Baumgarten, H.G., Holsten, A.F. and Stelzner, F. (1973) Nervous elements in the human colon of Hirschsprung's disease. *Virchows Arch. Alt. A Path. Anat.*, **358**, 113–136
7. Bennett, A., Garrett, J.R. and Howard, E.R. (1968) Adrenergic myenteric nerves in Hirschsprung's disease. *Br. Med. J.*, **1**, 487–489
8. Bentley, J.F.R. (1964) Some new observations on Hirschsprung's disease in infancy and childhood. *Dis. Colon Rectum*, **7**, 462–470
9. Bentley, J.F.R. (1966) Posterior excisional ano-rectal myotomy in the management of chronic faecal accumulation. *Arch. Dis. Child.*, **41**, 144–177
10. Berry, C.L. and Fraser, G.C. (1968) The experimental production of colitis in the rabbit with particular reference to Hirschsprung's disease. *J. Pediat. Surg.*, **3**, 36–42
11. Bill, A.H. Jr, and Chapman, N.D. (1962) The enterocolitis of Hirschsprung's disease. *Am. J. Surg.*, **103**, 70–74
12. Bishop, A.E., Polak, J.M., Zake, B.D., Bryant, H.G. and Bloom, S.R. (1981) Abnormalities of the colonic regulatory peptides in Hirschsprung's disease. *Histopathology*, **5**, 679–688
13. Bodian, M. and Carter, C.O. (1963) A family study of Hirschsprung's disease. *Ann. Hum. Genet.*, **26**, 261–277
14. Bodian, M., Carter, C.O. and Ward, B.C. (1951) Hirschsprung's disease. *Lancet*, **i**, 302–309
15. Bodian, M., Stephens, F.D. and Ward, B.C.H. (1949) Hirschsprung's disease. *Lancet*, **i**, 6–11
16. Bolande, R.P. (1974) The neurocristopathies. A unifying concept of disease arising in neural crest maldevelopment. *Hum. Pathol.*, **5**, 409–429
17. Bonham, J.R., Dale, G., Scott, D.J. and Wagget, J. (1987) A 7-year study of the diagnostic value of rectal mucosal acetylcholinesterase measurement in Hirschsprung's disease. *J. Pediat. Surg.*, **22**, 150–152
18. Boston, V.E. and Scott, J.E.S. (1976) Anorectal manometry as a diagnostic method in the neonatal period. *J. Pediat. Surg.*, **11**, 9–16
19. Boston, V.E., Dale, G. and Riley, K.W.A. (1975) Diagnosis of Hirschsprung's disease by quantitative biochemical assay of acetylcholinesterase in rectal tissue. *Lancet*, **ii**, 951–953
20. Bowring, A.C. and Kern, I.B. (1972) The management of Hirschsprung's disease in the neonate. *Aust. Paediat. J.*, **8**, 121–127
21. Brandt, C.T. (1983) Maturation of human enteric plexuses. PhD thesis, University of Liverpool
22. Bugaighis, A.G. and Lister, J. (1970) Incidence of diabetes in families of patients with Hirschsprung's disease. *J. Pediat. Surg.*, **5**, 620–621
23. Burnard, E.D. (1950) Hirschsprung's disease in infancy. *Br. Med. J.*, **1**, 151–156
24. Burnstock, G. (1971) Neuronal nomenclature. *Nature (Lond.)*, **229**, 282–283
25. Cameron, J.A.M. (1928) On the aetiology of Hirschsprung's disease. *Arch. Dis. Child.*, **3**, 210–211
26. Campbell, P.E. and Noblett, H.R. (1969) Experience

with rectal suction biopsy in the diagnosis of Hirschsprung's disease. *J. Pediat. Surg.*, **4**, 410–415

27. Caniano, D.A., Ormsbee, III, H.S., Polito, W., Sun, C.C., Barone, F.C. and Hill, L.J. (1985) Total intestinal aganglionosis. *J. Pediat. Surg.*, **20**, 456–460

28. Cannon, W.B. (1939) A law of denervation. *Am. J. Med. Sci.*, **198**, 737–750

29. Carter, C.O., Evans, K. and Hickman, V. (1981) Children of those treated surgically for Hirschsprung's disease. *J. Med. Genet.*, **18**, 87–90

30. Cass, D.T. and Myers, N. (1987) Total colonic aganglionosis. 30 years' experience. *Pediat. Surg. Int.*, **2**, 68–75

31. Causse, E., Vaysse, P., Tabre, J., Valdiguie, P. and Thouvenot, J. (1987) The diagnostic value of acetylcholinesterase/butyrylcholinesterase ratio in Hirschsprung's disease. *Am. J. Clin. Path.*, **88**, 477–480

32. Challa, V.R., Moran, R., Turner, C.S. and Lyerly, A.D. (1987) Histologic diagnosis of Hirschsprung's disease. *Am. J. Clin. Path.*, **88**, 324–328

33. Chow, C.W., Chan, W.C. and Yue, P.C.K. (1977) Histochemical criteria for the diagnosis of Hirschsprung's disease. *J. Pediat. Surg.*, **12**, 675–679

34. Clague, J.R., Sternini, C. and Brechan, N.C. (1985) Localization of calcitonic gene-related peptide-like immunoreactivity in neurons of the rat gastrointestinal tract. *Neurosci. Lett.*, **56**, 63–68

35. Cain, W.S. and Kiesewetter, W.B. (1965) Infant colostomy. *Arch. Surg.*, **91**, 314–320

36. Cremin, B.J. (1971) The delayed film in Hirschsprung's disease. *S. Afr. med. J.*, **45**, 67–69

37. Dalla Valla, A. (1924) Contributo alla conoscenza della forma famigliare del megacolon congenito. *Pediatria*, **32**, 569–599

38. De Brito, I.A. and Maksoud, (1987) Evolution with age of the acetylcholinesterase activity in rectal suction biopsy in Hirschsprung's disease. *J. Pediat. Surg.*, **22**, 425–430

39. Di Lorenzo, M., Yazbeck, S. and Brochu, P. (1985) Aganglionosis of the entire bowel: four new cases and review of the literature. *Br. J. Surg.*, **72**, 657–658

40. Dockray, G.J., Vaillant, C. and Walsh, J.A. (1979) The neuronal origin of bombesin-like immunoreactivity in the rat gastrointestinal tract. *Neuroscience*, **4**, 1562–1568

41. Dorman, G.W. (1957) Hirschsprung's disease. *Arch. Surg.*, **75**, 906–913

42. Duhamel, B. (1956) Une nouvelle operation pour le megacolon congénital. *Presse Méd.*, **64**, 2249–2250

43. Duhamel, B. (1963) Technique et indications de l'abaissement retrorectal et transanal en chirurgie colique. *Gaz. med. Fr.*, **70**, 599–608

44. Earlam, R. (1985) A vascular cause for Hirschsprung's disease? *Gastroenterol.*, **88**, 1274–1279

45. Eek, S. and Knutrud, O. (1962) Megacolon congenitum Hirschsprung. *J. Oslo Cy. Hosps.*, **12**, 245–270

46. Ehrenpreis, Th. (1946) Megacolon in the newborn. *Acta chir. scand.*, **94**, Suppl. 112

47. Ehrenpreis, Th. (1966) Some newer aspects on Hirschsprung's disease and allied disorders. *J. Pediat. Surg.*, **1**, 329–337

48. Ehrenpreis, Th. (1970) *Hirschsprung's Disease*. Year Book Medical Publishers, Chicago

49. Ehrenpreis, T. and Pernow, B. (1952) On the occurrence of substance P in the rectosigmoid in Hirschsprung's disease. *Acta Physiol. Scand.*, **27**, 380–387

50. Emanuel, B., Padorr, M.P. and Swenson, O. (1965) Familial absence of myenteric plexus (congenital megacolon). *J. Pediat.*, **67**, 381–386

51. Evans, W.A. and Willis, R. (1957) Hirschsprung's disease. *Am. J. Roent.*, **78**, 1024–1048

52. Ferreira-Santos, R. (1961) Megacolon and megarectum in Chagas' disease. *Proc. R. Soc. Med.*, **54**, 1047–1053

53. Ferri, G.L., Ali Rachedi, A., Tatemoto, K., Bloom, S.R. and Polak, J.M. (1984) Immunocytochemical localisation of neuropeptide Y-like immunoreactivity in extrinsic nonadrenergic and intrinsic gut neurons. *Front. Horm. Res.*, **12**, 81–84

54. Fisher, J.H., De Luca, F.G. and Swenson, O. (1965) Rectal biopsy in Hirschsprung's disease. *Z. Kinderchir.*, **2**, 67

55. Fock, G. and Kostia, J. (1963) Familial occurrence of Hirschsprung's disease. *Clin. Pediat.*, **2**, 371–373

56. Forshall, I., Rickham, P.P. and Mossman, D.B. (1951) Functional intestinal obstruction in the newborn. *Arch. Dis. Child.*, **26**, 294–299

57. Fraser, G.C. and Berry, C.L. (1967) Mortality in neonatal Hirschsprung's disease. *J. Pediat. Surg.*, **2**, 205–211

58. Fraser, G.C. and Wilkinson, A.W. (1967) Neonatal Hirschsprung's disease. *Br. Med. J.*, **3**, 7–10

59. Fujimoto, T. (1988) Natural history and pathophysiology of enterocolitis in the piebald lethal mouse model of Hirschsprung's disease. *J. Pediat. Surg.*, **23**, 237–242

60. Furness, J.B. and Costa, M. (1988) *The Enteric Nervous System*, 1st Edition, Churchill Livingstone, Edinburgh

61. Gannon, B.J., Noblett, H.R. and Burnstock, G. (1969) Adrenergic innervation of bowel in Hirschsprung's disease. *Br. Med. J.*, **3**, 338–340

62. Garrett, J.R., Howard, G.R. and Nixon, H.H. (1969) Autonomic nerves in rectum and colon in Hirschsprung's disease. *Arch. Dis. Child.*, **44**, 400–417

63. Garver, K.L., Law, J.C. and Gasrver, B. (1985) Hirschsprung's disease: a genetic study. *Clin. Genet.*, **28**, 503–508

64. Gershon, M.D., Dreyfus, C.F., Pickel, V.M. *et al.* (1977) Serotonergic neurons in the peripheral nervous system. *Proc. Natl Acad. Sci. USA*, **74**, 3086–3089

65. Gershon, M.D., Epstein, M.C. and Hegstrand, L. (1980) Colonization of the chick gut by progenitors of enteric serotonergic neurons. *Devel. Biol.*, **77**, 41–51

66. Gheradi, G.J. (1960) Pathology of the ganglionic-aganglionic junction in congenital megacolon. *A.M.A. Arch. Path.*, **69**,. 52/520–55/523

67. Gillis, D.A. and Grantmyre, E.B. (1965) The meconium plug syndrome and Hirschsprung's disease. *Can. Med. Ass. J.*, **92**, 225–227

68. Graivier, L. and Sieber, W.K. (1966) Hirschsprung's disease and mongolism. *Surgery*, **60**, 458–461

69. Guilleman, R. (1976) Somatostatin inhibits the release of acetylcholine induced electrically in the myenteric plexus. *Endocrinology*, **99**, 1653–1654

70. Hall, C.L. and Lampert, P.W. (1985) Immunohistochemistry as an aid in the diagnosis of Hirschsprung's disease. *Am. J. Clin. Pathol.*, **83**, 177–181

71. Hamada, Y., Bishop, A.E., Federici, G., Rivosecchi, M., Talbot, I.C. and Polak, J.M. (1987) Increased neuropeptide Y-immunoreactive innervation of aganglionic bowel in Hirschsprung's disease. *Virchows Arch. A.*, **411**, 369–377

72. Hanani, M., Lernan, O.Z., Zamir, O. and Nissan, S. (1986) Nerve mediated responses to drugs and electrical stimulation in aganglionic muscle segments in Hirschsprung's disease. *J. Pediat. Surg.*, **21**, 848–851

73. Harrison, M.W., Denby, D.M., Campbell, J.R. and Campbell, F.J. (1986) Diagnosis and management of Hirschsprung's disease. *Am. J. Surg.*, **152**, 49–56

74. Hawkins, H.P. (1907) Idiopathic dilatation of the colon. *Br. Med. J.*, **1**, 477

75. Hermann, R.E., Izant, R.J. and Bolade, R.D. (1963) Aganglionosis of the intestine in siblings. *Surgery*, **53**, 664–669

76. Hershlag, A., Arcel, I. and Lern, (1984) Cytomegalic inclusion virus and Hirschsprung's disease. *Z. Kinderchir.*, **39**, 253–254

77. Hiatt, R.B. (1951) The pathological physiology of congenital megacolon. *Ann. Surg.*, **133**, 313–320

78. Hirschsprung, H. (1888) Stuhltagheit Neugeborener in Folge von Dilatation und Hypertrophie des Colons. *Jb. Kinderheilk.*, **27**, 1–7

79. Hofman, S. and Rehbein, F. (1966) Hirschsprungsche Krankheit im Neugeborenenalter. *Z. Kinderchir.*, **3**, 182

80. Holschneider, A.M. (ed.) (1982) *Hirschsprung's Disease*, Hippokrates Verlag, Stuttgart: Thieme-Stratton Inc., New York

81. Holschneider, A.M., Kellner, E., Streibl, P. and Sippell, W.G. (1976) The development of anorectal continence and its significance in the diagnosis of Hirschsprung's disease. *J. Pediat. Surg.*, **11**, 151–156

82. Hope, J.W., Borns, P.F. and Berg, P.K. (1965) Roentgenologic manifestations of Hirschsprung's disease in infancy. *Am. J. Roent.*, **95**, 217–229

83. Howard, E.R. and Garrett, J.R. (1970) Electron microscopy of myenteric nerves in Hirschsprung's disease and in normal bowel. *Gut*, **11**, 1007–1014

84. Howard, E.R. and Garrett, J.R. (1983) Pathology of autonomic nerve – smooth muscle mechanisms in the gut of man. In *Somatic and Autonomic Nerve – Muscle Interactions* (ed. G. Burnstock), Elsevier Science Publishers, Amsterdam

85. Howard, E.R. and Nixon, H.H. (1968) Internal anal sphincter. Observations on development and mechanism of inhibitory responses in premature infants and children with Hirschsprung's disease. *Arch. Dis. Child.*, **43**, 569–578

86. Ikawa, H., Yokayama, J., Morikawa, Y. *et al.* (1980) A quantitative study of acetylcholine in Hirschsprung's disease. *J. Pediat. Surg.*, **15**, 48–52

87. Ikeda, K. G.T.S. (1986) Additional anomalies in Hirschsprung's disease. *Z. Kinderchir.*, **41**, 279–281

88. Joyle, F. (1909) La dilatation congénital idiopathique due colon. *Presse Med.*, **17**, 803

89. Kamijo, K., Hiatt, R.B. and Koelle, G.B. (1953) Congenital megacolon. *Gastroenterology*, **24**, 173–185

90. Karnovsky, M.J. and Roots, L. (1964) A 'direct coloring' chiocholine method for cholinesterases. *J. Histochem. Cyt. Chem.*, **12**, 219–221

91. Klein, M.D., Coron, A.G., Wesley, J.R. and Drongowski, R.A. (1984) Hirschsprung's disease in the newborn. *J. Pediat. Surg.*, **19**, 370–374

92. Klein, R.R. and Scarborough, R.A. (1954) Hirschsprung's disease in the newborn. *Am. J. Surg.*, **88**, 6–16

93. Kleinschmidt, H. (1926) Aetiologie des megacolon. *Arch. Dis. Chir.*, **142**, 91

94. Kluck, P., Van Muijen, G.N.P., Van der Kaap, A.W.M., Tibboel, D., Hoorn, W.A., Warnaar, S.O. and Molenaar, J.C. (1984) Hirschsprung's disease studied with monoclonal antineurofilament antibodies on tissue sections. *Lancet*, **i**, 652–653

95. Koberle, F. (1958) Megacolon. *J. Trop. Med.*, **61**, 21–24

96. Kumagota, S. and Donahoe, P.K. (1985) The effect of fibronection on cholinergic differentiation of the fetal colon. *J. Pediat. Surg.*, **20**, 307–314

97. Kurer, M.J.H., Lawson, J.O.A. and Pambakian, . (1986) Suction biopsy in Hirschsprung's disease. *Arch. Dis. Child.*, **61**, 83–84

98. Lake, B.D., Puri, P., Nixon, H.H. and Claireax, A.E. (1976) Hirschsprung's disease: an appraisal of histochemically demonstrated acetylcholinesterase activity in rectal suction biopsy specimens as an aid to diagnosis. *Arch. Pathol. Lab. Med.*, **102**, 244–247

99. Larsson, L.T. and Rehfeld, (1979) Localization and molecular heterogeneity of cholecystokinin in the central and peripheral nervous system. *Brain Res.*, **165**, 201–218

100. Larsson, L.T., Malmfors, G. and Sundler, F. (1983) Peptidergic innervation in Hirschsprung's disease. *Z. Kinderchir.*, **38**, 301–304

101. Larsson, L.T., Malmfors, G. and Sundler, F. (1988) Neuropeptide Y, calcitonin gene-related peptide and gelanin in Hirschsprung's disease. *J. Pediat. Surg.*, **23**, 342–345

102. Lawson, J.O.N. and Nixon, H.H. (1967) Anal canal pressure in the diagnosis of Hirschsprung's disease. *J. Pediat. Surg.*, **2**, 544–552

103. Le Dourin, N. (1980) Migration and differentiation of neural crest cells. *Curr. Top. Devel. Biol.*, **16**, 31–85

104. Le Quesne, G.W. and Reilly, B.J. (1975) Functional immaturity of the large bowel in the newborn infants. *Radiol. Clin. N. Am.*, **13**, 331–341

105. Leenders, E., Sieber, W.K., Girdany, B.R. and Kiesewetter, W.B. (1970) Aganglionic megacolon in infancy. *Surg. Gynec. Obstet.*, **131**, 424–430

106. Linnoile, R.I., Diangustina, R.P. *et al.* (1978) An immunohistochemical and radioimmunological study of the distribution of Met[5] and Len[5] encephalin in the gastrointestinal tract. *Neuroscience*, **3**, 1187–1196

107. Lipson, A.A. and Harvey, J. (1987) Three generation transmission of Hirschsprung's disease. *Clin. Genet.*, **32**, 175–178

108. Lister, J. (1966) Abnormal arteries in Hirschsprung's disease. *Arch. Dis. Child.*, **41**, 149

109. Lister, J., Webster, P.J. and Mirza, S. (1983) Colostomy complications in children. *Practitioner*, **227**, 229–237

110. Livaditis, A. (1976) Emergency colostomy in enterocolitis of Hirschsprung's disease. *Z. Kinderchir.*, **19**, 145

111. Loening-Baucke, V., Pringle, K.C. and Ekiro, G.G. (1985) Anorectal manometry for the exclusion of Hirschsprung's disease in neonates. *J. Pediatr. Gastroenterol. Nutr.*, **4**, 596–603

112. Louw, J.H. (1966) Colostomy in infants. *S. Afr. J. Surg.*, **4**, 39–41

113. McElhannon, F.M. (1959) Experimental production of megacolon resembling Hirschsprung's disease. *Surg. Forum*, **10**, 218–221

114. McKusick, V.A. (1973) Congenital deafness and Hirschsprung's disease. *New Engl. J. Med.*, **228**, 691

115. MacMahon, R.A., Cole, S.J. and Eckstein, H.B. (1963) Colostomy in infancy and childhood. *Arch. Dis. Child.*, **38**, 114–117

116. Martin, L.W. (1972) Surgical management of total colonic aganglionosis. *Ann. Surg.*, **176**, 343–346

117. Martin, L. and Perrin, E.V. (1967) Neonatal perforation of the appendix in association with Hirschsprung's disease. *Ann. Surg.*, **166**, 799–802

118. Meier-Ruge, W. (1971) Uber ein Erkrankungebild des Colons mit Hirschsprung Symptomatik. *Verk. Dtsch. Ges. Pathol.*, **55**, 506–510

119. Meier-Ruge, W. (1974) Hirschsprung's disease: its aetiology, pathogenesis and differential diagnosis. *Curr. Yop. Pathol.*, **59**, 131–179

120. Meier-Ruge, W. (1985) Ultrashort Hirschsprung's disease: a bioptically safely substantiated disease. *Z. Kinderchir.*, **40**, 146–150

121. Meier-Ruge, W., Lutterbeck, P.M., Herzog, B., Morger, R., Moser, R. and Scharli, A. (1972) Acetylcholinesterase activity in suction biopsies of the rectum in the diagnosis of Hirschsprung's disease. *J. Pediat. Surg.*, **7**, 11–17

122. Merkler, R.G., Solish, S.B. and Scherzer, A.L. (1985) Myelomeningocele and Hirschsprung's disease. *Pediatrics*, **76**, 299–300

123. Munakata, K., Okaba, I. and Monta, K. (1978) Histologic studies of rectocolic aganglionosis and allied disease. *J. Pediat. Surg.*, **13**, 67–75

124. Newman, B., Russbaum, A. and Kirkpatrick, Jr, J.A. (1987) Bowel perforation in Hirschsprung's disease. *Am. J. Roent.*, **148**, 1195–1197

125. Nirasawa, Y., Yokoyama, J., Ikawa, H., Monikawa, Y. and Katsunala, K. (1986) Hirschsprung's disease, catecholamine content, adrenoceptors and the effect of electrical stimulation in aganglionic colon. *J. Pediat. Surg.*, **21**, 136–142

126. Nixon, H.H. and Lake, B. (1982) Not Hirschsprung's disease – rare conditions with some similarities. *S. Afr. J. Surg.*, **20**, 97–103

127. Noblett, H.R. (1969) Rectal suction biopsy tube for use in the diagnosis of Hirschsprung's disease. *J. Pediat. Surg.*, **4**, 406–409

128. Okamoto, E. and Ueda, T. (1967) Embryogenesis of intramural ganglia of the gut and its relation to Hirschsprung's disease. *J. Pediat. Surg.*, **2**, 437–443

129. Okamoto, E., Iwasaki, T., Kakutani, T. and Ueda, T. (1967) Selective destruction of the myenteric plexus: its relation to Hirschsprung's disease, achalasia of the esophagus and hypertrophic pyloric stenosis. *J. Pediat. Surg.*, **2**, 444–454

130. Okesora, T. and Okamoto, E. (1982) Electrophysiological and pharmacological study on innervation of the aganglionic colon. *Z. Kinderchir.*, **41**, 93–96

131. Passarge, E. (1967) The genetics of Hirschsprung's disease. Evidence for heterogenous etiology and a study of sixty-three families. *New Engl. J. Med.*, **276**, 138–143

132. Payette, R.F., Tennyson, V.M., Phasu, T.D., Hawe, G.M., Pomerang, H.D., Rothman, T.P. and Gershon, M.D. (1987) Origin and morphology of nerve fibres in the aganglionic colon of the lethal spotted (ls/ls) mutant mouse. *J. Comp. Neurol.*, **257**, 237–252

133. Pease, P.W.B., Corkery, J.J. and Cameron, A.H. (1976) Diagnosis of Hirschsprung's disease by punch biopsy of the rectum. *Arch. Dis. Child.*, **51**, 541–543

134. Pellerin, D. (1966) La maladie de Hirschsprung chez l'enfant de moins de 2 mois. *Ann. Chir. Infant.*, **7**, 329

135. Pilling, G.P. and Cresson, S.L. (1962) Hirschsprung's disease. In *Pediatric Surgery* (ed. W.T. Mustard, M.M. Ravitch, W.H. Snyder, K.J. Welch and C.D. Benson), Year Book Medical Publishers, Chicago pp. 802–820

136. Pistor, G., Von Kapher, S.H., Grussner, R., Munakata, K. and Muntefering, H. (1987) Neuronal intestinal dysplasia. *Pediat. Surg. Int.*, **2**, 352–358

137. Porter, R. and O'Connor, M. (eds) (1982) *Substance P in the Nervous System*, Biba Foundation Symp. 91, Pitman, London

138. Puri, P. and Fujimoto, (1988) Diagnosis of allied functional bowel disorders using monoclonal antibodies and electronmicroscopy. *J. Pediat. Surg.*, **23**, 546–554

139. Rees, B.I., Azmy, A., Nigan, M. and Lake, B.D. (1983) Complications of rectal suction biopsy. *J. Pediat. Surg.*, **18**, 273–275

140. Robertson, H.E. and Kernohan, J.W. (1938) The myenteric plexus in congenital megacolon. *Proc. Staff Meet. Mayo Clin.*, **13**, 123–125

141. Rogawski, M.A., Goodrich, J.T., Gershon, M.D. and Touloukian, R.J. (1978) Hirschsprung's disease: absence of serotonergic neurons in the aganglionic colon. *J. Pediat. Surg.*, **13**, 608–615

142. Rosenfield, N.S., Ablow, R.C., Markowitz, R.I., Dipietro, M., Seashore, J.H., Touloukian, R.J. and Cicchetti, D.V. (1984) Hirschsprung's disease – accuracy of the barium enema examination. *Radiology*, **150**, 393–400

143. Roviralta, E. (1962) Nouvelle orientations chirurgicales dans le traitment de megacôlon congénital. *Ann. Chir. Infant.*, **3**, 155–158

144. Rudin, C., Jenny, P., Ohnacker, H. and Heitz, P.V.Z. (1986) Absence of the enteric nervous system in the newborn: presentation of three patients and review of the literature. *J. Pediat. Surg.*, **21**, 313–318

145. Said, S.I. (ed.) (1982) *Vasoactive Intestinal Polypeptide*, Raven Press, New York

146. Santulli, T.V. (1957) Intestinal obstruction in newborn. *Bull. N.Y. Acad. Med.*, **33**, 175–194

147. Scallen, C., Puri, P. and Reen, D.J. (1985) Identification of rectal ganglion cells using monoclonal antibodies. *J. Pediat. Surg.*, **20**, 37–40

148. Scharli, A.F. and Meier-Ruge, W. (1981) Localized and disseminated forms of neuronal intestinal dysplasia mimicking Hirschsprung's disease. *J. Pediat. Surg.*, **16**, 164–170

149. Schnaufer, L., Talbert, J.L., Haller, J.A., Reid, N.C.R.W., Toban, F. and Schuster, M.M. (1967) Differential sphincteric studies in the diagnosis of ano-rectal disorders of childhood. *J. Pediat. Surg.*, **2**, 538–543

150. Schuster, M.M., Hookman, P., Hendrix, T.R. and Mendeloff, A.I. (1965) Simultaneous manometric recording of internal and external anal sphincter reflexes. *Bull. Johns Hopkins Hosp.*, **116**, 79–88

151. Seldenrijk, C.A., Harten, H.J., Kluck, P., Tibboel, D., Moorman-Voestermans, K. and Meijer, C.J.L.M. (1986) Zonal aganglionosis. *Virchows Arch. A (Pathol. Anat.)*, **410**, 75–81

152. She, Y., Shi, C., Chen, J. and Wu, Y. (1984) Observation on erythrocyte acetylocholinesterase in infants and children with Hirschsprung's disease. *J. Pediat. Surg.*, **19**, 281–284

153. Shim, W.K.T. and Swenson, O. (1966) Treatment of congenital megacolon in 50 infants. *Pediatrics*, **38**, 185–193

154. Sieber, W.K. (1986) Hirschsprung's disease. In *Pediatric Surgery*, 4th Edition (ed. K.J. Welch, J.G. Randolph, M.M. Ravitch, J.A. O'Neill and M.I. Rowe) Year Book Medical Publishers Inc., Chicago, London, pp. 995–1020

155. Swenson, O. (1958) *Pediatric Surgery*, Appleton Century Crofts, New York

156. Swenson, O. and Bill, A.H. (1948) Resection of rectum and rectosigmoid with preservation of the sphincter for benign spastic lesions producing megacolon. *Surgery*, **24**, 212–220

157. Swenson, O., Rheinhard, H.F. and Diamond, I. (1949) Hirschsprung's disease. *New Engl. J. Med.*, **241**, 551–556

158. Taguchi, T., Tanaka, K. and Ikeda, K. (1985) Fibromuscular dysplasia of arteries in Hirschsprung's disease. *Gastroenterology*, **88**, 1099–1103

159. Taguchi, T., Tanaka, K. and Ikeda, K. (1985) Immunohistochemical study of neuron-specific-enolase and S-100 protein in Hirschsprung's disease. *Virchows Arch. (Pathol. Anat.)*, **405**, 399–409

160. Tam, P.K.H. (1984) Aspects of peptidergic innervation of human gut: normal distribution of substance P in the developing fetus and child and changes in infantile hypertrophic pyloric stenosis and Hirschsprung's disease. ChM Thesis, University of Liverpool

161. Tam, P.K.H. (1986) An immunohistochemical study with neuron-specific-enolase and substance P of human enteric innervation – the normal developmental pattern and abnormal deviations in Hirschsprung's disease and pyloric stenosis. *J. Pediat. Surg.*, **21**, 227–232

162. Tam, P.K.H. and Lister, J. (1986) Development profile of neuron-specific enolase in human gut and its implications in Hirschsprung's disease. *Gastroenterology*, **90**, 1901–1906

163. Tam, P.K.H. and Lister, J. (1986) Neuron-specific-enolase and Hirschsprung's disease. *Am. J. Surg. Pathol.*, **10**, 149–150

164. Tamate, S., Shiokawa, C., Yaneda, C., Takeuchi, S. and Nakahima, M. (1984) Manometric diagnosis of Hirschsprung's disease in the neonatal period. *J. Pediat. Surg.*, **19**, 285–286

165. Tatemoti, K., Rokaeus, A., Jornvell, H. *et al.* (1983) Galanin – a novel biologically active peptide from porcine intestine. *FEBS Lett.*, **164**, 124–128

166. Taxman, T.L., Yulish, B.S. and Rothstein, F.C. (1986) How useful is the barium enema in the diagnosis of infantile Hirschsprung's disease. *Am. J. Dis. Child.*, **140**, 881–884

167. Tennyson, V.M., Pham, T.D., Rothman, T.P. and Gershon, M.D. (1986) Abnormalities of smooth muscle, basal laminae, and nerves in the aganglionic segments of the bowel of lethal spotted mutant mice. *Anat. Res.*, **216**, 267–281

168. Thomas, D.F.M., Fernie, D.S., Bayston, R., Spitz, L. and Nixon, H.H. (1986) Enterocolitis in Hirschsprung's disease – a controlled study of the etiologic role of Clostridium difficle. *J. Pediat. Surg.*, **21**, 22–25

169. Tiffin, M.E., Chandler, L.R. and Farber, H.K. (1940) Localized absence of the ganglion cells of the myenteric plexus in congenital megacolon. *Am. J. Dis. Child.*, **59**, 1071–1082

170. Tittel, K. (1901) Uber eine angeborene Missbildung des Dickdarms. *Wien. Klin. Wschr.*, **14**, 903–907

171. Touloukian, R.J., Aghajanian, G. and Robert, H.R.

(1973) Adrenergic hyperactivity of the aganglionic colon. *J. Pediat. Surg.*, **8**, 191–195

172. Tsuto, T., Obato-Tsuto, H., Kawakami, F., Tukui, F., Iwai, N., Majima, S. and Ibata, Y. (1984) New application of catecholamine fluorescence histochemistry. *Z. Kinderchir.*, **39**, 250–252

173. Tsuto, T., Okamura, H., Fukui, K. *et al.* (1985) Immunohistochemical investigation of gut hormones in the colon of patients with Hirschsprung's disease. *J. Pediat. Surg.*, **20**, 266–270

174. Ueki, S., Okamoto, E., Kuwata, K., Toyosaka, A. and Nagai, K. (1985) Quantitative and quantitative analysis of muscarinic acetylcholine receptors in the piebald lethal mouse model of Hirschsprung's disease. *Gastroenterology*, **88**, 1834–1841

175. Van Campenhout, G. (1932) Further experiments on the origin of the enteric nervous system in the chick. *Physiol. Zool.*, **5**, 333–353

176. Van der Stoak, F.H.J. (1981) Reliability of the acetylcholinesterase reaction in rectal mucosal biopsies for the diagnosis of Hirschsprung's. *Z. Kinderchir.*, **54**, 36–43

177. Vanhoutte, J.J. (1969) Primary aganglionosis associated with imperforate anus. *J. Pediat. Surg.*, **4**, 463–472

178. Venugopal, S., Mancer, K. and Shandling, B. (1981) The validity of rectal biopsy in relation to morphology and distribution of ganglion cells. *J. Pediat. Surg.*, **16**, 433–437

179. Varmesh, M., Mayden, K.L., Confuco, E., Gigha, R.V. and Gleicher, N. (1986) Prenatal sonographic diagnosis of Hirschsprung's disease. *J. Ultrasound Med.*, **5**, 37–39

180. Walker, A.W., Kempson, R.L. and Ternberg, J.L.

(1966) Aganglionosis of the small intestine. *Surgery*, **60**, 449–457

181. Webster, W. (1973) Embryogenesis of the enteric ganglion in normal mice and mice that develop congenital megacolon. *J. Embryol. Exp. Morphol.*, **30**, 573–585

182. Wells, F.E. and Addison, G.M. (1986) Acetylcholinesterase activity in rectal biopsies. *J. Pediat. Gastroenterol. Nutr.*, **5**, 912–919

183. Weinberg, A.G. (1975) Hirschsprung's disease – a pathologist's view. *Perspect. Pediat. Pathol.*, **2**, 207–239

184. Whitehouse, F.R. and Kernohan, J.W. (1948) Myenteric plexus in congenital megacolon. *Archs intern. Med.*, **82**, 75–111

185. Wilson-Storey, D., Scobie, W.G. and Raeburn, J.A. (1988) Defective white blood cell function in Hirschsprung's disease – a possible predisposing factor to enterocolitis. *J.R. Coll. Surg. Edin.*, **33**, 185–188

186. Yanagihara, J., Tsuto, T., Iwai, N. and Takahashi, T. (1986) Anorectal electromyography in the diagnosis of Hirschsprung's disease. *Z. Kinderchir.*, **41**, 227–229

187. Yntema, C.L. and Hammond, W.S. (1954) The origin of intrinsic ganglia of trunk viscera from vagal neural crest in the chick embryo. *J. Comp. Neurol.*, **101**, 515

188. Yunis, E. and Sieber, W.K. (1983) Does zonal aganglionosis really exist. *Pediat. Pathol.*, **1**, 33–49

189. Zuelzer, W.W. and Wilson, J.C. (1948) Functional intestinal obstruction in a congenital neurogenic lesion in infancy. *Am. J. Dis. Child.*, **75**, 40–64

38

Anorectal malformations

R. C. M. Cook

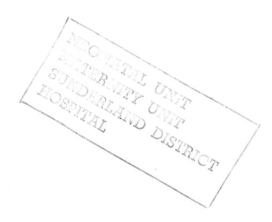

Introduction

'A properly functioning rectum is an unappreciated gift of the greatest price.' (Potts [92])

No one can start writing about congenital anorectal malformations without being both overawed by the great names of the past writers on this subject and also daunted by the complexity of the problems – a complexity reflected in continuing disagreement about the pathological anatomy and nomenclature of different forms, and about techniques of surgical correction.

In 1959, Potts wrote that 'atresia of the rectum is more poorly handled than any other congenital anomaly of the newborn' [92]. Thirty years later, it still cannot be claimed that the problem is universally well managed despite enormous advances in understanding and technique. We do well to heed Potts' warning [92] that 'the child who is so unfortunate as to be born with an imperforate anus may be saved from a lifetime of misery and social exclusion by the surgeon who, with skill and diligence and judgement, performs the first operation on the malformed rectum'.

Whilst an attempt has been made to include in this chapter all matter that is of immediate relevance to the management of a newborn child with one of the commonly described anorectal malformations, it must be recognized that other organ systems are involved, and that these may require specific and prior treatment.

Hindgut duplications [21,125] usually terminate in some form of 'imperforate anus' and may be part of a complex multisystem anomaly [26,136]. They will not be discussed further in this chapter. Similarly, exstrophy of the cloaca (vesico-intestinal fissure) is omitted here since it is dealt with in Chapter 51.

Historical notes

The chequered history of surgeons' attempts to deal with an infant born with an anorectal malformation is reviewed in fascinating detail by Webster [138]. The condition was undoubtedly recognized from earlier times but no record has been found of surgical intervention until the seventh century Byzantine physician Paul of Aegina opened the bowel by plunging a bistoury through the perineum and then dilating with bougies [65]. Such blind puncture followed by dilatations remained the method of treatment for the next 1000 years until, in 1787, Benjamin Bell carried out a dissection via the perineum to locate the rectal ampulla [12].

Amussat [2], recognizing that the severe complications of past methods resulted from 'the want of a protection which a mucous surface would afford the new passage', having found and opened the rectum, sutured it to the skin margins. Roux had already (1833) stressed the importance of keeping the perineal dissection strictly in the midline [65]. Splitting, dislocating or excising the coccyx were variously recommended as means of getting better exposure, and some surgeons deliberately opened the pelvic peritoneum to gain greater length of bowel. Neil McLeod in 1880 suggested [60] a combined abdominal and perineal exploration, and it was rapidly taken up and modified until in 1948, Rhoads et al. successfully tried one-stage abdominoperineal procedures in vigorous neonates [99].

A number of different operative techniques reflect attempts to make use of our greater understanding of the anatomical basis of continence. The first major breakthrough was Stephen's sacroperineal (or sacro-abdominoperineal) approach, first described in 1953 [113]. Rehbein [98] and Kiesewetter [52,53] independently advocated submucosal resection to avoid damaging pararectal nerves and muscles. Mollard's anterior dissection [55,69,70] to define the puborectalis muscle has proved another significant advance in the reconstruction of the anorectum, and deVries' and Pena's posterior sagittal approach [90,134] is currently very popular as it provides wide exposure by division of the entire pelvic floor, which must then be meticulously

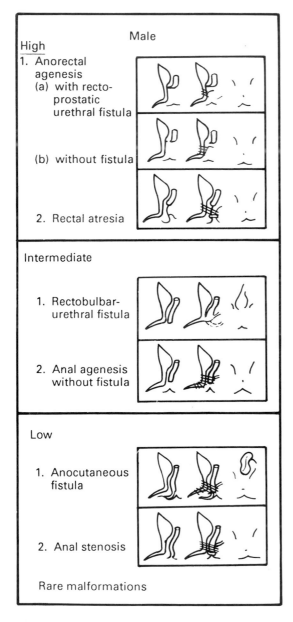

Figure 38.1 Wingspread classification of male anorectal anomalies showing visceral, sphincteric and perineal features [115] (Reproduced with permission of authors and publisher)

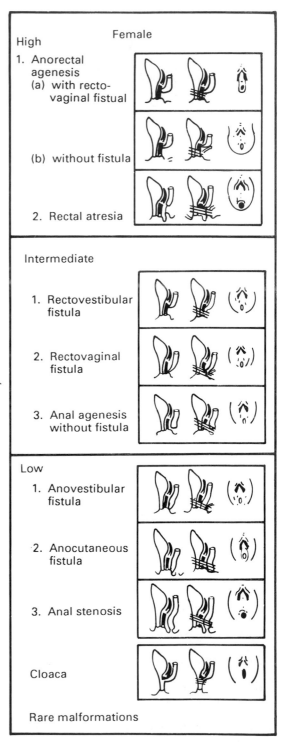

Figure 38.2 Wingspread classification of female anorectal anomalies showing visceral, sphincteric and perineal features [115] (Reproduced with permission of authors and publisher)

repaired around the pulled-down bowel. Such modifications of surgical technique have arisen from an increasing understanding of the normal neuromuscular mechanisms of continence and of the anatomy and embryology of the hindgut. Amussat (1835) [2], Bodenhammer (1860) [12] and Ball (1887) [6] all classified the main types of anomaly they found. Wood Jones (1904) [142] and Keith (1908) [50] devised embryological classifications. The Ladd and Gross classification (1934) [56] held sway for many years and various adaptations and modifications were proposed as knowledge of anatomy and embryology increased.

One of the great landmarks in the history of the surgery of these malformations will, no doubt, prove to be the Melbourne classification agreed at an international gathering at the Royal Children's Hospital, Melbourne, in 1970 [114]. In this classification, three main groups were distinguished from one another – high, intermediate and low. These were then subdivided to take into account the anatomical configurations (and in particular any fistula) and the sex of the infant. Nearly 40 named varieties appeared in this Melbourne classification, and its complexity made it difficult to use with sufficient accuracy to allow comparisons to be made between different surgical centres. Another international workshop developed the Wingspread classification in 1984 [115]. It omits many of the rarer anomalies, but adheres to the concept (now generally agreed to be of great importance) of distinguishing high, intermediate and low lesions in the two sexes (Figures 38.1 and 38.2). This classification was again put forward as a basis for study and discussion rather than as a final definitive answer. One of its merits is its close linkage to methods of later assessment of continence.

Pathological anatomy

The relationship of the termination of the bowel to the pelvic floor and to the sphincter muscle complex is the central factor not only in allotting a place in the classification, but more importantly in determining the management of each case. It also has a considerable bearing on the results of treatment. Where bowel terminates on the cranial side of the levator muscles, lesions are referred to as 'high'; those infants in whom the bowel extends through most of the muscle have 'low' lesions; whilst in a third 'intermediate' group, even though the fistula is embraced by these muscles, the bowel proper terminates above them.

The normal anatomy of the muscles of the pelvic floor and of those around the anorectum is complex, and recent history has seen a degree of polarization between the views of those who maintain that the all-important musculature is the puborectalis sling [114], and those who consider that the external sphincter muscles are intimately associated with the most medial part of the levator ani to form a 'striated muscle complex' but not a sling [90,134]. The truth undoubtedly lies in a fusion of these two concepts, which are not mutually exclusive [28]. It must be remembered that the relative proportions of muscle present in infants born with anorectal anomalies is very variable and much of our understanding of the anorectal musculature has been derived from dissections of pathological specimens or at surgery on infants with anomalies.

Posteriorly the midline of the pelvic floor (the postanal plate) is formed by the tendinous insertion of the pubococcygeus muscle, the raphe of iliococcygeus and the fibres of puborectalis that originate from the lateral part of the pubic bone and find insertion in the midline to the coccyx. The superficial external sphincter also sends fibres posteriorly to find support in the coccyx, while the deep external sphincter is in close relation with the most medial fibres of the puborectalis muscle which form a sling passing round the bowel at the recto-anal angle. The external sphincter muscle extends from the skin to the levator muscle in layers, some of which are circular and others elliptical with attachments to the perineal body and the coccyx. As stated above, the superficial external sphincter normally extends posteriorly to the coccyx and its subcutaneous portion has a similar and often well-marked coccygeal attachment (Figures 38.3 and 38.4).

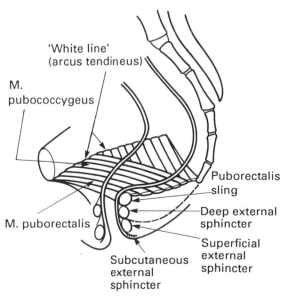

Figure 38.3 Diagrammatic representation of pelvirectal muscles

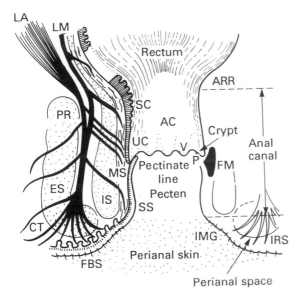

Figure 38.4 Composite diagram of the anal canal. AC, anal columns; ARR, anorectal ring; CT, 'coat-tails' of the conjoined longitudinal coat; ES, external sphincter; FBS, follicle-bearing skin; FM, zone of relatively fixed mucosa; IMG, intermuscular groove; IRS, ischiorectal space; IS, internal sphincter; LA, iliococcygeus portion of levator ani; LM, longitudinal smooth muscle of bowel wall; MS, musculus submucosae ani; P, anal papilla; PR, puborectalis; SC, specialized columnar epithelium with goblet cells and intestinal glands; SS, smooth stratified squamous epithelium of pecten; UC, unspecialized stratified columnar epithelium lacking goblet cells or intestinal glands; V, anal valve [28] (Reproduced with permission of the author and editor of the *Journal of Pediatric Surgery*)

The mass of muscle consisting of the external sphincter and the most medial part of the puborectalis, Pena and DeVries named the 'striated muscle complex' [134]. The close anatomical and functional relationship has been described [4,57,84,106] in modern anatomical and surgical texts, and the German anatomist Holl [43] emphasized this fact in 1881 when he claimed that the deep part of the striated external sphincter was intimately linked with the anterior group of muscles of the pelvic floor, which should properly be regarded as visceral rather than somatic muscles. Evidence for this comes now from three sources.

First, comparative anatomy [139] suggests that the puborectalis muscle is phylogenetically part of the sphincter complex – a part of that complex that in man has become tethered to the pubic bone. Second, histochemical studies [7] of the size and type of fibres show marked differences between the puborectalis portion of the levator ani and other parts of it, and a similarity between the puborectalis

and the external sphincter muscle. Third, the innervation of the puborectalis muscle is, like the external sphincter, usually accepted as being from below via the pudendal nerves, while the rest of the pelvic diaphragm is supplied from the sacral plexus by nerves entering the pelvic surface of the muscle. This source of innervation, however, has been questioned in recent electromyographic studies using microelectrodes to detect activity in various parts of the pelvic floor muscles when the sacral nerves are stimulated [111]. Despite this slight uncertainty there would seem to be plenty of evidence that the external sphincter muscle and the puborectalis muscle, part of which forms a sling, function in very close liaison.

Durham Smith [28] criticizes the term 'striated muscle complex' and would prefer the term 'sphincter muscle complex' as clearly the unstriated muscle of the anorectum is an important part of the mechanism of continence. The internal sphincter consists of a thickening of the circular muscle layer of the rectum. Even in high anorectal malformations there may be a condensation of circular muscle fibres found at the termination of the bowel just proximal to any fistula and this may show normal sphincteric responses [31,53,106]. Patients who have had corrective surgery for a high imperforate anus with preservation of this terminal portion of the rectum are said to have better long-term results than those in whom it has been discarded [121]. The ending of the longitudinal smooth muscle layer of the rectum has received little attention in recent years though Durham Smith [28] has stressed its significance and Milligan and Morgan's classic description [67] of the external sphincter muscle also includes a description of the bands of tissue that fan out from the outer smooth muscle coat of the rectum and interdigitate through the external sphincter muscle and even into the internal sphincter muscle to support it, and presumably to some extent pull it upwards into the pelvic floor.

Before moving to a brief description of the pathological anatomy in the more common forms of malformation it must be emphasized again that the classification of types of anomaly depends on the relationship of the termination of the bowel, and of any fistula that may be present, to the pelvic floor and to the sphincter muscle complex, and the ultimate prognosis depends on accurate identification and correct neonatal management of the child.

High malformations in the male infant

The commonest high deformity in the male in all reported series is *anorectal agenesis with a rectoprostatic urethral fistula*. There were 20 cases of this type identified in the Liverpool series between 1975 and 1985 out of a total of 98 boys (Table 38.1). The fistula is usually small and enters the posterior

Table 38.1 Incidence of types of anomaly in male infants according to the Wingspread classification, Liverpool 1975–85.

High	Males
(1) Anorectal agenesis	
(a) with rectoprostatic urethral fistula	20
(b) without fistula	8
(2) Rectal atresia	3
Intermediate	
(1) Rectobulbar urethral fistula	10
(2) Anal agenesis without fistula	2
Low	
(1) Anocutaneous fistula	36
(2) Anal stenosis	9
'Rare'	
(1) Anorectal agenesis with rectovesical fistula	8
(2) Shared colon in conjoined twins	2
Total	98

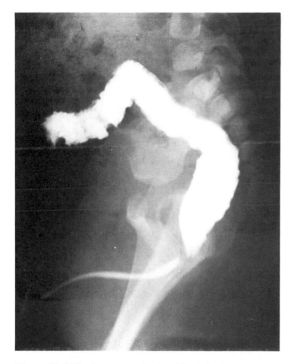

Figure 38.5 Urethrogram obtained by injecting contrast medium into the distal loop of a colostomy in an infant with a recto-urethral fistula

urethra, most commonly at the verumontanum, between the ejaculatory ducts (Figure 38.5). The levator muscle is usually well formed and normally innervated [109], unless there is an associated agenesis of three or more sacral vertebrae. In Stephen's and Smith's [114] original descriptions, which largely led on to the Melbourne classification,

the puborectalis muscle is described as a sling which is normally wrapped around the rectoanal junction, but in this malformation will be around the posterior urethra just caudal to the recto-urethral fistula. De Vries and Friedland [133] doubt the reality of the sling, but the puborectalis and external sphincter muscles are still described as forming their 'striated muscle complex' that is normally attached to and is intimately related to the recto-anal junction and the anal canal, and in this deformity lies below the bowel and posterior to the urethra.

There have been eight male infants with *anorectal agenesis without a fistula* in our current series, and the pathological anatomy is very similar to that found in the infant who has a recto-urethral fistula. The bowel is often connected to the wall of the urethra by a condensation of fibrous tissue.

Rectal atresia is a rare condition and is probably acquired later in development [61] than those deformities described as ageneses. The anus and anal canal are correctly sited and connected to the blind ending rectum by a cord of tissue which passes through the sphincter muscle complex.

Apart from the infant with rectal atresia, the appearance of the perineum in the newborn boy with a high malformation is variable and unrelated to the precise form of the anomaly except when the absence of a natal cleft together with flat buttocks points to the presence of sacral agenesis. No meconium will be visible, of course, in any anal dimple or prominent raphe that may be present (Figure 38.6), but may occasionally be seen issuing from the urethra (Figure 38.7).

Anorectal agenesis with a rectovesical fistula was omitted from the main named categories in the Wingspread classification as it was considered to be a relatively rare anomaly, but we have had eight infants with this serious malformation in the last 11

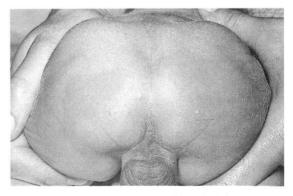

Figure 38.6 Perineal appearance of a male infant with anorectal agenesis. There is some pigmentation in thin skin immediately posterior to the scrotum

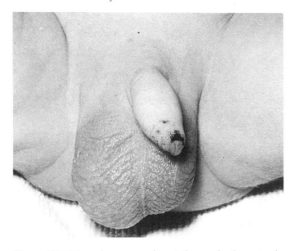

Figure 38.7 Meconium appearing at the urethral meatus in a male infant with a recto-urethral fistula

surrounded on its posterior aspect by a significant portion of the muscle complex. An abnormal perineum is common, with an absent or weak raphe, hypospadias or cleft scrotum. All these features provide evidence of abnormal development of the inner genital folds.

Low malformations in the male infant

In most low deformities, meconium is visible at the normal anal site or further forward in the perineum. Hypertrophied perineal tissues may cover the anus completely and an extravagant midline raphe may produce a 'congenital median band' (Figure 38.9) between a thinly covered pit on either side through which meconium is often visible or through which it leaks after disruption of the membrane.

By far the commonest lesion is the *anocutaneous fistula*. The anus is covered by an excessive posterior fusion of the genital folds and a fistula runs forward

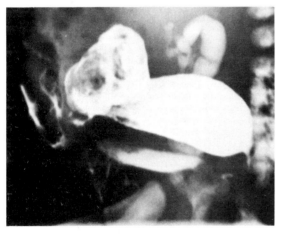

Figure 38.8 Cologram of an infant who had anorectal agenesis with a rectovesical fistula. Contrast medium has entered the bladder and also demonstrates the refluxing mega-ureter of a pelvic ectopic kidney

years (Table 38.1). There is a very high incidence of associated major anomalies of the urinary tract (Figure 38.8), vertebral column and cardiovascular system. These frequently prove lethal within a few days of birth [62,63].

Intermediate malformations in the male infant

These are rather more complex in that, although the bowel ends within the levator and 'striated muscle complex', any fistula is also embraced by this. The fistula, or any cord representing the remains of a fistula, descends to the bulbar urethra which may be

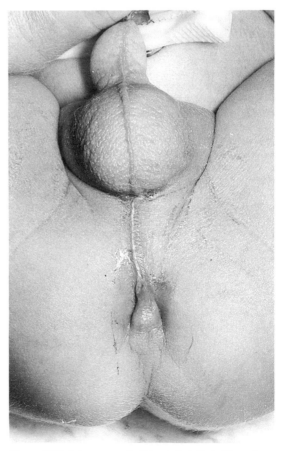

Figure 38.9 A low anomaly in a male infant. There is a prominent median band, and meconium has leaked from the thinly covered pits beside the band

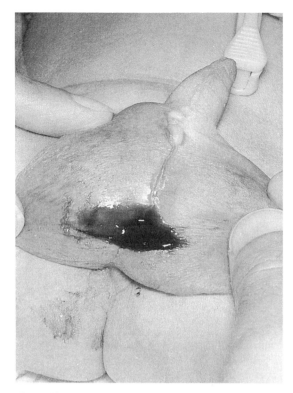

Figure 38.10 A male infant with a low lesion. An anocutaneous fistula tracks round the median raphe to discharge on the scrotum

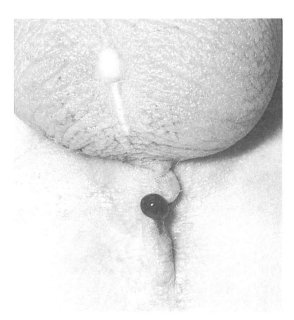

Figure 38.11 A male infant with an anocutaneous fistula running through a median band. Isolated portions of the fistula more anteriorly contain epithelial 'pearls'

subcutaneously [80] to open anywhere along the midline of the perineum, scrotum or penis (Figure 38.10 and 38.11).

High malformations in the female infant (Table 38.2)

These are less common than in boys and anorectal agenesis without a fistula is rare. Most of the high deformities have a fistulous opening into the upper vagina or a cloaca, and the bowel may decompress itself satisfactorily through this for some time after birth.

Table 38.2 Incidence of types of anomaly in female infants according to the Wingspread classification, Liverpool 1975–85.

High	*Females*
(1) Anorectal agenesis	
(a) with rectovaginal fistula	8
(b) without fistula	2
(2) Rectal atresia	0
Intermediate	
(1) Rectovestibular fistula	4
(2) Rectovaginal fistula	3
(3) Anal agenesis without fistula	0
Low	
(1) Anovestibular fistula	15
(2) Anocutaneous fistula	9
(3) Anal stenosis	5
Cloacal anomalies	7
Total	53

The *cloacal anomalies* are complex and represent a major embryological fault. There is only one external orifice (Figure 38.12) as the bladder drains into the cloaca also, through a urethra which may be so short as to be considered to be absent. Urinary incontinence or obstruction may result. As in the male, the puborectalis sling and muscle complex lie below the fistula, immediately posterior to the cloacal canal. The Wingspread classification puts all the cloacal malformations in a separate category and a descriptive classification of these was offered at Wingspread by Raffensperger [115] (Figure 38.13).

Anorectal agenesis with a high rectovaginal fistula should theoretically be distinguished from the *intermediate anal agenesis* with a *rectovaginal fistula* entering the *lower vagina*. In the neonate, the latter type of fistula may be visible on simple inspection, but since both lesions should be treated similarly in the neonatal period, early differentiation is not vital. type of fistula may be visible on simple inspection [10], but since both lesions should be treated similarly in the neonatal period, early differentiation is not vital.

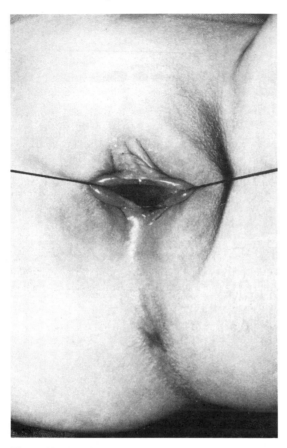

Figure 38.12 A single perineal orifice in a female infant with a cloacal anomaly

Figure 38.13 Raffensperger's descriptive classification of female cloacal anomalies. 1, 'Long' cloacal canal with junction of urethra, vagina and rectum at the apex a, without and b, with hydrocolpos; c, septate vagina; d, separate vaginas and rectovesical fistula; 2, cloaca with anorectal agenesis and urogenital sinus; 3, cloaca with vaginal atresia and recto-urinary sinus; 4, rectum joining vagina; vagina and urethra then form cloacal canal; 5, short cloaca; 6, cloaca with phallic urethra; 7, cloaca with double hydrocolpos and rectum joining one vagina; 8, cloaca with double vagina, one vagina with and one without obstruction; 9, cloaca with ultrashort cloacal segment [115] (Reproduced with permission of authors and publisher)

Intermediate malformations in the female infant

Apart from *anal agenesis with a low vaginal fistula* discussed above, intermediate deformities in the female are rare and include *anal agenesis without a fistula* (which we have not seen in recent years), and *anal agenesis with a rectovestibular fistula* (Figure 38.14). Anatomically they are similar to the equivalent lesions in the male infant. The rectovestibular fistula is relatively long and lies immediately posterior to the vagina for the whole of its course (Figure 38.15). It must be distinguished from the short subcutaneous anovestibular fistula (Figure 38.17).

Low deformities in the female infant

The low deformities are relatively more frequent in the female than high ones, with more varieties of

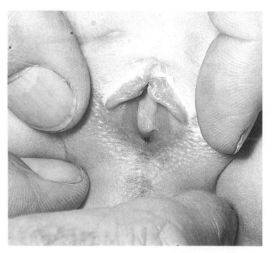

Figure 38.14 An infant with a rectovestibular fistula. The urethra and vagina could be separately identified

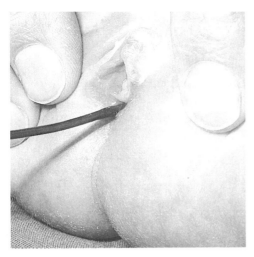

Figure 38.15 The same infant as in Figure 38.14, with a probe showing the direction of the fistula – parallel to the vagina (compare Figure 38.17)

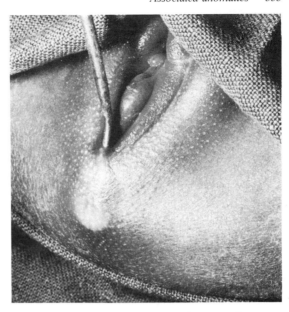

Figure 38.17 An infant with a probe demonstrating an anovestibular fistula – contrast Figures 38.14 and 38.15

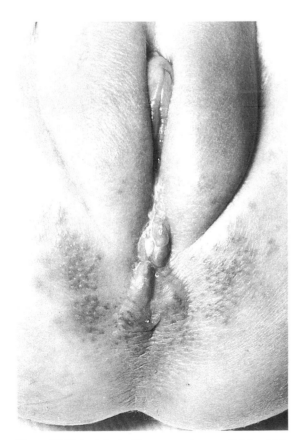

Figure 38.16 An infant with an anocutaneous fistula which had been adequate to pass meconium for a few days

site for the fistulous opening than in the male (Figures 38.16 and 38.17). The anatomy, however, is similar in most respects to the equivalent lesion in the male. The *anovestibular fistula* lies close to the vaginal orifice and a probe passed into it will run subcutaneously in contrast to the direction of a rectovestibular fistula (Figures 38.15 and 38.17).

Associated anomalies

It has long been recognized [9] that the infant born with an anorectal anomaly has a high risk of having other malformations. An appreciation of particular associations enables appropriate investigations to be carried out, and may well throw light on the embryogenesis of the malformations. It is logical to distinguish those conditions that are distinct even though frequently associated (such as oesophageal atresia or renal agenesis) from those that are an integral part of the primary malformation (such as recto-urinary fistula) and also from those that are a consequence or complication of it (such as urinary tract infection).

Genitourinary malformations form the major group of associated anomalies because of the closely integrated embryology of the systems. Other systems, however, need to be considered also (Table 38.6). Stephens and Smith [114] found that 60.6% (149 of 246 infants) had one or more associated anomalies and, collecting 3223 cases from other authors, computed an incidence of 43.4%. Of 151 infants recently admitted to Alder Hey Children's Hospital with 'imperforate anus' 99 (65.6%) were found to have other malformations.

A higher incidence is to be found in supralevator (high) lesions than in infralevator (low) lesions [82,87,89,140]. The associated anomalies in the high group are not only more common but also more severe. Significant lesions were found in 76.6% of infants with high and intermediate rectal anomalies in Liverpool and in 54.1% of low ones (Table 38.3). There were 12 deaths (15.6%) in the high and intermediate group and only four (5.4%) in the low. In both groups, this mortality was most frequently attributable to major anomalies of other systems (Table 38.4).

In the Liverpool series the incidence of associated anomalies was similar in the two sexes in both high and low lesions (Table 38.5). This contrasts with other reports [114] in which boys with high lesions have a higher incidence of associated anomalies than girls. Associated anomalies have been reported as being rare in female infants with low anal malformations also, but other series where large numbers have been studied show a significant number of female infants with other anomalies, as we have found in ours.

Urological anomalies and complications are common in children born with anorectal malformations (Tables 38.6 and 38.7). The incidence reported depends on the intensity of investigation and is considerable in children of both sexes, and in those with low as well as high lesions. The urinary tract anomalies in children with low lesions are usually discovered to be less serious than in those with high lesions [42,82,86,87,89,140]. Renal hypoplasia and unilateral agenesis are both common and bilateral renal agenesis also occurs. Hydronephrosis and hydroureter are also frequently found, both of

Table 38.3 Number of infants with one or more other anomalies

Low	40 out of 74	(54.1%)
High and intermediate	59 out of 77	(76.6%)

Table 38.4 Established causes of death

	Number of infants	
	Low lesions	High and intermediate lesions
Cardiac		4
Pulmonary		2
Obstructed tracheostomy (subglottic stenosis)	1	
Infective		2
Multiple anomalies	2	
Fetal alcohol syndrome	1	

Table 38.5 Sex and the incidence of associated anomalies

	Males with one or more other anomalies	Females with one or more other anomalies
Low	25 out of 45 infants (55.6%)	15 out of 29 infants (51.7%)
Intermediate and high (and cloacal)	40 out of 53 infants (75.5%)	21 out of 24 infants (87.5%)
Total	65 out of 98 infants (66.3%)	36 out of 53 infants (67.9%)

Table 38.6 Incidence of association of anomalies of major systems

	High and intermediate	Low	Total number of infants	Percentage affected
Urinary tract	38	13	51	33.8%
Vertebrae	23	5	28	18.5%
Heart and great vessels	14	3	17	11.3%
Oesophageal atresia	6	3	9	6.0%
Meckel's diverticulum	9	–	9	6.0%
Radial aplasia/hypoplasia	7	–	7	4.6%
Neural tube defects	2	4	6	4.0%
Lip, palate and mandible	2	3	5	3.3%
Down's syndrome	4	0	4	2.6%
Duodenal atresia	3	0	3	2.0%
Malrotation	3	–	3	2.0%
Exomphalos	1	1	2	1.3%

Table 38.7 Urinary tract anomalies

Associated anomaly	Number of infants	
	High and intermediate	Low
Horseshoe kidney	4	1
Renal agenesis	15	3
Renal hypoplasia	1	1
Hydronephrosis and hydroureter	14	4
Crossed ectopia	2	1
Duplex kidney	0	2
Persistent UG sinus	0	1
Prune belly	2	0

obstructive and refluxing origin (Figures 38.8 and 38.18). Many of these anomalies have a common embryological basis – faulty budding of the ureter from the Wolffian duct [14].

The presence of a recto-urinary fistula adds the very considerable hazard of acquired urinary infection. A rectovesical fistula (see Figure 38.8) produces infection readily and is commonly associated with severe urinary tract anomalies [63]. The combination carries a high mortality. A recto-urethral fistula may also lead to infection which may be difficult to eradicate if there is a structural anomaly of the urinary tract itself leading to urinary stasis [114].

Sacral agenesis (Figure 38.19) should not be forgotten as a cause of neurogenic bladder disturbance [24,101,114,140].

The urinary tract anomalies require treatment in their own right and may take precedence over the anorectal surgery once intestinal obstruction has

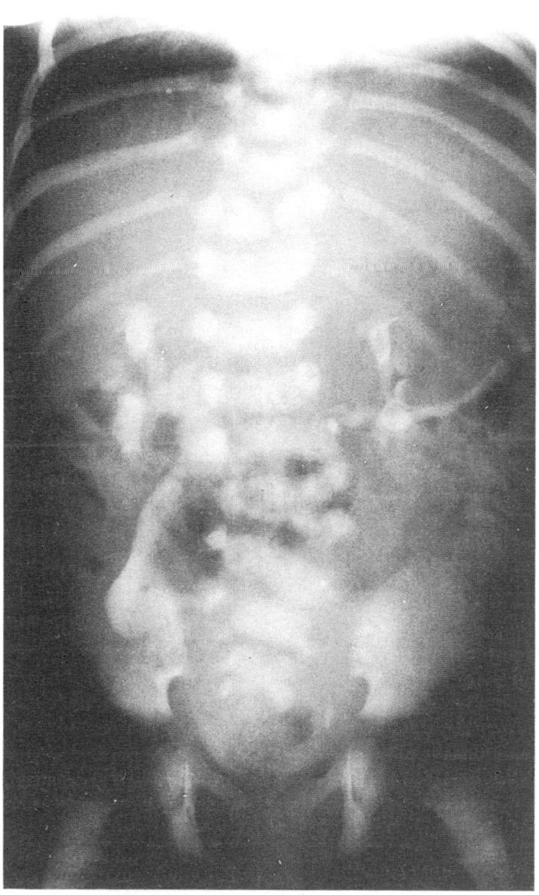

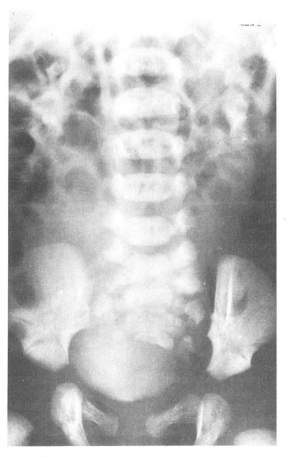

Figure 38.18 Pyelogram of a child who had anorectal agenesis with a rectoprostatic urethral fistula. There are thoracic and lumbar hemi-vertebrae and a right-sided refluxing mega-ureter

Figure 38.19 Radiograph of a boy with a low anomaly – an anocutaneous fistula. Note the deformities of the upper sacral vertebrae and agenesis of S.4 and 5

Table 38.8 Genital anomalies

Out of 98 boys	
Hypospadias	9
Undescended testis	12
Out of 53 girls	
Persistent urogenital sinus	2
Urethralization of phallus	1
Bicornuate uterus	6
Hydrometrocolpos	2

been relieved. The decompression of a loaded colon may allow spontaneous resolution of hydronephrosis [73]. The severity of the urinary tract anomalies may cause a very high mortality and may preclude useful treatment of the anorectal malformation.

Genital anomalies are common (Table 38.8). There were nine cases of hypospadias out of 98 boys in our series, but a reported compiled series [37] of 1272 revealed only 39 boys with hypospadias. Since the vas deferens and ureter both originate from the Wolffian duct at about the same level at first, separating later, it is not surprising to find persistence of the junction of the vas and ureter reported in association with anorectal anomalies [14].

Anomalous internal genitalia in female infants with high rectal lesions are common [29,85]. Absence of the vagina is said [34] to be rare but Hasse [37] found ten cases in 1272 infants. The external genitalia of female infants with low lesions are generally found to be normal apart from the possible fistulous opening, but one of our infants with an anterior ectopic anus had urethralization of the phallus [128]. The real incidence of internal anomalies is not known since laparotomy is rarely needed (Figure 38.29). The risk of complications at menarche is high with persistence of a urogenital sinus in association with an anorectal malformation [41,71,115].

Vertebral anomalies are now recognized [89] as commonly associated with anorectal malformations, but most reported figures of incidence are probably gross underestimates because few infants will have had full spinal radiography. Major anomalies causing kyphosis or other spinal deformity will usually be recognized clinically (Figure 38.20), and lumbosacral deformities will usually be apparent in the abdominal and pelvic radiographs taken to elucidate the pathology of the bowel or urinary tract (Figure 38.19). Hemivertebrae, absent and extra vertebrae, may occur at any level in association with both high and low anorectal malformations (Figure 38.21). Agenesis or hemi-agenesis of vertebrae is of special significance in relation to the ultimate attainment of faecal and urinary continence when the midsacral vertebrae (Figure 38.19) are affected

[18,24,101,114,140]. Fourteen infants are recorded in our series as having agenesis of some or all sacral vertebrae. Hemivertebrae and wedged vertebrae in the thoracolumbar region may lead to significant scoliosis. Eighteen of our infants were found to have vertebral anomalies above the sacral zone [36]. Where thoracic vertebrae are abnormal, deformities of the ribs will also be found.

Skeletal anomalies (other than vertebral ones) are also often reported. Pellerin and Bertin [89] noted malformations of the lower limbs, and Obenbergerova *et al.* [83] reported a 2% incidence of radial aplasia in infants with anorectal malformations. Radial aplasia (Figure 38.22) has been found more commonly in a previously reported Liverpool series as also have major abnormalities of the lower limbs (hypoplastic leg, absent tibia or fibula, ilial hypoplasia, arthrogryphosis) [36].

Anomalies of the heart and great vessels were found in 11.3% of the infants in the current

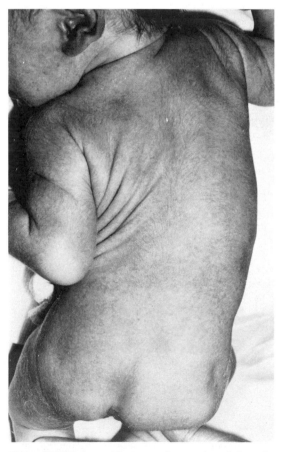

Figure 38.20 Infant with anorectal agenesis and thoracic hemi-vertebrae. The scoliosis was apparent at birth and fixed

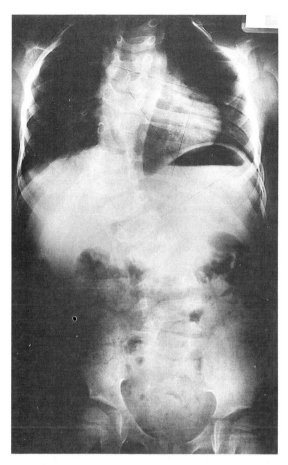

Figure 38.21 Radiograph of a 4-year-old boy born with anorectal agenesis without a fistula. He had multiple vertebral and costal anomalies leading to gross kyphoscoliosis

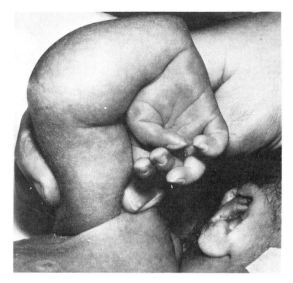

Figure 38.22 Arm of an infant with anorectal agenesis. There was aplasia of the radius. Note the hypoplastic pinna pinna – the pyelogram was, however, normal

Liverpool series. This is many times the incidence which would be expected for a purely random association and only a little smaller than the 12% of infants with imperforate anus whose cardiovascular malformations were analysed by Greenwood and his associates [35], although as many as 22% (15 out of 68) have been found [120]. Tetralogy of Fallot and large ventricular septal defects were the most frequently encountered malformations. Their mortality may be high and urgent cardiac surgery is often required.

A wide variety of anomalies of the *alimentary tract* are found in any large reported series, but the incidence of some is considerably higher than expected from their overall incidence in the live-born. Oesophageal atresia is increasingly reported [3] in association with 'imperforate anus'. Out of 151 infants with anorectal malformations in Liverpool, nine had oesophageal atresia – an incidence of 6.0%

compared with 10% in the Melbourne series [91], and 7% reported from Seattle [94].

The incidence of *Hirschsprung's disease* has been a source of controversy since Parkkulanian *et al.* [87] reported a 60% incidence of aganglionosis with high rectal anomalies. Kiesewetter *et al.* [54] reported only 3.4% by compiling figures from five centres, and Santulli *et al.* [101], in an even larger and wider survey, found only one case in 1166, while Hasse [37] found six cases out of 1420 infants. Takada *et al.* [117] describe two siblings with imperforate anus and aganglionosis extending up to the splenic flexure. Since aganglionosis may follow vascular compromise at surgery, it is essential to examine the neonatal bowel to prove an embryological association. It may well be that the fistula is always aganglionic [132]. The terminal bowel is normally aganglionic in the region of the internal sphincter and so the high termination of the bowel in rectal agenesis might be expected to show some degree of hypoganglionosis. This might add weight to the theory [11] that the malformation may arise as the result of a failure of migration of the terminal bowel. Whatever the theoretical possibilities, and whatever further histological studies of the bowel wall in anorectal anomalies will show, it remains clear that an extensive portion of aganglionic bowel is occasionally found in children who, clinically and radiologically, have Hirschsprung's disease as well as an anorectal anomaly. We have encountered only one such case.

A short *primitive colon* is sometimes associated with high anomalies [47,78,110,130,143]. It is found in conjunction with high vaginal or colovesical fistulae and the mortality is high.

Patterns of association

The tendency for certain defects to be allied together in a non-random manner has been extensively documented in recent years.

Say and colleagues [103,104,105] first put forward the idea of a specific syndrome of pre-axial polydactyly, imperforate anus and vertebral anomalies. Out of 186 index patients with polydactyly, they discovered ten with anorectal malformations and at least eight also had vertebral anomalies. In this same ten there were rib and long bone deformities, and one infant had oesophageal atresia. Others, looking at similar associations, found pre-axial deletion anomalies to be common as well as polydactyly [48,49,126].

There was a very high incidence of skeletal malformations in the Liverpool series of anorectal anomalies, especially where the anorectal malformation occurred together with oesophageal atresia [36]. Quan and Smith [94] coined the term VATER association – mnemonic for 'Vertebral defects, Anal atresia, Tracheo-Esophageal fistula with esophageal atresia, Radial and Renal dysplasia'. They did not suggest that this is a specific syndrome, but a non-random tendency for some defects to associate together. They expressed relative risks of association diagrammatically (Figure 38.23) but the figures

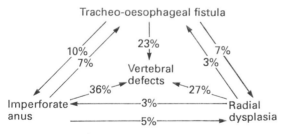

Figure 38.23 VATER association

will no doubt change as bigger series are analysed after full investigation [74].

Where there is a conjunction of alimentary malformations (e.g. oesophageal, duodenal and anorectal) the incidence of skeletal malformations reaches 40% [36].

In order to emphasize the additional frequent association of cardiac lesions, the term VACTERL has been put forward [5] ('Vertebral, Anal, Cardiac, Tracheal, Esophageal, Renal and Limb') while others [122] have recommended the slightly simpler expedient of making the 'V' of VATER stand for

Vascular as well as Vertebral! Children with such patterns of malformation often show significant growth retardation but normal mental development [122]. Mental retardation, however, is a specific feature of one familial complex of anomalies recently described.

Occasional reports [5,32,33] are to be found of familial cases with similar clusters of defects, and also of cases in which there have been suspicions that a teratogenic role has been played by oral contraceptives [5,48,81], maternal irradiation [122] or thalidomide [126]. It perhaps needs to be emphasized that apart from these sporadic reports there is little evidence that these groups of anomalies constitute specific syndromes with a single cause. Conversely, it should be borne in mind that the features of the VATER association form part of the list of defects of well-recognized syndromes (such as trisomy 18, 13q-deletion syndrome, etc.) which are specific chromosomal disorders [94]. Not only do such infants have a very different prognosis, but also their parents need accurate genetic counselling.

Embryology

By the ninth week of normal gestation, the structures of the rectum and anus and the urinary and genital tracts are laid down in their distinctive forms in considerable detail. To achieve this, a remarkable progression of coordinated changes has occurred which, despite extensive study, is still only partly understood. For detailed reviews of the literature and accounts of slightly differing views on morphogenesis, readers are referred to Chapter 5 of Stephens and Smith's book [114], and to de Vries and Friedland's report on their detailed study [133].

Three main phases of development are recognized.

(1) Formation of the cloaca.
(2) Division of the cloaca into the urogenital sinus and rectum.
(3) Development of the anal canal.

The cloaca

The cloaca is formed between 12 and 28 days (Streeter's age group VI–XIII). In the early embryo, endoderm and ectoderm are in contact without interplaced mesodermal cells between the caudal end of the primitive streak and the body stalk. The allantois grows out of the caudal end of the gut ventrally into the body stalk and as the dorsal portion of the embryo grows, the allantoic duct and the cloacal membrane are displaced ventrally. There is some caudal extension of the hindgut to form the tailgut. At the beginning of age group XIV (32 days), the cloaca is thus a terminal

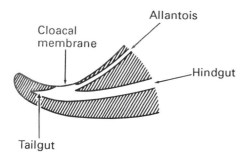

Figure 38.24 The cloaca complete at age group XIV

expansion of the hindgut (Figure 38.24) into which enter the allantois, the gut and the tailgut, and, also, by the end of the third week, the Wolffian or mesonephric ducts. The whole structure lies in the hollow of the tailfold of the embryo and the cloacal membrane faces ventrally. Later growth of the abdominal wall and unfolding and disappearance of the tail cause the cloacal membrane to recede caudally.

Development of urogenital sinus and rectum

In age group XIV and XV (32–33 days) the cloacal membrane thickens and is displaced downwards and rotated to face caudally rather than ventrally by new growth of mesoblast beneath the body stalk. Mesoblastic proliferation between the entry of the hindgut and the allantois into the cloaca and lateral to the cloaca constricts the cloacal lumen and forms a horseshoe-shaped fold, the urogenital fold, which in its craniocaudal descending portion is the Tourneux fold [123], and laterally, the lateral plicae of Rathke [96,97] (Figure 38.25). The cloaca thus becomes divided into an anterior urogenital sinus and posterior rectum when these folds coalesce with the

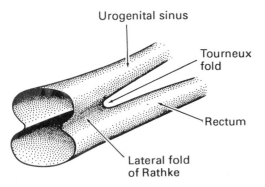

Figure 38.25 Representation of the combined effect of the development of the lateral plicae of Rathke and the Tourneux fold

inner surface of the cloacal membrane. This is complete by about the middle of the seventh week (age group XIX). The last part to close will be the central area just above the membrane. When the fusion is complete, the cloacal membrane breaks down, first in the urogenital portion and then the anal membrane.

Development of the anal canal

There is a fundamental disagreement between the description by Stephens and Smith [114], and that by de Vries and Friedland [133] over this area. Stephens and Smith consider that the build-up of the genital tubercle and folds forms an external cloaca into which the posterior rectum and anterior urogenital sinus both open when the cloacal membrane breaks down. The external cloaca is then subdivided partly by further caudal extension of the urorectal septum and partly by inward migration of the genital folds which in the male will tent over the urogenital sinus to form the bulbous urethra while further infolding builds up the perineal raphe and scrotum. De Vries and Friedland, however, in the embryos they studied, demonstrated that there was no external cloaca at the time the anal membrane broke down, and found that even before this, the anal tubercles had formed a prominent fold dorsal and lateral to the cloaca, while an evagination of the dorsal wall of the cloaca became the bulbus analis portion of the anorectal wall which is thus formed from endoderm.

Pathogenesis

The complex and lengthy process of formation of the rectum and anus occupies a good deal of the embryonic period and is simultaneously closely related to the development of the vertebrae and the renal tract [82]. Folic acid antagonists exhibited prior to age group VI (33 days post-ovulation) are known to cause urogenital, skeletal and vertebral anomalies [133]. The simple mechanical factor of excessive embryonic folding is also put forward to explain the multisystem anomalies of the VATER association [91]. The rare rectal atresia may develop because of vascular compromise of a previously normal anorectum [61], and an even rarer H-type recto-urinary fistula associated with renal ectopia may be explained by failure of fusion of the urorectal septum and cloacal membrane [133].

Aetiology

Genetic factors

Most cases appear sporadically with no evidence of any increased risk in siblings [75]. We have no familial cases in Liverpool and only two siblings with imperforate anus were found in 1166 affected infants in a large American study [101], but a survey of 186 patients in Manchester revealed 15 with a family history of similar anorectal anomalies [13]. More than 25 families with multiple affected members have been described in the literature [5,22,32,46,64,79,124,131,141]. Most of these studies point to an autosomal recessive type of inheritance. When such families have been identified, the risk of recurrence is of course 25%. A dominant gene seemed to be involved in some families [107], and an autosomal dominant syndrome affecting anus, hands and ears was described in two families by Townes and Brocks [124].

Uniovular twins with identical malformations have been described [22,114], but where anorectal anomalies occur in twins, it is usually only one who is affected.

Genetic factors may be more important in some forms of anorectal anomaly (e.g. anorectal stenosis) than in others [22].

Environmental factors

Birth rate and maternal age do not seem to influence the incidence. Maternal ingestion of thalidomide [44,127] and of oral contraceptives [48,81] has been implicated, and, theoretically, folic acid inhibitors or folic acid deficiency could cause multiple system anomalies of vertebral, urogenital and anorectal structures. Mechanical factors have also been blamed [91], with the suggestion that excessive ventral folding of the embryo may distort the tubular hindgut (and foregut) and deflect the developing urogenital septum to meet the posterior wall rather than the cloacal membrane.

The frequent association of other anomalies, in predictable patterns in any individual, but arising sporadically in the population, has been taken to conform to the concept of intrinsic mutagenesis – random mutations due to errors of DNA replication [100]. This is not to say, however, that teratogens should not be searched for in cases of congenital malformation.

Incidence

Estimates of the overall incidence of anorectal malformations vary from 1 in 1800 births in South Africa [59] to 1 in 10 000 in France, but the generally quoted [114,141] figure is 1 in 5000. Louw [59] found the highest incidence in both Caucasian and coloured racial groups, while in the Bantu the incidence was not so high – 1 in 2260. High lesions are not likely to be overlooked but the overall incidence may be higher than reported since low lesions may not appear in hospital statistics.

The sex incidence in all comprehensive reported series shows a preponderance of boys. Stephens and Smith [114] collated 36 published reports and in more than 3000 cases there were 57% males and 43% females. In Liverpool, from 1953 to 1985, 351 boys were admitted and 184 girls (65.6% boys). The frequency of occurrence of the different forms of anomalies is difficult to determine from publications before 1970 when confused nomenclature makes comparisons and summations impossible. The incidence of the main types of anomaly found recently in Liverpool is shown in Tables 38.1 and 38.2. The greater incidence of high lesions in male infants and low lesions in female infants is agreed by most authors, although an equal number of high and low anomalies in male infants has been reported from India [119].

Clinical features

Many of the clinical features of the infant with 'imperforate anus' will be apparent from the descriptions of the pathological anatomy given above. Other factors, however, need to be stressed. Most of the infants with imperforate anus are of good birth weight [101], but a proportion, especially those with high lesions and with other major malformations, are found to be of low birth weight [23]. The weight and the gestational age should be noted because of the special needs of the premature and dysmature infant.

In most instances the lesions will have been noticed immediately after birth by simple inspection, but the perineum may look remarkably normal to the casual attendant and the abdominal distension of low intestinal obstruction may, in these circumstances, be the presenting feature. If the fistula is of large size the bowel may, however, decompress itself adequately for a considerable period of time.

In both male and female infants, exact identification of the nature of any fistula to the surface can be determined by inspection and by probing (Figures 38.16 and 38.17), with the occasional necessary addition of special investigations.

Male infant

In the male infant the presence of a perineal opening should enable a precise diagnosis to be made. If there is no external opening then the infant has a high or intermediate lesion (or the rare complete covered anus).

Urine must be examined and if it contains obvious meconium, or microscopic examination shows the presence of squamous cells, there must be a rectovesical or recto-urethral or rectobulbar fistula and the lesion is not a low one. Meconium may be seen to issue from the urethral meatus even when urine is not being passed (see Figure 38.7).

Female infant

In the female, neonatal assessment is again primarily made from perineal inspection. If only one orifice can be identified (Figure 38.12), it will be a cloaca and the malformation must be a high one with a rectocloacal or rectovesical fistula. If there are two orifices (urethra and vagina) then the lesion is most likely to be a high or intermediate one with a rectovaginal fistula. If there are three orifices (Figures 38.16 and 38.17), the malformation must be low except for a rectal atresia with a normal anus and the intermediate rectovestibular fistula (Figures 38.14 and 38.15).

In both sexes it is important to know whether or not the child has passed urine because of the possibility of renal agenesis and obstructive uropathies and it should be recorded whether or not the bladder is expressible and whether the anal and cremasteric reflexes are present and whether perineal sensation seems to be normal [28].

Radiological features

Early X-rays of the lumbosacral spine are important to assess the normality of the sacral vertebrae. We still find an invertogram of great use (Figure 38.26). The technique was first described by Wangensteen and Rice [137] and subsequently the details of technique necessary to avoid erroneous results have gradually been clarified. While the important measurement used to be thought to be the distance between the most caudal gas shadow and the perineal skin, it is now considered more important to relate this to bony pelvic landmarks. The radiograph should be centred on the trochanters and the hips must be extended so that the pubic ossification centres are not obscured by the femora. If films are taken in very young infants, gas may not have reached the terminal portion of the gut. Durham Smith [27] suggests that the child should be at least 24 h old. The infant should also be held upside down for at least 3 min prior to the exposure of the film and a minimum of two films should be taken – an attempt being made to expose one of them when the infant is not straining. Even so, the gas shadows may be anatomically higher than the true termination of the gut because of slowness of passage of gas, viscous meconium filling the termination [9], or active contraction of the puborectalis muscle emptying the lower rectum [114]. Transperineal injection of water-soluble contrast medium into the rectal pouch has been suggested to give more precise

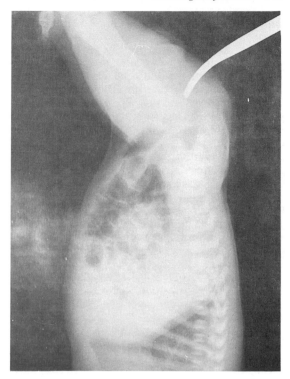

Figure 38.26 Radiograph of a neonate in inverted position. The gas bubble does not reach below the pubococcygeal line. The bladder is filled with air. There was a rectoprostatic urethral fistula

definition of its termination and of any fistula [28,72,76,135].

Stephens suggested and developed the concept of the pubococcygeal (PC) line – a line from the centre of the pubis to the inferior margin of the fifth sacral vertebral body (the lowest ossification point). This was shown in dissections to be the position of the lateral portions of the puborectalis sling. Kelly [51] defined the ischial point (or I point) showing that the inferior end of the comma-shaped ischial shadow on a correctly centred pertrochanteric X-ray corresponds to the level at which the central fibres of the puborectalis muscle embrace the rectum or fistula or, in the absence of both, surround the cloaca, vagina or urethra. This radiological landmark has been confirmed by others [66]. Durham Smith [27] considers lesions above the PC line to be high, between the PC line and the I point to be intermediate and below the I point to be low.

It is not necessary to suspend the infant in the inverted position. Equally good radiological results can be obtained by nursing him prone with the pelvis high and then to take a cross-table lateral view of the pelvis, again with the trochanters superimposed so that the bony landmarks can be accurately defined [77]. Durham Smith [28] recommends that a voiding cysto-urethrogram should be combined with the invertogram to determine the presence and site of the fistula.

Ultrasonography can also be used to determine the distance between the skin and the rectal pouch. It is a non-invasive and basically simple investigation but the interpretation of the result demands a good deal of experience on the part of the ultrasonographer.

Where computed tomography is available valuable confirmatory evidence can be obtained but it is in no way essential to the initial management of the infant. The blind rectal end can, however, be easily identified by the meconium/tissue interface and the fistula can be identified and an accurate measurement of the distance of the bowel from the skin level can be made. An assessment of the pelvic muscles is also possible. Transverse 'cuts' of the pelvis are not easy to interpret and direct sagittal scans are obtainable in the neonate who can be positioned transversely in the relatively large aperture of most CT scanner gantries [118].

The satisfaction of elucidating the exact anatomy of a complex anorectal malformation may divert attention from other urgent and life-threatening problems. It must be emphasized that thorough clinical examination of the baby is essential and the urinary tract and cardiovascular system deserve especial attention. Initial examination and investigation should be planned with a view to relieving intestinal obstruction in order to allow normal nutrition, and to rule out other life-threatening conditions. The neonatal treatment of the infant

with an anorectal anomaly can be planned accurately by careful clinical examination and the minimum of investigation. The ultimate correction of the anorectal anomaly demands careful and detailed assessment of the infant's pelvis. Some of this may be appropriately done in the neonatal period but some may best be deferred.

Treatment

From the preceding discussion, it will be clear that the surgeon's initial responsibility is to identify the level of the malformation and choose the appropriate management. Various 'flow charts' have been devised to assist in this. The principle is that low lesions can be managed by relatively simple cutback procedures or anoplasties; intermediate or high lesions are best treated by an initial colostomy, and definitive reconstructive surgery is deferred until 6–9 months of age. While this is still our view and that of many others [27], some consider an immediate abdominoperineal pull-through to be the treatment of choice in male infants of good birth weight and without other major anomalies [112,116]. The long-term results are reportedly as good, in some surgeons' experience, with early as with later operations [30,98]. In some cultures, a colostomy is unacceptable and is made as a very short-term expedient to relieve obstruction and allow radiological investigation of the infant in preparation for a pull-through at a few weeks of age [1].

In male or female infants with an anocutaneous fistula a cutback procedure is simple and effective.

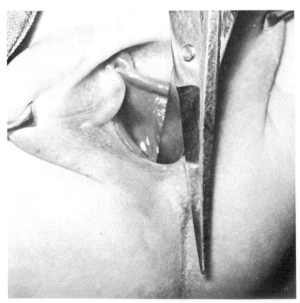

Figure 38.27 The 'cutback' operation. One blade of the scissors has been inserted along the anovestibular fistula

This was first described by Denis Browne [15] in 1951 and, although some modifications are practised, it has remained virtually unaltered [20]. One blade of a pair of straight scissors is placed along the horizontal fistula and the perineal tissues cut back in the midline to the site of the external sphincter (Figure 38.27). The mucosa is sutured to the skin with interrupted sutures. Dilatation is done from the fifth day onwards.

An anterior ectopic anus [108] is sometimes said to require no treatment unless it is stenotic, but even if not stenosed it is often associated with severe and protracted constipation [40,58,129]. While a neonatal operation may not be necessary, the child should be followed carefully and an anoplasty carried out if need be [16,40].

The female infant with an anovestibular fistula can also be treated with a simple cutback but an anoplasty to transfer the anus to a more normal position and build a perineal body is preferred by some [95,102].

The site of the colostomy for an infant with an intermediate lesion is often vigorously debated. The neonatal construction of a transverse colostomy will leave an adequate length of distal colon and rectum for the definitive operation without disturbance of the colostomy. It does, however, lead to loose stools and greater problems of skin care, and makes cleansing of the distal defunctioned loop of colon and rectum difficult. If the proximal loop of the sigmoid colon is used the length of bowel distal to it is usually adequate for the 'pull-through' [20] and yet not too difficult to clean out [27]. The stools will be better formed and colostomy care easier.

The technique of the procedure should ensure that the colostomy is a defunctioning one and at Alder Hey a skin bridge is used to hold it out (see Chapter 37). Others advocate the production of a fairly high spur to protrude well beyond skin level or even complete separation of the stomata by a very wide skin bridge.

While the infant is on the operating table, or as soon as practicable afterwards, the distal colon must be washed free of meconium with warm normal saline. Where there is a recto-urinary fistula the washout should be repeated at intervals until the definitive surgery is done, in order to minimize the risks of urinary tract infection. Stephens and Smith [114] claim that good colostomy care will prevent urinary tract infection unless there is an obstructive urinary tract anomaly. If there is, this should be dealt with in its own right. Closure of a recto-urethral fistula should thus not need to be expedited because of urinary infection.

When the infant has recovered from the construction of the colostomy, additional investigations are undertaken to determine the specific anatomy of the anorectal anomaly and to establish the nature and the significance of any associated malformations.

While it is essential to discover major and life-threatening anomalies early, investigations such as colonograms, to provide exact identification of the site of the fistula, may be better deferred until the child is older, prior to the definitive surgery. As short a period of separation as possible from the mother in the neonatal period is desirable.

Results

For low lesions, treated by dilatations or simple cutback procedures, the mortality should be very small. Deaths in this group in our recent experience have been related to other anomalies. In high lesions the mortality was again related to gross cardiac or pulmonary pathology and not to colostomy construction, nor even later reconstructive surgery. Where the peritoneal cavity is opened and where procedures are staged, the risk of complications and mortality are increased. Some older series [88] reported an alarmingly high mortality rate from colostomy construction alone. This is one reason occasionally put forward for a single stage procedure in the newborn.

In terms of the ultimate result, when simple dilatation or a cutback is done on appropriate low anomalies, the functional result should be excellent [16,114]. In girls, separation of the rectum and vagina usually occurs spontaneously as the child grows (Figure 38.28, cf. Figure 38.16). Some children, however, remain constipated and may have overflow incontinence, or the anal orifice may remain so close to the vulva that hygiene is difficult and recurrent urinary infection occurs (Figure 38.29). Some of these imperfect results follow an inadequate cutback or are in children who were not recognized to have an intermediate lesion – a rectovaginal fistula. The late results of the cutback are not good in some children with anovestibular fistulae if a perineal body is not present. Operations to separate the anal and vaginal orifices after such cutbacks are described [17] and should be considered, though in our experience the functional results after a simple cutback are better than after perineal anoplasties. A perineal approach and anal transplant is recommended by some for both low and intermediate lesions [40]. The matter is discussed at length in the literature, but for the genuinely low lesion, such complex procedures seem to be quite unnecessary, and for the intermediate lesion endanger the neuromuscular basis of continence.

No comprehensive later assessment has been carried out here on children with intermediate and high lesions. They have been treated mostly by Stevens' sacroperineal or sacro-abdominoperineal procedures and more recently some have had posterior sagittal anorectoplasties [90]. In company with other centres [25,38,39,52] the results are

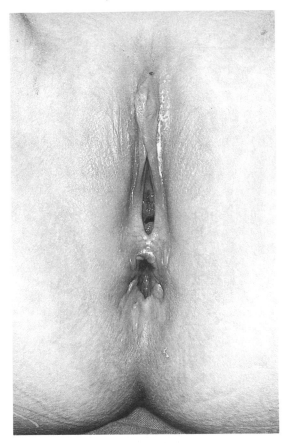

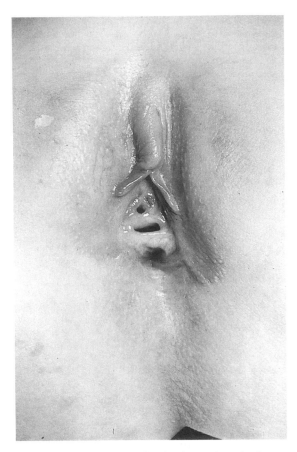

Figure 38.28 The perineal appearance 10 years after the 'cutback' procedure for an anocutaneous fistula. The child was fully continent and had no problems with perineal hygiene (same patient as Figure 38.16)

Figure 38.29 Later result of an inadequately cutback anovulvar fistula. A residual posterior shelf led to severe constipation. Note the double vagina with an apparently transverse septum. The septum was lying in the more usual sagittal plane internally. The uterus and one Fallopian tube were later discovered to be absent

disappointing in terms of absolute continence, but most children seem to cope increasingly well as they themselves mature [19]. This is often in spite of very deranged neuromuscular function as judged by electromyography [8], and other sophisticated tests [45,68]. The assessment formula proposed in association with the Wingspread classification [115] should provide a simple basis for late assessment of results and the comparison of different procedures in relation to the pathological anatomy of the malformation.

References

1. Adeyemi, S.D. and Da Rocha-Afodu, J.T. (1982) Management of imperforate anus at the Lagos University Teaching Hospital, Nigeria: a review of ten years' experience. *Prog. Pediat. Surg.*, **15**, 187–194

2. Amussat, J. (1835) Observation sur une opération d'anus artificiel pratiquée avec succès par un nouveau procédé. *Gaz. med. Paris*, **28**, 8

3. Aszodi, A. (1974) Imperforate anus combined with esophageal atresia and agenesis of the right kidney. *Am. J. Proctol.*, **25**, 59–61

4. Ayoub, S.F. (1979) Anatomy of the external anal sphincter in man. *Acta Anat.*, **105**, 25–36

5. Balci, S., Say, B., Pirnar, T. and Hicsonmez, A. (1973) Birth defects and oral contraceptives. *Lancet*, **ii**, 1098

6. Ball, C. (1887) *The Rectum and Anus. Their Diseases and Treatment*, Cassell, London

7. Beersiek, F., Parks, A.G. and Swash, M. (1979) Pathogenesis of anorectal incontinence. A histometric study of the anal sphincter musculature. *J. Neurol. Sci.*, **42**, 111–127

8. Berger, D., Schneider, L.C., Landry, M. and Genton, N.Z. (1977) Functional and prognostic evaluation of anorectal malformations. *Z. Kinderchir.*, **22**, 286–312

9. Berman, J.K. (1938) Congenital anomalies of rectum and anus. *Surg. Gynec. Obstet.*, **66**, 11–22

10. Bill, A.H. Jr (1975) Position of the rectal fistula in relation to the hymen in 46 girls with imperforate anus. *J. Pediat. Surg.*, **10**, 361–365

11. Bill, A.H. Jr and Johnson, R.J. (1958) Failure of migration of the rectal opening as the cause for most cases of imperforate anus. *Surg. Gynec. Obstet.*, **106**, 643–644

12. Bodenhammer, W. (1860) *A practical treatise on the etiology, pathology and treatment of the congenital malformation of the anus and rectum*, Samuel S. and William Wood, New York

13. Boocock, G.R. and Donnai, D. (1987) Anorectal malformations: familial aspects and associated anomalies. *Arch. Dis. Child.*, **62**, 576–579

14. Borger, J.A. and Belman, A.B. (1975) Uretero-vas deferens anastomosis associated with imperforate anus: an embryologically predictable occurrence. *J. Pediat. Surg.*, **10**, 255–257

15. Browne, D. (1951) Some congenital deformities of the rectum, anus, vagina and urethra. *Ann. Roy. Coll. Surg. Engl.*, **8**, 173–177

16. Bryndorf, J. and Madsen, C.M. (1960) Ectopic anus in the female. *Acta Chir. Scand.*, **118**, 466–468

17. Burrington, J.D. (1975) Recto-vaginal separation operation after a 'cut-back' procedure for ano-rectal anomalies. *Arch. Surg.*, **110**, 471–475

18. Carson, J.A., Barnes, P.D., Tunell, W.P., Smith, E.I. and Jolley, S.G. (1984) Imperforate anus: the neurologic implications of sacral abnormalities. *J. Pediat. Surg.*, **19**, 838–842

19. Cook, R.C.M. (1985) Faecal incontinence. In: *Coloproctology and the Pelvic Floor* (ed. M.M. Henry and M. Swash), Butterworths, London, pp. 242–252

20. Cook, R.C.M. (1987) Anorectal malformations. In: *Rob and Smith's Operative Surgery, Paediatric Surgery*, 4th Edition, (ed. L. Spitz and H.H. Nixon), Butterworths, London, pp. 348–369

21. Cooksey, G. and Wagget, J. (1984) Tubular duplication of the rectum treated by mucosal resection. *J. Pediat. Surg.*, **19**, 318–319

22. Cozzi, F. and Wilkinson, A.W. (1968) Familial incidence of congenital ano-rectal anomalies. *Surgery*, **64**, 669–671

23. Cozzi, F. and Wilkinson, A.W. (1969) Intra-uterine growth rate in relation to ano-rectal and oesophageal anomalies. *Arch. Dis. Child.*, **44**, 59

24. Currarins, G., Coln, D. and Votteler, T. (1981) Triad of anorectal, sacral and presacral anomalies. *Am. J. Roent.*, **137**, 395–398

25. Cywes, S., Cremin, B.J. and Louw, J.H. (1971) Assessment of continence after treatment for anorectal agenesis: a clinical and radiologic correlation. *J. Pediat. Surg.*, **6**, 132–136

26. Daorong, Z. (1983) Rectal duplication. *Chin. J. Pediatr. Surg.*, **4**, 5–7

27. Durham Smith, E. (1976) The identification and management of ano-rectal anomalies. The factors ensuring continence. *Prog. Pediat. Surg.*, **9**, 7–40

28. Durham Smith, E. (1987) The bath water needs changing, but don't throw out the baby: an overview of anorectal anomalies. *J. Pediat. Surg.*, **22**, 335–384

29. Fleming, S.E., Hall, R., Gysler, M. and McLovie, G.A. (1986) Imperforate anus in females: frequency of genital tract involvement, incidence of associated anomalies and functional outcome. *J. Pediat. Surg.*, **21**, 146–150

30. Freeman, N.V. and Bulut, M. (1986) 'High' anorectal anomalies treated by early (neonatal) operation. *J. Pediat. Surg.*, **21**, 218–220

31. Frenckner, B. (1985) Use of the recto-urethral fistula for reconstruction of the anal canal in high anal atresia. *Z. Kinderchir.*, **40**, 312–314

32. Fuhrmann, W. (1968) A new polydactyly/imperforate anus/vertebral anomalies syndrome? *Lancet*, **II**, 918–919

33. Fuhrmann, W., Rieger, A. and Vogel, F. (1958) Zwei Beabachtungen zur Genetik der Atresia ani. *Arch. Kinderheilk.*, **158**, 264–270

34. Fujiwara, Y., Ohizumi, T., Sasahara, M., Kato, E., Kakizaki, G., Ishidate, T. and Fujiwara, T. (1974) Imperforate anus with absence of vagina incurring hematometra and hematosalpinx. *J. Pediat. Surg.*, **9**, 555–556

35. Greenwood, R.D., Rosenthal, A. and Nada, A.S. (1975) Cardiovascular malformations associated with imperforate anus. *J. Pediat.*, **86**, 576–579

36. Gruchalski, J., Irving, I.M. and Lister, J. (1976) Skeletal anomalies associated with oesophageal, duodenal and ano-rectal atresias. *Lancet*, **ii**, 517

37. Hasse, W. (1976) Associated malformation with anal and rectal atresiae. *Progr. Pediat. Surg.*, **9**, 99–101

38. Hecker, W.C.L. and Holschneider, A.M. (1979) Long term follow-up in congenital anomalies. *Paed. Surg. Symp., Pittsburg*, pp. 54–55

39. Hecker, W.C.L., Holschneider, A.M. and Kraeft, H. (1980) Complications, deaths and long-term results after surgery of ano-rectal atresia. *Z. Kinderchir.*, **29**, 238–244

40. Hendren, W.H. (1978) Constipation caused by anterior location of the anus, and its surgical correction. *J. Pediat. Surg.*, **13**, 505–512

41. Hendren, W.H. (1980) Urogenital sinus and anorectal malformation: experience with 22 cases. *J. Pediat. Surg.*, **15**, 628–641

42. Hoekstra, W.J., Scholtmeijer, R.J., Molenaar, J.C. *et al.* (1983) Urogenital tract abnormalities associated with congenital anorectal anomalies. *J. Urol.*, **130**, 962–963

43. Holl, M. (1881) Uber den Verschluss des mannlichen Beckens. Archiv fur Anatomie und Physiologie, Leipzig. *Anat. Abt.*, 225–271

44. Imdahl, H., Koch, W. and Hermans, A. (1963)

Thalidomid in der Fruhschwangerschaft und end darmmissbildungen. *Bull. Soc. Chir.*, **22**, 602–611

45. Iwai, N., Yanagihara, J. and Tsuto, T. (1984) Results of anorectal manometry following surgery for anorectal malformation. *Ann. Paediat. Surg.*, **1**, 77–82

46. Kaijser, K. and Malmstrom-Groth, A. (1957) Anorectal abnormalities as a congenital familial incidence. *Acta Pediat. Scand.*, **46**, 199

47. Kalani, B.P. and Sogani, K.C. (1984) Short colon associated with anorectal agenesis: Treatment by colonorraphy. *Ann. Paediat. Surg.*, **1**, 83–85

48. Kaufman, R.L. (1973) VACTERL associated with oral contraceptives. *Lancet*, **i**, 1396

49. Kaufman, R.L., Quinton, B. and Ternberg, J.L. (1970) Polydactyly/imperforate anus/vertebral anomalies syndrome. *Lancet*, **i**, 841

50. Keith, A. (1908) Three demonstrations on malformations of the hind end of the body. I. Specimens illustrating malformations of the rectum and anus. *Br. Med. J.*, **2**, 1736–1741

51. Kelly, J.H. (1969) The radiographic anatomy of the normal and abnormal neonatal pelvis. *J. Pediat. Surg.*, **4**, 432–444

52. Kiesewetter, W.B. and Chang, J.H.T. (1977) Imperforate anus: A 5–30 year follow-up prospective. *Prog. Pediat. Surg.*, **10**, 111–121

53. Kiesewetter, W.B. and Nixon, H.H. (1967) Imperforate anus. I. Its surgical anatomy. *J. Pediat. Surg.*, **2**, 60–63

54. Kiesewetter, W.B., Sukarochana, K. and Sieber, W.K. (1965) The frequency of aganglionosis associated with imperforate anus. *Surgery*, **58**, 877–880

55. Laberge, J.M., Bosc, O., Yazbeck, S., Youssef, S., Ducharme, J.U.C., Guttman, F.M. and Nguyen, L.T. (1983) The anterior perineal approach for pull-through operations in high imperforate anus. *J. Pediat. Surg.*, **18**, 774–778

56. Ladd, W.E. and Gross, R.E. (1934) Congenital malformations of the anus and rectum; report of 162 cases. *Am. J. Surg.*, **23**, 167–183

57. Lawson, J.O.N. (1974) Pelvic Anatomy I, Pelvic floor muscles. *Ann. Roy. Coll. Surg. Eng.*, **54**, 244–252

58. Leape, L.L. and Ranenofsky, M.L. (1978) Anterior ectopic anus: a common cause of constipation in children. *J. Pediat. Surg.*, **13**, 627–630

59. Louw, J.H., Cywes, S. and Cremin, B.J. (1971) The management of ano-rectal agenesis. *S. Afr. J. Surg.*, **9**, 21–26

60. McLeod, N. (1880) Case of imperforate rectum with a suggestion for a new method of treatment. *Br. Med. J.*, **2**, 657–658

61. Magnus, R.V. (1965) Rectal atresia as distinguished from rectal agenesis. *J. Pediat. Surg.*, **3**, 593–598

62. Magnus, R.V. (1972) Congenital rectovesical fistula and its associated anomalies. *Aust. N.Z. J. Surg.*, **42**, 197–200

63. Magnus, R.V. (1974) Urinary abnormalities in children with congenital rectovesical fistula. *Aust. Pediat. J.*, **10**, 82–84

64. Manny, J., Schiller, M., Horner, R., Stein, H. and Luttwak, E.M. (1973) Congenital familial ano-rectal anomaly. *Am. J. Surg.*, **125**, 639–640

65. Matas, R. (1897) The surgical treatment of congenital ano-rectal imperforation considered in the light of modern operation procedures. *Trans. Am. Surg. Ass.*, **15**, 453–553

66. Mendoza, F.M. and Gough, E.C.S. (1969) The radiologic anatomy of the puborectalis muscle. *J. Pediat. Surg.*, **18**, 172–173

67. Milligan, E.T.C. and Morgan, C.N. (1934) Surgical anatomy of the anal canal. *Lancet*, **ii**, 1150–1156; 1213–1217

68. Molander, M. and Frenckner, B. (1985) Anal sphincter function after surgery for high imperforate anus – a long term follow-up investigation. *Z. Kinderchir.*, **40**, 91–96

69. Mollard, P., Marechal, J.M. and de Beaujeu, M.J. (1975) Le reperage de la sangle du releveur au cours du traitement des imperforations ano-rectales hautes. *Ann. Chir. Inf.*, **16**, 461–468

70. Mollard, P., Marechal, J.M. and de Beaujeu, M.J. (1978) Surgical treatment of high imperforate anus with definition of the puborectalis sling by an anterior perineal approach. *J. Pediat. Surg.*, **13**, 499–504

71. Mollitt, D.L., Schullinger, J.N., Santulli, T.V. and Hensle, T.W. (1981) Complications at menarche of urogenital sinus with associated anorectal malformations. *J. Pediat. Surg.*, **16**, 349–352

72. Motovic, A., Kovalivker, M., Man, B. and Krausz, L. (1979) The value of transperineal injection for the diagnosis of imperforate anus. *Surgery*, **190**, 668–670

73. Munn, R. and Schillinger, J.F. (1983) Urologic abnormalities found with imperforate anus. *Urology*, **21**, 260–264

74. Muraji, T. and Mahour, G.H. (1984) Surgical problems in patients with VATER-associated anomalies. *J. Pediat. Surg.*, **19**, 550–554

75. Murken, J.D. and Albert, A. (1976) Genetic counselling in cases of anal and rectal atresia. *Prog. Pediat. Surg.*, **9**, 115–118

76. Murugasu, J.J. (1970) A new method of roentgenological demonstration of ano-rectal anomalies. *Surgery*, **68**, 706–712

77. Narasimharao, K.L. (1983) Prone cross-table lateral view: an alternative to the invertogram in imperforate anus. *Am. J. Radiol.*, **140**, 227–229

78. Narasimharao, K.L., Yadav, K. and Mitra, S.K. (1984) Congenital short colon with imperforate anus (pouch colon syndrome). *Ann. Paediat. Surg.*, **1**, 159–167

79. Naudi, Y. and Friedman, A. (1976) Familial imperforate anus. *Am. J. Dis. Child.*, **130**, 441–442

80. N'Guessan, G. and Stephen, F.D. (1986) Covered anus with anocutaneous fistula: the muscular sphincters. *J. Pediat. Surg.*, **21**, 33–35

81. Nora, J.J. and Nora, A.H. (1973) VACTERL associated with oral contraceptives. *Lancet*, **i**, 941–942

82. Obeid, M.L. and Corkery, J.J. (1974) Importance of the urinary tract in imperforate anus. *Proc. R. Soc. Med.*, **67**, 203–204

83. Obenbergerova, D., Tosovsky, V. and Zitkova, M. (1975) Coincidence of atresias of the alimentary tract – in particular of the oesophagus – with skeletal malformations. *Z. Kinderchir.*, **16**, 268

84. Oh, C. and Kark, A.E. (1972) Anatomy of the external anal sphincter. *Br. J. Surg.*, **59**, 717–723

85. Palken, M., Johnson, R.J., Derrick, W. and Bill, A.H. (1972) Clinical aspects of female patients with high anorectal agenesis. *Surg. Gynec. Obstet.*, **135**, 411–414

86. Parkkulainen, K.V. (1957) Sacro coccygeal and urological anomalies in connection with congenital malformations of anus and rectum. *Ann. Paediat. Fenn.*, **3**, 51–57

87. Parkkulainen, K.V., Hjelt, L. and Sulamaa, M. (1959) Anal atresia combined with aganglionic megacolon. *Acta Chir. Scand.*, **118**, 252–256

88. Partridge, J.P. and Gough, M.H. (1961) Congenital abnormalities of the anus and rectum. *Br. J. Surg.*, **49**, 37–50

89. Pellerin, D. and Bertin, P. (1967) Genito-urinary malformations and vertebral anomalies in ano-rectal malformations. *Z. Kinderchir.*, **4**, 375

90. Pena, A. and De Vries, P.A. (1982) Posterior sagittal anorectoplasty: important technical considerations and new applications. *J. Pediat. Surg.*, **17**, 638–643

91. Piekarski, D.H. and Stephens, F.D. (1976) The association and embryogenesis of tracheo-oesophageal and ano-rectal anomalies. *Progr. Pediat. Surg.*, **9**, 63–76

92. Potts, W.J. (1959) *The Surgeon and the Child*, W.B. Saunders, Philadelphia

93. Puri, P. and Nixon, H.H. (1977) The results of treatment of ano-rectal anomalies: a 13–20 year follow-up. *J. Pediat. Surg.*, **12**, 27–37

94. Quan, L. and Smith, D.W. (1973) The VATER Association. *J. Pediat.*, **82**, 104–107

95. Raffensperger, J.G. (1980) Anorectal anomalies. In: *Swenson's Pediatric Surgery*, 4th Edition, Appleton Century Crofts, New York, pp. 538–580

96. Rathke, M.H. (1832) *Abhardlungen zur Bildings – und Entwickelungs – Geschichte des Menschen und de Thiere*, Pt. 1, Vogel, Leipzig

97. Rathke, M.H. (1861) *Entwickelungs-geschichte de Wirbelthiere*, Engelman, Leipzig, pp. 144–174

98. Rehbein, F. (1959) Operation for anal and rectal atresia with recto-urethral fistula. *Chirurgie*, **30**, 417–419

99. Rhoads, J.E., Piper, R.L. and Randall, J.P. (1948) A simultaneous abdominal and perineal approach in operations for imperforate anus with atresia of rectum and recto-sigmoid. *Ann. Surg.*, **127**, 552–556

100. Roberts, C.J. and Powell, R.G. (1975) Interrelation of the common congenital malformations. Some aetiological implications. *Lancet*, **i**, 848–850

101. Santulli, T.V., Schullinger, J.N., Kiesewetter, W.B. and Bill, A.H. Jr (1971) Imperforate anus: a survey from the members of the surgical section of the American Academy of Pediatrics. *J. Pediat. Surg.*, **6**, 484–487

102. Saxena, N., Bhattacharyya, N.C., Katariya, S., Mitra, S.K. and Pathak, K. (1981) Perineal anal transplant in low ano-rectal anomalies. *Surgery*, **90**, 464–467

103. Say, B., Balci, S., Pirnar, T. and Hicsonmez, A. (1971) Imperforate anus/polydactyly/vertebral anomalies syndrome: a hereditary trait? *J. Pediat.*, **79**, 1033–1034

104. Say, B., Balci, S., Pirnar, T. and Tuncbilek, E. (1971) A new syndrome of dysmorphogenesis: imperforate anus associated with polyoligodactyly and skeletal (mainly vertebral) anomalies. *Acta Paediat. Scand.*, **60**, 197–202

105. Say, B. and Gerald, P.S. (1968) A new polydactyly/imperforate anus/vertebral anomalies syndrome? *Lancet*, **ii**, 688–689

106. Schuster, M.M. (1975) The riddle of the sphincters. *Gastroenterology*, **69**, 249–262

107. Schwoebel, M.G., Hirsig, J., Schinzel, A. and Stauffer, U.G. (1984) Familial incidence of congenital anorectal anomalies. *J. Pediat. Surg.*, **19**, 179–182

108. Scott, J.E.S. (1966) The microscopic anatomy of the terminal intestinal canal in ectopic vulval anus. *J. Pediat. Surg.*, **1**, 441–443

109. Scott, J.E.S. and Swenson, O. (1959) Imperforate anus, results in 63 cases and some anatomical considerations. *Ann. Surg.*, **150**, 477–487

110. Singh, S. and Pathak, I.C. (1972) Short colon associated with imperforate anus. *Surgery*, **71**, 781–786

111. Snooks, S.J. and Swash, M. (1986) The innervation of the muscles of continence. *Ann. Roy. Coll. Surg. Engl.*, **68**, 45–49

112. Soave, F. (1969) Surgery of rectal anomalies with preservation of the relationship between the colonic muscular sleeve and the pubo-rectalis muscle. *J. Pediat. Surg.*, **4**, 705–712

113. Stephens, F.D. (1953) Imperforate rectum: a new surgical technique. *Med. J. Aust.*, **2**, 202–203

114. Stephens, F.D. and Durham Smith, E. (1971) *Anorectal Malformations in Children*, Year Book Medical Publishers, Chicago

115. Stephens, F.D. and Durham Smith, E. (1986) Classification, identification and assessment of surgical treatment of anorectal anomalies. *Pediat. Surg. Int.*, **1**, 200–205

116. Swenson, O. and Donnellan, W.L. (1967) Preservation of the puborectalis sling in imperforate anus. *Surg. Clin. N. Am.*, **47**, 173–193

117. Takada, Y., Aoyama, K., Goto, T. and Mori, S. (1985) The association of imperforate anus and

(depending on the gestational age). Unconjugated serum bilirubin levels greater than 220 μmol/l in full-term infants (and 255 μmol/l in preterm) are not 'physiological'. Haemolytic and metabolic causes then need to be excluded [75]. Infection, hypothyroidism, dehydration, low calorie intake and meconium retention are all problems which we have seen as causes of jaundice in 'surgical' infants.

It is, however, *conjugated hyperbilirubinaemia* which is of particular surgical significance. A few rare conditions deserve mention before more detailed consideration of infantile obstructive cholangiopathy.

Extrinsic obstructions of the bile duct

Pressure from outside the bile duct, causing obstruction to the flow of bile, is a common cause of obstructive jaundice in adults, but excessively rare in infancy. Obstruction in association with duodenal malformation [33] and pancreatic haemangio-endothelioma [113] has been reported. In the past 25 years we have encountered only one neonate with obstruction of biliary flow due to external pressure. This was an infant with gradually increasing jaundice from birth and a large cystic abdominal mass which, at laparotomy, was found to be an enormous left hydronephrosis causing compression of the porta hepatis [91].

Jaundice associated with hypertrophic pyloric stenosis

This used to be considered to be an extrahepatic obstructive jaundice due to pressure of the pyloric tumour on the bile ducts. The hyperbilirubinaemia is, however, largely due to an excess of unconjugated, indirect, bilirubin. A low level of activity of hepatic glucuronyl transferase seems to be the specific causative factor in a starved child. The condition need not really be included any more in discussions of obstructive jaundice (see Chapter 28).

Spontaneous perforation of the common bile duct

This is a rare condition with relatively few case reports in the literature [22,45,51,63,83,88]. The early symptoms include vomiting, increasing jaundice, obstructive in type, with pale stools and dark urine. The infant fails to thrive and develops ascites, which may occasionally lead to bile-stained inguinal herniae [45]. There is a higher bilirubin level in the ascitic fluid than in the serum [51], and the infant may develop severe toxaemia. The perforation, usually in the wall of the common bile duct, is usually explained as being due to local weakness and/or distal obstruction [63]. The perforation may

be repaired if it is accessible, and if a cholecystogram excludes obstruction to the distal common duct. More often, local inflammatory oedema precludes safe identification of the perforation and its repair, and a cholecystojejunostomy is made. Choledochal cysts have occurred (or been recognized) several years after spontaneous perforation [119].

Hepatic neoplasms

These are rare in the neonatal period and it must be very uncommon for them to cause biliary obstruction. We have records of only one such case with diffuse haemangiomatosis of the liver. This type of lesion may be rapidly fatal [117], but the infant in question recovered spontaneously, and must therefore have been an example of the benign type.

Cholestasis associated with intravenous feeding

Obstructive jaundice is often described in infants receiving total parenteral nutrition. The changes in biliary physiology may well be due to absence of enteral feeding rather than the components of the intravenous feed. Our own experience has led us to believe that the jaundice of infants on parenteral nutrition is almost always explained by finding complications such as infection (see Chapter 5).

The inspissated bile syndrome

This condition was first described [50] by Ladd in 1935 as jaundice caused by a plug of inspissated bile obstructing the common duct. Studies of the liver biopsies, has, however, revealed that most of these cases show evidence of parenchymal liver damage and fall into the group now more usually described as neonatal hepatitis. There are, nevertheless, occasional cases where inspissated bile seems to be the only abnormal finding. An operative cholangiogram washes out the system and the jaundice fades rapidly afterwards. Cases have been described where the inspissated material was actually removed from the common duct at surgery [85].

Infantile obstructive cholangiopathy (hepatitis syndrome of infancy)

This has been described as a lesion in search of a name [57]. Clinically the affected infant has an increased (conjugated) bilirubin level in the serum, bile in the urine, pale stools, hepatomegaly and evidence of hepatocellular damage and vitamin K deficiency. Pathologically, all have variable proportions of cholestasis, giant cell transformation, inflammatory infiltration, proliferation of bile ductules and fibrosis. Disease probably begins in a morphologically complete hepatobiliary system late

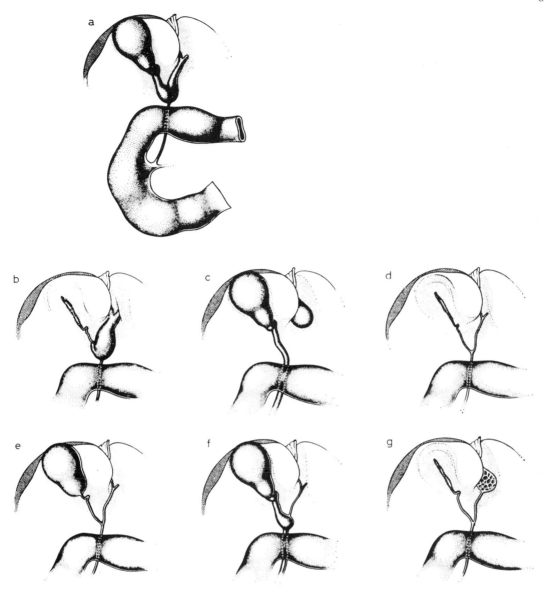

Figure 39.1 Types of biliary atresia encountered in Liverpool

in pregnancy or after delivery. It often progresses or persists even if bile drainage is later re-established.

Landing [61] considered that a single pathological process could lead to neonatal hepatitis, biliary atresia and choledochal cysts. Biliary hypoplasia should probably be included in this list. They all have some histological features in common, though in varying degrees.

In the fully developed condition of *biliary atresia* the bile ducts may be obstructed distally with dilated proximal ducts in the lesser omentum. This is

sometimes described as correctable extrahepatic atresia (Figure 39.1a–c). Rarely, a simple and easily correctable membranous obstruction is found in an otherwise normal duct system [86]. Another surgically correctable form has no major length of patent extrahepatic ducts but, while the major ducts are obstructed, dilated ducts are accessible in the porta hepatis. In the 'non-correctable' forms of biliary atresia (Figure 39.1d–g), the extrahepatic ducts are either entirely absent or any patent remnants are not connected to the intrahepatic biliary tree. The

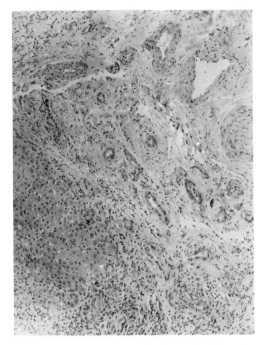

Figure 39.2 Photomicrograph of a section from the porta hepatis. No bile ducts were identifiable at surgery but tiny bile ductules are visible microscopically. The infant became anicteric after porto-enterostomy

hepatic duct is atretic and often hepatic radicles cannot be identified at surgery, though histological examination of the tissue from the porta hepatis may show tiny bile ductules (Figure 39.2). Relief of jaundice can be achieved in some of the forms previously described as 'non-correctable' by porto-enterostomy [29]. In 1959 Kasai described [54,55] a

new operation based on his experience of the development of an internal biliary fistula following the suturing of the duodenal wall to the porta hepatis to control haemorrhage.

Detailed histological studies of the remnants of the bile ducts have been reported from Japan [65,72]. The ducts are replaced by dense fibrous tissue with some inflammatory cell infiltration (Figure 39.3). Occasional isolated islands of epithelium may remain while in other sites small cystic spaces may contain bile-stained material but lack any epithelial lining. In Kasai's sections of the porta hepatis some of the bile ducts were obstructed by proliferating epithelium.

Within the liver itself, fibrosis of the portal areas, proliferation of bile ductules and plugging of interlobar bile ducts with bile pigment are the diagnostic histological features [11] (Figure 39.4); but features more typical of 'hepatitis' may also be found, namely, degenerative changes in the hepatic parenchyma and giant cell transformation [38,56,61].

Later in the disease process, marked hepatic cirrhosis may supervene. Bile stasis is probably the cause of this and its continuation beyond 3 months of age is assumed to render the process hopelessly irreversible. Some claim, however, that the cirrhosis can resolve, others give evidence that it persists or progresses even when bile is drained [36].

'Neonatal hepatitis' was first defined as a clinical entity by Craig and Landing in 1952 [19]. It is still, in many senses, a diagnosis reached by exclusion [39,50]. Infective, metabolic and endocrine causes need to be excluded (Table 39.1). While the histological picture is variable, a specific feature is well-marked giant cell transformation of the parenchymal cells (Figure 39.5). There is an increase in free iron, intracellular and intracanalicular bile retention, and inflammatory infiltration and fibrosis

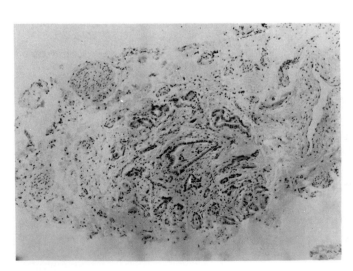

Figure 39.3 Photomicrograph of tissue from site of extrahepatic ducts. Instead of one large duct, there are numerous minute channels with a much reduced overall lumen. The amount of inflammatory and fibrous tissue is less marked in this specimen than usual

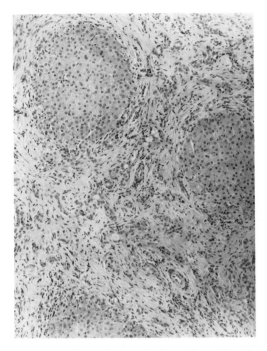

Figure 39.4 Photomicrograph of a section of liver from an infant with biliary atresia. There is portal fibrosis and proliferation of bile ductules. Precipitated bile pigment plugs are not obvious in this section

Table 39.1 Commoner causes of conjugated hyperbilirubinaemia

Infective	*Metabolic*	*Endocrine*
Septicaemia	Galactosaemia	Hypothyroidism
Urinary infection	Fructosaemia	Hypopituitarism
Toxoplasmosis	Alpha-1-antitrypsin	Hypoadrenalism
Hepatitis B	deficiency	
Syphilis	Cystic fibrosis	

of the portal tracts. Bile duct proliferation may occur, as in atresia, but it is usually not such a prominent feature.

The pregnancy history of infants with 'hepatitis' is often abnormal and birth weight may be low. In most infants, the jaundice, and evidence of liver disease, fades over a few months, but a mortality rate of 15% is recorded, and some show progressive cirrhosis [38].

Intrahepatic bile duct hypoplasia is easily confused with hepatitis or atresia, but is a distinct entity [58,87]. The diagnosis depends on the histological recognition of the small size or paucity of the intralobar ducts. The condition can be divided into 'syndromic' or 'non-syndromic' forms. In the former, certain extrahepatic features may lead to the early recognition of Alagille's syndrome [2] (Table 39.2). The non-syndromic forms have a worse

Table 39.2 Extrahepatic features of Alagille's syndrome

Pulmonary stenosis
'Butterfly' vertebrae
Embryotoxon in anterior chamber of eye
Abnormal facies
Growth retardation
Mental retardation

prognosis, even though the pathology is isolated to the liver. There is often a marked degree of hepatic fibrosis. It can be familial as in alpha-1-antitrypsin deficiency, or related to infections such as cytomegalovirus or rubella. It is of great importance [39,64] to diagnose hepatitis and intrahepatic hypoplasia without recourse to open surgery, since laparotomy (or perhaps anaesthesia) is said to aggravate the hepatitis, and exploration of the extrahepatic ducts cannot help and may well lead to total obstruction in the infant with hypoplasia [77].

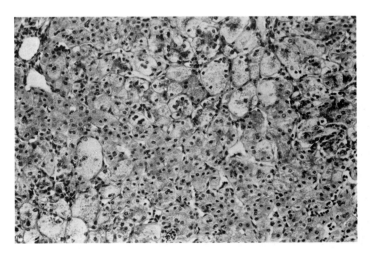

Figure 39.5 Photomicrograph of a section of liver from an infant with 'neonatal hepatitis'. There are numerous multinucleate giant cells. The infant made an uneventual recovery

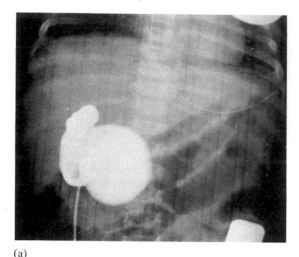

(a)

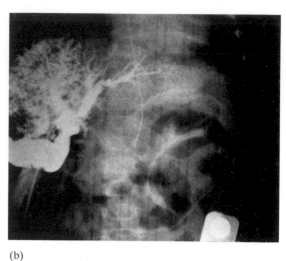

(b)

Figure 39.6 Radiographs of an infant showing (a) filling of the gall bladder and choledochal cyst, and (b) reflux into right and left hepatic ducts after clamping the inferior portion of the cyst. The infant had been jaundiced from the tenth day of life and was presumed to have atresia. The cyst was not palpable

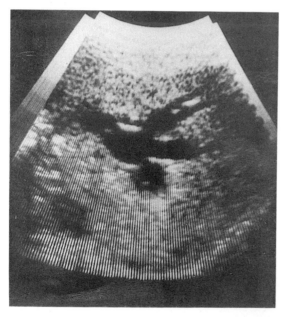

Figure 39.7 Ultrasound scan of a jaundiced infant showing marked dilatation of the common bile duct and distal hepatic ducts

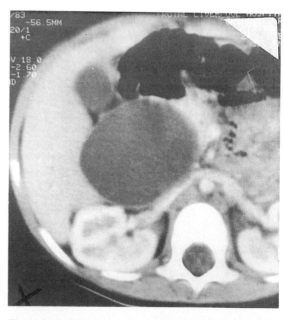

Figure 39.8 CT scan (contrast enhanced) of a jaundiced infant showing a large choledochal cyst and distended gall bladder

Choledochal cysts (Figures 39.6, 39.7 and 39.8), although relatively rare, have been widely reported and reviewed [17,93,105,119,122]. They may present at any age [118], and occasionally are discovered in the neonate with obstructive jaundice. As with other neonatal biliary obstructions, the hepatic pathology is relatively non-specific but there is less severe plugging of interlobar ducts and usually less fibrosis than in atresia, and most authors consider it to be part of the same disease process that leads to hepatitis or atresia. Lilly [66] believes it to be a true malformation rather than an acquired lesion like atresia, but it has also been described [120] as occurring late after spontaneous perforation of the common bile duct. Where it is looked for, an anomalous choledochopancreatic duct junction is found [48,93,114], and the extramural inflow of pancreatic enzymes refluxing up the bile ducts may be the important factor in the aetiology. Choledochal cysts are commoner in females than males [93,105] and familial cases have been described [18].

The classic description is of a recurrent obstructive jaundice, associated with pain and fever, and a mass in the right hypochondrium. In the neonatal period, the first 'attack' may be observed and ultrasound and isotope scans should lead to an early, correct diagnosis (Figure 39.7).

The treatment of choice [20,65,70,71,85,93] is excision of the cyst, and internal drainage via a long Roux-en-Y loop of jejunum. The simpler expedient of making a cystojejunostomy is associated with a considerable risk of complications – recurrent cholangitis, stone formation, malignant change in the cyst wall and pancreatitis.

Intrahepatic cystic changes of the bile ducts are also recognized [7,102]. Caroli originally described [16] intrahepatic cysts in isolation, but they have been reported as multiple [114] and in association with extrahepatic biliary atresia and with extrahepatic cystic changes of the main bile ducts. It should be remembered that the intrahepatic biliary system will become dilated in the presence of extrahepatic duct obstruction, while in biliary atresia the intrahepatic ducts are not dilated, but are often narrow and irregular.

Associated anomalies

A large number of variations in the pattern of the biliary tree are recognized, but these should probably not be considered as anomalies since function is not impaired, and the infantile obstructive cholangiopathies are not associated with any particular pattern of branching of the ducts, although the relationship of the distal duct to the pancreatic duct and the sphincters may well be of importance [93,114,118].

Duodenal malformations are not commonly associated with biliary atresia [89], but polysplenia and splenic hypoplasia are, whether or not there is co-existent situs inversus. Abnormalities of the subdiaphragmatic venous system, and cyanotic heart disease are also described with biliary atresia.

Embryology

The liver and biliary tract are formed from a diverticulum that arises from the ventral surface of the primitive gut – from the portion destined to become the duodenum. Later rotation and differential growth of the duodenal wall move the orifice of this diverticulum posteriorly and ultimately to its left-sided position. The diverticulum gives two lateral branches, one to form the ventral anlage of the pancreas, and the other the cystic duct and gall bladder. By the fifth week all the elements of the biliary tree are recognizable and considerable elongation of the ducts is occurring together with plugging of the lumen by epithelial cells. Cell proliferation of the terminal portion takes place very rapidly to produce masses of cells which invade the septum transversum to form the primordium of the liver parenchyma [101]. These cells surround the vitelline veins and lateral umbilical vessels and, later, the umbilical veins. The veins break up into numerous small sinusoids lined by parenchymal cells.

Bile canaliculi differentiate from hepatic cells [26], and the development of an intrahepatic duct system is complete by the tenth week. Recanalization of the extrahepatic ducts occurs in parallel with the duodenum [97], beginning at about the sixth week, although the gall bladder does not redevelop a lumen until the 12th week, by which time bile is found in the duct system and reaches the intestine by the fifth month [34].

Aetiology

Biliary atresia is now generally considered not to be a developmental anomaly in the sense of one arising from a failure of the normal embryological processes. Agenesis of the bile ducts would lead to agenesis of the liver. Failure of recanalization is feasible but almost certainly not the cause of biliary atresia, since the meconium is always bile stained, and many infants who ultimately are proved to have biliary atresia are known not to have been jaundiced at birth [53]. Experimental total obstruction of the bile flow in fetal puppies leads to the birth of jaundiced animals [42].

It is therefore concluded that some obliterative process takes place in formed extrahepatic ducts [30,36]. The process is inflammatory, and could be chemical due to pancreatic juice flowing into the biliary system. The anatomy of the hepatopancreatic junction has been studied extensively [72,118], particular interest being focused on variations in the site of the sphincter muscle. The sclerosing inflammatory process could be infective. Rubella and hepatitis A and B viruses have been suggested, but the best evidence is for a perinatal infection with Reovirus type III [6,74].

Whether the causative agent produces hepatitis, hypoplasia or atresia or choledochal cyst may depend on the susceptibility of the biliary epithelium and the liver parenchyma, and this in turn could be related to age and maturity, or to sex and other genetic factors. The syndromic type of hypoplasia

[2] (Alagille's syndrome) seems to be an autosomal dominant disease, and the non-syndromic type associated with alpha-1-antitrypsin deficiency is sometimes familial also.

Incidence

Biliary atresia occurs in about 1 in 10 000 live births [1,44], and despite the well-established belief that it is more common in Japanese than in Caucasian infants, the incidence is probably similar. It may be much higher in infants of Chinese descent according to a study published in 1974 [104].

Atresia is said to be less common in negro infants, but there is no difference in the incidence of hepatitis in white and coloured racial groups. Biliary atresia and choledochal cysts are commoner in females, but males have a higher incidence of hepatitis [11,94].

Clinical features

Clinical features and laboratory findings must be precisely defined in relation to the stage of the disease. Biliary atresia usually progresses inexorably from obstructive jaundice in an otherwise thriving infant, to death within 1 or 2 years from hepatic failure, though some children survive for several years to become deeply bronzed with generalized wasting and massive abdominal distension from hepatosplenomegaly and ascites, and sometimes exhibiting peripheral cyanosis and finger clubbing. The infant with neonatal hepatitis or biliary duct hypoplasia often shows some degree of failure to thrive, and the extrahepatic features of the syndromic forms of hypoplasia should be looked for – cardiac murmurs, butterfly vertebrae, and embryotoxon in the anterior chamber of the eye, as well as the characteristic facies (Table 39.2).

The neonate who will ultimately be proved to have biliary atresia may be of smaller birth weight than average [104] and may not be jaundiced at first. Kimura [56] found that only 35% of infants with atresia were jaundiced at birth. Jaundice is usually apparent in the first few days and certainly within the first 4 weeks, though Rickham [90] described a child who was perfectly normal for the first 6 months of life and then, following a further 2 months of jaundice was found to have atresia. At the other extreme, the diagnosis has been made antenatally and surgery done on the fourth day of life [35].

Stools may be similarly acholic in atresia and hepatitis, and the urine dark with bile. Liver enlargement is common to both conditions; the liver remains soft for the first couple of months, but is increasingly obviously cirrhotic later. Vitamin K deficiency may lead to haemorrhages at an early

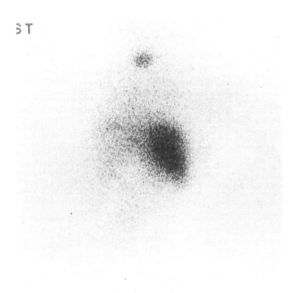

(a)

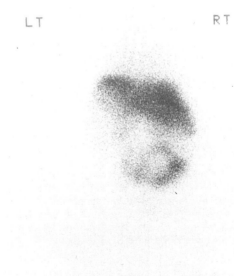

(b)

Figure 39.9 (a) Gamma camera scan of infant 24 h after injection of ^{123}I-bromsulphthalein. There has been no excretion into the intestine and isotope is retained in the liver. Biliary atresia.

(b) Similar scan 4 h after injection of isotope. The amount of retention in the liver suggests poor function, but isotope has been excreted into the gut. Hepatitis

age, and hepatocellular damage is evidenced by raised transaminases in both conditions. Considerable effort used to be expended, and valuable time lost, by attempting to differentiate hepatitis and atresia biochemically. It was usually a fruitless exercise and an operative cholangiogram and exploratory laparotomy were required to reach a diagnosis. Isotope scans, combined perhaps with a percutaneous needle biopsy [3,69], have made an almost certain diagnosis possible by the age of 6 weeks, so that the surgeon can avoid operating on infants with hepatitis, and can approach a laparotomy for the infant with atresia with a considerable degree of certainty about what will be found at surgery [40].

Different isotopes are favoured by different centres [27,69,82,106], ^{123}I bromsulphthalein (rose bengal) is made more reliable by measuring faecal excretion as well as using simple abdominal scanning (Figure 39.9). If more than 10% of the isotope is excreted into the faeces in 72 h the child has not got atresia. DISIDA (diisopropyl iminodiacetic acid) labelled with 99m-technetium is said [21] to be quicker than rose bengal, by noting not only excretion into the gut, but also the ratio of hepatic to cardiac distribution. Phenobarbitone may enhance excretion and clarify the picture [3].

Management

Conjugated hyperbilirubinaemia in the early weeks of life needs to be regarded with considerable suspicion and the infant investigated urgently [14,75]. Initial screening for infection is done, and urinalysis for non-glucose reducing substances. The prothrombin time should be measured and parenteral vitamin K started. Alpha-1-antitrypsin deficiency is excluded (by determining the phenotype rather than the concentration). Ultrasonography may give some idea of the gross pattern of the liver, but, more usefully, will reveal a choledochal cyst – or perhaps demonstrate a normal biliary system. Our local preference is then to arrange an isotope scan ([131]-I rose bengal), and only to do a needle biopsy of the liver if the diagnosis is in doubt and a laparotomy is not obviously essential. Where surgery is needed, the chances of success fade rapidly after the 60th day of life [25], and we aim to operate by the sixth or seventh week of life if at all possible.

As already stated, surgery is usually undertaken with a firm diagnosis based on an isotope scan and perhaps a needle biopsy. The operation should be planned so that only a cholangiogram is done if the patency of the ducts is proved. Preparation should be made, and the parents' agreement obtained to proceed to full exploration and porto-enterostomy if necessary. Vitamin K is given parenterally and blood crossmatched. Under general anaesthesia the

infant is placed supine with a small towel under the left side to roll him a little so that the gall bladder, and biliary system, if present, will not be overlying the vertebral column if an X-ray is taken. A small (4-cm) muscle-cutting transverse incision is made in the right upper quadrant over the gall bladder. With suitable moist packs and malleable retractors the inferior surface of the liver can be inspected easily with minimal disturbance of the intestines. If the gall bladder is present, its fundus is opened between stay sutures and the contents noted. A fine catheter (filled with saline) is introduced and the aqueous contrast medium is injected gently and the film exposed. Further films may be required with more contrast medium injected or with the inferior end of the free edge of the lesser omentum gripped by a bulldog clamp to encourage intrahepatic filling. The catheter is removed and the gall bladder closed with catgut. A small wedge of liver is taken from its diaphragmatic surface and, after haemostasis is secured, the abdomen is closed, if the cholangiogram is normal.

In our hands (or perhaps more truthfully, with the anaesthetic technique used by our colleagues) no significant risk is involved in this procedure. We have not found any case of hepatitis which has deteriorated abruptly following this, though our experience contrasts with the reports of others [56].

If there is no lumen to the gall bladder the transverse abdominal wound is extended and the bile ducts explored. The gall bladder is dissected from its bed and the cystic duct followed to the hepatic duct (Figure 39.10). The peritoneum along the free edge of the lesser omentum is opened and the remains of the hepatic and common bile ducts are identified. They are usually represented by a distinct fibrous track. We consider it wise to identify, and usually to put slings around, the hepatic artery and to ligate its cystic branch after the right hepatic branch has been defined. At the upper border of the duodenum, the fibrous remnant of the common bile duct is ligated and divided, and then the other remnants of the ducts are dissected right up into the porta hepatis. If any major and patent biliary ducts are discovered then clearly the dissection need proceed no further provided bile is seen to drain or cholangiograms demonstrate good connections with the intrahepatic biliary system. In the more usual case no macroscopically identifiable extrahepatic ducts are found and the mass of scar tissue is excised from within the porta hepatis, continuing the dissection for a short distance into the liver substance (Figure 39.2).

Kasai's original operation involved the construction of a Roux-en-Y loop of jejunum [53,54,55]. The end of the jejunal loop was closed and anastomosis between the porta hepatis and the jejunal loop made through the antimesenteric border of the proximal end of this loop (Figure 39.10). A variety of

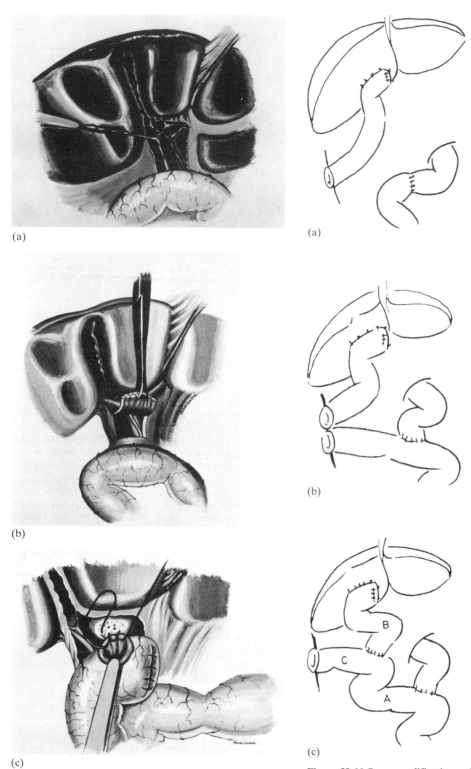

(a)

(b)

(c)

Figure 39.10 Stages of porto-enterostomy (from Kasai [53])

(a)

(b)

(c)

Figure 39.11 Some modifications of the simple porto-enterostomy (from Kasai [53]): (a) Sawaguchi [95], (b) Suruga [107], (c) Kasai [53]

modifications of the intestinal drainage system have been devised [15,53,96,108] in the hope of preventing postoperative cholangitis (Figure 39.11).

The hepatic ducts lie in close relationship to the branches of the portal vein [4]. Suruga and his co-workers reported [107] in 1976 considerably improved results when the dissection at the porta hepatis is done with the aid of an operating microscope to ensure that the right and left ducts are dissected out without damage to the surrounding small blood vessels, lymphatics and liver parenchyma. They later listed [108] the operative factors that they considered to be of particular importance, and apart from the continued recommendation to use magnification, they listed frozen section for the verification that dissection had proceeded far enough, a jejunal anastomosis very close to the margins of the opened ducts at the porta hepatis and then drainage to a cutaneous stoma.

Diversion of the jejunal conduit to the surface, while it allows clear observation of any bile flow, is found not to affect the long-term outcome [13], has a considerable morbidity – a 43% incidence of stomal haemorrhage – and has not reduced the incidence of ascending cholangitis [41,44]. An anti-reflux Roux-en-Y has been tried experimentally and with a few children [28,103,111]. Hepatic portogastrostomy has also been recommended [46].

Phenobarbitone is often recommended postoperatively to potentiate the liver enzymes that conjugate bilirubin. No clear benefit has been demonstrated in its use [115]. Cholestyramine appears to reduce serum bile acid levels and to improve liver function [52]. Experimental studies on bile flow after a diverting portenterostomy have been reported, and do not provide firm evidence for the effectiveness of any of the so-called cholagogues [47,115].

Broad-spectrum antibiotics, active against Gram-negative and anaerobic organisms should be given at operation and postoperatively [10,62]. Their long-term prophylactic administration is probably not effective in preventing cholangitis which is a common complication and one which probably leads to increasing liver damage. Recurrent cholangitis is common [67,80,109], and is probably best treated with high dose/short duration antibiotic therapy [62]. The simultaneous administration of corticosteroids is said [52] to be associated with a more rapid drop in temperature, a quicker return to normal serum bilirubin and alkaline phosphatase levels. Immunoglobulin (IgA) may play a protective role [95].

Re-operation is now an accepted procedure, and has many exponents [37,78,110]. Cessation of bile flow after an initially successful porto-enterostomy is an absolute indication for re-exploration [78]. Blockage is said to be due to granulation tissue over the dissected area of the porta hepatis. It can be removed by curettage or by further dissection and trimming of the tissues. Insufficient flow of bile after the initial operation may also be improved by further exploration, but the indications for re-exploration in this situation are not so clear [84,110].

Results

Untreated, only 2% of infants with extrahepatic biliary atresia will survive for 4 years; most will die within the first 2 years. The results of porto-enterostomy for atresia are expressed in rather different terms from different centres. Schweizer lists [98,99] five criteria for success:

(1) operation is performed before 6 weeks of age,
(2) there is no cirrhosis at this time,
(3) there are no morphological changes in the intrahepatic bile ducts,
(4) duct diameters at the porta hepatis are >450 μm,
(5) no cholangitis occurs after surgery.

Kasai [53], and later Miyano *et al*. [72], had earlier set a lower limit of duct size at 200 μm, but Suruga found no correlation between duct size and long-term survival [109].

Some bile flow is reported in most published series in about two-thirds of infants operated on, with a 5-year survival rate of 30–35%. Schweizer found that 66% of those patients with 'good' criteria at surgery were well at 5 years of age [98,99]. The Japanese paediatric surgeons, however, continue to obtain much better success rates (90% 10-year survival rates in those operated on before 60 days of age). In Europe and North America, it seems that, although some bile flow is very often obtained following the initial surgery, only about one-third of the children become free of jaundice, and rather fewer are alive and well in late childhood. Our own experience in Liverpool accords with this.

Apart from persistent jaundice, other long-term problems are commonly reported. Recurrent cholangitis has been discussed above, and is likely to lead to further biliary obstruction, and increasing liver damage. Histological evidence of cirrhosis will be found, if looked for, in perhaps as many as 90% of survivors [31.32]. Portal hypertension may develop because of damage to the portal vein at surgery, or because of the developing cirrhosis [68,79,81]. Variceal haemorrhage has been reported in 23% of survivors, occurring as early as 5 months of age.

When Kasai's operation fails to allow any bile drainage, or when it is inadequate and cirrhosis is early and rapid, the only alternative to early death is liver transplantation. This is now a proven procedure [12,49], and practised in an increasing number of centres. A limiting factor is the difficulty in obtaining sufficient numbers of small donor organs [76]. The technique of liver transplantation is made more difficult [84] by previous abdominal surgery, particularly if complex drainage techniques with stomata have been used, but this does not make the survival rate poorer. One-year survival rates of up to 90% are obtainable. The 5-year survival rate is 60%. Transplantation is not usually done in children under 2 years of age, but there is no absolute contraindication to transplantation in younger or smaller infants. It is important to ensure that, during the time that they are waiting for a transplant, they are kept in as good a state of nutrition as possible. Feeds with medium chain triglycerides in place of fats are needed, and the fat soluble vitamins must be provided [73].

The treatment of children with biliary atresia – and indeed with most forms of liver disease – is still far from satisfactory. Elucidation of the exact aetiology could possibly lead to prevention. Medical or surgical intervention after the onset of the process that destroys the ducts is unlikely ever to produce 'cures', but refinements of technique have led to improvement in length and quality of life in a proportion of children with an otherwise fatal condition.

References

1. Alagille, D. (1984) Extrahepatic biliary atresia. *Hepatology*, **4**, 7–10
2. Alagille, D., Odièvre, M., Gautier, M. and Dommergues, J.P. (1975) Hepatic ductular hypoplasia associated with characteristic facies, vertebral malformations, retarded physical, mental and skeletal development and cardiac murmur. *J. Pediat.*, **86**, 63–71
3. Altman, R.P. and Levy, J. (1985) Biliary atresia. *Pediat. Ann.*, **14**, 481–485
4. Ando, H., Ito, T. and Nagaya, M. (1984) Ultrasonographic studies of intrahepatic bile ducts: a contribution to operation of biliary atresia. *J. Jap. Soc. Pediat. Surg.*, **20**, 1199–1206
5. Arey, L.B. (1965) *Developmental Anatomy: a Textbook and Laboratory Manual of Embryology*, 7th Edition, W.B. Saunders, Philadelphia
6. Banjura, B., Morecki, R., Glaser, H., Gartner, L.M. and Horwitz, H.S. (1980) Comparative studies of biliary atresia in the human newborn and Reo virus-induced cholangitis in weanling mice. *Lab. Invest.*, **43**, 456–461
7. Barros, J.L., Polo, J.R., Sanabia, J., Garcia-Sabrido, J.L. and Gomez-Lorenzo, F.J. (1979) Congenital cystic dilatation of the intrahepatic bile ducts (Caroli's disease): report of a case and review of the literature. *Surgery*, **85**, 589–592
8. Bill, A.H. (1974) Introduction: biliary atresia and choledochal cyst. *Progr. Pediat. Surg.*, **6**, 1–3
9. Bill, A.H., Brennon, W.S. and Huselay, T.L. (1974) Biliary atresia; new concepts of pathology, diagnosis and management. *Arch. Surg.*, **109**, 367–369
10. Brook, I. and Altman, R.P. (1984) The significance of anaerobic bacteria in biliary tract infection after hepatic portoenterostomy for biliary atresia. *Surgery*, **95**, 281–283
11. Brough, A.J. and Bernstein, J. (1969) Liver biopsy in the diagnosis of infantile obstructive jaundice. *Pediatrics*, **43**, 519–526
12. Burdelski, M., Jurgens, K. and Budde, M. (1985) Indications for liver transplantation in childhood. *Z. Kinderchir.*, **40**, 268–269
13. Burnweit, C.A. and Coln, D. (1986) Influence of diversion on the development of cholangitis after hepatoportoenterostomy for biliary atresia. *J. Pediat. Surg.*, **21**, 1143–1146
14. Campbell, D.P., Poley, J.R., Alaupovic, P. and Ide Smith, E. (1974) The differential diagnosis of neonatal hepatitis and biliary atresia. *J. Pediat. Surg.*, 699–705
15. Canty, T.G., Self, T.W., Collins, D.L. and Donaldi, L. (1985) Recent experience with a modified Sawaguchi procedure for biliary atresia. *J. Pediat. Surg.*, **20**, 211–216
16. Caroli, J., Soupault, R. and Kossakowski, J. (1958) La dilatation polikistique congénitale de voies biliaries intrahépatique. Essai de classification. *Sem. Hôp. Paris.*, **34**, 488–495
17. Chang, M.H., Wang, T.H., Cheu, C.C. and Hung, W.T. (1986) Congenital bile duct dilatation in children. *J. Pediat. Surg.*, **21**, 112–117
18. Chiba, T. (1981) Congenital bile duct dilatation in siblings. *Z. Kinderchir.*, **32**, 118–190
19. Craig, J.M. and Landing, B.H. (1952) Form of hepatitis in neonatal period simulating biliary atresia. *Arch. Path.*, **54**, 321–333
20. Crittenden, S.L. and McKinley, M.J. (1985) Choledochal cyst – clinical features and classification. *Am. J. Gastroenterol.*, **80**, 643–647
21. Dick, M.C. and Mowat, A.P. (1986) Biliary scintigraphy with DISIDA. *Arch. Dis. Child.*, **61**, 191–192
22. Donahoe, P.K. and Hendren, W.H. (1976) Bile duct perforation in a newborn with stenosis of the ampulla of Vater. *J. Pediat. Surg.*, **11**, 823–825
23. Donop, C.F. (1828) De ictero speciation neonatorum. Inaugural Dissertation, Berlin
24. Douglas, A.H. (1852) Case of dilatation of the common duct. *Month. J. med. Sci.,* **14**, 97–101
25. Editorial (1980) Biliary atresia. Lessons from Japanese experience. *Lancet*, **ii**, 1283–1284
26. Elias, H. (1955) Origin and early development of the liver in various vertebrates. *Acta Hepat.*, **3**, 1
27. El Tumi, M.A., Clarke, M.B., Barrett, J.J. and Mowat, A.P. (1987) Ten minute radiopharmaceutical test in biliary atresia. *Arch. Dis. Child.*, **62**, 180–184
28. Endo, M., Sanbonmatsu, T. and Hagane, K. (1985) Non refluxing draining conduit for biliary atresia: an intussuscepted ileocolic conduit and the conduit-duodenostomy. *Jap. J. Pediat. Surg.*, **17**, 41–49

29. Gans, S.L. (1983) Correctable or not correctable: biliary atresia. *J. Pediat. Surg.*, **18**, 107–108

30. Gautier, M. and Elliot, N. (1981) Extrahepatic biliary atresia: morphological study of 94 biliary remnants. *Arch. Path. Lab. Med.*, **105**, 397–504

31. Gautier, M., Moitier, G. and Odièvre, M. (1980) Uncorrectable extrahepatic biliary atresia: relationship between intrahepatic bile duct pattern and surgery. *J. Pediat. Surg.*, **15**, 129–132

32. Gautier, M., Valayer, J., Odièvre, M. and Alagille, D. (1984) Histological liver evaluation 5 years after surgery for extrahepatic biliary atresia, a study of 20 cases. *J. Pediat. Surg.*, **19**, 263–268

33. Gillespie, J.B. and Rogers, J.C.T. (1940) Enterogenous cyst of duodenum. *Archs Pediat.*, **57**, 652–658

34. Gray, S.W. and Skandalakis, J.E. (1972) *Embryology for Surgeons*, W.B. Saunders, Philadelphia

35. Greenholz, S.K., Lilly, J.R., Shikes, R.H. and Hall, R.J. (1986) Biliary atresia in the newborn. *J. Pediat. Surg.*, **21**, 1147–1148

36. Haas, J.E. (1978) Bile duct and liver pathology in biliary atresia. *World J. Surg.*, **2**, 561–569

37. Hata, Y. Uchino, J. and Kasai, Y. (1985) Revision of portoenterostomy in congenital biliary atresia. *J. Pediat. Surg.*, **20**, 217–220

38. Heathcote, J., Deodhar, K.P., Scheuer, P.J. and Sherlock, S. (1976) Intrahepatic cholestasis in childhood. *New Engl. J. Med.*, **295**, 801–805

39. Henriksen, N.T., Drablos, P.A. and Aagenaes, O. (1981) Cholestatic jaundice in infancy. The importance of familial and genetic factors in the aetiology and prognosis. *Arch. Dis. Child.*, **56**, 622–627

40. Hirsig, J. and Rickham, P.P. (1980) Early differential diagnosis between neonatal hepatitis and biliary atresia. *J. Pediat. Surg.*, **15**, 13–15

41. Hirsig, J., Kara, D. and Rickham, P.P. (1978) Experimental investigations into the etiology of cholangitis following operation for biliary atresia. *J. Pediat. Surg.*, **78**, 55–58

42. Holder, T.M. and Ashcraft, K.W. (1967) Effects of bile duct ligation and inflammation in the fetus. *J. Pediat. Surg.*, **2**, 35–40

43. Holmes, J.B. (1916) Congenital obliteration of the bile duct: diagnosis and suggestions for treatment. *Am. J. Dis. Child.*, **11**, 405–431

44. Howard, E.R. (1983) Extra-hepatic biliary atresia: A review of current management. *Br. J. Surg.*, **70**, 193–197

45. Howard, E.R., Johnstone, D.I. and Mowat, A.P. (1976) Spontaneous perforation of the common bile duct in infants. *Arch. Dis. Child.*, **51**, 883–886

46. Ikeda, K. and Suita, S. (1975) Hepatic portogastrostomy using a gastric tube for the treatment of congenital biliary atresia. *Z. Kinderchir.*, **17**, 360

47. Isenberg, J.N. and Schwatz, M.Z. (1984) Stimulation of bile output by gastrointestinal hormones following portoenterostomy for biliary atresia. *J. Pediat. Surg.*, **19**, 471–475

48. Ito, T., Ando, H. and Nagaya, M. (1984) Congenital dilatation of the common bile duct in children – the etiologic significance of the narrow segment distal to the dilated common bile duct. *Z. Kinderchir.*, **39**, 40–45

49. Iwatsuki, S., Shaw, B. and Starzl, T. (1984) Liver transplantation for biliary atresia. *World J. Surg.*, **8**, 51–56

50. Japan Medical Research Foundation (1980) Cholestasis in infancy – its pathogenesis, diagnosis and treatment. University of Tokyo Press, Tokyo

51. Johnston, J.H. (1961) Spontaneous perforation of the common bile duct in infancy. *Br. J. Surg.*, **48**, 532–533

52. Karrer, F.M. and Lilly, J.R. (1985) Corticosteroid therapy in biliary atresia. *J. Pediat. Surg.*, **20**, 693–695

53. Kasai, M. (1974) Treatment of biliary atresia with special reference to hepatic portoenterostomy and its modifications. *Prog. Pediat. Surg.*, **6**, 5–52

54. Kasai, M., Kimura, S., Asakura, Y., Suzuki, H., Taira, Y. and Ohashi, E. (1968) Surgical treatment of biliary atresia. *J. Pediat. Surg.*, **3**, 665–675

55. Kasai, M. and Suzuki, S. (1950) A new operation for 'non-correctable' biliary atresia: hepatic portoenterostomy. *Shujitsu*, **13**, 733–739 (in Japanese)

56. Kimura, S. (1974) The early diagnosis of biliary atresia. *Progr. Pediat. Surg.*, **6**, 91–112

57. Koop, C.E. (1975) Progressive extrahepatic biliary obstruction of the newborn. *J. Pediat. Surg.*, **10**, 169–170

58. Krant, S.M. and Swenson, O. (1973) Biliary duct hypoplasia. *J. Pediat. Surg.*, **8**, 301–307

59. Ladd W.E. (1928) Congenital atresia and stenosis of the bile ducts. *J. Am. Med. Ass.*, **91**, 1082–1085

60. Ladd, W.E. (1935) Congenital obstruction of the bile ducts. *Ann. Surg.*, **102**, 742–751

61. Landing, B.H. (1974) Considerations of the pathogenesis of neonatal hepatitis, biliary atresia and choledochal cyst – the concept of infantile obstructive cholangiopathy. *Progr. Pediat. Surg.*, **6**, 113–139

62. Leblanc, A., Lambert-Zechovsky, N., Proux, M.-Chr. and Odièvre, M. (1983) Bacteriological analysis of jejunostomy fluid after surgery for extrahepatic biliary atresia. *J. Pediat. Gastroenterol. Nutr.*, **2**, 307–310

63. Lees, W. (1966) Bile peritonitis in infancy. *Archs Dis. Child.*, **41**, 185–192

64. Lilly, J.R. (1976) The surgery of biliary hypoplasia. *J. Pediat. Surg.*, **11**, 815–821

65. Lilly, J.R. (1979) The surgical treatment of choledochal cyst. *Surg. Gynec. Obstet.*, **149**, 36–42

66. Lilly, J.R. (1985) Choledochal cyst and 'correctable' biliary atresia. *J. Pediat. Surg.*, **20**, 299–301

67. Lilly, J.R. and Hitch, D.C. (1978) Postoperative ascending cholangitis following portoenterostomy for biliary atresia: measures for control. *World J. Surg.*, **2**, 581–587

68. Lilly, J.R. and Stellin, G. (1984) Variceal haemorrhage in biliary atresia. *J. Pediat. Surg.*, **19**, 476–479

69. Manolaki, A.G., Larcher, V.F., Mowat, A.P., Barrett, J.J., Portman, B. and Howard, E.R. (1983) The pre-laparotomy diagnosis of extrahepatic biliary atresia. *Arch. Dis. Child.*, **58**, 591–594

70. Miyano, T. and Suruga, K. (1983) Choledochal cyst. *J. Jap. Soc. Pediat. Surg.*, **19**, 1061–1068

71. Miyano, T. and Suruga, K. (1984) The importance of early excision of primarily drained choledochal cysts. *Ann. Paediat. Surg.*, **1**, 89–91

72. Miyano, T., Suruga, K., Tsuchiya, H. and Suda, K. (1977) A histopathological study of the remnant of the extrahepatic bile duct in so-called uncorrectable biliary atresia. *J. Pediat. Surg.*, **12**, 19–25

73. Miyano, T., Yamashiro, Y., Shimizu, T., Arai, T. and Hayasawa, H. (1986) Essential fatty acid deficiency in congenital biliary atresia: successful treatment to reverse deficiency. *J. Pediat. Surg.*, **21**, 277–281

74. Morecki, R., Slaser, J. and Cho, S. (1982) Biliary atresia and Reovirus type 3 infection. *New Engl. J. Med.*, **307**, 481–484

75. Mowat, A.P. (1986) Disorders of the liver and biliary system. In: *Textbook of Neonatology* (ed. N.R.C. Robertson), Churchill Livingstone, Edinburgh, pp. 394–406

76. Mowat, A.P. (1987) Liver transplantation – a role for all paediatricians. *Arch. Dis. Child.*, **62**, 325–326

77. Odièvre, M., Hadchouel, M., Landrieu, C., Alagille, D. and Elliot, N. (1981) Long-term prognosis for infants with intrahepatic cholestasis and patent extrahepatic biliary tract. *Arch. Dis. Child.*, **56**, 373–376

78. Ohi, R., Hanamatsu, M., Mochizuki, I., Ohkohchi, N. and Kasai, M. (1985) Reoperation in patients with biliary atresia. *J. Pediat. Surg.*, **20**, 256–259

79. Ohi, R., Mochizuki, I., Komatsu, K. and Kasai, M. (1986) Portal hypertension after successful hepatic portoenterostomy in biliary atresia. *J. Pediat. Surg.*, **21**, 271–274

80. Ohi, R., Shikes, R.H., Stellin, G.P. and Lilly, J.R. (1984) In biliary atresia duct histology correlates with bile flow. *J. Pediat. Surg.*, **19**, 467–470

81. Ohuchi, N., Ohi, R., Takaheshi, T. and Kasai, M. (1986) Postoperative changes of intrahepatic portal veins in biliary atresia – a 3-D reconstruction study. *J. Pediat. Surg.*, **21**, 10–14

82. Padhy, A.K., Gopinath, P.G. and Basu, A.K. (1984) Role of hepatobiliary scintigraphy in the evaluation of infantile jaundice using Tc-99M-N-Butyl Iminodiacetic Acid (BULIDA). *Ann. Paediat. Surg.*, **1**, 101–105

83. Petterson, G. (1955) Spontaneous perforation of the common bile duct in infants. *Acta Chir. Scand.*, **110**, 192–201

84. Pettitt, B.J., Zitelli, B.J. and Rowe, M.I. (1984) Analysis of patients with biliary atresia coming to liver transplantation. *J. Pediat. Surg.*, **19**, 779–785

85. Pickett, L.K. (1969) The liver and biliary tract. In: *Pediatric Surgery* (ed. W.T. Mustard, M.M. Ravitch, W.H. Snyder, K.J. Welch and C.D. Benson) Year Book Publishers, Chicago

86. Pinter, A., Pilaszanovich, I., Schafer, J. and Weisenbach, J. (1975) Membranous obstruction of the common bile duct. *J. Pediat. Surg.*, **10**, 839–840

87. Porter, S.D., Soper, R.T. and Tidrick, R.T. (1968) Biliary hypoplasia. *Ann. Surg.*, **167**, 602–608

88. Prévot, J. and Babut, J.M. (1971) Spontaneous perforation of the biliary tract in infancy. *Prog. Pediat. Surg.*, **1**, 187–208

89. Reid, I.S. (1973) Biliary tract abnormalities associated with duodenal atresia. *Arch. Dis. Child.*, **48**, 952–957

90. Rickham, P.P. (1976) Editorial: Gallengangsatresia. *Helv. Paed. Acta*, **31**, 283–286

91. Rickham, P.P. and Lee, E.Y.C. (1964) Neonatal jaundice: surgical aspects. *Clin. Pediat.*, **3**, 197–208

92. Rolleston, H.D. and Hayne, L.B. (1901) A case of congenital hepatic cirrhosis with obliterative cholangitis. *Br. Med. J.*, **1**, 758–760

93. Saing, H., Tam, P.K.H., Lee, J.M.H. and Pe-Nyun (1985) Surgical management of choledochal cysts: a review of 60 cases. *J. Pediat. Surg.*, **20**, 443–448

94. Saito, S. and Ishida, M. (1974) Congenital choledochal cyst (cystic dilation of the common bile duct). *Prog. pediat. Surg.*, **6**, 63–90

95. Sasaki, K., Miyano, T., Ogawa, T. (1985) IgA as a protective factor against ascending cholangitis in postoperative biliary atresia patients *J. Jap. Soc. Pediat. Surg.*, **21**, 433–438

96. Sawaguchi, S., Akiyama, Y., Saeki, M. and Ohia, Y. (1972) The treatment of congenital biliary atresia, with special reference to hepatic port-entero-anastomosis. Fifth Annual Meeting of Pacific Association of Pediatric Surgeons, Tokyo, Japan

97. Schwegler, R.A. and Boyden, E.A. (1937) The development of the pars intestinalis of the common bile duct in the human fetus, with special reference to the origin of the ampulla of Vater and the sphincter of Oddi. *Anat. Rec.*, **67**, 441–467; **68**, 17–41

98. Schweizer, P. (1985) Long-term results in the treatment of extrahepatic bile duct atresia. *Z. Kinderchir.*, **40**, 263–267

99. Schweizer, P. (1986) Treatment of extrahepatic bile duct atresia: results and long term prognosis after hepatic portoenterostomy. *Paediat. Surg. Int.*, **1**, 30–36

100. Seneque, J. and Tailhefer, A. (1920) Les dilatations congénitales du cholédoque. *J. Chir. Paris*, **33**, 154

101. Severn, C.B. (1968) The morphological development of the hepatic diverticulum in staged human embryos. *Anat. Rec.*, **160**, 427

102. Shangen, X. (1983) Congenital cystic dilatation of the intrahepatic biliary duct in children. *Chin. J. Pediat. Surg.*, **4**, 28–30

103. Shim, W.K.T. and Jin-Zhe, Z. (1985) Antirefluxing Roux-en-Y biliary drainage valve for hepatic portenterostomy: animal experiments and clinical experience. *J. Pediat. Surg.*, **20**, 689–692

104. Shim, W.K.T., Kasai, M. and Spence, M.A. (1974) Racial influence on the incidence of biliary atresia. *Prog. Pediat. Surg.*, **6**, 53–62

105. Somasundaram, K., Wong, T.J. and Tan, K.C. (1985) Choledochal cyst: a review of 25 cases. *Aust. N.Z. J. Surg.*, **55**, 443–446

106. Sty, J.R. (1981) Technetium-99m biliary imaging in paediatric surgical problems. *J. Pediat. Surg.*, **16**, 686–690

107. Suruga, K., Kono, S., Miyano, T., Kitahara, T. and Soul-Chin, C. (1976) Treatment of biliary atresia: microsurgery for hepatic portoenterostomy. *Surgery*, **80**, 558–562

108. Suruga, K., Miyano, T., Arai, T., Ogawa, T. and Deguchi, E. (1984) Crucial points of our hepatic portoenterostomy. *J. Pediat. Surg.*, **19**, 171

109. Suruga, K., Miyano, T., Arai, T., Ogawa, T., Sasaki, K. and Deguchi, E. (1985) A study of patients with long-term bile flow after hepatic portoenterostomy for biliary atresia. *J. Pediat. Surg.*, **20**, 252–255

110. Suruga, K., Miyano, T., Kimura, K., Ogawa, T. and Deguchi, E. (1986) The criteria for repeat hepatic portoenterostomy. *J. Pediat. Surg.*, **21**, 275–276

111. Tanaka, K., Matsukawa, Y. and Inomata, Y. (1985) Jejunal interposition hepatic portoduodenostomy with intestinal valve for treatment of biliary atresia. *Jap. J. Pediat. Surg.*, **17**, 65–71

112. Thomson, J. (1891) On congenital obliteration of bile ducts. *Edinb. Med. J.*, **37**, 523–531

113. Tunell, W.P. (1976) Hemangioendothelioma of the pancreas obstructing the common bile duct and duodenum. *J. Pediat. Surg.*, **11**, 827–830

114. Upadhyaya, P. and Upadhyaya, P. (1984) Choledochal cyst: a report of fifteen cases. *Ann. Paediat. Surg.*, **1**, 181–186

115. Vajro, P., Couturier, M., Lemonnier, F. and Odièvre, M. (1986) Effects of post-operative cholestyramine and phenobarbital administration on bile flow restoration in infants with extrahepatic biliary atresia. *J. Pediat. Surg.*, **21**, 362–365

116. Waller, E. (1917) Idiopathic choledochus cyst. *Ann. Surg.*, **66**, 446–463

117. Winters, R.W., Robinson, S.J. and Bates, G. (1954) Haemangioma of the liver with heart failure. *Pediat., Springfield*, **14**, 117–121

118. Wong, K.C. and Lister, J. (1981) Human fetal development of the hepato-pancreatic duct junction – a possible explanation of congenital dilatation of the biliary tract. *J. Pediat. Surg.*, **16**, 139–145

119. Yamaguchi, M. (1980) Congenital choledochal cyst. Analysis of 1,433 patients in the Japanese literature. *Am. J. Surg.*, **140**, 653–657

120. Yano, H. and Matsumoto, H. (1983) Choledochal cyst developed after drainage for idiopathic perforation of the bile duct. *Jap. J. Surg.*, **13**, 441–445

121. Yllpo, A. (1913) Zwei falle von Kongenitalen gallengansverschluss: fett – und bilirubin – stoffwechselversuche bei einum derselben. *Z. Kinderheilk.*, **9**, 319

122. Zinniger, C. (1932) Congenital cystic dilatation of the common bile duct. *Arch. Surg.*, **24**, 77–105

123. Zukin, D.D., Liberthson, R.R. and Lake, A.M. (1981) Extrahepatic biliary atresia associated with cyanotic congenital heart disease: three case reports and a review. *Clin. Pediat.*, **20**, 64–66

Part VII

Central nervous system

Hydrocephalus

R. E. Cudmore and P. K. H. Tam

Historical notes

Hippocrates (462–377 BC) was the first to recognize that fluid was responsible for the enlargement of the head in hydrocephalus [163]. Galen (131–201 AD) described cases of 'water on the brain' and was aware how thin the brain and skull became in this condition. He also noted how minimal the symptoms might be in children with hydrocephalus. He threw light on the anatomy of the ventricular system, suggesting that the ventricles communicate with each other. He believed that the ventricles were inhabited by the *spirit animalis*, the soul [186], and this doctrine was held valid until the Middle Ages. Leonardo da Vinci determined the shape of the cerebral ventricles with a wax mould. In 1543, Vesalius denied the existence of the *spirit animalis* and described internal hydrocephalus in detail [183]. In 1762, Morgagni [130] showed that the cerebrospinal fluid originated in the ventricles. Hydrocephalus resulting from tuberculosis was outlined by Whytt [191] in 1768. Monro [129], Magendie [117] and Luschka [112] enlarged the understanding of the anatomy of the cerebrospinal fluid pathways.

In 1854, Faivre [51] carried out further work on the production of cerebrospinal fluid from the choroid plexus and this was extended and amplified by Key and Retzius in 1875 [92]. The malformation described by Arnold [11] and Chiari [28] in 1894 and 1891 respectively was first noted by Cleland [30] in 1883.

The first known description of the treatment of hydrocephalus was given by Fabricius Hildanus [74] in 1646 when he removed the fluid by incision of the skull and insertion of a tube. Boinet [23] tried injecting iodine after aspiration, with disastrous results. Blane [22] in 1821 tried to cure hydrocephalus by compression of the head and repeated aspirations which remained the treatment of choice until the middle of the nineteenth century.

Wernicke in 1881 [190] reported the use of permanent external ventricular drainage; Illingworth in 1891 [85] modified the approach to temporary external drainage for a duration of 8 days. Closed ventricular drainage was pioneered by Mikulicz [123] who unsuccessfully attempted decompression of the ventricles into the subdural and subarachnoid spaces in 1896; efforts by Sutherland and Cheyne [175] in 1898 similarly failed. At the turn of the century, Gartner [61] suggested that the most physiological way of correcting the excess fluid would be by drainage into the blood or lymphatic stream. About this time, Ferguson [52] drained the spinal subarachnoid space to the peritoneum. A few years later Payr [145], in 1908, attempted to drain fluid from the lateral ventricles to the longitudinal sinus. The first ventriculoperitoneal shunt is said to have been performed by Kausch in 1908 [91] using a rubber tube but the patient died 20 h after the procedure, probably from overdrainage. Other surgeons also had unsatisfactory experiences with ventriculoperitoneal shunting and the procedure lost favour. Ventriculoperitoneal shunting was revived by Cone [33] but he did not publish his results. Scarff [170] in 1963 reported the results of ventriculoperitoneal shunting in 230 patients: hydrocephalus was arrested in 55% of the cases. Use of the pleural cavity for drainage was first outlined by Heile [72]. A direct attack on cerebrospinal fluid production by coagulation of the choroid was first introduced by Lespinasse [104] in 1910. Torkildsen [179] in 1939, showed how excess fluid could best be drained by ventriculocisternotomy. Various shunting operations for congenital hydrocephalus and that associated with myelomeningocele were tried in the postwar years, culminating in the introduction of the subcutaneous valve by Nulsen and Spitz [136] in 1952. Holter [154], a precision machinist whose child had a myelomeningocele with hydrocephalus, worked tirelessly to develop a valve for shunting into the internal jugular vein or right atrium and his work culminated in the introduction of the Holter valve in 1957 which has since been used universally for atrial and peritoneal shunting. Subsequent developments have been directed towards improvement of valves and draining mechanisms but the principles of controlled drainage of cerebrospinal fluid from the lateral ventricles to the venous system or a body cavity remain unchanged.

Physiological considerations

Hydrocephalus is an abnormal enlargement of the cerebral ventricles, caused by an increased pressure gradient between the intraventricular fluid and the brain [19]. Before discussing the pathology of the condition, the physiology of the formation and absorption of the cerebrospinal fluid (CSF) must be described briefly [25]. Unfortunately, our understanding of CSF is still incomplete [68].

The widely accepted view is that under normal conditions, most of the CSF is secreted by the choroid plexus; the CSF flows through the ventricular system emerging from the fourth ventricle to enter the subarachnoid space where it is absorbed by the arachnoid villi to drain into the venous sinuses. In hydrocephalus, compensatory pathways which normally only play minor roles in CSF absorption may be opened up [122].

Cerebrospinal fluid formation

The major site of CSF formation is the choroid plexus. The choroid plexus consists of an epithelial covering and a stromal core. Most of the choroid plexus is attached to the medial wall of the lateral ventricles; some hangs from the roofs of the third and fourth ventricles. Cerebrospinal fluid formation probably occurs in two phases: hydrostatic pressure results in ultrafiltration of plasma from the choroidal capillary; the ultrafiltrate is then transformed into a secretory product (i.e. CSF) by active metabolic processes within the choroidal epithelium [189].

The classic work of Dandy and Blackfan [36] in 1914 suggested that the choroid plexus was the sole producer of CSF. Recent studies of the isolated choroid plexus has demonstrated that 35–70% of derived from this source alone [127]. On the other hand, perfusion studies of the ventricles without choroid plexus has demonstrated that 35–70% of CSF may be non-choroidal in origin [149], most of which probably is derived from the extracellular fluid. The rate of human cerebrospinal fluid formation has been estimated to be up to 20 ml/h or

800 ml/day [111] which is equivalent to a threefold turnover of CSF daily. Most physical and chemical changes tend to decrease CSF formation. Drugs that reduce CSF secretion act by interfering with cellular metabolism; however, reduced CSF production has only a transient effect on intraventricular pressure. Intraventricular changes can affect the first phase of CSF production (ultrafiltration) but the effect is only slight except at high pressures.

Cerebrospinal fluid absorption

Cerebrospinal fluid is absorbed from the subarachnoid space into the venous sinuses by a hydrostatic gradient and most of this takes place at the arachnoid villi. The arachnoid villi are structures which project from the subarachnoid space through the dura into the venous sinuses and their endothelial linings are continuous with those of the venous sinuses. There are endothelial lined tubules in the villi which open into the venous sinuses to allow one-way passage of CSF into the sinuses when a pressure gradient exceeding 25 cm of water is reached. Under normal physiological conditions, little CSF is absorbed by other sites. Hydrocephalus with the rare exception of CSF overproduction in choroid plexus papilloma, occurs as a result of impaired CSF absorption. As there is no reduction of CSF formation in hydrocephalus, a baby's head would explode within a few days if no CSF were absorbed [19]. Since there is only gradual enlargement of a baby's head, most CSF must be absorbed. It is likely that the arachnoid villi are still the site of most CSF absorption even in non-communicating hydrocephalus since the obstruction is usually not complete and compensatory pathways will open up to allow ventricular CSF to pass into the subarachnoid space. It is possible that some compensatory CSF absorption may occur via the lymphatics or choroid plexus [42].

Cerebrospinal fluid circulation

Cerebrospinal fluid moves in bulk from sites of origin to sites of absorption in a true circulatory current unaffected by body position and physical activities [41]. The most important factor for driving the CSF forward is the pressure gradient across the arachnoid villi; other possible contributory factors include the continuous output of newly formed CSF, ciliary action of the ventricular ependyma, the ventricular pulsations transmitted from arterial pulsatile flow and a 'suction pump' action of the dural sinuses as a result of the high velocity of blood flow through the non-collapsable venous sinuses [126].

Pathology

Hydrocephalus is nearly always a result of impaired CSF absorption; we have not encountered the rare entity of CSF overproduction by choroid plexus papilloma in Alder Hey in the past 10 years. Hydrocephalus can be classified into communicating lesions and non-communicating lesions.

In non-communicating hydrocephalus, obstruction occurs in the ventricular system, thereby preventing free exit of CSF from the ventricles. In communicating hydrocephalus, obstruction occurs at the subarachnoid space and there is free flow of CSF out of the ventricles.

Post-haemorrhagic hydrocephalus

Ventricular dilatation following intraventricular/periventricular haemorrhage in low birthweight infants was first observed by Larroche [99] in 1972 in an autopsy study. Its occurrence was soon confirmed in clinical studies [94]. With improved survival of low birthweight babies and major advances in non-invasive imaging studies including computed tomography initially and portable cranial ultrasonography subsequently, the magnitude of the problem became increasingly apparent.

The usual site of haemorrhage is in the germinal matrix which is in an area of proliferation of neuronal and glial precursors and is situated in a subependymal location. Haemorrhage usually involves immature vessels termed 'immature vascular rete' [141], supplied by distinctive arteries which are abnormally large in preterm infants. The area is also characterized by a high fibrinolytic activity which is most prominent between 22 and 30 weeks' gestation [63]. The pathogenesis of periventricular-intraventricular haemorrhage is probably multifactorial and most factors are associated with prematurity and hyaline membrane disease. Alteration of cerebral blood flow as a result of stress factors such as hypoxia and systemic blood pressure changes is probably a key event in this process [4]. Coagulation defects in premature infants have to be considered at least as a contributory factor, especially for the progression in the severity of haemorrhage [20]. Table 40.1 shows the gestational ages of 55 infants with post-haemorrhagic hydrocephalus treated in Alder Hey in 1976–85.

Table 40. 1 Gestational age of 55 infants with post-haemorrhagic hydrocephalus

Gestational age (weeks)	Number of infants
25–28	20
29–32	19
33–36	6
>37	5
Unknown	5
Total	55

The pathological studies of Larroche [99] suggested that chronic post-haemorrhagic ventricular dilatation occurs most commonly as a result of obliterative arachnoiditis in the posterior fossa. A less common cause of post-haemorrhagic hydrocephalus is obstruction of CSF flow in the ventricular system at the foramen of Monro, the aqueduct of Sylvius or the outlets of the fourth ventricle by clots or necrotic debris. In rare instances where early ventricular dilatation occurs following intraventricular haemorrhage, plugging of arachnoid villi by small particulate matter has been postulated [76].

Congenital hydrocephalus without spina bifida

Apart from rare causes such as congenital absence of arachnoid granulations, most lesions causing congenital ventricular dilatation occur proximal to the outlets of the fourth ventricle, to produce a non-communicating type of hydrocephalus [54,57,100,124,150]. Aqueduct obstructions can be demonstrated in approximately 70% cases; this may be caused by gliosis, forking, true narrowing or septum. Simple stenosis or septum of the aqueduct is rare. Aqueductal forking consists of two greatly narrowed channels, one behind the other, the channels separated by normal nervous tissue [167,169]. Aqueductal gliosis is a progressive condition due to overgrowth of densely fibrillary subependymal neuroglia [86]. There is also evidence that some cases of aqueductal obstruction are the result rather than the cause of hydrocephalus [192]: compression and angulation of the upper brain stem by the enlarged lateral ventricles can convert a communicating hydrocephalus into a non-communicating one.

Congenital obstruction or absence of the foramina of Monro, Magendie and Luschka are rare causes of hydrocephalus in the neonatal period. Atresia of the foramina of Luschka and Magendie produces the Dandy–Walker syndrome with a characteristic cystic lesion in the posterior fossa [54,71]. In cases of obstruction in the roof of the fourth ventricle, the hydrocephalus usually develops very gradually [176].

Recently it has been postulated that some cases of 'congenital' hydrocephalus may be due to prenatal intracranial haemorrhage and at least one such case has been reported [88].

Hydrocephalus with spina bifida cystica

In the so-called Arnold–Chiari [146] malformation there is a herniation of a tongue-like process of cerebellum and the lower part of the medulla oblongata through the foramen magnum. The cervical spinal cord is therefore displaced downwards and

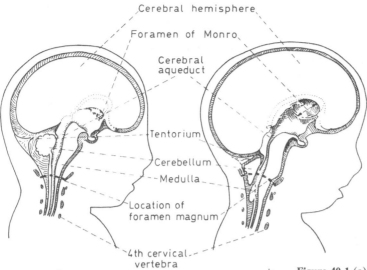

Cerebral hemisphere

Foramen of Monro

Cerebral aqueduct

Tentorium

Cerebellum

Medulla

Location of foramen magnum

4th cervical vertebra

a
b

Figure 40.1 (a) Normal. (b) Arnold–Chiari malformation

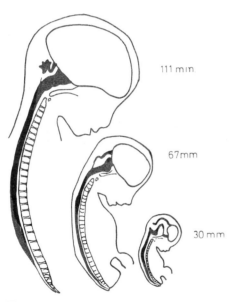

111 mm

67mm

30 mm

Figure 40.2 Diagrammatic representation of differential growth of spinal cord and vertebral column in the fetus

the cervical nerve roots run upwards and laterally to their respective interspinal foramina. The cerebellar 'tongue' is bound down to the medulla and may obstruct the flow of CSF through the foramina in the roof of the fourth ventricle (Figure 40.1).

During embryonic development the longitudinal growth of the vertebral column is much greater than that of the spinal cord (Figure 40.2). As the cephalic end of the cord is fixed and as, in cases of spina bifida cystica, the spinal cord is fixed caudally to the

vertebral column, it used to be assumed that the Arnold–Chiari malformation was due to abnormal traction pulling the medulla and cerebellum down through the foramen magnum. This mechanical explanation of the genesis of the malformation has been questioned by a number of authorities [2,140,176]. Patten [144] showed that in the Arnold–Chiari malformation there is local overgrowth of the neural tube and it is now known that the malformation affects the whole brain. The cerebral hemispheres are enlarged partly because of the developing hydrocephalus, but also because there is an actual increase in cerebral tissue. The surface of the cerebral hemispheres is excessively folded, forming microgyri, and the occipital lobes of the hemispheres herniate through the incisura of the tentorium cerebelli [37].

In our experience, some degree of the Arnold–Chiari malformation is present in practically every case of spina bifida cystica but this does not mean that hydrocephalus develops in all cases. It has been observed [167] that in the Arnold–Chiari malformation the CSF escapes from the fourth ventricle and is prevented from passing upwards by the tongue of cerebellum in the foramen magnum. We have, however, frequently seen cases with this malformation in which air injected into the ventricle escaped into the posterior cranial fossa. MacNab [114] has suggested that in these cases the block is at the tentorial notch and is produced by pressure of the hindbrain and arachnoiditis, but this cannot be the whole explanation as in our experience the injected air can be made to pass freely to the top of the cranium.

In the normal embryo the increasing pressure of CSF bursts the membranous caudal part of the roof of the fourth ventricle thus forming the foramina, and subsequently the lower pole of the cerebellar vermis is turned inwards. In open myelomeningocele the CSF escapes into the amniotic cavity, pressure does not increase, and hence the caudal part of the roof of the fourth ventricle is not perforated but remains as a tight membrane which hampers the inward rotation of the cerebellum and causes the lower pole of the vermis to be pulled downwards.

It has often been assumed that excision of a myelomeningocele may cause the sudden development of hydrocephalus and it was thought that this was due to the fact that the sac of the myelomeningocele actively absorbed CSF [169]. It has, however, been shown that in all such cases the hydrocephalus is already present at birth [107]. Rapid increase in the rate of growth of the head after operation may be brought about by sudden obstruction of the CSF pathways caused by meningeal reaction to bleeding or by shifting of the hindbrain due to sudden pressure changes following release of CSF. Recent alternative theories of the aetiology of hydrocephalus in myelomeningocele are discussed in Chapter 41.

Family history

About 2% of cases of congenital hydrocephalus without spina bifida have X-linked recessive inheritance [6]. Family data on uncomplicated congenital hydrocephalus excluding cases of X-linked inherited hydrocephalus has revealed an incidence of 1.1–1.9% of hydrocephalus in sibs, representing a recurrence risk of about 26 times the population incidence [1,110]. The recurrence risk is approximately 1 in 40 after an affected male and 1 in 80 after an affected female. Lorber [110] has also suggested that there is an increased risk of neural tube defects (2.0%) in sibs of patients with uncomplicated congenital hydrocephalus but such an association has not been confirmed in several other studies [1,101].

Incidence

The most frequent cause of neonatal hydrocephalus used to be the Arnold–Chiari malformation associated with spina bifida. However, in recent years the incidence of spina bifida has decreased substantially as a result of improved antenatal diagnosis and other reasons (see Chapter 41). The prevalence of congenital hydrocephalus without spina bifida has remained relatively constant in the past two decades occurring 1 per 2500 live births in the Liverpool area. On the other hand, post-haemorrhagic hydrocephalus has assumed greater importance in the past decade as a result of improved survival of low birthweight babies. The annual incidence of various types of hydrocephalus without spina bifida treated in Alder Hey Children's Hospital from 1976 to 1985 is shown in Figure 40.3.

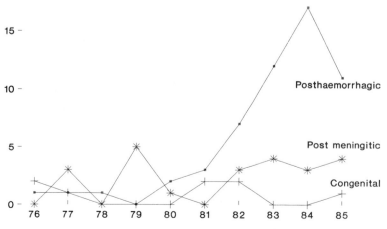

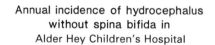

Figure 40.3 Annual incidence of neonatal hydrocephalus without spina bifida in Royal Liverpool Children's Hospital, Alder Hey

Clinical picture

Symptoms of raised intracranial pressure include vomiting, lethargy, drowsiness, irritability and constant crying but these are often not apparent initially in babies with hydrocephalus [93]. Early diagnosis depends on a high index of awareness and the recognition of increasing head circumference. Low birthweight infants, especially those with hyaline membrane disease, are particularly prone to develop hydrocephalus. In 1976–85 we treated 55 low birthweight infants with post-haemorrhagic hydrocephalus. Their gestational ages are listed in Table 40.1. Other infants requiring special attention include infants with myelomeningocele, infants who had meningitis and siblings of hydrocephalic patients. It is important to note in the birth history whether there has been any difficulty in delivery, because moulding of the larger than normal head may produce intraventricular or subdural haemorrhage in addition to the hydrocephalus. Intraventricular haemorrhage due to birth trauma is particularly severe in such children. In addition, there is also a relation between the degree of hypoxia or birth asphyxia and periventricular-intraventricular haemorrhage. Antenatal diagnosis of congenital hydrocephalus with or without spina bifida is now possible and this will be further discussed in the section on ultrasonography.

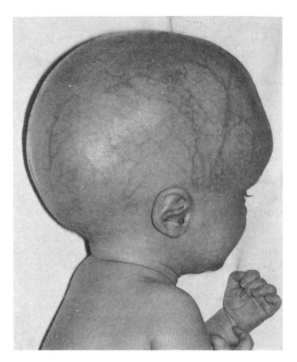

Figure 40.4 Obvious hydrocephalus with distended scalp veins and bulging fontanelle

Examination

In advanced hydrocephalus, the head is large and the scalp veins are distended (Figure 40.4). The shape of the head may suggest the type of lesion present. Communicating hydrocephalus produces a generalized roundness of the head whilst aqueductal stenosis tends to produce a more anterior 'bossing'. On the other hand, there may be very obvious occipital enlargement in the presence of a Dandy–Walker cyst or other posterior fossa lesion.

'Setting sun' sign

This characteristic sign is generally ascribed to the expanding brain causing depression of the orbital roof and downward displacement of the eyeball. As a result, the white of the sclera can be seen beneath the upper eyelid, giving the typical 'setting sun' appearance (Figure 40.5). Displacement alone as a cause of this sign has been questioned [10] because not only does it occur before there is much enlargement of the head but it soon disappears after shunting. A more likely explanation is that of pressure on the oculomotor nerves by the dilating third ventricle [115].

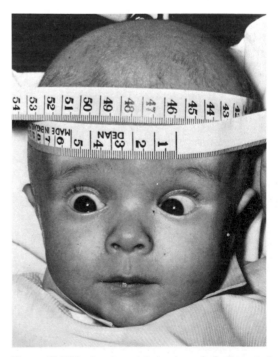

Figure 40.5 The 'setting sun' sign in early hydrocephalus. Note that the head circumference is measured along the occipitofrontal axis

Bulging fontanelle

Fontanelle pressure is a useful guide to intracranial tension and, in assessing it, various fontanometers have been devised as a means of constant monitoring. Hydrocephalus may be developing in the presence of a fontanelle that feels normal on palpation. By the time the hydrocephalus is advanced, however, the fontanelle is very tense and bulging (Figure 40.4).

Cranial nerve paralyses

These are common and should be looked for in every examination of the hydrocephalic baby. Commonest is the sixth nerve palsy presenting as a squint in the older baby but it is very difficult to observe in the newborn as the baby does not focus [31].

Cord paralyses are not uncommon and an obvious stridor may be present. If there is bilateral cord paralysis, tracheostomy may be necessary although this problem is quite rare in our experience. There may be difficulties with sucking and swallowing, so palatal movement should be carefully assessed.

Papilloedema

Papilloedema is due to increased pressure on the central retinal vein as it crosses the subarachnoid space to enter the cavernous sinus. With a block to cerebrospinal flow at ventricular or subarachnoid level the fluid does not reach the optic sheath and the vein cannot be compressed; hence papilloedema rarely occurs in congenital hydrocephalus [115]. Nevertheless, the fundi should be examined because there may be an associated subdural haematoma producing the characteristic 'flame shaped' haemorrhages.

Attempts should be made to ascertain whether the baby will follow a light or whether a corneal reflux is present, as some babies with hydrocephalus may be blind. Blindness, however, is more common at a later date following sudden shunt blockage, or progressing insidiously in the older hydrocephalic child with fused cranial sutures.

Progressive enlargement of the skull circumference

This is the most important feature and regular periodic measurement of head size in cases of marginal hydrocephalus will be the most useful guide as to whether or not further investigation is necessary. It is better if the measurement is undertaken by the same observer on each occasion as we have noted frequently that there is variation of 1 cm or more in measurements taken by different clinicians or nurses. The measurement is plotted on a chart which should be weight and age related so that allowance can be made for prematurity or dysmaturity (Figure 40.6).

Other signs

Percussion of the skull in the older baby may give a characteristic 'cracked pot' sound (MacEwen's sign); transillumination of the skull in a darkened room will give a guide to cortical thickness. Estimate of the degree of dilatation of the ventricles, however, depends on special investigation.

Investigation

A plain skull X-ray is a useful initial procedure in order that the size, shape and thickness of the bones can be assessed. The pattern of suture separation may suggest the type of lesion [125] present whilst intracranial calcification or the presence of a lacunar skull defect is noted. Lacunar skull deformity or 'Luckenschadel skull' (Figure 40.7) is not uncommon in cases associated with myelomeningocele and can be a guide to eventual intellectual status [106]. Multiple lacunae may also be present in the skull of premature babies with post-haemorrhagic hydrocephalus.

Ultrasonography

The advent of ultrasonography has revolutionized the diagnosis and assessment of hydrocephalus [29,79,89,102]. The detection of ventricular dilatation by ultrasonography allows the diagnosis of congenital hydrocephalus to be made antenatally. Antenatal ultrasonography can also detect fetuses with myelomeningocele – in some cases the neural tube defect can be seen; in others a lemon-shaped head will raise the suspicion (Figure 40.8).

In neonates, the anterior fontanelle provides the perfect access for intracranial imaging with ultrasound examination. The availability of portable ultrasound machines with high resolution allows rapid, inexpensive and repeated assessment of the neonatal brain at the bedside.

Cranial ultrasonography has now become a routine practice in special care baby units for surveillance of the premature population at risk for periventricular-intraventricular haemorrhage and for follow-up of those affected. The site and extent of haemorrhage can be identified allowing the severity of haemorrhage to be graded as mild (subependymal), moderate (intraventricular) or severe (parenchymal) [18,96], (Figure 40.9). Porencephalic cysts or cysts of periventricular leucomalacia detected before hydrocephalus is established represent cerebral atrophy and are associated with a poor long-term prognosis [34]. Serial cranial imaging studies are valuable because following

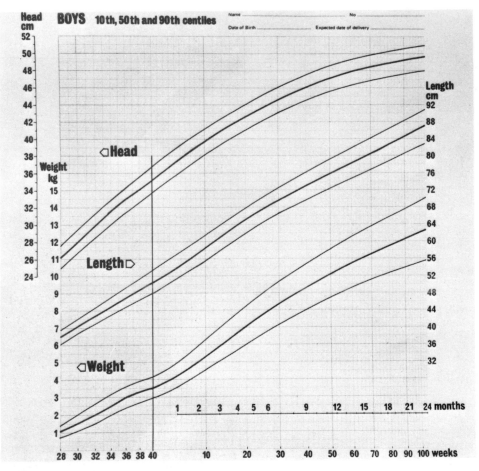

Figure 40.6 A useful head circumference chart, as the measurement can be weight and age related. (From Gairdner and Pearson [59])

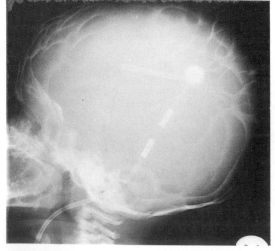

Figure 40.7 Plain X-ray of 'Luckenshadel skull' in an infant with hydrocephalus (shunt inserted)

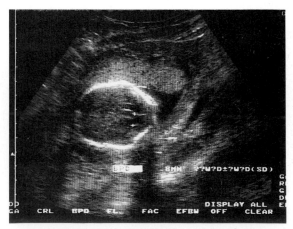

Figure 40.8 Ultrasonography showing 'lemon-shaped' head of fetus suggesting spina bifida

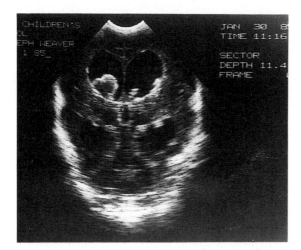

Figure 40.9 Cranial ultrasonograph of premature infant with intraventricular haemorrhage and hydrocephalus

neonatal intracranial haemorrhage ventricular dilatation may precede rapid head growth [184,185]. In some cases, there is even an absence of increased intracranial pressure [75] and ultrasonographic evidence of progressive ventriculomegaly may be the only positive finding to indicate the necessity for intervention.

For congenital hydrocephalus, ultrasound examination can reveal the aetiology and the site of the block by defining whether the lateral ventricles alone are dilated or the third and/or the fourth ventricles are also involved. Knowledge of the anatomy of the dilated ventricular system also aids the surgeon in the optimal placement of the shunt catheter.

The thickness of the cerebral cortex has been used as a guide to the necessity of valve insertion and this information can now be obtained non-invasively with cranial ultrasonography thus avoiding invasive air ventriculography. Lorber [107] defined four grades of cortical thickness as measured with ventriculogram studies in the days before ultrasonography was available:

Grade 1:   cortical thickness 15 mm – valve certainly necessary
Grade 2a   cortical thickness 15–25 mm – valve almost certainly necessary
Grade 2b   cortical thickness 25–35 mm – valve may be necessary
Grade 3   cortex 35 mm – valve is probably not necessary.

Patients in grades 2b and 3 should have regular head circumference measurement with careful follow-up to plot progress.

Cortical thickness was thought to be a guide to prognosis and cerebral function but this relationship is not always reliable and a thickness of 5 mm or less can be compatible with a normal IQ [108].

Computed tomography

Computed tomography (CT) is another useful non-invasive investigation giving an accurate outline of intracranial anatomy (Figure 40.10). Before the refinements of ultrasound technology in the late 1970s, computer tomography represented the most

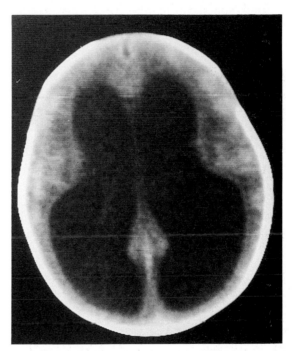

Figure 40.10 CT scan of head showing dilated lateral ventricles

exciting advance in the diagnosis and assessment of hydrocephalus. Much of the knowledge of the growing problem of periventricular-intraventricular haemorrhage in low birthweight infants was initially gained from CT scan studies and the earliest grading system of periventricular-intraventricular haemorrhage was based on CT scan findings [143]. The anterior fontanelle, an anatomical feature unique to the neonate, however, provides ultrasonography with a window to the baby's brain. Compared with CT scan, cranial ultrasonography has the following advantages: (i) it is less expensive, (ii) it does not involve even a small radiation dose, (iii) it is portable and therefore is ideal for use in sick low birthweight infants on ventilation, (iv) the resolution of its images is not dependent on the thickness of the sections as in CT scans. On the other hand, the accuracy of ultrasonography is operator-dependent. Provided expertise is available, cranial ultrasonography is the investigation of choice for neonates with hydrocephalus and usually gives sufficient information; not infrequently a CT scan can be complementary. In addition to demonstrating dilated ventricles, intracranial imaging may show up additional pathologies such as agenesis of corpus callosum [97], a condition which is often associated with proneness to seizures and delayed development. Encysted cerebrospinal fluid collections and isolated third and/or fourth ventricles may also be shown (Figure 40.11); these may be the cause of

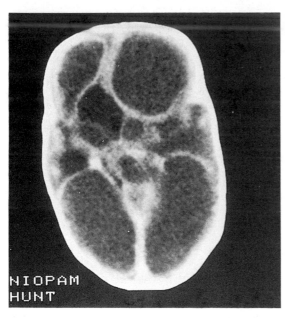

Figure 40.11 CT scan of head showing complex cystic dilatation of brain

persistent symptoms in infant despite apparently uncomplicated shunting procedures [138]. Very rarely, CT scan may reveal a brain tumour to be the true cause of hydrocephalus.

After infancy when the fontanelle is closed, cranial ultrasonography is not possible and CT scan is required for accurate cranial imaging. Computed tomography has been found to be particularly helpful in the management of shunt complications [46]. A baseline CT scan for a child with hydrocephalus after shunt insertion when he/she is asymptomatic is often useful as it allows future comparison should symptoms of shunt blockage occur.

Intracranial pressure measurement

Intracranial pressure may be measured invasively by direct ventricular puncture or in cases of communicating hydrocephalus by lumbar puncture. Until non-invasive imaging techniques became available, routine investigation of the newborn with hydrocephalus included a ventricular tap which would provide a sample of CSF for examination as well as a recording of intraventricular pressure. This invasive procedure is now rarely indicated for diagnosis alone. Serial lumbar or ventricular punctures for temporary control of post-haemorrhagic hydrocephalus is discussed later. In some instances when ultrasonography and computed tomography give equivocal information as to whether a shunting procedure is indicated, direct intracranial pressure measurement may be helpful. Ventricular puncture is best performed in the operating theatre under strictly aseptic techniques. With the baby lying supine and held firmly by the attendant nurse, the ventricle is punctured after skin preparation, at the lateral border of the anterior fontanelle. For this procedure, a 20 or 22 gauge spinal needle is best. There is a characteristic feel once the ventricle has been entered. The stilette is removed and the manometer attached. Fluid should be taken for culture, microscopy and biochemistry. Xanthochromic fluid with high protein content is not uncommonly found in infants with post-haemorrhagic or post-meningitic hydrocephalus.

It is also possible to measure anterior fontanelle pressure non-invasively by the application of a pressure sensor known as the Ladd monitor (Ladd Research Laboratories, Burlington, VT, USA) [147] or similar device. The procedure, sometimes known as 'fontanometry', allows intermittent or continuous recording of the fontanelle pressure and several studies suggest a good correlation of fontanelle pressure readings with ventricular fluid pressure measurements [90,187]. There are, however, fundamental technical problems such as the external pressure applied, tension in the fontanelle, etc. which make this method unsuitable for routine clinical practice [128].

It is important to realize that there is a wide range of normal values of intracranial pressure in neonates and the normal values in preterm infants are usually lower than those in full-term infants [148]. In addition, progressive ventricular dilatation may occur without accompanying raised intracranial pressure. Hence pressure measurements should not be interpreted in isolation but should be considered in conjunction with information provided by cranial imaging studies.

Isotope studies

Isotope studies are mainly used for research purposes and can give information about the production, circulation and absorption of cerebrospinal fluid in hydrocephalus [40,124,188]. These methods are of limited value in routine clinical practice.

Differential diagnosis

The diagnosis of hydrocephalus is usually obvious. Some normal babies have 'large heads' a trait which can run in families; imaging studies confirming the absence of dilatation will be reassuring to both the parents and the clinician. Subdural haematomas, usually resulting from birth trauma, may also cause enlargement of the infant's head and the diagnosis can again be established by imaging studies.

Treatment

'Whilst shunt therapy is undoubtedly good palliation, it carries a high morbidity. One day, the treatment or control of hydrocephalus will become a pharmacological rather than a surgical matter.'

(*Lancet*, 1971, **i**, 587)

Nearly two decades after this prophecy was made, the research for a consistently effective method to avoid shunt surgery for hydrocephalus remains elusive. There have been anecdotal reports of success with head wrapping [49,157] but no large series exists to validate such claims and the method has not been adopted generally. Acetazolamide [83], a carbonic anhydrase inhibitor, has been shown to be capable of reducing CSF production by 35–90% in animal studies [171] but its action in humans is uncertain and, to produce any significant effect, severe acid-base imbalance is also produced. Enhanced efficacy in controlling hydrocephalus had been claimed with the combined use of acetazolamide and frusemide [172] but even its advocates admitted that this approach was generally ineffective in neonates with hydrocephalus secondary to myelomeningocele who became symptomatic during the first 20 days of life.

Lorber [109] and Shurtleff [84,173] introduced isosorbide which is a dihydric alcohol derived from sorbitol. This osmotic agent is supplied as a 45% solution and can be given orally, or by nasogastric tube (as it has an unpleasant taste) in a dose of 2–2.5 g/kg body weight every 4–6 h. Its action is more on the extraventricular intracerebral fluid than on the ventricular CSF. Intraventricular pressure falls and the head circumference growth rate slows but there is associated hypernatraemic dehydration, increased blood urea and acidosis. Hence the electrolytes and Astrup levels have to be monitored frequently.

Lorber concluded that isosorbide was a useful adjunct to hydrocephalus therapy but could not replace shunting. Indeed, because of the large volumes of isosorbide needed in the older child, it is as yet only suitable for treatment of the neonate. Infants with a cerebral mantle less than 15 mm do not, however, respond well and its use in congenital hydrocephalus is only indicated when there is a thick cortex or when temporary control is desired before surgery. Glycerol, another osmotic agent, has similarly been used [184]. There is as yet no controlled clinical studies to confirm the efficacy of these medical methods of controlling hydrocephalus.

In recent years, increasing interest has been focused on the management of post-haemorrhagic hydrocephalus. As it results from periventricular-intraventricular haemorrhage, a logical approach would be to aim at the prevention of haemorrhage. A multicentre, placebo-controlled, double-blind trial [18] showed that ethamsylate, a non-steroidal drug that limits small vessel bleeding, given parenterally to very low birthweight infants immediately after birth and thereafter for 4 days resulted in a statistically significant reduction in the incidence of intraventricular and parenchymal haemorrhage from 29.8% in the control group to 18.5% in the ethamsylate group. However, as a substantial number of very low birthweight infants will develop intraventricular haemorrhage irrespective of treatment, post-haemorrhagic hydrocephalus remains an unsolved problem. Serial lumbar punctures have been used successfully for at least temporary amelioration of the hydrocephalus until the infant is fit for shunt surgery [95]. The efficacy of serial lumbar punctures in the prevention of hydrocephalus after intraventricular haemorrhage and the treatment of established post-haemorrhagic hydrocephalus is more controversial. Papille [142] reported that arrest in the progression of hydrocephalus was achieved in 11 out of 12 infants who had serial lumbar punctures but there was no control group in the study and it is possible that spontaneous arrest of hydrocephalus has occurred [7]. In two studies evaluating the efficacy of repeated lumbar punctures in preventing hydrocephalus after periventricular-intraventricular haemorrhage, no difference in eventual requirement for ventricular shunts was found between the treatment group and the control group [9,119]. It is important to realize that repeated CSF drainage may result in hyponatraemia as CSF is rich in electrolytes, and appropriate preventive measures should be taken [116].

Other methods for temporary CSF removal have also been reported. Harbaugh [70] reported the use of external ventricular drainage via a subcutaneous tunnelled catheter in 11 infants with periventricular-intraventricular haemorrhage for a mean of 20.7 days and avoided shunt surgery in two patients.

Some authors have also reported the use of a subcutaneous ventricular catheter reservoir for repeated CSF removal in post-haemorrhagic hydrocephalus [8,103] but these procedures are not without complications and it is doubtful if they offer any particular clinical advantage over other methods of intermittent removal of CSF such as repeated lumbar punctures or ventricular taps.

Antenatal decompression of congenital hydrocephalus remains an experimental procedure [21,32] and its clinical value has not been established.

The historical evaluation of shunt therapy has already been outlined but a wide variety of techniques have been used including drainage of the CSF into the cisterna magna [179], middle ear [134], pleura [158], peritoneum [52,113], ureter [121] and fallopian tube. Another method of controlling CSF production has been by destruction of the choroid plexus [72,156,169], which had very poor results.

Shunt therapy

The greatest advance in the treatment of hydrocephalus was the introduction of a drainage system incorporating a non-return valve allowing CSF to flow directly from the ventricles to the blood stream [98]. The first valve of this type was introduced by Nulsen and Spitz [135] in 1952, but it was not until 1956 that the engineer Holter modified the valve and introduced the silicone rubber Silastic into its manufacture. The Holter system has withstood the test of time and although modifications have been introduced, including a new mini-valve, the basic design remains the same. It is important that 'medical grade' Silastic is used for the tubing and valve components as it is inert and causes no tissue reaction except that a fibrous sheath is laid down around the Silastic [87,174]. Medical grade Silastic

is made from high viscosity polydimethyl siloxane to which is added silica for strengthening plus a vulcanizing agent.

Since the introduction of the Holter valve, various other shunting systems have been devised and there is now a plethora of shunting systems available [17,153,178,181,193]. This has tended to produce considerable confusion in assessing results and techniques [39,67].

In Liverpool, we now routinely use the Cordis integral shunt system which has incorporated the Hakim mechanism (Cordis Corporation, Miami, FL, USA). Ventriculo-peritoneal shunting is our operation of choice; on occasions when this is undesirable or impossible, e.g. in the presence of intraperitoneal pathology, ventriculo-atrial shunting is performed.

Shunt system

The Cordis integral shunt system for ventricular shunting is an implantable device containing the Hakim valve mechanism to provide continuous controlled drainage of CSF from the ventricles to an internal drainage site and helps to control intraventricular pressure. The system consists of a straight ventricular catheter with introducing rod, a burr hole reservoir and an integral shunt assembly (Figure 40.12). Silicone elastomer, impregnated with barium sulphate, and stainless steel are used for construction of the system, allowing radiological visualization. Unlike older systems, the integral nature of this system minimizes connections between various components and hence reduces the future risk of disconnection of parts of the system. The unidirectional valve unit consists of two valves incorporating the Hakim mechanism, which is a

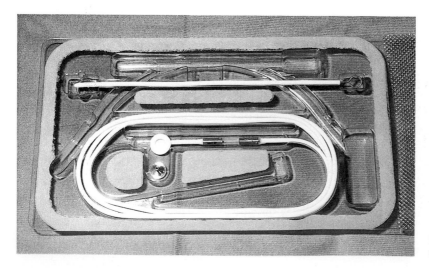

Figure 40.12 The Cordis integral shunt system

ball-in-cone design. Compression of the silastic tube between the two valves against the skull allows the valve unit to be 'pumped'. The ball-in-cone valves are designed to open at a constant pressure and they close as soon as the pressure falls below a certain level. Although the pressure range is labelled in each product these values should only be used as a rough guide. *In vitro*, tests on valves give varying results depending on fluid viscosity, temperature and other factors [159,182]. It seems certain that bench studies of valve function bear little relation to function in the patient which would account for so much variation in actual shunt performance in children [56,64]. Many surgeons prefer to use a low-pressure valve [43] especially in the neonate where the intracranial pressure is low; over-draining, however, can cause severe symptoms and may be followed by cranial synostosis [164]; a medium-pressure valve avoids these risks and should certainly be used when the intraventricular pressure exceeds 200 mmH$_2$O. In low birthweight infants, intracranial pressure is usually lower than that of term infants and a low pressure valve is advisable.

The upper end of the valve is in continuity with a reservoir cap which can be fitted onto a burr hole reservoir. The reservoir is connected to the ventricular catheter and serves as a needlestop for obtaining cerebrospinal fluid samples, measurement of intraventricular pressure to diagnose shunt blockage and, if necessary, injection of antibiotics to control ventriculitis [160,162,177]. The lower end of the valve is in continuity with a drainage catheter (107 cm long), transporting CSF from the valve unit to the peritoneal cavity or other drainage site.

Operation for valve insertion

Meticulous cleanliness is essential because shunt colonization is initiated most commonly at the time of shunt insertion [13]. It is impossible to sterilize normal skin completely, but we shave the scalp and apply chlorhexidine gluconate (Hibitane) soaks under a bandage for 2 days pre-operatively if at all possible. There is some debate as to whether a shunt should be inserted if the protein level is greater than 2 g/litre (200 mg/100 ml). The objection to insertion is that fibrin may be deposited in the valve parts and cause malfunction, but in practice there does not seem to be a significant danger of this and we have certainly inserted valves with CSF protein up to 10 g litre (1 g/100 ml) without complications. It is not necessary to cross-match blood if the baby's haemoglobin level is satisfactory. A blood loss of greater than 20–30 ml at valve insertion should be rare.

Our operation of choice at present is ventriculo-peritoneal shunting. If the peritoneal cavity is not suitable for use as a drainage site, e.g. in neonates with active necrotizing enterocolitis, the alternative operation of ventriculo-atrial shunting is performed. The baby is placed on the operating table on a water blanket with the head turned to the left and a small rolled up towel placed under the shoulders (Figure 40.13); an X-ray table is used if a ventriculo-atrial shunting procedure is planned. While this is being done it is convenient to test the valve: first for patency; secondly to ensure there is no reflux – a meniscus of saline should be convex and not collapse at the lower end; and thirdly to check the flow by holding a vertical column of saline in a manometer attached to the proximal end. A crude idea of flow rate can then be determined. The main function of this last test is to ensure that saline does not flow too quickly or slowly through the system. Detailed pre-operative bench testing of valves is unnecessary in our opinion for the reasons stated above. Valve and tubing are placed in a bowl containing saline.

Skin preparation is carried out on the right scalp,

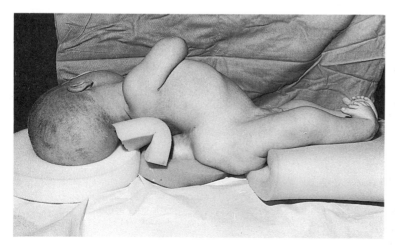

Figure 40.13 Position of the body on the operating table before valve insertion. The head is turned to the left and the shoulders extended over padding

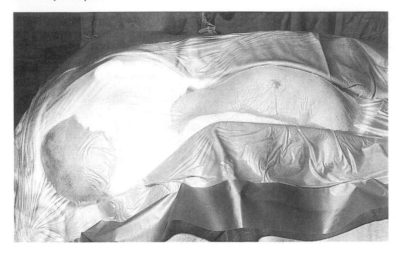

Figure 40.14 Operating site after preparations

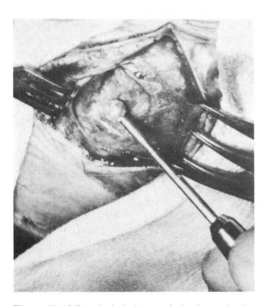

Figure 40.15 Burr hole being made in the parietal area. If the bone is very thin it is easier to nibble away with bone forceps

neck, chest and upper abdomen. Abdominal packs soaked in chlorhexidine are placed around the operation site. Skin towels are then applied and a large steridrape is placed to cover the entire operating area (Figure 40.14).

A curved C-shaped incision is made just posterior to and around the parietal eminence. The edge of the flap must be sufficiently far away from the reservoir when placed to prevent wound tension at closure, and similarly the lower part of the incision must not overlie the eventual valve position. The skin flap is reflected, the periosteum incised in a

cruciate fashion and a burr hole is made. For this, a dental or compressed air drill is best, using a suitable diamond burr to give a 0.5 cm diameter hole (Figure 40.15). Occasionally there is such a degree of lacunar skull defect that dura is prolapsing through the bone and such sites provide a site for the ventriculostomy without much bone removal.

Attention is now turned to the abdomen where a small transverse incision is made in the right upper quadrant. The fascia is incised and the abdominal muscle is split. The peritoneum is picked up with two pairs of artery forceps and a small opening is made. A subcutaneous tunnel is created between the incisions of the scalp and the abdomen using a valve introducer (Figure 40.16). Sometimes the tunnel has to be made in two stages making an extra stab incision in the lower neck. A strong thread is tied to the introducer and passed from scalp wound to the abdomen, and used to draw the system down through the tunnel. Alternatively if a hollow introducer has been used the peritoneal catheter can be threaded down it. To avoid kinking of the catheter at its final entry into the peritoneal cavity from the subcutaneous tunnel, an artery forceps can be used to make an oblique passage through peritoneum and muscle picking up the catheter 0.5–1.0 cm above the main abdominal incision (Figure 40.17).

A small incision is made in the dura with diathermy and the ventricular catheter is inserted into the ventricle using the introducer and aiming towards the right orbit (Figure 40.18). There is a characteristic feeling of 'give' when the ventricle is entered and CSF will flow out of the catheter. The introducer is removed and a sample of CSF is taken for analysis. The catheter is trimmed proximally to leave a catheter length of 5–7 cm. To prevent excessive CSF loss a small bulldog clamp is placed near the proximal catheter end which is then tied to

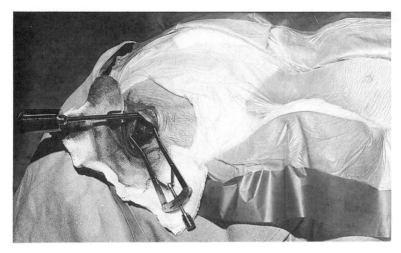

Figure 40.16 Subcutaneous tunnelling using a valve introducer

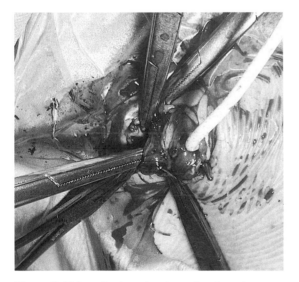

Figure 40.17 Introduction of peritoneal catheter into peritoneal cavity

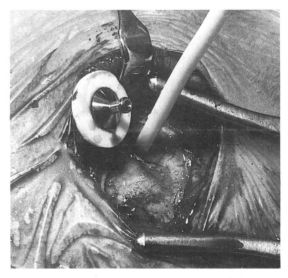

Figure 40.18 Ventricular catheter being passed

the reservoir attached to the integral shunt system using a linen suture (Figure 40.19). The shunt system is positioned to lie snugly in the subcutaneous tunnel. The valve is pumped several times to confirm patency and function (Figure 40.20). The peritoneal catheter is placed in the subhepatic region inside the peritoneal cavity. Closure of the wounds is carried out in the usual way. It is not our custom to give routine postoperative antibiotics as we feel this masks rather than removes the risk of infection [14,27].

For the alternative procedure of ventriculo-atrial shunting, instead of an abdominal incision, a horizontal incision is made in the neck at the junction of the middle and lower thirds of the sternomastoid and should overlie that muscle. This line may be marked with methylene blue in a skin crease so that a cosmetically acceptable scar is obtained. Often, ugly scars result from a badly placed neck incision.

After dividing the skin and platysma, the body of the sternomastoid muscle is split in the line of its fibres until the internal jugular vein comes into

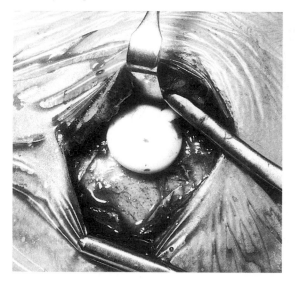

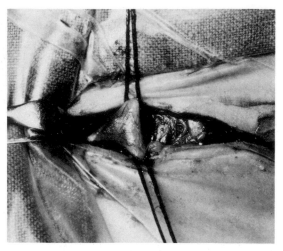

Figure 40.21 The internal jugular vein being held up by stay sutures to demonstrate its junction with the facial vein

Figure 40.19 Ventricular catheter connected to the reservoir and its attached integral shunt system

view. At this point, the common facial vein is encountered and both it and the jugular vein are freed and thread stay sutures are passed round them (Figure 40.21).

Cannulation of the internal jugular vein via the facial vein has been recommended as a means of preserving the flow of blood in the jugular vein and preventing thrombosis. In practice, at re-exploration, it is rare to find a patent vein at the site of original insertion and it seems there is nothing to choose between cannulating the facial vein, tying off the internal jugular or cannulating the internal jugular vein via a purse-string suture in its wall (Figure 40.22).

Accurate placement of the distal catheter is, however, important and various techniques have

been described to achieve this end. A crude method, but one that is reasonably accurate, is to measure from the neck incision to the xiphisternum which is the anatomical surface marking of the right atrium. The bead in the catheter is then adjusted to this length. It is our practice to shorten the fine distal tubing of the C-type catheter to 2 cm, which seems less likely to kink in the vein or the heart than the original 4 cm length. A rather more precise method is to use the saline-filled distal catheter as an electrode and identify the right atrium by the ECG pattern obtained when the catheter lies in it [165]. This method may be time consuming and is not necessary if the position of the tube is checked by X-ray on the table and this we perform routinely; the silver-impregnated catheter makes this simple [161]. Despite these checks, accurate placement may be difficult because allowance must be made for

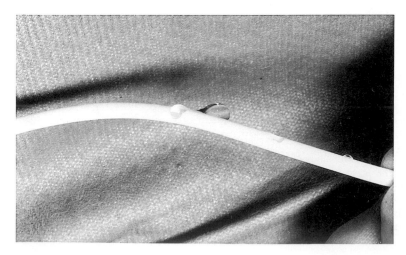

Figure 40.20 Cerebrospinal fluid flowing out of peritoneal catheter on 'pumping'

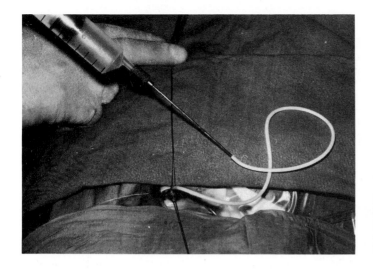

Figure 40.22 The distal C-type catheter has been passed down the vein and its patency is being checked. It is important to ensure that not only can saline be injected but also that blood can be aspirated

a downwards movement of the tube of as much as the depth of one vertebral body when the head is returned to the central position from being turned to the left postoperatively. Repeat X-rays are therefore taken postoperatively since, if the distal catheter should pass into the right ventricle, the system is unlikely to function normally. Having placed the lower catheter satisfactorily, a tie around the vein secures the bead and tubing at the venotomy.

Nixon [131] first described ventriculopleural shunts and we have used these from time to time. The disadvantage is that in time a pleural effusion develops so that it is almost always necessary to change from a pleural to venous or peritoneal shunt.

The technique is exactly the same as for the venous shunt except that the distal tube is inserted into the pleural cavity through the second or third intercostal space. This is most conveniently done by retracting the pectoralis muscle via a small incision and then inserting a trocar and cannula through the space into the pleural cavity. As it is inserted, the anaesthetist halts the anaesthetic for a moment to allow the lung to fall away from the trocar – lung perforation is rare. Via the cannula, a 5–10 cm length of A-type catheter with a few small side holes cut in the end is introduced. The lung is re-inflated and the catheter attached to the pleura by a circumscribing catgut suture loosely tied. Connection of the valve is made by threading the introducer through the neck to the chest wall, care being taken not to damage the external jugular vein or enter the chest through the neck.

Of 86 neonates with hydrocephalus not associated with spina bifida seen in the neonatal surgical unit in Royal Liverpool Children's Hospital Alder Hey in the period 1976–85, 80 had a shunting procedure: ventriculoperitoneal shunt 68, ventriculo-atrial shunt 11, ventriculopleural shunt one. Prior to this period, the common procedure performed was ventriculo-atrial shunting. Several large series [53,65,139] comparing the results of ventriculo-atrial and ventriculo-peritoneal shunting have shown that whilst complication rates of the two procedures are similar, complications from ventriculo-atrial shunts are often more severe and result in a higher mortality rate.

Postoperative care

It is advisable to nurse the baby with a head-up tilt in order to promote drainage. Sometimes, over-drainage occurs so that the fontanelle becomes very depressed, the baby vomits and may even collapse, in which case the head-down position is indicated. In practice, most babies can be nursed prone with the head turned to the left in order that to minimize pressure over the valve.

Normal feeding can be commenced as soon as it is tolerated. It is not necessary to pump the valve for it is designed to open and close at appropriate pressures; indeed, regular pumping may cause skin necrosis over the valve if done too vigorously. Only if there is sluggish drainage is pumping advised or allowed.

Morbidity and mortality

Not surprisingly, the implantation of a foreign body does cause complications [5]. Complications in our series of 80 patients treated with a shunting operation in 1976–85 included: shunt infection eight, wound infection two, early shunt blockage one. There were five deaths in the 10-year period: one patient died without surgery for hydrocephalus, two patients died from hyaline membrane disease, one patient had cardiac arrest with no apparent cause and one patient died of shunt infection and ventriculitis.

Infection

This is the most serious postoperative complication and can occur immediately after operation or later [78]. Infections which reveal themselves later can frequently be traced back to the early postoperative days and have presumably lain dormant in the system. The main infecting organism is *Staphylococcus albus* [27] which gets into the system at operation [13] and colonies become adherent to the Silastic of the valve by means of a mucoid substance produced by the organism [12].

The duration of the operation may well have a bearing on the infection rate – undue prolongation doubtless increases the chances of an intra-operative infection.

Infection rates are quoted from 2–39% [58,66,137]. Our experience of 10% shunt infection rate is in accordance with these figures. Recently there have been reports suggesting that prophylactic antibiotics may prevent shunt infection [3,15]. Malis [118] reported a series of 1732 consecutive major neurosurgical operations in which intra-operative prophylactic tobramycin, vancomycin and streptomycin were given with no postoperative infections. Gardner and Gordon [60] however, reported similarly impressive results of only 1.5% postoperative infection in 200 consecutive shunt operations without prophylactic antibiotics. All the infective complications in their series were attributed to inexperience of the operating surgeon and they suggested that scrupulous surgical technique alone should be enough to prevent shunt infection. Most of their patients, however, were outside the neonatal age group. Our neonatal patients probably have a higher risk of infection: ascending infection can occur in patients with open myelomeningocele and introduction of skin organisms into the CSF system is theoretically possible when repeated taps have been performed for neonates with post-haemorrhagic hydrocephalus. We agree that meticulous surgical technique is probably the most important factor but in high risk patients the possible benefits of prophylactic antibiotics should be investigated with further studies.

Any pyrexia in the postoperative period should be regarded with suspicion. General symptoms such as irritability or reluctance to feed are often present.

We have found serum C-reactive protein estimation to be a useful guide, a rising level strongly suggesting shunt infection. Blood cultures and ventricular reservoir aspiration should be carried out. The latter is best done using a Huber needle which has a non-bevelled tip with a side opening and does not punch a hole out of the Silastic [177]. If infection is found then treatment should commence with intrathecal gentamicin daily until the fluid becomes sterile, and parenteral gentamicin and penicillin. If the infecting organism is resistant to gentamicin, intrathecal vancomycin has been found to be effective [16].

It is important to monitor the blood and CSF antibiotic levels and adjust the dosage accordingly. Despite apparent sterilization of the system, complete eradication of infection is rarely possible, due to adherence mentioned above. Repeated cultures are indicated and in the event of recurrence, exteriorization of the system and replacement will be required [45].

Blockage of the system

Contrary to the common usage of the term 'blocked valve' the valve itself rarely if ever blocks. The ventricular catheter, however, is frequently the site of blockage [82,168], usually by choroid plexus (Figure 40.23) even in the first few weeks after valve insertion. Alternatively, the catheter may be either too long so that brain tissue impinges on the drainage holes in the catheter as the ventricular size decreases [69], or too short so that it comes out of the ventricle altogether. Sometimes a block with choroid plexus may be relieved by syringing the upper catheter [44,55] but this is not a procedure to be repeated and it is not without problems as too forcible a pressure may dislodge the catheter.

Lower end blockage can also occur. The peritoneal catheter may become kinked, or blocked by omentum. The atrial catheter, similarly, may become kinked or the lower end may have been misplaced in the inferior vena cava so that blood tends to flow up the tube [77].

In our experience, a much more reliable diagnosis of shunt blockage can be made by needling the reservoir than by palpation of the valve [177]. Imaging studies including ultrasound and CT scans [46] are useful adjunctive investigations.

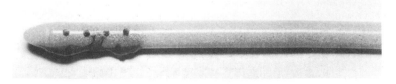

0   1   2   3   4

Figure 40.23 Ventricular catheter occluded by choroid plexus

Other complications

Abdominal complications of ventriculoperitoneal shunts include pseudocyst formation [26,133,166], peritonitis [81], pseudotumour, ascites, perforated viscus [38], inguinal hernia [120] and hydrocele [62], and catheter migration [152]. Vascular complications of ventriculo-atrial shunts include cardiac perforation [180], pulmonary emboli [47,50,132] leading to pulmonary hypertension [48] and superior vena cava thrombosis. Other possible complications include tube disconnections which should become rarer with the use of integral shunt systems, intrinsic pressure changes [31,35,151], epilepsy [80] and hemiparesis [24]. These complications are rare in the neonatal period.

Results

As shunting procedures using valves have only been available for three decades, it is difficult to obtain accurate and meaningful assessment of the eventual outcome. The problem is compounded by the multiplicity of valves available and the varied techniques of insertions, which makes comparison tedious if not impossible. In addition underlying or associated pathology such as spina bifida and prematurity will affect the outcome of the child.

It is clear that there are many problems in relation to both shunt insertion and long-term shunt dependency. For example, an increasing number of young people, having had no 'valve symptoms' for years, are presenting with raised intracranial pressure from valve malfunction during adolescence. It would seem likely that once a shunt has been inserted, it is there for life. 'Once a shunt, always a shunt?' (Hemmer) [73]; whether this statement holds true for children with post-haemorrhagic hydrocephalus is too early to tell as treatment for this condition has been undertaken only in the past decade: our impression however has been that arrest of the hydrocephalus does occur in some cases as channels reopen.

The IQ in many patients with treated hydrocephalus falls within the normal range but there is a wide scatter and few are of high ability. Indeed, the IQ would seem to deteriorate consequent upon the number of valve revisions [105]. In a series [155] 182 survivors of shunted hydrocephalus not due to periventricular-intraventricular haemorrhage, 11.5% had epileptic fits; 55% of those with primary hydrocephalus had normal verbal skills. Children with post-haemorrhagic hydrocephalus often have major handicap which is related to the brain injury associated with severe periventricular-intraventricular haemorrhage rather than to the management of their hydrocephalus [34].

References

1. Adams, C., Johnston, W.P. and Nevin, W.C. (1982) Family study of congenital hydrocephaly. *Dev. Med. Child Neurol.*, **24**, 493–498
2. Adams, R.D., Schatzki, R. and Scoville, W.B. (1941) The Arnold-Chiari malformation. *New Engl. J. Med.*, **225**, 125–131
3. Ajir, F., Levin, A.B. and Duff, T.A. (1981) Effect of prophylactic methicillin on cerebrospinal fluid shunt infection in children. *Neurosurgery*, **9**, 6–8
4. Allan, W.C. and Volpe, J.J. (1986) Periventricular haemorrhage. *Pediat. Clin. N. Am.*, **36**, 47–63
5. Anderson, F.M. (1973) Ventriculo-cardiac shunt; identification and control of practical problems in 143 cases. *J. Pediat.*, **82**, 222–227
6. Anonymous (1962) Sex-linked hydrocephalus with severe mental defect. (editorial). *Br. Med. J.*, **1**, 168
7. Anonymous (1985) Post-haemorrhagic ventricular dilatation in infants: who and how to treat (editorial). *Lancet*, **ii**, 1280–1281
8. Anwar, M.J., Doyle, A.J., Kadim, S., Hiatt, I.M. and Hegyi, T. (1986) Management of post-haemorrhagic hydrocephalus in the preterm infant. *J. Pediat. Surg.*, **21**, 334–337
9. Anwar, M., Kadam, S., Hiatt, I.M. and Hegyi, T. (1985) Serial lumbar punctures in prevention of post-haemorrhagic hydrocephalus in preterm infants. *J. Pediat.*, **107**, 446–450
10. Aronson, N. (1962) Hydrocephalus. In *Pediatric Surgery* (ed. W.T. Mustard, M.M. Ravitch, W.H. Snyder, K.J. Welch and C.D. Benson), Year Book Medical Publishers, Chicago
11. Arnold, J. (1894) Myelocyste. *Beitr. Path. Anat.*, **16**, 1–28
12. Bayston, R. and Penny, S.R. (1972) Excessive production of mucoid substance in staphylococcus S II A. *Dev. Med. Child Neurol.*, (Suppl.), **27**, 25–28
13. Bayston, R. and Lari, J. (1974) A study of the sources of infection in colonised shunts. *Dev. Med. Child Neurol.*, (Suppl.), **32**, 16–22
14. Bayston, R. (1975) Antibiotic prophylaxis in shunt surgery. *Devl. Med. Child Neurol.*, (Suppl.), **35**, 99–103
15. Bayston, R. and Milner, R.D.G. (1981) Antimicrobial activity of silicone rubber used in hydrocephalus shunts, after impregnation with antimicrobial substances. *J. Clin. Pathol.*, 1057–1962
16. Bayston, R., Barnicoat, M., Cudmore, R.E., Guiney, E.J., Gurusinghe, N. and Norman, P.M. (1984) The use of intraventricular vancomycin in the treatment of CSF shunt-associated ventriculitis. *Z. Kinderchir.*, **39**, (Suppl. II), 111–113
17. Becker, D.P. and Nulsen, F.E. (1968) Control of hydrocephalus by valve regulated shunt. Avoidance of complications in prolonged shunt maintenance. *J. Neurosurg.*, **28**, 215–226
18. Benson, J.W.T., Drayton, M.R., Hayward, C. *et al.* (1986) Multicentre trial of ethamsylate for prevention

of periventricular haemorrhage in very low birth-weight infants. *Lancet*, **ii**, 1297–1300

19. Bering, E.A. (1965) Pathophysiology of hydrocephalus. In *Workshop in hydrocephalus* (ed. K. Shulman), Children's Hospital, Philadelphia

20. Beverley, D.W., Chance, G.W., Inwood, M.J., Schaus, M. and O'Keefe, B. (1984) Intraventricular haemorrhage and haematosis defects. *Arch. Dis. Child.*, **59**, 444–448

21. Birnholz, J.C. and Frigoletto, F.D. (1981) Antenatal treatment of hydrocephalus. *New Engl. J. Med.*, **304**, 1021–1023

22. Blane, G. (1821) On the effect of mechanical compression of the head as a preventive and cure in certain cases of hydrocephalus. *London Med. Phys.*, **46**, 353

23. Boinet, A.A. (1810) *De l'alimentation iodée comme moyen preventife et curatif dans toutes les maladies on l'iode est employé a l'interieur comme médicament.* Masson, Paris

24. Boltshauser, E., Hirsig, J., Isler, W. and Rickham, P.P. (1980) Hemiparesis – an uncommon symptom of hydrocephalus or shunt dysfunction. *Z. Kinderchir.*, **30**, 191–197

25. Bowsher, D. (1956) *Cerebrospinal Fluid Dynamics in Health and Disease.* Charles C. Thomas, Springfield

26. Briggs, J.R., Hendry, G.M.A. and Minns, R.A. (1984) Abdominal ultrasound in the diagnosis of cerebrospinal fluid pseudocysts complicating ventriculoperitoneal shunts. *Arch. Dis. Child.*, **59**, 661–664

27. Callaghan, R.P., Cohen, S.J. and Stewart, G.T. (1961) Septicaemia due to colonisation of Spitz Holter valves by staphylococci. *Br. Med. J.*, **1**, 860–863

28. Chiari, H. (1891) Ueber veraenderungen des kleinhirns infolge von hydrozephalien des grosshirns. *Deutsch. Med. Wschr.*, **17**, 1172–1175

29. Chiswick, M.L. (1984) Ultrasound brain scanning in the newborn. *Br. Med. J.*, **289**, 337–338

30. Cleland, J. (1883) Contribution to the study of spina bifida encephalocele and anencephalus. *J. Anat. Physiol.*, **17**, 257–292

31. Clements, D.B. and Kaushal, K. (1970) A study of the ocular complications of hydrocephalus and meningomyelocele. *Trans. Ophthal. Soc. UK*, **99**, 383–390

32. Clewell, W.H., Johnson, M.L. and Meier, P.R. *et al.* (1982) A surgical approach to the treatment of fetal hydrocephalus. *New Engl. J. Med.*, **306**, 1320–1325

33. Cone, W.V., Lewis, R.D. and Jackson, I.J. (1949) Shunting of cerebrospinal fluid into the peritoneal cavity. Presented at the meeting of the American College of Physicians, Montreal, Canada

34. Cooke, R.W.I. (1987) Determinants of major handicap in post-haemorrhagic hydrocephalus. *Arch. Dis. Child.*, **62**, 504–506

35. Corkery, J.J. and Zachary, R.B. (1967) Increased resistance in valves. *Lancet*, **ii**, 1331–1333

36. Dandy, W.E. and Blackfan, K.D. (1914) Internal hydrocephalus. *Am. J. Dis. Child.*, **8**, 406–482

37. Daniel, P.M. and Stich, S.J. (1950) Some observation on the congenital deformity of the central nervous system known as the Arnold-Chiari malformation. *J. Neuropath.*, **17**, 255

38. Davidson, R.I. (1976) Peritoneal bypass in the treatment of hydrocephalus: historical reviews and abdominal complications. *J. Neurol. Neurosurg. Psychiat.*, **39**, 640–646

39. Dawson, B.H., Dervin, E. and Heywood, O.B. (1975) The problems of design and implantation of shunt systems for the treatment of hydrocephalus. *Dev. Med. Child. Neurol.* (Suppl.), **35**, 78–84

40. Di Chiro, G. (1964) Movements of the cerebrospinal fluid in human beings. *Nature (Lond.)*, **204**, 290–291

41. Di Chiro, G., Reames, R.M. and Matthews, W.B. (1964) RISA ventriculography and RISA cisternography. *Neurology*, **14**, 185–191

42. Dodge, P.R. and Fisman, M.A. (1970) The choroid plexus – two way traffic? *New Engl. J. Med.*, **283**, 316–317

43. Eckstein, H.B. (1965) Management of hydrocephalus. In *Proceedings of a Symposium on Spina Bifida*. National Foundation for Research into Poliomyelitis and Other Crippling Diseases, London

44. Eckstein, H.B. and MacNab, G.H. (1966) Myelomeningocele and hydrocephalus. *Lancet*, **i**, 842–845

45. Nicholas, J.L., Kamal, I.M. and Eckstein, H.B. (1970) Immediate shunt replacement in the treatment of bacterial colonisation of Holter valves. *Dev. Med. Child Neurol.*, (Suppl.) **22**, 110–113

46. El-Gohary, M.A., Forrest, D.M. and Starer, F. (1988) The role of the CT scan in the management of blocked ventricular shunt. *Pediat. Surg. Int.*, **4**, 247–251

47. Emery, J.L. (1964) Fibrin and thrombosis in the central nervous system in children with particular reference to congenital hydrocephalus. *J. Clin. Path.*, **17**, 348–352

48. Emery, J.L. and Hilton, H.B. (1961) Lung and heart complications of the treatment of hydrocephalus by ventriculo-auriculostomy. *Surgery*, **50**, 309–314

49. Epstein, F.H., Hochwald, G.H., Wald, A. and Ransohoff, H. (1975) Avoidance of shunt dependency in hydrocephalus. *Dev. Med. Child Neurol.* (Suppl), **35**, 71–77

50. Erdohazi, M., Eckstein, H.B. and Crome, L. (1966) Pulmonary embolisation as a complication of ventriculo-atrial shunts inserted for hydrocephalus. *Dev. Med. Child Neurol.* (Suppl), **11**, 36–44

51. Faivre, E. (1854) Recherches sur les structure du conarium et des plexus chorides chez l'homme et les animaux. *C.R. Acad. Sci.*, **39**, 42

52. Ferguson, A.H. (1898) Intraperitoneal diversion of the cerebrospinal fluid in cases of hydrocephalus. *NY Med. J.*, **67**, 902

53. Fernell, E., Wendt, L.V., Serlo, W., Heikkinen, E.

and Anderson, H. (1985) Ventriculoatrial or ventriculoperitoneal shunts in the treatment of hydrocephalus in children? *Z. Kinderchir.*, **40**, (Suppl. I), 12–14

54. Fischer, E.G. (1973) Dandy-Walker syndrome; an evaluation of surgical treatment. *J. Neurosurg.*, **39**, 615–621

55. Foltz, E.L. (1965) The first seven years of a hydrocephalus project. In *Workshop in Hydrocephalus* (ed. K. Shulman), Children's Hospital, Philadelphia

56. Forrest, D.M. (1962) Flow characteristics of the Holter valve. *Dev. Med. Child Neurol.*, **14**, 295–297

57. Forrest, D.M., Hole, R. and Wynne, J.M. (1966) Treatment of infantile hydrocephalus using the Holter valve. *Devl. Med. Child Neurol.*, (Suppl.), **11**, 27–35

58. Forrest, D.M. and Cooper, D.G.W. (1968) Complications of ventriculoatrial shunts. A review of 455 cases. *J. Neurosurg.*, **29**, 506–512

59. Gairdner, D. and Pearson, J. (1971) A growth chart for premature and other infants. *Arch. Dis. Child.*, **46**, 783–787

60. Gardner, B.P. and Gordon, D.S. (1982) Postoperative infection in shunts for hydrocephalus: are prophylactic antibiotics necessary? *Br. Med. J.*, **284**, 1914–1915

61. Gartner. Cited by Kausch, W. (1908) Die Behandlung des Hydrozephalus der Kleinen Kinder. *Arch. klin. Chir.*, **87**, 709–796

62. Georgacoulo, P., Franchella, A. and Massarotti, M. (1979) Inguinal hernia and hydrocele: a complication of ventriculoperitoneal shunting procedure. *Z. Kinderchir.*, **27**, 28–30

63. Gilles, F.H., Price, R.A. and Kevy, S.V. *et al.* (1971) Fibrinolytic activity in the ganglionic eminence of the premature human brain. *Biol. Neonat.*, **18**, 426–432

64. Go, K.G., Van der Veen, P.H. and Van der Berg, J. (1970) Detection of CSF flow in ventriculoatrial shunts by cold transfer. *Dev. Med. Child Neurol*, (Suppl.), **22**, 69–72

65. Gruber, R. (1979) Therapy of hydrocephalus in childhood: comparison of ventriculoperitoneal and ventriculoatrial shunt and their complications. *Z. Kinderchir.*, **28**, 212–225

66. Haines, S.J. (1980) Systemic antibiotic prophylaxis in neurological surgery. *Neurosurgery*, **6**, 355–361

67. Hakim, S. (1973) Hydraulic and mechanical mismatching of valve shunts used in the treatment of hydrocephalus; the need for a servo-valve shunt. *Dev. Med. Child Neurol.*, **15**, 646–653

68. Hammock, M.K. and Milhorat, T.H. (1973) Recent studies on the formation of cerebrospinal fluid. *Devl. Med. Child Neurol.*, (Suppl.), **29**, 27–34

69. Hammock, M.K., Milhorat, T.H. and McClenathan, J.G. (1975) Expanding ventricular shunts for the detection of valve blockage in hydrocephalus. *Devl. Med. Child Neurol.* (Suppl.), **35**, 89–93

70. Harbaugh, R.E., Saunders, R. and Edwards, W.H. (1981) External ventricular drainage for control of posthaemorrhagic hydrocephalus in premature infants. *J. Neurosurg.*, **58**, 766–770

71. Hart, M.N., Malamud, N. and Ellis, W.G. (1972) The Dandy-Walker syndrome. A clinico-pathological study. *Neurology*, **22**, 771–780

72. Heile, B. (1914) Zur chirurgischen des Hydrozephalus internus. *Arch. klin. Chir.*, **105**, 501–516

73. Hemmer, R. and Bohm, B. (1976) Once a shunt, always a shunt? *Dev. Med. Child Neurol.* (Suppl.), **37**, 69–73

74. Hildanus, F.G. (1946) Observationen et curationum medico chirurgicarum. Franco-forti ad Moenum; J. Beyeri.

75. Hill, A. and Holpe, J.J. (1981) Normal pressure hydrocephalus in the newborn. *Pediatrics*, **68**, 623–629

76. Hill, A., Shackelford, G.D. and Volpe, J.J. (1984) A potential mechanism of pathogenesis for early posthemorrhagic hydrocephalus in the premature newborn. *Pediatrics*, **73**, 19–21

77. Hooper, R. (1969) A lengthening procedure for VA shunts. *J. Neurosurg.*, **30**, 93–96

78. Holt, R.J. (1970) Bateriological studies on colonised ventriculo-atrial shunts. *Devl. Med. Child Neurol.*, (Suppl.), **22**, 83–87

79. Horbar, J.D., Waters, C.L., Philip, A.G.S. and Lucey, J.F. (1980) Ultrasound detection of changing ventricular size in posthemorrhagic hydrocephalus. *Pediatrics*, **66**, 674–678

80. Hosking, G.P. (1974) Fits in hydrocephalic children. *Arch. Dis. Child.*, **49**, 633–635

81. Hubschmann, O.R. and Countee, R.W. (1980) Acute abdomen in children with infected ventriculoperitoneal shunts. *Arch. Surg.*, **115**, 305–307

82. Hummel, E.G., Ono, H. and Galo, A.E. (1974) Percutaneous management of ventricular catheter obstruction. *J. Neurosurg.*, **41**, 511–512

83. Huttenlocher, P.R. (1965) Acetazolamide in hydrocephalus. *J. Pediat.*, **66**, 1023–1030

84. Hayden, P.W., Foltz, E.L. and Shurtleff, D.B. (1968) Effect of an oral osmotic agent on ventricular fluid pressure of hydrocephalic children. *Pediatrics*, **41**, 955–967

85. Illingworth, C.R. (1891) Tapping the ventricles. *Br. Med. J.*, **11**, 755

86. Ingraham, F.D. and Matson, D.D. (1955) *Neurosurgery of Infancy and Childhood*. Charles C. Thomas, Springfield

87. Irving, I.M., Castilla, P. and Hall, E.G. (1971) Tissue reaction to pure and impregnated Silastic. *J. Pediat. Surg.*, **6**, 724–729

88. Jackson, J.L. and Blomhagen, J.D. (1983) Congenital hydrocephalus due to prenatal intracranial hemorrhage. *Pediatrics*, **72**, 344–346

89. Johnson, M.L., Mack, L.A., Rumack, C.M., Frost, M. and Rashbaum, C. (1979) C-mode echoencepha-

lography in the normal and high risk infants. *Am. J. Roent.*, **133**, 375–381

90. Kaiser, G. and Minibus, H. (1985) Simultaneous measurement of ventricular fluid and fontanelle pressure in neonates and infants with hydrocephalus. *Z. Kinderchir.*, **40**, 3–6

91. Kausch, W. (1908) Die Behandlung des Hydrocephalus der klein. *Kinder. Arch. Klin. Chir.*, **87**, 709–796

92. Key, A. and Retzius, G. (1872) *Studier i nervystemets anatomi*. P.A. Norstedt, Stockholm

93. Kirkpatrick, M., Engleman, H. and Minns, R.A. (1989) Symptoms and signs of progressive hydrocephalus. *Arch. Dis. Child.*, **64**, 124–128

94. Korobkin, R. (1975) The relationship between head circumference and the development of communicating hydrocephalus following intraventricular hemorrhage. *Pediatrics*, **56**, 74–77

95. Kreusser, K.L., Tarby, T.J., Kovnar, E., Taylor, D.A., Hill, A. and Volpe, J.J. (1985) Serial lumbar punctures for at least temporary amelioration of neonatal posthemorrhagic hydrocephalus. *Pediatrics*, **75**, 719–724

96. Kuban, K. and Teele, R.L. (1984) Rationale for grading intracranial hemorrhage in premature infants. *Pediatrics*, **74**, 358–363

97. Lacey, D.J. (1985) Agenesis of the corpus callosum. *Am. J. Dis. Child.*, **139**, 953–955

98. Lange, S.A. (1966) *Surgical Treatment of Progressive Hydrocephalus*. North-Holland, Amsterdam

99. Larroche, J.C. (1972) Post-haemorrhagic hydrocephalus in infancy: Anatomical study. *Biol. Neonate*. **20**, 287–299

100. Laurence, K.M. (1959) The pathology of hydrocephalus. *Ann. R. Coll. Surg. Engl.*, **24**, 388–401

101. Laurence, K.M. (1984) Genetic aspects of 'uncomplicated' hydrocephalus and its relationship to neural tube defects. *Z. Kinderchir.*, **39**, 96–99 (Suppl. 2)

102. Lees, R.F., Harrison, R.B. and Sims, T.L. (1978) Grey scale ultrasonography in the evaluation of hydrocephalus and associated abnormalities in infants. *Am. J. Dis. Child.*, **132**, 376–378

103. Leomhardt, A., Steiner, H.H. and Linderkamp, O. (1989) Management of posthaemorrhagic hydrocephalus with a subcutaneous ventricular catheter reservoir in premature infants. *Arch. Dis. Child.*, **64**, 24–28

104. Lespinasse. Quoted by Davis, L. (1936). *Neurological Surgery*, Lea and Febiger, Philadelphia

105. Lister, J., Zachary, R.B. and Brereton, R. (1977) Open myelomeningocele – a ten year review of 200 consecutive closures. *Progr. Pediat. Surg.*, **11**, 161–176

106. Lonton, A.P., Barrington, N.A. and Lorber, J. (1975) Lacunar skull deformity related to intelligence in children with myelomeningocele and hydrocephalus. *Devl. Med. Child Neurol.* (Suppl.), **35**, 58–64

107. Lorber, J. (1961) Systematic ventriculography studies in infants born with myelomeningocoele and encephalocoele. *Arch. Dis. Child.*, **36**, 381–389

108. Lorber, J. (1969) Ventriculocardiac shunt in the first week of life; results of a controlled trial in the treatment of hydrocephalus in babies with spina bifida. *Devl. Med. Child Neurol.* (Suppl.), **20**, 13–22

109. Lorber, J. (1973) Isosorbide in the medical treatment of hydrocephalus. *J. Neurosurg.*, **39**, 702–711

110. Lorber, J. (1984) The family history of 'simple' congenital hydrocephalus. *Z. Kinderchir.*, **39**, 94–95

111. Lorenzo, A.V., Page, L.K. and Walters, G.V. (1970) Relationship between cerebrospinal fluid formation, absorption and pressure in human hydrocephalus. *Brain*, **93**, 679–692

112. Luschka, H. von (1851) *Die struktur des serosen Haute des Menschan* Laupp and Siebeck, Tubingen, p. 98

113. Luyendijk, W. and Noordijk, J.A. (1959) Surgical treatment of internal hydrocephalus in infants and children. *Acta neurochir.*, **7**, 483–501

114. MacNab, G.H. (1963) *Recent Advances in Paediatric Surgery* (ed. A.W. Wilkinson), Churchill, London

115. MacNab, G.H. (1966) The development of knowledge and treatment of hydrocephalus. *Dev. Med. Child Neurol.*, (Suppl.), **11**, 1–9

116. Macmahon, P. and Cooke, W.I. (1983) Hyponatraemia caused by repeated cerebrospinal fluid drainage in posthaemorrhagic hydrocephaly. *Arch. Dis. Child.*, **58**, 385–386

117. Magendie, F. (1842) *Recherches philosophiques et cliniques sur le liquide cephalorachidien un cerebrospinal*. Paris, Mesquinon, p. 40

118. Malis, L.I. (1979) Prevention of neurosurgical infection by intraoperative antibiotics. *Neurosurgery*, **5**, 339–343

119. Mantovani, J.F., Pasternak, J.F., Matthew, O.P., Allan, W.C., Mills, M.T., Casper, J. and Volpe, T.J. (1980) Failure of daily lumbar punctures in prevention of posthemorrhagic hydrocephalus in preterm infants. *J. Pediat.*, **107**, 446–450

120. Maozam, F., Glenn, J.D., Kaplan, B.J., Jalbert, J.L. and Mickle, J.P. (1984) Inguinal hernias after ventriculoperitoneal shunt procedures in pediatric patients. *Surg. Gynec. Obstet.*, **159**, 570–572

121. Matson, D.D. (1951) Ventriculo-ureterostomy. *J. Neurosurg.*, **8**, 398–404

122. McComb, J.G. (1982) Cerebrospinal fluid formation and absorption. In *Pediatric Neurosurgery* (ed. R.L. McLaurin), Grune & Stratton Inc., New York, pp. 171–182

123. Mikulicz, J. (1896) Beitrag zur Pathologie und Therapie des Hydrozephalus. *Mitt. Grenzgeb. Med. Chir.*, **1**, 264

124. Milhorat, T.H. and Hammock, M.K. (1971) Isotope ventriculography interpretation of ventricular size and configuration in hydrocephalus. *Arch. Neurol.*, **25**, 1–8

125. Milhorat, T.H. (1972) *Hydrocephalus and the Cerebrospinal Fluid*. Williams and Wilkins, Baltimore

126. Milhorat, T.H. (1982) Circulation of the cerebrospinal fluid. In *Pediatric Neurosurgery* (ed. R.L.

McLaurin) Grune & Stratton Inc., New York, pp. 1893–195

127. Miner, L.C. and Reed, D.J. (1972) Composition of fluid obtained from choroid plexus tissue isolated in a chamber *in situ. J. Physiol. (Lond.)*, **227**, 127–139

128. Minns, R.A. (1984) Intracranial pressure monitoring. *Arch. Dis. Child.*, **59**, 486–488

129. Monro, A. (1783) *Observations on the structure and function of the nervous system*. William Creech, Edinburgh

130. Morgagni, J.B. (1762) *De Sedibus et causis morborum*, Typographia Simoniana, Naples

131. Nixon, H.H. (1962) Ventriculo pleural drainage with a valve. *Dev. Med. Child Neurol.*, **4**, 301–302

132. Noble, T.C., Lassman, L.P., Urquhart, W. and Aherne, W.A. (1970) Thrombotic and embolic complications of ventriculo atrial shunts. *Dev. Med. Child Neurol.*, (Suppl.), **22**, 114–122

133. Norfray, J.F., Henry, H.M., Givens, J.D. and Sparberg, M.S. (1979) Abdominal complications from peritoneal shunts. *Gastroenterology*, **77**, 337–340

134. Nosik, W.A. (1950) Treatment of hydrocephalus by ventriculomastoidostomy. *J. Pediat.*, **37**, 190–194

135. Nulsen, F.E. and Spitz, E.B. (1952) Treatment of hydrocephalus by direct shunt from ventricle to jugular vein. *Surg. Forum*, **2**, 399–403

136. Nulsen, F.E. and Becker, D.P. (1965) The control of progressive hydrocephalus in infancy by valve-regulated venous shunt. In *Workshop in Hydrocephalus* (ed. K. Shulman), Children's Hospital, Philadelphia

137. Odio, C., McCracken, G.H., Jr. and Nelson, J.D. (1984) CSF shunt infections in pediatrics. *Am. J. Dis. Child.*, **138**, 1103–1108

138. O'Hare, A.E., Brown, J.K. and Minns, R.A. (1987) Specific enlargement of the fourth ventricle after ventriculo-peritoneal shunt for post-haemorrhagic hydrocephalus. *Arch. Dis. Child.*, **62**, 1025–1029

139. Olsen, L. and Frykberg, T. (1983) Complications in the treatment of hydrocephalus in children. *Acta Paediat. Scand.*, **72**, 385–390

140. Orryzlo, M.A. (1942) The Arnold-Chiari malformation. *Arch. Neurol. Psychiat.*, **48**, 30

141. Pape, K.E. and Wigglesworth, J.S. (1979) Hemorrhage, ischaemia and the perinatal brain. *Clinics in Developmental Medicine*. Nos. 69/70. SIMP, J.B. Lippincott, Co., Philadelphia

142. Papile, L.A., Burstein, J., Burstein, R., Koffler, H., Koops, B.L. and Johnson, J.D. (1980) Posthemorrhagic hydrocephalus in low-birth-weight infants: treatment by serial lumbar punctures. *J. Pediat.*, **97**, 273–277

143. Papile, L.A., Burstein, J., Burstein, R. *et al.* (1978) Incidence and evolution of subependymal and intraventricular hemorrhage: a study of infants with birth weights less than 1,500 gms. *Pediatrics*, **92**, 529–534

144. Patten, B.M. (1953) *Human Embryology*. McGraw-Hill, New York

145. Payr, E. (1908) Drainage des Hirnventrikel Mittels frei transplantierter Blutgefaesse. *Arch. Klin. Chir.*, **87**, 801–855

146. Penfield, W. and Coburn, D.F. (1938) Arnold-Chiari malformation and its operative treatment. *Archs Neurol. Psychiat.*, **40**, 328–336

147. Philip, A.G.S. (1979) Noninvasive monitoring of intracranial pressure: a new approach to neonatal clinical pharmacology. *Clin. Perinatal.*, **6**, 123–137

148. Philip, A.G.S., Long, J.G. and Donn, S.M. (1981) Intracranial pressure: sequential measurements in full-term and pre-term infants. *Am. J. Dis. Child.*, **135**, 521–524

149. Pollay, M. and Curl, F. (1967) Secretion of cerebrospinal fluid by the ventricular ependyma of the rabbit. *Am. J. Physiol.*, **213**, 1031–1038

150. Potter, E.C. (1952) *Pathology of the Fetus and the Newborn*. Year Book Medical Publishers, Chicago

151. Potthoff, P.C. and Hemmer, R. (1969) Valve insufficiency with ventriculo-atrial shunts. *Dev. Med. Child Neurol.*, (Suppl.), **20**, 38–41

152. Prabhu, S., Cochran, W. and Azmy, A.F. (1985) Wandering distal ends of ventriculo peritoneal shunts. *Z. Kinderchir.*, **40**, 80–81

153. Pudenz, R.H., Russel, F.E., Hurd, A.H. and Shelden, C.H. (1957) A technique for shunting cerebrospinal fluid into the right auricle. *J. Neurosurg.*, **14**, 171–179

154. Pudenz, R.H. (1981) The surgical treatment of hydrocephalus in a historical review. *Surg. Neurol.*, **15**, 15–26

155. Puri, P., Dorner, S. and Eckstein, H.B. (1979) The results of treatment of hydrocephalus with the Holter valve: a six to eighteen year follow-up. *Z. Kinderchir.*, **22**, 14–21

156. Putnam, T.J. (1934) Treatment of hydrocephalus by endoscopic coagulation of choroid plexus. *New Engl. J. Med.*, **210**, 1373–1380

157. Quinn, R.J.M. and Adhikari, M. (1978) Compressive head wrapping: treatment of neonatal hydrocephalus. *Clin. Pediat.*, **17**, 464–466

158. Ransohoff, J. (1954) Ventriculo-pleural anastomosis in treatment of midline obstructional neoplasm. *J. Neurosurg.*, **11**, 295–298

159. Rayport, M. and Reiss, J. (1969) Hydrodynamic studies of certain shunt assemblies available for the treatment of hydrocephalus. *J. Neurosurg.*, **30**, 455–467

160. Rickham, P.P. (1964) A ventriculostomy reservoir. *Br. Med. J.*, **2**, 173

161. Rickham, P.P. (1968) A new silver impregnated Silastic catheters in the Holter valve operation. *Devl. Med. Child Neurol.*, (Suppl.), **15**, 14–16

162. Rickham, P.P. and Penn, I.A. (1965) The place of the ventriculostomy reservoir in the treatment of myelomeningoceles and hydrocephalus. *Dev. Med. Child. Neurol.*, **7**, 296–301

points to close are situated at either end and are called neuropores [81].

In the 18–19 somites embryo, at the end of the third week of intrauterine life, the neural tube is completely formed and extends along the entire length of the embryo's body and tail. The primitive mesoderm now starts to organize to form the vertebrae, skull and meninges, enclosing the neural tube [71].

The concept of a primary inhibiting influence on the embryo as a cause of myelomeningocele [77] was to a certain extent confirmed by experimental production of the condition by the introduction of noxious substances into animal embryos [55,102], but an early overgrowth of the neural plate was also suggested [78] and serial sections of embryos with myelomeningoceles showed that the bulk of the neural plate tissue was much greater in the region of the spinal defect than in adjacent normal segments of the spinal cord [79]. Examination of an 8-mm embryo showed a neural tube defect established prior to the spina bifida, suggesting that vertebral deformities were a secondary phenomenon; and in the chick, slitting open of the roof plate of the neural tube caused considerable increase in the bulk of the spinal cord and subsequent myelomeningocele [35].

Since the classic work of Dandy and Blackfan in 1913 [19] it has traditionally been accepted that the frequently associated hydrocephalus is the result of arachnoiditis and adhesions around the hindbrain which combine with downward displacement of cerebellum and medulla (Arnold–Chiari malformation) through the foramen magnum, which is present in practically every case, to obstruct the flow of cerebrospinal fluid. Further obstruction is brought about by aqueduct abnormalities secondary to the hindbrain crowding. An alternative suggestion has been that the hydrocephalus could be a primary lesion [7]; a 'late opening' of the foramina of Luschka and Magendi could result in an increase in pressure within the cerebral ventricles and the central canal of the spinal cord, and the neural tube deformity would then be due not to failure of closure but to rupture of a formed neural tube with consequent damage to overlying mesoderm and hydromyelia [26,64]. The Arnold–Chiari malformation could also be explained by alterations in pressure differential after rupture of the tube. However, the malformed medulla and cerebellum are not only displaced downwards but also appear large in relation to surrounding structures [22], and this disproportion seems more likely to be the primary lesion [25].

The split notochord syndrome and myelomeningocele

Occasionally, embryos develop with partial duplication of the notochord. It is then possible for the ventrally placed yolk sac to herniate through the gap between the two segments of the split notochord, to adhere to the dorsal ectoderm or even to rupture into the amniotic cavity [2] (Figures 41.4, 41.5 and 41.6).

This syndrome may give rise to a number of malformations. Isolated visceral malformations, such as duplication cysts [5,34], are discussed in Chapter 33. If the intestinal fistula persists and traverses the spinal canal (Figures 41.7, 41.8) endodermal structures will be intimately associated with myelomeningocele. This type of lesion used to be described as a teratoma occurring in conjunction

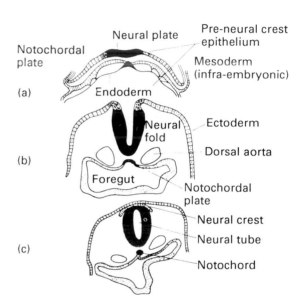

Figure 41.4 Formation of the neural tube

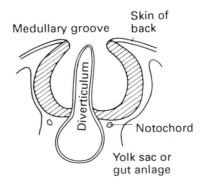

Figure 41.5 Split notocord. Yolk sac hernia

with a myelomeningocele [46], but it is now gene-rally accepted that these tumours arise from endodermic fistulae or sinuses.

Fusion of the medial pedicles of a pair of hemivertebrae to form a bony spur which lies between the split halves of the spinal cord is another malformation commonly associated with the split notochord syndrome [5,28]; this condition is called diastematomyelia [42] (Figure 41.9, 41.10). Vesico-intestinal fissure [99], or exstrophy of the cloaca, is usually associated with a myelomeningocele and is a severe variation of the split notochord syndrome. It is discussed in Chapter 51.

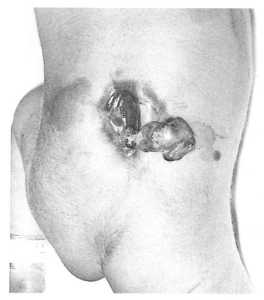

Figure 41.8 Split notocord syndrome. Endodermic structure projecting as 'teratoma' from myelomeningocele

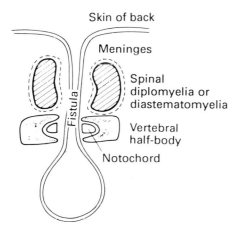

Figure 41.6 Split notocord. Yolk sac fistula

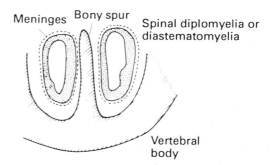

Figure 41.9 Split notocord. Diastematomyelia

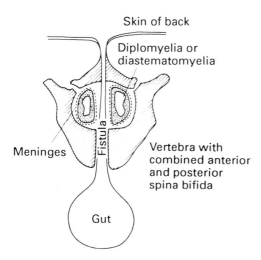

Figure 41.7 Split notocord

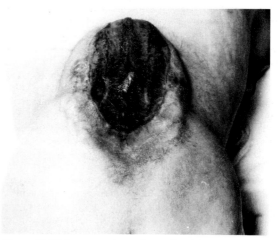

Figure 41.10 Open myelomeningocele with diastematomyelia

Aetiology

It is probable that in myelomeningocele as in all neural tube abnormalities there is both an environmental and a genetic factor. Only a few clues are available [19].

Genetic

Sex differences, ethnic variations and increased incidence where there is parental consanguinity [10,14,115] all suggest a polygenically inherited predisposition. In several large series of sibships studied, the proportion of siblings affected has varied from 3% to 6% which is 7–15 times the incidence in the general population of the areas studied [12,66,118]. The incidence of myelomeningoceles in first cousins of the patient is about twice that of the general population. In the UK, the risk of a mother having a second affected child after the birth of one child with myelomeningocele is about 1 in 25 and after two affected children, about 1 in 10 [13]. The affected siblings may have any neural tube malformation from a small meningocele to anencephaly, and thus the chances of having two surviving severely handicapped children to bring up are quite small. Studies of the children of affected patients [11] suggest an incidence similar to that in siblings.

Environmental

Whilst the genetic predisposition may be presumed from the above clues, the environmental insult is even more difficult to identify [117]. Migration affects ethnic differences and in a country such as the UK with little ethnic variation there can be striking geographical variations in incidence; the rates for South Wales are two and a half times and those for Northern Ireland are three times the rates for London [48]. Steady declines [37,62,67] and unexpected peaks [4,63] in incidence have been reported.

There is a well-recognized increased frequency of neural tube abnormalities in social class 5 (unskilled labour), and there are high rates for babies conceived in March, April and May in England and Wales, but no specific factor has been positively identified [14,54].

Dietary factors have been suggested. The blighted potato hypothesis of Renwick [83] has proved to be untenable [6], and the relation of incidence to other foods awaits substantiation though a significantly high incidence of defective folate metabolism in the mothers of infants born with central nervous system malformations has been reported [106]. Smithells [105,107,108] related the widely observed social class gradient in the incidence of neural tube defects to a possible nutritional contribution to causation. Multicentre trials [109] strongly suggest that periconceptual vitamin supplementation given to women at risk (who had already had a child with a neural tube defect) reduced the incidence of recurrence of a neural tube defect: a double blind placebo trial is required to confirm this suggestion but is difficult to mount for ethical reasons.

The fact that the pregnancy immediately preceding the birth of a child with a neural tube defect terminated in abortion nearly three times as frequently, and in stillbirths nearly twice as frequently, as that preceding normal controls [106] has led to another unsubstantiated hypothesis that the defect is brought about in some way by retained products of the previous conception [15].

Incidence

There is a very wide variation in the incidence of spina bifida cystica reported from different centres. The term 'spina bifida cystica' comprises both meningoceles and myelomeningoceles [22] and the differentiation between the two deformities is difficult, and varies from observer to observer; the true incidence of myelomeningocele is, therefore, somewhat in doubt. Spina bifida cystica appears to be very uncommon in Japan; Neel [74] reported an incidence of 0.32 per 1000 births. The incidence is a little higher in Australia; in Melbourne [16] it was estimated to be 0.56 per 1000. Several reports from the USA [76,80] suggest that the incidence is generally thought to be in the neighbourhood of 3 per 1000 but there are considerable local variations. In Birmingham [82] it was found to be 3 per 1000, in Liverpool [106] 3.5 per 1000 and in South Wales [48] 4.1 per 1000 total births. Richards *et al.* [85] even showed a variation between the valleys of east and west Glamorgan and Monmouth where the incidence was considerably higher than in the rest of those two counties. However, most of these reports of incidence were made some years ago and there is a remarkable waxing and waning of frequency which is now becoming apparent.

Table 41.1 Birth rate and admission to Neonatal Surgical Unit, Alder Hey Hospital in 3-year periods

	1963–65	*1973–75*	*1983–85*
Birth rate (per 1000 population)	17.7	13.9	12.9
Total admissions	688	531	484
Myelomeningocele	268	190	70
Encephalocele	12	16	9
Primary hydrocephalus	13	7	11

Lorber reported the virtual disappearance of spina bifida births in Sheffield between 1974 and 1984: the incidence of neural tube anomalies in all parts of the UK had fallen by more than 50% during the same time. In the 3 years from 1973 to 1975, 190 children with myelomeningocele were admitted to the Neonatal Surgical Unit in Alder Hey, whereas only 70 were admitted in the 3 years 1983–85 (Table 41.1). Only a part of this remarkable reduction can be accounted for by antenatal diagnosis and pregnancy termination. There is a slight preponderance of females born with this malformation [22,65,106] and there appears to be a particular susceptibility of mothers between the ages of 20 and 24 to give birth to such a child.

Clinical picture

General condition

A detailed examination is first required to assess the general condition of the infant and to exclude the possibility of severe intracranial damage and any associated major congenital abnormalities.

Local lesion

The diagnosis of an open myelomeningocele or an encephalocele can rarely be in doubt; skin-covered sacral myelomeningoceles which may occasionally be mistaken for sacrococcygeal teratomata (see Chapter 14) do not concern us here, as there is usually no immediate urgency for treatment. Occasionally, there may be more than one myelomeningocele or a myelomeningocele and an encephalocele in the same patient.

On examining the spine the extent of the bony defect can be palpated. In addition, a marked kyphosis and/or scoliosis due to absent or wedged vertebrae is often observed. The Klippel–Feil syndrome is frequently observed in association with a cervical myelomeningocele. In the flat, open myelocele-type of lesion with kyphosis the defective vertebral laminae often form a marked bony ridge on each side of the defect. These lesions are frequently difficult to close and this observation is, therefore, of significance in the prognosis. Transillumination of a myelomeningocele sac has been advised in order to discover whether nerves traverse the sac [46]. The nerves show up as dark strands in the brilliantly transilluminating sac. In our experience fibrous strands and thickenings in the covering membranes may, however, also appear as dark strands on transillumination.

Neurological complications

Open myelomeningocele will almost invariably be accompanied by some degree of paralysis and anaesthesia below the level of the lesion, though the extent of the neurological involvement will not always bear an accurate relationship to the level of the lesion; it may be more extensive than expected because of abnormalities in the cord beyond the exposed neural plaque, or on occasion the cord may, surprisingly, have been spared and function may be much better than expected, especially in the case of lesions confined to the dorsal spine. Future bladder function can be related better to the neurological activity of the legs than to the level of the lesion [113].

Motor disturbances of skeletal muscles

Partial or complete paralysis of the muscles of the buttocks, thighs, legs and feet is common, as is paralysis of the pelvic floor. Paralytic deformities such as dislocation of the hips, talipes equinovarus and genu recurvatum may be seen where paralysis is incomplete; stiffness of the lower limbs with arthrogryposis is less often observed. The paralysis is usually flaccid but spastic paraplegia may occur in myelomeningocele [40,94], especially in high lesions and sometimes as a result of the associated hydrocephalus. The best time to observe voluntary movement in the newborn infant with myelomeningocele is immediately after birth, and prolonged observation is necessary. The differentiation between voluntary and reflex movement is difficult [21] and spinal reflexes are frequently anomalous. Once the child has been allowed to get cold, and the child with myelomeningocele does so very easily, then voluntary movement may disappear temporarily though paralysis is not present. Response to faradic stimulation in the hands of an experienced observer may give a better assessment of eventual clinical function than simple clinical examination but accurate interpretation of findings is difficult [101].

Sensory disturbances

Sensory disturbances, producing areas of anaesthesia over the lower limbs, the perineum and buttocks, are also very common, but are even more difficult to demonstrate in the newborn than the motor deficiencies; in a warm relaxed infant the patient observer can map out the response to pinprick, and Brocklehurst [8] suggests that the true sensory level at which the infant responds to pinprick will correspond with the myotome level to which upper motor neuron control persists.

Trophic lesions tend to appear in the older child but such lesions on the ankles and heels, and particularly in the nappy area, may occur in the newborn, emphasizing the importance of skilled nursing care.

Neurological disturbances of the pelvic organs

Partial or complete paralysis of the bladder and pelvic floor is a frequent complication. Weakness of the anal sphincter may be demonstrated by an evident lax anus, an absent anal reflex or even a prolapse of the rectal mucosa (Figure 41.11). Less severe degrees of rectal incompetence are very difficult to assess in early life.

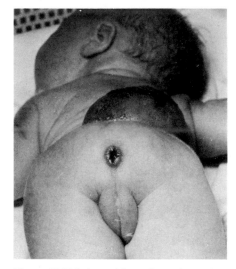

Figure 41.11 Infant with myelomeningocele and paralysed anus

Essentially, there are three types of bladder function.

(1) If there is a normal spinal cord, even on one side as in hemimyelocele [23], it is likely that there will be normal micturition. These account for about 10%.
(2) Where there is a complete lower motor neuron lesion there is a constant dribble of urine from an empty bladder. This condition is very rare and has been shown to be due to frequent detrusor contractions with virtually no bladder outlet compression [120]. These are rare.
(3) Where there is imbalance between detrusor and sphincter due to an incomplete lower motor neuron lesion or a complete or mixed upper motor neuron lesion, there is consequently a tendency to urinary stasis. These form the majority of cases. Bladder trabeculation may already be present at birth [96].

The vast majority of cases have a normal upper urinary tract at birth but hydroureter and hydronephrosis may occasionally already be present and vesicoureteric reflux has been demonstrated [89].

The general examination of the child in relation to the level of the neural plaque, the degree of paralysis of the legs [110,112], perineal sensation [103] and the activity of the anal sphincter may combine to give an indication of the degree of innervation of the bladder [32]. Observation of the pattern of micturition and palpation of the bladder is extremely important; if urine can be expressed by suprapubic compression (as distinct from a spontaneous contraction of the detrusor being stimulated by the cold hand on the abdomen) then bladder innervation can be presumed to be abnormal. Minor neurological involvement of the bladder, however, may not become evident for many years, and conversely minor degrees of detrusor/sphincter imbalance may be overcome when the child is 8–10 years old so that normal control of micturition is achieved [59].

Hydrocephalus

At least 80% of children with myelomeningocele have hydrocephalus [24,33,90]. This subject is discussed in detail in Chapter 40.

Special investigations

Radiography

Radiography of the spine will demonstrate the extent of the bony defect and any associated abnormalities of the axial skeleton, including particularly hemivertebrae and rib defects and the extent of any kyphoscoliosis present. Except in those cases where the severity of the deformity suggests that operative closure will be difficult and may involve bone surgery, the baseline views of the axial skeleton may conveniently be obtained at the time of the routine IVP which will be done during the child's first admission.

Treatment

Timing of operation

Sharrard and his colleagues [100,101] suggested that closure of the myelomeningocele within the first 24 h of life resulted in some improvement of the neurological status but this has not been accepted by other writers [38,95] and has not occurred in our experience. Some authors have shown that in their hands early closure has no advantage over non-closure with respect to mortality and the incidence of hydrocephalus and ventriculitis [20]: others point out that early operation may be an important preventive measure against the late complications of scoliosis and neurological deterioration due to a tethered cord [39]. Desiccation and infection of the exposed nervous tissue may result in extension of the paralysis below the myelomeningocele unless that paralysis is already complete: there seems no reason therefore why an open myelomeningocele should be treated any way differently from any other open wound, by early closure, unless there are positive contraindications. It has already been stated that infants who seem likely to die within 24–48 h should not have the back closed as an emergency; but those who have some movement below the hip flexors, should be closed urgently in order to preserve that movement. Between these two extremes come a considerable number of children who have no movement below the hip flexors and who do not seem likely to die. In these cases early closure is not mandatory since there is no useful movement to preserve; if closure seems to be easy then the child will be more easily managed, and will be discharged home sooner if the back is closed, but if closure seems likely to be difficult then conservative management allowing epithelialization to occur over the lesion is justifiable.

Pre-operative management

As soon as a baby is born with a myelomeningocele or encephalocele the lesion should be covered with a non-adherent dressing to prevent drying out of the nerve plaque or membranous covering. Sterile gauze moistened with 2% chlorhexidine (Hibitane) in water may be used provided the dressing is kept moist by dripping Hibitane onto it and appropriate measures can be taken to avoid cooling the child.

Melolin (Smith and Nephew) non-stick dressing protects the plaque without providing an evaporating cooling surface and is more suitable for use if the baby has to travel some distance.

The routine pre-operative management as described in Chapter 5 is applied.

Operation for myelomeningocele

The child is placed prone on the operating table with the head rotated to the right through 90 degrees. Heat loss is minimized in the usual way. Bacterial swabs are taken from the exposed plaque and surrounding skin (which are likely to be negative if Hibitane dressings have been applied) and cerebrospinal fluid is aspirated from the sac (if present) for culture. The neural plaque is cleansed with 2% Hibitane dressings have been applied) and cerebrospinal fluid is aspirated from the sac (if present) for spirit. The plaque is protected with a small Hibitane swab and the whole back of the child from head to feet covered with skin drape (Figure 41.12).

The gauze swab covering the myelomeningocele is now removed and the lesion is again gently cleansed with a 2% watery Hibitane solution. The membrane between the edge of the skin defect and the neural plaque is now removed. It has been pointed out that it is very important to remove every vestige of this membrane, as the burying of even a small segment of membrane beneath the skin may cause the formation of epidermoid cysts which can cause late paralysis due to pressure on the cord. When the dissection approaches the neural plaque,

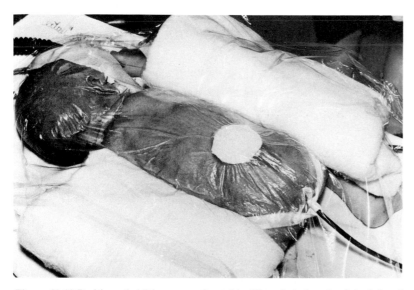

Figure 41.12 Position of child on operating table. The whole length of the infant is covered by transparent skin drape. Note the electric thermometer lead which has been placed in the anus

it is helpful to stimulate the edges of the plaque with faradic current in order to identify functional motor nervous tissue. The transparent skin drape sheeting over the buttocks and legs allows for accurate observation of any muscle contraction in these parts. The neural plaque is completely freed and can now be seen in the centre of the wound with the spinal nerves coursing from its undersurface (Figure 41.13). If possible, the neural plaque is now folded over and closed along its axis. The dura is incised on both sides of the plaque, leaving a thin strip of dura at the outer side attached to the skin. The dural sac is then closed with a running suture of 3/0 silk (Figure 41.14). The thick, tough, fibrous layer overlying the deformed spinal laminae on each side of the defect is now freed from the bone by diathermy dissection (Figure 41.15).

In infants with a pronounced kyphos the prominent laminae may prevent satisfactory skin closure or cause pressure necrosis under the tight skin flaps after closure. The tips of the projecting laminae should therefore be removed with bone nibbling forceps; troublesome bleeding may occur from the cut bone ends and should be controlled by the application of bone wax. The muscles are now freed from the spine by deep, blunt dissection (Figure 41.16), and the musculofascial layer is approximated using interrupted 3/0 silk sutures (Figure 41.17). When this layer has been closed completely, it forms a tough cover for the spinal cord without having to resort to wide separation of the musculofascial layer from the subcutaneous tissue. The skin of the back receives its main blood supply from small arteries which, running straight backwards, perforate the spinal muscles and fascia to reach the skin. Wide mobilization of the skin flaps by dissecting them off the deep fascia destroys most of this blood supply.

The skin flaps are now approximated by putting interrupted 3/0 silk sutures through the dural strip which was left attached to the skin (Figure 41.18), placing the knots inside. It is thus possible to approximate the skin completely without putting a

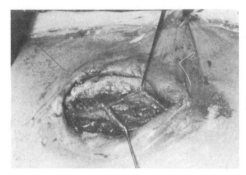

Figure 41.14 The dura is closed by a running suture

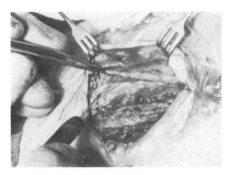

Figure 41.15 Freeing the fibrous layer from the spine with the aid of diathermy

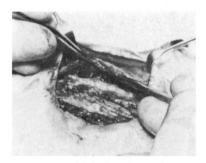

Figure 41.16 The muscles are dissected off the spine

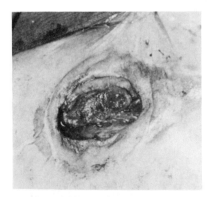

Figure 41.13 The neural plaque has been completely freed

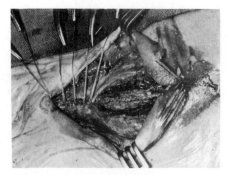

Figure 41.17 The musculofascial layer is approximated with interrupted sutures. Superficial fascia and skin being still attached to the deep fascia are thus displaced medially

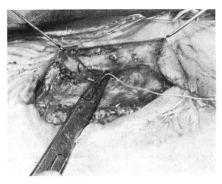

Figure 41.18 The skin is approximated by placing sutures through the dural strip which was left attached to the skin

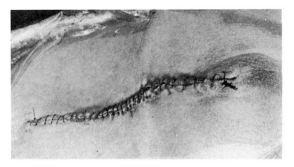

Figure 41.20 Closure of skin with a continuous suture

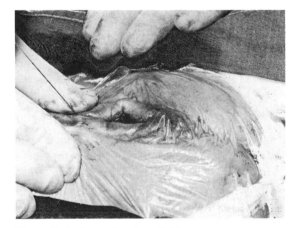

Figure 41.19 Approximation of skin

suture through the actual skin and without having to mobilize it extensively from the underlying muscle and deep fascia (Figure 41.19). Any excess of skin is now trimmed off and the approximated skin edges are then sutured loosely with interrupted or continuous nylon sutures (Figure 41.20). This modification of the Zachary procedure [106] has allowed us to close most defects without having to resort to undermining of the skin, rotation flaps, delayed closure or free skin grafts – methods which have been freely advocated in the literature, but have, in our hands at any rate, been followed frequently by breakdown of the wound.

Postoperative treatment

The infant is returned to the incubator where he is nursed prone, a corset of orthopaedic strapping having been applied which pulls the abdominal skin backwards as the child is slung from a special frame (Figure 41.21). These infants are prone to vomit during the first 12–24 h after operation and it is

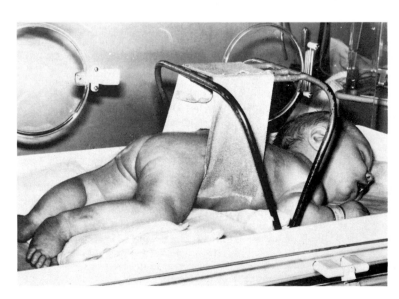

Figure 41.21 Child suspended by orthopaedic strapping on special frame fitting into incubator – tension on wound edges reduced

therefore wise to keep a gastric catheter *in situ* and to aspirate the stomach at regular intervals. Feeding is then commenced, but the child remains suspended prone until the skin sutures are removed on the 10th to 14th day after operation. Nursing of the infants in this manner not only prevents tension on the suture line, but greatly facilitates the disposal of urine or faeces, which are collected beneath the child and cannot contaminate the operation wound.

Hydrocephalus

When the back is healed, a shunt can be established if indicated (see Chapter 40).

Urinary tract

Urinary tract care in the neonatal period is mainly directed to nursing care and basic assessment which includes observation of bladder function, repeated urine cultures, ultrasound assessment of the urinary tract and intravenous urography.

Preservation of the upper urinary tract depends on the early recognition of deviation from the normal, particularly with regard to urinary stasis; a few children in the neonatal period have a neuropathic bladder outlet obstruction which cannot be overcome by suprapubic expressions and these patients will require urethral dilatation or possibly bladder catheterization.

Management of complications

Wound infection

Wound infection is not uncommon [93]: swabs taken from the plaque at operation, and cerebrospinal fluid aspirated, are usually sterile on culture but thin strips of skin excised at the junction with the membranous coverings not infrequently show a significant bacterial growth. If organisms have been grown and their sensitivity to antibiotics has been reported, the appropriate antibiotic can be vigorously exhibited at the first sign of infection of the wound or of meningitis.

An even more frequent cause of wound infection is undue tension on the skin edges and subsequent skin necrosis. Provided the musculofascial layer beneath the slough remains intact, this is an annoying, but not too serious complication, but if the infection penetrates the dural coverings spreading meningitis results. *Staphylococcus*, *Escherichia coli*, *Pseudomonas aeruginosa* and *Bacillus proteus* are the most common infecting organisms. These infections must be treated with the appropriate antibiotics both locally and systemically [75]. Where sloughs occur, frequent dressing of the wound with eusol or trypsin or streptokinase preparations (Varidase, Trypure) at 4-h intervals is required.

Cerebrospinal fluid leak

Wound leaks of cerebrospinal fluid occasionally occur, especially when there is marked increase of the intracranial pressure with rapidly enlarging hydrocephalus. Small leaks can often be stopped by dressing the leaking wound with gauze soaked in a 2% watery solution of mercurochrome and applying pressure dressings. Persistent leaks in the presence of hydrocephalus may necessitate repeated ventricular tapping or, in some cases, the insertion of a Holter valve prior to the complete healing of the wound (see Chapter 40).

Results

Results of operation for spina bifida cystica and encephalocele have been published from many centres but comparisons become increasingly difficult. The published views of various authors on 'selection' for treatment or non-treatment must influence the cases referred to these authors [58]; the severe cases will not be referred to those centres where only the less handicapped children are vigorously treated and the smaller number of children involved may well be better treated. Conversely, in those centres where the majority of children will be vigorously treated, 'preselection' will result in larger numbers of more severely affected children being referred with the consequent increase in the proportion of poor long-term results. Furthermore, series reported do not always refer to exactly similar groups of cases.

The classic studies of the natural history of spina bifida cystica are from Laurence [48,49,52]. In 1966 a group of 426 cases born between 1956 and 1962 showed a 15.5% survival where no initial treatment had been carried out; these figures did not distinguish between open and closed myelomeningocele and included encephaloceles.

In Liverpool city [70,92] a series of cases born between 1960 and 1963, most of them operated upon in the first days of life, were reviewed in 1967; 64% of operated patients were surviving and 49% of all patients. This group, however, included open myelomeningoceles and encephaloceles, and excluded stillbirths and children who died of gross associated abnormalities within a few hours of birth.

In an unselected series of 200 consecutive closures of open myelomeningocele in Sheffield in 1963 and 1964 [59] there were 117 (58.5%) survivors at 5 years and 106 (53%) traced at 10 years. Only two cases admitted during that period died before closure of the back. Of the 88 deaths in the first 10 years of life, 48 occurred in the first 6 weeks, another 20 under 1 year and a further 15 under 5 years. This series included every myelomeningocele born in the region: such an unselected series is never likely to be available for study again.

Doran and Guthkelch [22] in 1961 reviewed 243 patients with open myelomeningocele, of whom 136 were operated upon and 107 were not; at 2½ years or more 70% of the operated cases survived and 75% of the unoperated ones. But this series was selected because cases were not referred to hospital until 3 months of age or so and the overall survival of 43% probably represents something nearer Laurence's 15.5% when wastage in the first 3 months is allowed for.

Keys and Durham Smith [104] in 1973 reported on 295 patients born between 1961 and 1969, of whom 73% were operated on and 79 received no active surgical treatment; only two of the unoperated cases survived whilst 169 (79%) of those actively treated survived. There was a total survival rate of 58%. However, 87 of the 214 children operated on had the back closed when they were more than 48 h old and this may have indicated delayed referral and some natural wastage.

Stark and Drummond [113] from 163 patients, almost all seen within 12 h of birth, selected 78 children (47.8%) for surgery. Almost all the unoperated children were dead within 3 months and 70% of the operated ones survived 6 years – a total survival rate of 33%.

Lorber [61], out of 37 patients referred under 24 h old, rejected 25 from surgical treatment, all of whom died. Of the 12 treated, ten were early survivors. He thus had a total survival rate of 27% but this was a highly selected group since 78 other cases were referred to another unit in the same hospital during the same period of time.

As indicated above the pendulum continues to swing both with regard to referral and to early treatment [111]. In the 10 years from 1976–85 250 newborns with myelomeningocele were admitted – about a quarter of those admitted 10 years earlier; 193 had their backs closed early and 67 had delayed closure or no closure at all; 16 of the early closures died before they were a year old (8.3%) and 28 of the late or no closures (41.8%). The overall mortality of 17.6% is a great deal lower than in many earlier series: infection is better controlled but an entirely unselected series of cases will never be seen again. Even so, at least three of the deaths were from major associated anomalies – two Edwards trisomy 18 and another child with multiple anomalies including a severe heart defect.

Quality of life for survivors

It is clear that modern treatment of open myelomeningocele will increase the 5-year survival rate from around 10% in the untreated to around 70–80% when all are treated. But the increasing number of survivors will include an ever-increasing number of children handicapped by locomotion difficulties, incontinence and renal failure, mental retardation, severe spinal deformities and trophic disturbances.

Further studies of the Liverpool group of children [69] born between 1960 and 1963, showed that, of 133 survivors with operated myelomeningoceles, 56 (42%) were normal or near normal, but 63 (47%) had major handicaps and a further 14 children had considerable mental handicap.

Of the Sheffield group of 200 consecutive closures [59], 59 (56%) of the 106 survivors at 10 years were considered acceptable and able to fit into society but 47 (44%) were not.

These figures of up to 50% severely handicapped survivors are the explanation of attempts to recognize the severe cases in the neonatal period and exclude them from treatment [31,45,50,57,60,104,113].

It is not difficult to recognize the child with the high lesion, with severe kyphosis or scoliosis, with severe hydrocephalus or in poor general state; serious congenital malformations in other systems can be searched for and found. Few of these situations, however, are clearly incompatible with immediate survival and predictions have been shown to depend to some extent on the optimism or pessimism of the observer [53]. Follow-up studies of adult spina bifida cases [29,51] have shown a number of severely paralysed patients who do not have hydrocephalus, who are self-supporting and living competitive lives. It seems that paralysis and incontinence can be tolerated; but hydrocephalus with a degree of mental retardation often confounded by shunt problems presents a much more formidable obstacle to a useful life. A series of 26 babies admitted to Alder Hey in 1973 whose backs were not closed, was studied by Robards et al. [95]; eight survived for more than 1 year. All babies had hydrocephalus and, of the 18 who died in the first year, only three had valved shunts established whilst, of the eight who survived 1 year, seven had shunts and the only one without a shunt died at 13 months. This suggests that control of the hydrocephalus plays a major part in the saving of life, though it is possible that those children who did not have shunts established were being treated less vigorously [97].

Provided a baby receives normal care it would appear that the hydrocephalus is the factor which will most influence its long-term survival and also its future ability to fit into society. Stein et al. [102] have taken this concept a little further and modified their predictive criteria by looking for lacunar skull deformities in the neonatal skull X-ray, which they found closely related to later IQ.

In summary, of 100 children born with myelomeningocele, 5–10% will have intracranial haemorrhage or severe associated congenital anomalies which will make them almost certain to die within a few days; these children should not be operated on in the neonatal period. About 50–60% will have some active movement below the hips; these children should have the back closed urgently, recognizing that their total care must be undertaken in half of them for many years to come. There remain 25–30% of children with complete paralysis below the hips for whom closure of the back presents no possibility of preservation of function, since function is already lost, and therefore operative closure is indicated only if it is considered that nursing will be made easier.   The concern of the surgeon is to achieve the best possible result for his patient: but he cannot assume that society will provide unlimited funds for the long-term treatment of multiple congenital malformations (see Chapter 1). If funds are not going to be available for the treatment of such diseases then money must be devoted to methods for their prevention [41,47]. It must be accepted that in those parts of the world where resources are severely limited, the expensive and highly sophisticated care of the specialist neonatal surgical centre, if available, should be reserved for those children to whom ongoing specialist care for the hydrocephalus, urinary tract and orthopaedic problems will be available and of benefit.

In these circumstances, the last group of babies mentioned above should be given custodial care only, away from the specialist centre, in the expectation that very few will survive for more than a few months.

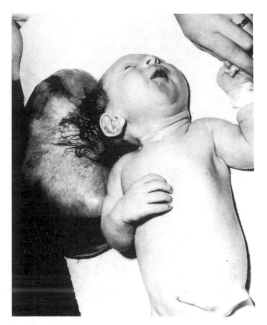

Figure 41.22 Large encephalocele and microcephalus

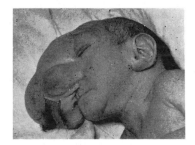

Figure 41.23 Large anterior encephalocele

Encephalocele

Encephalocele is a neural tube deformity related to anencephaly and spina bifida but it has attracted far less attention than myelomeningocele possibly because of the gloomy prognosis. Of 270 papers presented in 9 years (1968–1976) at the Society for Research into Hydrocephalus and Spina Bifida only two were concerned with cranium bifidum. It is often stated that Richter [86] was the first to describe this abnormality in 1813 but it is such an obvious one it seems unlikely that it had not been observed before that date. Certainly Corvinius [18] incised and drained a large anterior encephalocele and Bayer [1] advocated his musculofascial flap closure technique in 1892 for covering encephalocele defects as well as those resulting from myelomeningocele. Cranial defects occur about one-tenth as commonly as spinal ones and usually are associated with a circular or oval defect in the occipital bone; the swelling may be quite small or very large and both types usually contain brain tissue – cerebellum or parts of the occipital lobes. Not infrequently they are associated with microcephaly (Figure 41.22) and severe cerebral dysplasia, but the degree of cerebral abnormality is not closely related to the size of the

lesion. Anterior encephaloceles (Figure 41.23) also occur but are excessively rare [68].

The content of the encephalocele varies in relation to its site: the anterior lesions do not usually have direct communication with cerebral tissue though the meninges penetrate the skull, whilst the posterior lesions contain nubbins of brain tissue which is in direct continuity with cerebral cortex and/or cerebellum [27]. It appears that although the condition seems related to spinal dysraphism, the nature of the lesion differs somewhat: the frequent appearance of cerebral cortex and cerebellum in the occipital encephalocele is probably due to a herniation late in development since the primary break in the covering of the midbrain occurs before cerebellum is developed to any degree and the cerebral hemispheres are lying well cephalad to the defect. Emergy and Kalhan [27] suggest that herniation of the caudal part of the cerebral hemispheres into the encephalocele would push the midbrain caudally and account for the frequent necrosis of the cerebellum which is found.

Associated congenital abnormalities are common; amongst our 103 patients, there were eight with myelomeningocele, five with Klippel-Feil abnormalities, three with congenital heart disease and one each with duodenal atresia, anorectal anomalies and cystic disease of kidney and pancreas.

The aetiology of encephalocele is related to that of spina bifida but no more clearly understood. Of our 103 cases, 12 had affected siblings – eight with myelomeningoceles, two with anencephaly and two with congenital heart disease. These and other family histories suggest that there is a genetically determined predisposition to the condition and there are racial differences not only in the incidence of neural tube abnormalities but also in their type; anterior cranial meningocele and encephalocele are much commoner in mongoloid races [8]. To the inherited predisposition is added an unidentified environmental insult which results in an abnormality which may vary according to the time as well as the nature of the teratogenic insult.

Encephalocele accounts for about 10% of all congenital anomalies of the neural tube admitted to a neonatal surgical unit [27]; 103 cases were admitted to the Alder Hey unit over a period of 22 years during which 1406 cases of myelomeningocele were admitted.

Clinical picture

The lesion may vary from a small skin-covered nodule to a large cystic swelling bigger than the baby's head. The covering is sometimes quite thin, and warning of imminent rupture of a large sac may be given by drops of cerebrospinal fluid 'weeping' through the stretched membrane. The face of the child and a receding forehead may suggest microcephaly but the size of the lesion is not necessarily related to the severity of the condition. Hydrocephalus occurs with this lesion as often as it does with myelomeningocele. Neurological disturbances are largely confined to those attributable to cerebral damage. Blindness may be suspected in the neonatal period but is difficult to assess unless there is primary optic atrophy or a clearly absent light reflex.

Treatment

It has been shown [3] that of those children who are operated on for encephalocele, closure without removal of brain tissue can be achieved in about one-third, and in the other two-thirds where brain tissue has been excised there is a higher incidence

of blindness and retardation; however, these facts cannot be proved to be related. The anterior lesions are usually small and do not contain vital tissue; although they are a potential portal of entry for infection to the meninges, they are not neonatal emergencies and, like small posterior lesions, may be excised at a convenient time. The large posterior lesions, however, do demand urgent repair since the thin membranes are easily traumatized and may become infected [87]; haemorrhage into or rupture of the sac may occur. These lesions usually contain vital brain tissue which should be preserved as far as possible. CT scans (Figure 41.24) have at least made it possible to recognize brain tissue in the

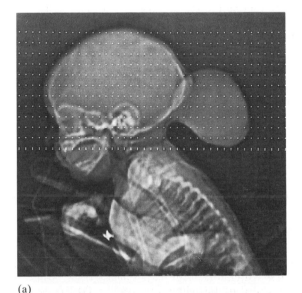

(a)

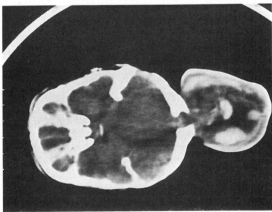

(b)

Figure 41.24 CT scan showing occipital encephalocele with brain tissue and large vessels protruding into the sac

encephalocele and also to give warning of major blood vessels that may lie within or around the sac.

The operation for encephalocele is performed with the baby placed prone on the operating table with a rolled-up towel under his chest so that the head can be flexed forwards. After sterilizing the skin, a circular incision is made through the skin of the neck of the encephalocele, leaving enough skin to permit its closure later without undue tension. The incision is deepened until the dura is reached, and the neck of the encephalocele is then dissected free to the point where the dura passes through the bony defect. Care must be taken not to injure extradural veins near the bony defect. Many large, thin-walled abnormal veins may be encountered which, if injured, will retract inside the skull behind the bony rim and cause bleeding which may be very profuse and difficult to control.

The encephalocele sac is then opened at a point where no brain matter appears to adhere to the sac and the inside of the sac is carefully inspected. If there is a large amount of brain present in the sac it may have to be amputated with the diathermy needle, because attempts at reducing the brain into the skull may cause a fatal acute rise of intracranial pressure. Smaller knuckles of brain tissue can be left *in situ*, provided a firm watertight closure of dura can be carried out. The distal part of the sac is amputated and the dural neck of the encephalocele is then closed with a continuous suture of 3/0 silk. If possible, this first suture is invaginated by a second continuous 3/0 silk suture of Lembert's stitches. The repair is further strengthened by raising a musculofascial flap from the neck or a flap of cranial aponeurosis and periosteum from the skull and suturing it over the defect with interrupted 3/0 silk sutures. Throughout the operation all bleeding must be meticulously stopped. The skin is then sutured, using first interrupted 3/0 catgut sutures for the subcutaneous tissues and then nylon skin sutures.

Postoperatively, the child is nursed prone and great care is taken to watch for any signs of increase in intracranial pressure (see Chapter 40). The postoperative management is otherwise similar to that of repaired myelomeningoceles, including a careful watch for developing hydrocephalus.

Results

Encephalocele carries a high early mortality and the prognosis for survivors is poor. In a series of 103 cases admitted to Alder Hey over a period of 22 years, 30 died under 6 months of age: of these, 11 were children with large lesions who were not operated upon and mostly died within a few hours of birth from major cerebral problems or from associated abnormalities. There were 19 other deaths, 17 of them having had brain tissue removed

and two meninges only; five of these died of ventriculo-atrial shunt malfunction, the remainder of associated abnormalities or the severity of the lesion.

Of the 103 patients, 57 had significant hydrocephalus and 45 of these had shunts established for drainage of the cerebrospinal fluid; 35 of those operated on for hydrocephalus had had brain tissue removed, the remainder meninges only.

Of 73 survivors, 38 are known to be mentally retarded, 17 of them severely so and 15 of them in permanent care institutions. Eighteen survivors have severely impaired vision or are totally blind, 32 are spastic to a greater or less degree and 27 have convulsions. Seventeen children had only one of these handicaps and ten of them lead near normal lives – two with hydrocephalus, two with some muscular incoordination and one blind. Nine children had two of these handicaps, seven had three and five had four. Only 15 out of the original 72 are normal.

These 15 children include two children with skin-covered anterior lesions, one unoperated small skin covered occipital encephalocele and 12 other small lesions. If surgical correction involves only resection of meninges, though some neural cells are usually found in the sac, then moderate mental retardation and minor physical defects may be anticipated. In the large lesions with a considerable amount of herniated brain, however, the prognosis is extremely gloomy – though even in this condition there is an occasional surprise.

References

1. Bayer, L. (1892) Zur Technik der Operation der Spina Bifida und Encephalocele. *Prag. med. Wschr.*, **17**, 317, 332 and 345
2. Bentley, J.L. and Smith, J.R. (1960) Developmental posterior enteric remnants and spinal malformations. *Arch. Dis. Child.*, **35**, 76–86
3. Blaze, J.B., Eckstein, H.B. and Tsingoglu, S. (1971) Cranium bifidum: a review of 93 cases. *Devl. Med. Child. Neurol.*, **13**, (suppl. 25), 134
4. Boris, M., Blumberg, R., Feldman, D.B. and Sellers, J.E. (1963) Increased incidence of myelomeningocele. *J. Am. Med. Ass.*, **184**, 768
5. Bremer, J.L. (1952) Dorsal intestinal fistula, accessory neurenteric anal, diastematomyelia. *Arch. Path.*, **54**, 132–138
6. *Br. Med. J.* (1975) Leading article: End of the potato avoidance theory. **4**, 308–309
7. Brocklehurst, G. (1971) The pathogenesis of spina bifida: a study of the relationship between observation hypothesis and surgical incentive. *Devl. Med. child Neurol.*, **13**, 147–163
8. Brocklehurst, G. (1976) *Spina Bifida for the Clinician*, Spastics International Medical Publications,

William Heinemann, London; J.B. Lippincott, Philadelphia

9. Bucy, P.C. and Siqueira, E.B. (1966) In *Practice of Pediatrics*, (ed. J. Brennerman) Prior, Hagerstown, Maryland

10. Carter, C.O. (1965) Genetics of spina bifida. In: *Proceedings of a Symposium on Spina Bifida*. Christopher Foss, London

11. Carter, C.O. (1974) Clues to the aetiology of neural tube malformations. *Devl. Med. Child Neurol.*, **16**, (suppl. 32), 3–15

12. Carter, C.O. and Evans, K. (1973) Spina bifida and anencephalus in Greater London. *J. Med. Genet.*, **10**, 209–234

13. Carter, C.O. and Fraser Roberts, J.A. (1967) The risk of recurrence after two children with central nervous system malformations. *Lancet*, **i**, 306–308

14. Carter, C.O., David, P.A. and Laurence, K.M. (1968) A family study of major central nervous system malformations in South Wales. *J. Med. Genet.*, **5**, 81–106

15. Clarke, C., Hobson, D. and McKendrick, O. (1975) Spina bifida and anencephaly: miscarriage as a possible cause. *Br. Med. J.*, **4**, 743–746

16. Collman, R.D. and Stoller, A. (1962) Epidemiology of congenital anomalies of the central nervous system with special reference to patterns in the State of Victoria, Australia. *J. Ment. Defic. Res.*, **6**, 22

17. Cooper, A. (1811) Some observations on spina bifida. *Med.-chir. Trans. Lond.*, **2**, 322

18. Corvinious, J.F.C. (1755) *Dissertation medicochirurgica de hernia cerebri*. Lausannae; Sumpibus, Marci-Michael Bousquet and Socior

19. Dandy, W.F. and Blackfan, K.D. (1913) An experimental and clinical study of internal hydrocephalus. *J. Am. Med. Ass.*, **61**, 2216–2218

20. Deans, G.T. and Boston, V.E. (1988) Is surgical closure of the back lesion in open neural tube defects necessary? *Br. Med. J.*, **296**, 1441–1442

21. Donovan, D.E., Coves, P. and Paine, R.S. (1962) Prognostic implications of neurological abnormalities in the neonatal period. *Neurology*, **12**, 910–914

22. Doran, P.A. and Guthkelch, A.N. (1961) Studies in spina bifida cystica. *J. Neurol. Neurosurg. Psychiat.*, **24**, 331–345

23. Duckworth, T., Sharrard, W.J., Lister, J. and Seymour, N. (1968) Hemimyelocele. *Devl. Med. Child Neurol.*, (suppl.), **16**, 69–75

24. Eckstein, H.B. and MacNab, G.H. (1966) Myelomeningocele and hydrocephalus. *Lancet*, **i**, 842–845

25. Emery, J.L. (1974) Deformity of the aqueduct of Sylvius in children with hydrocephalus and myelomeningocele. *Devl. Med. Child Neurol.*, **12**, (suppl. 22), 51–64

26. Emery, J.L. (1976) Personal communication

27. Emery, J.L. and Kalhan, S.C. (1970) The pathology of exencephalus. *Devl. Med. Child Neurol.*, **12**, (suppl. 22), 51–64

28. Emery, J.L. and Lendon, R.G. (1972) Clinical implications of cord lesions in neurospinal dysraphism. *Devl. Med. Child Neurol.*, **27** (suppl.), 45–51

29. Evans, K., Hickman, V. and Carter, C.O. (1974) Handicap and social status of adults with spina bifida cystica. *Br. J. Prev. Soc. Med.*, **28**, 85

30. Evans, R.C., Tew, B., Thomas, M.D. and Ford, J. (1985) Selective surgical management of neural tube malformations. *Arch. Dis. Child.*, **60**, 415–419

31. Finlay, H.V.L. (1971) Selecting cases of myelomeningocele for surgery. *Br. Med. J.*, **3**, 429

32. Forrest, D. (1976) Management of bladder and bowel in spina bifida. In: *Spina Bifida for the Clinician* (ed. G. Brocklehurst), Heinemann Medical, London

33. Forrest, D.M., Hole, R. and Wynne, J.M. (1966) Treatment of infantile hydrocephalus using the Holter valve. *Devl. Med. Child Neurol.*, **11** (suppl.), 27–35

34. Forshall, I. (1961) Duplication of the intestinal tract. *Postgrad. med. J.*, **37**, 570–589

35. Fowler, I. (1953) Response of the chick neural tube in mechanically produced spina bifida. *J. Exp. Zool.*, **123**, 115

36. Gardiner, W.J. (1968) Myelocele: rupture of the neural tube. *Clin. Neurosurg.*, **15**, 57

37. Gittelsohn, A. and Milham, S. (1964) Statistical study of twins. *Am. J. Publ. Hlth*, **54**, 286–294

38. Guthkelch, A.N. (1965) Thoughts on the management of spina bifida cystica. *Acta Neurochir.*, **13**, 407–418

39. Guthkelch, A.N. (1986) Aspects of the surgical management of myelomeningocele: a review. *Dev. Med. Child. Neurol.*, **28**, 525–532

40. Hassin, G.B. (1925) Spina bifida occulta cervicales. *Arch. Neurol. Psychiat.*, **14**, 813–818

41. Haynes, B.F., Cheek, W.R. and Mintz, A.A. (1974) Treatment of myelomeningocele in indigent and nonindigent patients. *Am. J. Dis. Child.*, **127**, 182–186

42. Herren, R.Y. and Edwards, J.E. (1940) Diplomyelia. *Archs Path.*, **30**, 1203–1214

43. Hippocrates (1825) *In medicorum graecorum opera quae extant*, C. Cnoblochius, Leipzig

44. Holtzman, N.A. (1983) Prenatal screening for neural tube defects. *Pediatrics*, **71**, 658–660

45. Hunt, G.H., Lewin, W., Gleave, J. and Gardiner, D. (1973) Predictive factors in open myelomeningocele. *Br. Med. J.*, **4**, 197–201

46. Ingraham, F.D. and Matson, D.D. (1955) *Neurosurgery of Infancy and Childhood*. Charles C Thomas, Springfield, IL

47. Lange, S.A. (1976) Introduction studies in hydrocephalus and spina bifida. *Devl. Med. Child Neurol.*, **18** (Suppl. 37)

48. Laurence, K.M. (1964) The natural history of spina bifida cystica. *Arch. Dis. Child.*, **39**, 41–57

49. Laurence, K.M. (1966) The survival of untreated spina bifida cystica. *Devl. Med. Child Neurol.*, **11** (suppl.), 10–19

50. Laurence, K.M. (1974) Effect of early surgery for

Part VIII

Urogenital system

42

Renal failure

T. McKendrick

Normal renal function in the neonate has been described in Chapter 3. With the glomerulotubular imbalance noted therein, dramatic effects may occur in sick infants. Infants are normally strongly anabolic and little urea is produced for excretion. Nevertheless, even mild dehydration may lower the already low glomerular filtration rate sufficiently to permit rapid accumulation of urea, and blood urea levels of up to 60 mmol/l (360 mg/100 ml) may occur in the absence of any renal pathology. It is only when the infant is well hydrated that blood urea levels give any indication of renal function.

For a similar reason, following debilitating illness, some infants may quickly increase their protein intake (if permitted) to catch up with lost growth. The increased urea production may be reflected in blood urea levels sustained at higher than normal levels (e.g. 8–12 mmol/l (50–70 mg/100 ml)) for several weeks.

Neither of these states necessarily implies true renal failure although they may indicate the need for a higher water intake.

The distinction between acute failure which may recover if therapy enables the patient to survive and chronic renal failure which implies non-recoverable renal pathology is important but it may not be possible to make the distinction when the baby presents.

The major causes of pathological acute renal failure are summarized in Table 42.1.

Causes

The traditional classification into prerenal, renal and postrenal types is not always satisfactory, especially in babies. Some lesions such as pyelonephritis may act prerenally because of dehydration and vomiting, renally because of extensive renal parenchymal damage, and postrenally if there is extensive tubular obstruction. With some causes it is uncertain where or how the lesion acts (e.g. intrarenal haemorrhage). Table 42.1 gives the causes of acute renal failure, taking into account

Table 42.1 Causes of renal failure in newborn

Infection
Prerenal:
    Septicaemia
    Extensive localized infection, e.g. pneumonia
Renal:
    Pyelonephritis

Obstruction
Infravesical:
    Posterior urethral valves
    Urethral stenosis
    Ectopic ureterocele
    Tumours, e.g. rhabdomyosarcoma
Upper tract:
    Pelvi-ureteric obstruction
    Ureteric stricture
    Ureteric valve

Vascular lesions
Aortic and/or renal artery thrombosis
Renal venous thrombosis
Intrarenal haemorrhage due to asphyxia
Haemolytic disease of the newborn
Thrombocytopenic purpura

Acute tubular necrosis
Peripheral circulatory failure:
    Trauma
    Asphyxia
    Haemorrhage
    Cardiorenal failure with respiratory infection
    Dehydration, especially with hypernatraemia
Pigment excretion:
    Mismatched transfusion
Toxic nephropathy:
    Antibiotics
    Contrast media

underlying pathology and site of action. Rare causes and those which are theoretically possible but of no practical importance are omitted. Most of the causes listed may progress to chronic renal failure. To this list may be added other causes of chronic renal failure which may be found in infancy. Various forms of congenital hypoplasia or dysplasia have been described [7]. Some remain quite unexplained.

The term 'septicaemia' is a loose one, including not only the infant with true blood-borne infection involving urinary tract, liver, meninges and occasionally the pericardium, but also the infant in whom no bacterial infection can be demonstrated and who may subsequently develop gastroenteritis. Acute pyelonephritis in the newborn is not uncommon. Although usually not severe it may sometimes cause renal failure and, if so, it is more likely to be a complication of lower urinary tract obstruction. Of the listed obstructive causes, posterior urethral valves and ectopic ureterocele are by far the commonest. The vascular lesions are almost all associated with delivery and nearly always appear to be due to asphyxia whether intra- or postpartum, or to local haemorrhage in the kidney [8].

Clinical features

As the neonate normally lives with little or no renal reserve, it is probably of no value to think in terms of incipient renal failure or the prodromal stage of renal failure, certainly as regards symptoms. In the presence of the factors listed in Table 42.1, careful observation should be instituted. The early signs are common to so many illnesses in the newborn that they are of little diagnostic value [6]. The observation of anorexia, vomiting, diarrhoea, weight loss, malaise or drowsiness should lead to more formal examination. Some estimate of urinary output or frequency is essential; retrospective enquiries about this are seldom of value. Pallor, loss of muscle tone, twitching and altered state of hydration may be important pointers to renal failure but they are not early signs. In practice, the falling urinary output is the cardinal clinical observation and the importance of the accurate recording of micturition or wet napkins in sick neonates cannot be over-stressed on their attendants.

The degree of dehydration should be assessed clinically, as follows:

(1) 5% weight loss
    restless and apparently thirsty infant, dry tongue, skin slightly inelastic
(2) 10% weight loss
    dry tongue, sunken fontanelle, eyes dull and sunken, hyperpnoea
(3) 15% weight loss

the above signs, with apathy, inertia, pallor, slight cyanosis, distended abdomen, cardiac irregularity, hypotonia

In any dehydrated baby a turgid or 'doughy' skin suggests hyperelectrolytaemia.

Chemical pathology

As noted above, the urine is scanty. There is always some proteinuria. Usually blood is present, but this may be seen on microscopy only. There is also an abnormal number of leucocytes even in the absence of infection. Careful search will usually reveal granular, epithelial or cellular casts. The osmolality is low, often 200–300 mOsm/kg, and urea concentration is low, usually below 70 mmol/l (420 mg/100 ml) and sometimes below 30 mmol/l (180 mg/100 ml). These low figures must be interpreted with caution for, in health, the neonatal urea and solute output depend greatly on diet and figures not much greater than these may be observed for short periods. Both they and the urine sodium concentration must be considered with blood levels taken at the same time. The latter are dependent on intake and gastrointestinal loss as well as on the degree of renal failure. Sodium levels vary greatly. They are often low but, if feeds with high electrolyte content have been continued, very high plasma levels of sodium may be found. When this happens a low urine sodium concentration (e.g. 20 mmol/l (20 mEq/l)) would be inappropriately low and would tend to confirm the presence of renal failure. The same level, however, could be inappropriately high if the infant had low plasma values following vomiting or diarrhoea.

The plasma potassium level is nearly always high and rises progressively. In the first 2 days of life levels of up to 8.0 mmol/l (8.0 mEq/l) are normal [1] and infants as a rule seem less susceptible to the dangers of high plasma levels. Hyperkalaemia is seldom a primary indication for therapy but it often responds to measures directed against the likely precipitating features such as hypercatabolism, sodium deficiency and acidosis.

Acidosis is always present and may be profound. Plasma bicarbonate levels down to 4 mmol/l (4 mEq/l) and pH values down to 6.9 are sometimes seen. Two factors are concerned: (1) there is a rise in sulphate and phosphate anions as well as various organic acids [22]; (2) the plasma chloride may remain normal or may be low due to vomiting – during which more chloride than sodium may be lost. In infants rendered hyperelectrolytaemic by excessive water loss and partial replacement with hypertonic feeds there may also be marked hyperchloraemia and relatively little change in the anions referred to above. These changes with the relatively poor tubular function described above produce the dramatic alteration in acid-base balance which will prevent recovery of renal function unless corrected.

Haematology

Anaemia is usual. It may be masked by dehydration but as a rule the haemoglobin level and haematocrit fall progressively while renal failure is present. Anaemia may, however, be associated with the reason for the failure; for example, haemolytic disease of the newborn, haemorrhage, etc. Examination of a blood film usually reveals a few 'cocked hat' or fragmented cells. Leucocytosis is always present. As with anaemia, this may be associated with the cause (e.g. sepsis) and it should be remembered that in the first few days of life the infant usually has a high white cell count.

Various coagulation defects may be found. The prothrombin concentration, normally low in the neonatal period, is likely to be even lower. There may be increased capillary fragility and thrombocytopenia. Even when platelets are present in normal numbers they do not apparently function normally. Except in terminal stages, such coagulation defects do not often appear to cause severe clinical effects.

Diagnosis

The first and perhaps most important diagnosis is between anuria or oliguria and lower urinary obstruction (remembering that both can be present). Inability to palpate the bladder suprapubically does not necessarily eliminate the possibility of obstruction. If there are any doubts an ultrasound scan of the infant's abdomen should be carried out.

Second, it is important to determine whether the oliguric infant has merely an accentuation of the 'physiological' renal failure (see above) due to dehydration or whether there is true renal pathology. Concomitant clinical features may indicate the diagnosis, but in their absence the differentiation is of less immediate urgency for the early management is common to both types of failure. The character of such urine as can be obtained may be the most useful diagnostic feature. Frequently an improved urine composition (as regards urea excretion, osmolality and sodium-regulating ability) over 24 or 48 h in response to rehydration clarifies the situation. It has been suggested that the response of the blood urea to rehydration gives a good indication as to the presence or absence of renal disease [4]. If the initial blood urea level is halved within 24 h, it is less likely that renal disease is present.

Management

As a prodromal or incipient stage of renal failure is seldom recognized in neonates, the question of early preventive therapy does not often arise. Postoperative therapy (dealt with in Chapter 5) is probably the only situation where prophylaxis is practicable. Attempts to expand the circulation, alkalinize the urine or promote excretion by diuretics are never successful in the first few days and may be dangerous. After the first week it is sometimes worth stimulating urine production after rehydration, using frusemide (Lasix) 1–5 mg or mannitol 1–3 g by intravenous injection.

When renal failure is established, therapy can be considered under four headings:

(1) Management of the underlying pathology.
(2) Control of water and electrolyte balance.
(3) Control of nitrogenous waste retention.
(4) Control of other effects such as heart failure, hypertension, anaemia.

Management of underlying cause of acute renal failure

When severe infection is suspected, or clinically manifest, antibiotic therapy should be started as soon as relevant specimens have been taken for bacteriological examination. These will usually include samples of blood and cerebrospinal fluid for culture, swabs of any septic lesions found and urine if available. The blood white cell count is seldom of value but plasma electrolyte concentrations may be most important, for septicaemia may be mimicked by congenital adrenal hyperplasia, when the finding of low plasma sodium and chloride with very high potassium levels may provide an important clue.

The initial antibiotic treatment of severe infection must be empirical pending the results of bacteriological investigation. The choice of antibiotic will vary both in time and place with predominant flora but a wide spectrum should be covered. Thus, suitable regimens include gentamicin (4 mg/kg body weight) given once daily with penicillin (20 000 units/kg body weight) given 6-hourly, both intravenously. Some common suitable regimens appear in Table 42.2.

Control of water and electrolyte balance

When the baby is severely ill with circulatory collapse the circulating blood volume must be restored as quickly as possible. This is best done by intravenous infusion of plasma, 20 ml/kg body weight. Such infants are always acidotic and the acidosis can be temporarily controlled by injecting 5–10 ml of 8.4% sodium bicarbonate.

Table 42.2 Antibiotic dosage in renal failure

	Initial dose (per kg)	Maintenance dose (per kg)	Frequency (hourly)	Removal by PD	Removal by HD	Intraperitoneal dose per l fluid	Risks
Penicillin G		15–30 mg	12	No	Yes	30 mg	Sodium load
Ampicillin		20–50 mg	12	No	Yes	25 mg	Sodium load
Flucloxacillin		25 mg	12	No	No	50 mg	
Erythromycin		12.5 mg	12	No	No	25 mg	Transient deafness Local irritation
Cephradine	50 mg	8 mg	24	Yes	Yes	50 mg	
Cefuroxime	35 mg	35 mg	24	Slight	Yes	25–50 mg	Neurotoxicity
Cefotaxime	25 mg	25 mg	24	Slight	Yes	50 mg	Neurotoxicity
Ceftazidime	20 mg	20 mg	24	Slight	Yes	50 mg	Bleeding
Gentamicin Tobramycin Netilmicin	3 mg	~3 mg	24	Yes	Yes	5–10 mg	Ototoxic Nephrotoxic
Vancomycin[4]	15		? weekly[5]	No	No	10–25 mg	Nephrotoxic
Amphotericin	100 μg	up to 1 mg	24	No	No	not used	Nephrotoxic, Hepatotoxic
Flucytosine[4]	25 mg	4 mg	24–48	Yes	Yes	50 mg	
Miconazole	5–10 mg	5–10 mg	8	No	No	10–25 mg	

Based on Bennett *et al.* [2], Lee *et al.* [5] and Bennett [3]
Notes (1) Drugs which are removed by haemodialysis should be given after dialysis
   (2) Penicillins and aminoglycosides should not be mixed
   (3) Aminoglycoside dosage should be based on serum level assays at 1, 12 and 24 h
   (4) Vancomycin and flucytosine should be given over 1 h and amphotericin over 6 h
   (5) Second dose should be based on serum level assayed at about 1 week. Often one dose is adequate
PD = peritoneal dialysis
HD = haemodialysis

The body water must then be replaced. Although this entails the administration of electrolyte solutions, electrolyte imbalance cannot be stabilized until most of the intra- and extracellular water has been restored. Dehydration is of two types, depending on the relative deficiency of electrolyte and water.

Hypertonic dehydration

When fluid loss is either not replaced or is replaced with hypertonic fluids such as cows' milk, hyperelectrolytaemia results. Plasma sodium levels rise and may reach 180 mmol/l (180 mEq/l) with commensurate rises in chloride and potassium levels. There is nevertheless a total deficit of these substances. Replacement is most safely carried out with N/5 saline. Knowing the baby's weight and approximate state of dehydration, the amount of fluid required can be calculated and should be given over 24–48 h. Rapid or generous replacement should not be done. The danger is that while plasma hyperosmolality can be quickly corrected (e.g. with 5% dextrose) and the extracellular water will quickly equilibrate with it, intracellular electrolyte cannot quickly escape so that water will pass into cells, causing cerebral oedema. It is likely that a hydrogen ion gradient is also created.

Hypotonic dehydration

This occurs when fluid loss is replaced in early stages with water. Low plasma electrolyte levels result. Change in plasma osmolality, however, is likely to be very slight because retained urea compensates for loss of sodium and chloride. Replacement with intravenous N or N/2 saline can be rapid. The quantity required is estimated from the weight of the infant and his estimated loss of fluid. Table 42.3 summarizes the rates of replacement with varying losses. The total amount given may include sodium bicarbonate. Some units use Hartman's solution in place of saline.

Table 42.3 Fluid replacement in small babies

Weight loss	Plasma Na (mmol/l)	Saline strength	Rate (ml/kg per h)
5%	145	N/5	1
	130–145	N/2	2
	130	N	2
10%	145	N/5	2
	130–145	N/2	4
	130	N	4
15%	145	N/5	3
	130–145	N/2	6
	130	N	8

When the water is being thus replaced some electrolyte correction occurs but in severe losses this is unlikely to be complete with these regimens. In renal failure the kidney cannot carry out its normal function of adjusting electrolyte balance, so careful calculation of deficiencies must be made. This is estimated from the infant's body weight (of which about 40% is extracellular fluid and plasma) and the difference between normal and observed plasma electrolyte levels. As a rule small quantities of normal saline or 8.4% sodium bicarbonate are required.

The potassium level is likely to be high (i.e. more than 8.0 mEq/l) but rehydration, correction of hyponatraemia and acidosis will usually lower the plasma potassium level. Indeed, in neonates hyperkalaemia is seldom a great problem. There is likely to be a total body deficit of potassium and as a rule 2 ml of potassium chloride, 20% solution, should be added to infusion solutions after the initial rehydration.

Control of nitrogenous waste retention

After the first 24 h of renal failure the calorie intake becomes important because starvation increases tissue breakdown and hence intensifies acidosis, ketosis and uraemia. This effect is of little importance in the first 2 or 3 days of life when the infant is unable to break down protein but will metabolize fat and carbohydrate. Carbohydrate is thenceforth necessary to promote the cellular uptake of potassium. Electrolyte solutions such as N/5 saline with 4.3% dextrose are totally inadequate for this purpose for the requirement is not less than 420 kJ/kg (100 kcal/kg) body weight per 24 h. If the infant cannot tolerate oral feeding, tube feeds may be vomited and therefore intravenous nutrition may be required. Several mixtures of fat, carbohydrate and amino acids are available. Two such regimens are presented in Table 42.4. It will be noted that the volumes of water entailed are greater than those required by the anuric infant (Table 42.5) but most

such infants will also require dialysis (see below). If the flow of urine is such that larger quantities of fluid are permissible, it is better to use 10% fat suspension with amino acid solutions, best run simultaneously. It is customary to add heparin, 800 units/l of fluid.

Oral feeding should be restarted as soon as the baby will tolerate it. Unless renal function has recovered very quickly (as judged by urine urea concentration and osmolality) it is important to offer a milk with low electrolyte content. For this purpose SMA (scientific milk adaptations), Cow & Gate V Formula or Babymilk Plus and Ostermilk Complete Formula are all suitable (see Table 42.6).

Table 42.5 Management of fluid balance in acute renal failure: minimal daily fluid requirement

Age (days)	Weight (kg)	(ml/kg per h)	(ml/kg per 24 h)	(ml/24 h)
0–4	1–3	0.4	10	10–30
4–10	1–3	0.5	12	12–36
10 and over	1–5	0.6	15	15–75

Table 42.6 Demineralized whey-based formulas

Preparation	Protein (g/l)	Sodium (mOsm/l)	Potassium (mOsm/l)
Human milk	12	6.5	14
Cows' milk	33	25.2	35.6
Gold cap SMA	15	6.5	14.3
Cow and Gate Premium	15	7.8	16.7
Osterfeed Baby Milk	14.5	8.3	14.6
Aptamil	15	7.9	21.7

Table 42.4 Intravenous feeding for neonates

Regimens	Volume (ml/kg per 24 h)	Water (ml)	Joules (calories)	
1. Dextrose 10%	25	25	42	(10)
Aminosol-fructose-ethanol	60	50	231	(55)
Intralipid 20%	20	13	168	(40)
Total	105	88	441	(105)
This regimen introduces only 6 mmol (6 mEq) of sodium in 24 h				
2. Vamin	90	80	252	(60)
Intralipid 20%	20	13	168	(40)
Total	110	93	420	(100)

Control of other effects

Hyperkalaemia

As indicated above, hyperkalaemia is seldom a problem in neonates but occasionally levels of more than 9 mmol/l (9 mEq/l) may be encountered even after rehydration. This will usually only occur when there is severe renal disease and will be an indication for dialysis. Temporary lowering may follow the administration of insulin (0.5–1.0 units) and glucose (10–20 ml of 50% solution) by intravenous injection. It should be remembered, however, that infants with hyperelectrolytaemia often have hyperglycaemia, blood glucose levels of about 35 mmol/l (630 mg/100 ml) being not uncommon. Such infants are likely to be unusually sensitive to insulin.

Infection

If the neonate developing renal failure is not already infected he is likely to become so. Prevention of secondary infection is important because it is one of the commoner causes of death. Aseptic techniques in blood sampling must be rigorous especially when an indwelling line is used. If the infant is anuric a urethral catheter becomes no more than a foreign body and should be removed. The place of prophylactic antibiotics is debatable but an antifungal agent (usually Nystatin) should be given especially to those on dialysis. Repeated cultures of all effluents – endotracheal aspirate, peritoneal fluid, stool, wound drainage, etc., should be done.

Oedema

The response to diuretics, e.g. frusemide, chlorothiazide, or ethacrynic acid, is unpredictable. Although in adults large doses can result in continuing diuresis, such a result is rare in infants and there is often no demonstrable effect. Undesirable intercompartmental fluid changes may be produced. Rarely a diuresis follows the raising of plasma albumin by intravenous transfusion of low salt content albumin but care must be exercised because of the danger of precipitating acute left ventricular failure. Usually retained fluid can only be removed by dialysis (see below).

Hypertension

There is little information about hypertension in neonates, probably because it is technically difficult to measure blood pressure at this age. Most reports on the treatment of renal failure in neonates make no mention of hypertension. It appears to be either mild or transitory, requiring no specific therapy.

Anaemia

Anaemia may develop rapidly if there is sepsis or concomitant bone marrow depression (e.g. due to asphyxia). It is important to correct this by transfusion of blood, for renal function is much less likely to recover if the haemoglobin level is less than 8 or 9 g/100 ml.

Dialysis in neonates

In spite of the measures described above, some neonates require dialysis. Precise indications for instituting dialysis cannot easily be laid down but the commoner reasons are as follows:

(1) Persistent oliguria (less than 50 ml urine/24 h) with oedema following rehydration.
(2) Blood urea continuing to rise over 50 mmol/l (300 mg/100 ml).
(3) Persistent acidosis (blood pH below 7.25), plasma bicarbonate below 15 mmol/l (15 mEq/l) or hyperkalaemia (plasma K greater than 7.5 mmol/l (7.5 mEq/l) with oliguria.

The procedure may also be required for certain metabolic disorders producing hyperammonaemia and has been used in the therapy of respiratory distress syndrome.

Although haemodialysis has been used for small babies, peritoneal dialysis is so much safer and easier to perform that it is the method of choice. The peritoneum is used as a semipermeable membrane between the blood plasma and fluid introduced into the peritoneal cavity, and other soluble substances and water will equilibrate across this membrane. The dialysate is similar in composition to protein-free plasma and the transfer of electrolyte from the plasma is therefore minimal. It is available commercially in sterilized litre packs (see Table 42.7).

The hypertonic solution is used when large quantities of water have to be removed. It is advisable to add heparin (1000 units/l of solution) during the first 24 h, especially if the introduction of the cannula has caused bleeding. An antibiotic such as gentamicin (2 mg/l of solution) may be added but should not be necessary with experienced staff. Meticulous sterile technique in changing containers of fluid and the use of a sealed circuit (see Figure 42.1) will prevent the ingress of infection. Potassium chloride (4 mmol/l) is usually required, especially if the baby has been digitalized. This is not necessary if the baby is taking milk feeds or if the dialysis lasts less than 24 h.

A Teflon catheter (gauge 14 Ch)* is introduced percutaneously under local anaesthesia at about the level of the umbilicus. This site is preferred to the

---

*Wallace Paediatric Peritoneal Dialysis Cannula (Guy;s Hospital Pattern), Vygon Paediatric Dialysis Unit (296.04) or Pendlebury pattern (Cambruae Instruments) are suitable.

Table 42.7 Solutions available in the UK for peritoneal dialysis

	Na content (mmol/l; mEq/l)	*Osmolality* (mOsm/kg)	*Dextrose* (%)
Dialaflex 61	140	365	1.36
Dialaflex 62	140	640	6.36
Dialaflex 63	130	345	1.36
Dianeal B5204	140	365	1.36
Dianeal B5204	130	345	1.36
Dianeal B5204[a]	140	500	3.86
Dianeal B5961[a]	130	345	1.36

[a] Contains potassium 2.5 mmol/l (2.5 mEq/l)
Note there may be slight variation between batches

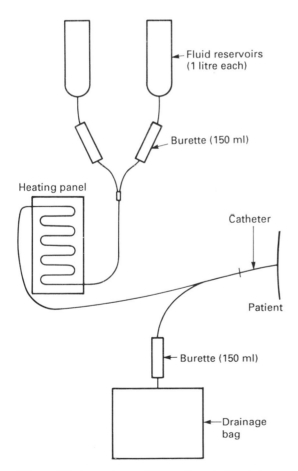

Figure 42.1 Apparatus used for peritoneal dialysis in infants

more commonly used lower site in bigger subjects in order to ensure that the entire perforated end of the catheter is within the peritoneal cavity. The midline above the umbilicus should be avoided as the ligamentum venosum is prominent. As the catheter tip fits over the trochar its blunted rim creates a 'shoulder' which is difficult to introduce through the skin unless a small incision is first made preferably with a pointed scalpel blade. If this is slightly too long, bleeding may occur and therefore when the catheter is *in situ* a purse-string suture should be used to secure it. With experience, a tight fit can be obtained without the need for a suture.

Dialysate is then introduced, having been warmed to about 35°C (94.5°F). Up to 40 ml/kg body weight can be used but 20 ml/kg is usually enough and is less likely to cause respiratory embarrassment. It is left in the peritoneum for about 45 min and then allowed to drain by gravity into the collecting chamber. Although it is feasible to repeat this cycle twice an hour this is seldom necessary and an hourly cycle is adequate. During dialysis the plasma creatinine, urea, electrolyte and water concentrations will approach normal unless too much water is removed by excessive use of high osmolality dialysate. Usually only about one cycle in four should be of the hyperosmolar solution.

Little supervision is required. A specimen of the effluent fluid should be cultured daily. The plasma urea and electrolyte concentrations may be helpful in assessing the efficiency of the process.

Complications

Complications are few and uncommon. Turbidity of the effluent fluid may indicate peritonitis. This is usually due to coliform organisms and may be clinically mild. Such peritonitis does not interfere with dialysis and is not an indication to stop the procedure.

Bleeding around the site of insertion of the cannula is seldom troublesome. Leakage of fluid around the cannula or into the abdominal wall should not occur within 48 h if the cannula has been inserted correctly. After that time, however, the track may tend to gape slightly. If this occurs, infection will follow and the cannula should therefore be resited.

Occasionally the baby appears to experience discomfort, usually when dialysate is flowing in. This may be due to the tip of the cannula impinging on bowel or abdominal wall. Altering the direction of the catheter is difficult but, if successful, may relieve the symptoms. Infusion of cold fluid is uncomfortable. Discomfort is rarely severe enough to warrant resiting the cannula.

Much the commonest complication is slowness or even cessation of drainage, while infusion remains satisfactory. This is nearly always due to the flap valve effect produced when omentum becomes wrapped round the cannula. The only remedy is to resite the cannula. Interruption of syphon drainage by intraperitoneal air has been described, but with the technique described above does not occur.

There is always some loss of protein and amino acid in the dialysate and this should be replaced in the diet or by intravenous infusion if dialysis has to be continued for more than a few days.

Haemodialysis

Acute renal failure can usually be managed by peritoneal dialysis. Occasionally, however, haemodialysis may be required. Indications for using this are as follows:

(1) Recent extensive intra-abdominal surgery.
(2) Uncontrolled peritonitis, e.g. monilia or staphylococcal infection in the severely debilitated baby.
(3) Excessive waterlogging of the baby due to hypercatabolism following extensive surgery or to large amounts of fluid infused for therapeutic reasons.

The small artificial kidneys are available commercially and when used with paediatric lines ensure that the extracorporeal blood volume need not exceed around 50 ml. Standard haemodialysis monitors can be used and even in infants as small as 2 kg, effective and repeated dialysis can be carried out using a single line of internal diameter 1.6 mm approx. inserted by the Seldinger technique into one subclavian vein.

A useful alternative is to use haemofiltration when it is mainly water which needs to be removed. A simple circuit for artery via the filter to vein requires less expert supervision and may remove up to about 100 ml of water/h if required. The extracorporeal volume with such a system is about 20 ml.

References

1. Acharya, P.T. and Payne, W.W. (1965) Blood biochemistry of normal full term infants in the first forty eight hours of life. *Arch. Dis. Child.*, **40**, 430–435
2. Bennett, W.M., Singer, I. and Coggins, C.J. (1974) A guide to drug therapy in renal failure. *J. Am. med. Ass.*, **230**, 1544–1553
3. Bennett, W.M. (1983) Drug prescribing in renal failure: dosing guidelines for adults. *Am. J. Kid. Dis.*, **3**, 155–193
4. Brill, C.B., Uretsy, S. and Gribetz, D. (1973) Indications of intrinsic renal disease in azotenic infants with diarrhoea and dehydration. *Pediatrics*, **52**, 197–205
5. Lee, R.V., Black, H.R. and Finkelstein, F.O. (1974) Treating peritonitis in patients with indwelling peritoneal catheters. *Dialysis Transplant.*, **3**, 52
6. Lloyd-Still, J.O. and Atwell, J.D. (1966) Renal failure in infancy. *J. Pediat. Surg.*, **1**, 466–475
7. Manley, G.L. and Collipp, P.J. (1968) Renal failure in the newborn. *Am. J. Dis. Child.*, **115**, 107–110
8. Mauer, S.M. and Mogrady, M.B. (1969) Renal papillary and cortical necrosis in a newborn infant. *J. Pediat.*, **74**, 750–754
9. Scott, D.K. and Roberts, D.E. (1985) Drugs and continuous ambulatory peritoneal dialysis. *Pharm. J.*, **234**, 592–593 and 621–624

43

Infection in the urinary tract

T. McKendrick

Although the first month of life is the time when urinary tract infection is most likely to begin, little attention has been given to it until recently.

In 1925 Sauer [30] described 15 babies with 'pyelitis'. He drew attention to the male preponderance and stressed the non-specific clinical features – poor colour and muscular tone, anorexia, vomiting and diarrhoea. Craig (1935) [3] recorded a larger series of 61 infants. He pointed out that symptoms sometimes preceded abnormal urinary findings by several days and that fever was found in only about half the babies. He also emphasized that pyuria was an unreliable diagnostic feature for it was totally absent from three ill babies and variable in others. James [9] in 1959 observed that about 1% of all the babies in a maternity unit developed urinary infection. She recorded failure to gain weight or loss of

weight and apathy as common less obvious clinical features. The babies in this series were, on the whole, mildly ill, as were those of Littlewood et al. [16]. Symptomless infection is probably not uncommon and it seems likely [12,22] that it may clear spontaneously.

Incidence

There are widely differing estimates of the frequency of urinary tract infection in the newborn. These are summarized in Table 43.1. Comparison of the various figures is unjustified because the criteria of diagnosis vary greatly. Thus James included babies suspected on clinical grounds and confirmed by bacteriological investigation but did not examine

Table 43.1 Reported infections in neonates

Author	Year	No. of babies		No. infected		%
Craig [3]	1935					0.9
James [9]	1959		NS	32		1.5
McCarthy and Pryles [18]	1963	M	100	2	2.0 }	1.0
		F	100	0	0 }	
Lincoln and Winberg [13]	1964	M	298	8	2.7 }	1.5
		F	286	1	0.3 }	
Smellie et al. [31]	1964		NS	34		0.3
O'Brien et al. [22]	1968		1000	1	0.1	
O'Doherty [23]	1968	M	410	9	2.2 }	1.1
		F	420	0	0.0 }	
Littlewood et al. [16]	1969	M	309	7	2.3 }	1.3
		F	291	1	0.3 }	
Bergstrom et al. [1]	1972		57 000	80 + ?36	0.14–0.2	
Edelmann et al. [5]	1973		836 term	6		0.7
			206 premature	5		2.4

the others for infection. James and Smellie [31] relied only on urine voided into plastic bags. Littlewood relied partly on similar specimens but confirmed doubtful infections by suprapubic aspiration. To some extent the incidence varied with the enthusiasm with which infection was sought as well as the method of collection (see below) and of counting bacteria.

Clinical features

The commonest early feature is an unusually large weight loss following birth before any symptoms are noted. The earliest symptoms are usually lethargy and a poor feeding performance so that weight gain is unsatisfactory. Vomiting may occur but is such a common symptom in young babies that it can hardly be considered a presenting symptom. Craig [3] and Littlewood [15] recorded diarrhoea as commonly present. Dehydration as a consequence of these features may ensue.

Pallor is a very common feature. The baby is said to have a grey hue. Cyanosis may also be seen. When the infection is severe and recognition is delayed, jaundice may be the presenting feature [2,21]. In such babies there is usually coliform septicaemia [15]. The liver may be enlarged 2–6 cm below the costal margin. Abdominal distension not due to enlargement of liver, kidneys or bladder may be seen as part of a generalized septicaemia.

There may be no localizing signs indicating urinary tract involvement. Not infrequently both kidneys are more easily palpable than normal and sometimes they are greatly enlarged. In severely ill infants, especially if there is urinary suppression, such swelling may suggest hydronephrosis or renal venous thrombosis. As this swelling usually subsides completely with adequate medical therapy it is presumably not due to anatomical obstruction. Distension of the bladder should raise the suspicion of underlying lower urinary tract obstruction; for example, due to posterior urethral valves or ectopic ureterocele.

As in most neonatal infections, fever is seldom found in the first few days. In severely ill babies hypothermia may occur. After the first week, however, some fever is usual.

The possibility of urinary tract infection must be considered when other infection such as meningitis is found.

Other presenting features seen less commonly include convulsions, irritability and sweating.

Pathology

Contrary to a long-held view, urinary tract infection in neonates is not commonly associated with malfor-

mation in the urinary tract. In more than 90% no anatomical abnormality can be demonstrated and malformation does not explain the greater frequency of infection in boys. There is, however, a commoner association with sepsis or septicaemia as noted by Ginsburg and McCracken [6]. Blood culture is a more important investigation in this context in neonates than in older children.

In the acute phase one or both kidneys may be swollen and hyperaemic. Inflammation usually extends to the calyces and pelvis, and may involve the lower urinary tract but this is less common in neonates. When it does occur, it usually denotes urinary stasis or obstruction.

Microscopic appearances vary with the duration and severity of the infection. When the illness has been of short duration, the changes are similar to those seen at any age. There are varying degrees of polymorphonuclear leucocyte infiltration of the renal parenchyma. Some areas may be necrotic. In the cortex there may be abscesses which destroy glomeruli and tubules. Organisms can be demonstrated in them. In less severely involved areas the brunt of the disease falls on the tubules, which are dilated and full of pus. The interstitial tissue is oedematous and may show polymorph infiltration. In these areas the glomeruli may be uninvolved but occasionally they, too, are invaded by polymorphs, the appearance being that of an acute glomerulitis.

When the illness has continued for more than a few weeks, e.g. because of delayed or ineffective therapy, chronic changes appear [25]. The interstitium is infiltrated with lymphocytes, plasma cells and eosinophils. The tubules are dilated and filled with 'colloid' casts. The glomeruli are reduced in number, and some of those remaining show pericapsular fibrosis, crescent formation (of epithelial cells) and adhesions between tuft and capsule. The smaller arteries have developed endarteritis.

Microbiology

Although viruses and other organisms such as protozoa and fungi have caused urinary tract infections in babies, the great majority are due to bacteria. A large variety of bacteria have been incriminated. The common urinary pathogens are as follows:

Escherichia coli
Other coliform bacilli
Klebsiella
Proteus vulgaris and *Mirabilis*
Streptococcus faecalis
Pseudomonas aeruginosa

Of these *E. coli* is by far the commonest and accounts for more than 90% of uncomplicated infections. When infection is a complicating factor (e.g. with meningomyelocele, posterior urethral valves, trauma, etc.), a wider selection of organisms may be found and these will reflect the pattern predominant in the hospital population at the relevant time.

Few studies of the serological types of *E. coli* found in babies have been published. Bergstrom *et al.* [1] observed that about 70% of nearly 50 strains which had been typed were of the common O types; i.e. 1, 2, 4, 6, 7, 8, 18 and 75. This was a pattern similar to the pattern recorded in adults in the north London [7] area although there are minor variations within this area. It can be inferred that the infection is probably transmitted from mother to baby, for it is unlikely that neonates harbour these organisms in the bowel – the only other likely source of infection. Craig's observation that symptoms sometimes preceded bacterial evidence of bowel colonization tends to confirm this view [3].

Sometimes lactobacilli or diphtheroids are isolated from urine cultures, often as a mixed growth and usually a light growth. These usually originate from the urethra and are seldom significant.

In recent years there has been much interest in the study of virulence and other factors which affect the host/parasite interactions. Although studies have involved infants and children, neonates have not so far been studied but there is no reason to suspect that the fundamental interactions between them and invading organisms are different.

Virulent strains of *E. coli* tend to have increased ability to adhere to uroepithelium, to increase haemolysis and aerobactin production and to resist the natural killing power of serum. The increased adherence is due to production of an adhesin which is found in fimbriated organisms and which binds to a disaccharide as part of a glycolipid on the uroepithelial surface [17]. There is some correlation between adherence and inflammation [19]. There is less correlation, however, between virulence and subsequent scarring of the kidney [33].

Diagnosis

The diagnosis of urinary tract infection depends to a large extent on the isolation of the causative organism from the urine. In order to obtain useful and reliable information from this, certain conditions should be met:

(1) The specimen should be uncontaminated by organisms from bowel, vagina or preputial sac.
(2) A quantitative bacterial examination should be made.
(3) More than one specimen should be examined.
(4) Specimens should be examined as soon as possible after collection.

(5) Antibacterial activity in the urine should be assayed.

These conditions will be discussed in more detail.

When bacteriological examination of urine is indicated, it is more important to exclude contamination than to obtain a large quantity. One or 2 ml suffices for culture and microscopy.

The mid-stream urine

This is also known as the 'clean specimen' or 'clean catch'. It is the simplest method in theory but unfortunately the most time-consuming and specimens tend to be lost if the collector fails to concentrate his or her attention for the vital relevant few seconds. The genitalia are carefully cleansed with a weak antiseptic (e.g. chlorhexidine) followed by water and then left exposed. In baby boys the foreskin should, if possible, be gently retracted. A sterile receptable is then held ready to intercept the next stream of urine while the infant is supported in the semirecumbent position with legs held apart. A variation of this is to hold the infant in one hand in the ventral position and stroke the lower part of the back in order to stimulate the micturition reflex while an assistant catches the resultant urine. While suitable for well-staffed wards, both these methods are too uncertain and frustrating for routine use in postnatal wards or clinics. Premature micturition during cleansing and faecal contamination of the receptacle are the most obvious hazards It is doubtful if cleansing the genitalia is necessary and it is probably of no value at all if the infant does not micturate within the following few minutes. Some contamination with genital secretion is likely, in boys from the preputial sac and in girls, who often have some vaginal reflux on micturition, from the vagina.

Collecting appliances

Several patterns of adhesive plastic bags are now on the market and have largely replaced a variety of rubber and moulded plastic appliances. None is entirely satisfactory because, unless the interval between application and removal with the specimen is very short (i.e. less than 20 min), contamination is usual. Only when gross urinary tract infection is present is bacterial culture reliable. A light or mixed growth from a bag specimen is of no diagnostic significance. In girls it is often difficult to seal such bags to the skin at the posterior end of the vulva.

Catheterization

Apart from being technically difficult in small boys, catheterization carries a risk, in all babies, of introducing infection. It should be avoided unless careful sterile precautions, as practised in operating theatres, can be taken.

Suprapubic aspiration

In infancy the bladder is mainly an abdominal organ and is easily palpable when containing urine. It is not usually difficult to introduce a gauge 23 needle through the skin 1–2 cm above the symphysis pubis into the bladder and to aspirate 1–5 ml of urine [20,27]. Local anaesthesia is unnecessary. In order to prevent micturition during the procedure, the urethra may be occluded by an assistant, either by grasping the penis or by compressing the urethra against the back of the symphysis with a finger inserted into the rectum. The procedure should be successful in 80–90% of attempts. It is safer than catheterization and obviates any possibility of contamination by genital, urethral or bowel organisms. There is little risk of subsequent leakage of urine through the puncture. Subsequent mild transient haematuria [18] and inadvertent puncture of the bowel [24] have been reported.

Suprapubic aspiration is indicated:

(1) when there is urgency in obtaining urine from a sick neonate;
(2) when there is doubt about the presence of infection following the examination of one or more mid-stream or bag specimens;
(3) when an uncontaminated specimen cannot be obtained.

The main contraindication is evidence that the infant has recently voided.

At all ages, many voided specimens of urine contain bacteria and most authorities agree that up to 10 000 bacteria/ml is not abnormal, particularly if the growth is of mixed organisms. Counts of more than 100 000 organisms/ml nearly always indicate infection [26], especially if of a single pure growth. Numbers between these two levels are inconclusive. Urine obtained by bladder aspiration is normally sterile. Pryles [27] suggests that any number of Gram-negative organisms is abnormal but a light growth of Gram-positive organisms may occur from contamination of the aspirating needle with skin organisms.

From these observations, therefore, it is better to examine two or three specimens of urine, preferably not within 24 h of each other. This can be done only if the baby's clinical condition permits. When the bacterial count is in the inconclusive range of 10 000–100 000/ml, the baby is not usually ill and repeated examination is feasible.

When urine is allowed to stand at room temperature, organisms multiply, cells begin to degenerate and the chemical composition changes. In 2 h the bacterial population may have multiplied ten times

and the cell count may be halved. It is important, therefore, that examination of urine should be carried out as soon as possible after collection. This should normally be within 30–40 min, but if a longer interval is unavoidable, steps should be taken to inhibit bacterial proliferation. Refrigeration at 4°C, or the addition of 3% benzoic acid, permits examination to be postponed for up to 24 h. In such specimens, however, white cell estimations cannot be relied upon. If antibacterial activity is demonstrated in urine, bacterial growth may have been diminished. This may lead to a suspicion that the bacterial count should be higher than it appears. Thus a count of (say) 50 000/ml, not normally diagnostic of infection, may be a significant growth. In newborn babies such antibacterial activity may have been transmitted from the mother, may be due to the cleansing technique used during collection or may be caused by the administration of barbiturates to the baby.

Pyuria

The presence of strands of pus in voided urine is incontrovertible evidence of infection. A little less convincing is a leucocyte count of more than 100/mm^3 of uncentrifuged urine. Epithelial cells, which may be present in large numbers, should be excluded from cell counts for they do not necessarily relate to infection. It is the presence of a few cells which causes difficulty. Most healthy neonates pass urine with fewer than 2 cells/mm^3. There is no unanimity of opinion about the upper limit of cell counts. Stansfield [32] and others [11,28] suggest 10/mm^3, but James [9] and Lincoln and Winberg [13] accept up to 25/mm^3 in baby boys and 40/mm^3 in baby girls. The discrepancy may be due to different collecting techniques [14]. With counts between 10 and 100/mm^3 the 'pyuria' may be due to contamination from preputial sac or vulva, although with normal social cleanliness this is less likely with counts of more than 50/mm^3.

Specimens obtained by suprapubic aspiration should normally contain no leucocytes. Occasional epithelial or red cells may be seen.

The estimation of pyuria by 'high power field' examination of a centrifuged deposit is less reliable. Whilst some factors involved such as speed and radius of centrifugation and volume of specimen can be standardized, others such as transfer of deposit to slide and placing of coverslip cannot [8]. Large variations in degree of pyuria can result so that, for the many specimens containing more than the 'very occasional cell per high power field', a leucocyte count of uncentrifuged urine in a counting chamber is desirable.

Whilst the correlation between pyuria and bacteriuria is high provided care is taken with collection [10], pyuria may also result from non-infective causes such as cystinuria, cystinosis, hypercalcaemia, renal acidosis or renal dysplasia. It should be stressed, therefore, that in the diagnosis of urinary tract infection prompt bacterial culture of an uncontaminated specimen of urine is the most important step. Microscopic leucocyte counts are, at best, confirmatory only and reliance should not be placed on them.

Management

The infant with urinary tract infection may be severely ill due to derangement of fluid and electrolyte balance as well as to the toxicity of local or generalized infection. He may also have anatomical abnormalities requiring correction. Four things, therefore, may need to be done:

(1) correction of fluid and electrolyte balance;
(2) eradication of the infecting organism;
(3) assessment of the anatomy of the urinary tract;
(4) assessment of the renal function when the infection is over.

Problems of fluid and electrolyte balance and assessment of renal function are discussed in Chapters 3 and 5 and will not be considered further here. The initial assessment of the urinary tract anatomy is predominantly clinical. Examination, combined with ultrasonic scan of the abdomen, will determine whether or not lower urinary tract obstruction is present. In the early stages catheter drainage per urethram, suprapubically or by nephrostomy may be urgently indicated. Abnormalities can be expected in up to half of neonates with urinary infections [4]. Some of these will have been appreciated by prenatal ultrasonography [29]. Subsequent surgical management is discussed in Chapter 45.

When the nature and antibiotic sensitivity of the infecting organism are known, effective therapy can be given. Table 43.2 summarizes the dosage of the commoner agents at present in use.

As a substantial proportion of neonatal urinary tract infections accompany infection elsewhere in the body, it is often important to use antibiotics which achieve effective tissue concentrations rather than those which are concentrated in the urine. When the latter are used it is possible to sterilize the urine without sterilizing the kidney. It is usually not necessary except in severely ill infants to give more than one antibiotic, but when this is necessary it is probably better not to mix bacteriostatic and bactericidal substances.

Therapy may have to be started before the antibiotic sensitivity of the organism is known. For this purpose, ampicillin and kanamycin are at present the most useful antibiotics, but local knowledge of prevalent organisms may indicate alternatives.

It is usually not difficult to sterilize the urinary tract. Indeed, the first dose of relevant antibiotic may achieve this. It is of some value to demonstrate the rapidity with which bacterial clearance is attained, for delay beyond a day or two may indicate obstruction or reflux within the urinary tract.

References

1. Bergstrom, T., Larson, M., Lincoln, K. and Winberg, J. (1972) Studies of urinary tract infection in infancy and childhood. XII. Eighty consecutive patients with neonatal infection. *J. Pediat.*, **80**, 858–866
2. Bernstein, J. and Brown, A.K. (1962) Sepsis and jaundice in early infancy. *Pediatrics*, **29**, 873–882
3. Craig, W.S. (1935) Urinary disorders occurring in the neonatal period. *Arch. Dis. Child.*, **10**, 337–354
4. Drew, J.H. and Acton, C.M. (1976) Radiological findings in infants with urinary infection. *Arch. Dis. Child.*, **51**, 628–630
5. Edelmann, C.M., Ogwo, J.E., Fine, B.P. and Martinez, A.B. (1973) The prevalence of bacteriuria in full term and premature newborn infants. *J. Pediat.*, **82**, 125–132

Table 43.2 Antibiotic dosage for neonates with urinary tract infection

	Route	*Dose* (mg/kg per dose)	*Frequency*
Ampicillin	Oral or i.v.	25	12 hourly if < 7 days age 8 hourly if > 7 days age
Gentamicin	i.v.	3 2	12 hourly if <14 days age 8 hourly if >14 days age
Trimethoprim[a]	Oral or i.v.	4	12 hourly
Augmentin	i.v.	30	12 hourly if < 7 days age 8 hourly if > 7 days age
Cephradine	Oral or i.v.	50	12 hourly if < 7 days age 8 hourly if > 7 days age

[a] As there may be interference with folate metabolism and haematopoiesis this is probably not a first choice drug in neonates

6. Ginsburg, C.M. and McCracken, G.H. (1982) Urinary tract infection in young infants. *Pediatrics*, **69**, 409–412

7. Gruneberg, R.N., Leigh, D.A. and Brumfitt, W. (1968) *Escherichia coli* serotypes in urinary tract infection: studies in domiciliary, ante-natal and hospital practice. In: *Urinary Tract Infection* (ed. F. O'Grady and W. Brumfitt), Oxford University Press, London, p. 68

8. Houston, I.B. (1963) Pus cells and bacterial counts in the diagnosis of urinary tract infections in childhood. *Arch. Dis. Child.*, **38**, 600–605

9. James, U. (1959) Urinary infection in the newborn. *Lancet*, **ii**, 1001–1002

10. Lam, C.N., Bremner, A.D., Maxwell, J.D., Murphy, A.V. and Low, W.J. (1967) Pyuria and bacteriuria. *Arch. Dis. Child.*, **42**, 275–280

11. Lawson, J.S. and Hewstone, A.S. (1964) Microscopic appearance of urine in the neonatal period. *Arch. Dis. Child.*, **39**, 287–288

12. Lincoln, K. and Winberg, J. (1964) Studies of urinary tract infection in infancy and childhood. I. Quantitative estimation of bacteria in unselected neonates with special reference to the occurrence of asymptomatic infections. *Acta Paediat. Scand.*, **53**, 307–316

13. Lincoln, K. and Winberg, J. (1964) Studies of urinary tract infection in infancy and childhood. II. Quantitative estimation of cellular excretion in unselected neonates. *Acta Paediat. Scand.*, **53**, 447–453

14. Littlewood, J.M. (1971) White cells and bacteria in voided urine of healthy newborns. *Arch. Dis. Child.*, **46**, 167–172

15. Littlewood, J.M. (1972) 66 infants with urinary tract infection in first month of life. *Arch. Dis. Child.*, **47**, 218–226

16. Littlewood, J.M., Kite, P. and Kite, B.A. (1969) Incidence of neonatal urinary tract infection. *Arch. Dis. Child.*, **44**, 617–620

17. Lomberg, H., Hellström, M. and Jodal, V. (1986) Renal scarring and non-attaching *Escherichia coli*. *Lancet*, **ii**, 1341

18. McCarthy, J.M. and Pryles, C.V. (1963) Clean voided and catheter neonatal urine specimens. *Am. J. Dis. Child.*, **106**, 473–478

19. Marild, S., Wettergren, B., Hellström, M., Jodal, V., Lincoln, K., Orskov, I. and Svanborg-Eden, C. (1988) Bacterial virulence and inflammatory response in infants with febrile urinary tract infection or screening bacteriuria. *J. Pediat.*, **112**, 348–354

20. Nelson, J.D. and Peters, P.C. (1965) Suprapubic aspiration of urine in premature and term infants. *Pediatrics*, **36**, 132–134

21. Ng, S.J. and Rawsthorn, J.R. (1971) Urinary tract infections presenting with jaundice. *Arch. Dis. Child.*, **46**, 173–176

22. O'Brien, N.G., Carroll, R., Donovan, D.E. and Dundon, S.P. (1968) Bacteriuria and leucocyte excretion in the newborn. *J. Ir. Med. Ass.*, **61**, 267–268

23. O'Doherty, N.J. (1968) Urinary tract infection in the neonatal period and later infancy. In *Urinary Tract Infection* (ed. F. O'Grady and W. Brumfitt), Oxford University Press, London, p. 113

24. Polnay, L., Fraser, A.M. and Lewis, J.M. (1975) Complication of suprapubic bladder aspiration. *Arch. Dis. Child.*, **50**, 80–81

25. Porter, K.A. and Giles, M.M. (1956) A pathological study of 5 cases of pyelonephritis in the newborn. *Arch. Dis. Child.*, **31**, 303–309

26. Pryles, C.V. (1960) The diagnosis of urinary tract infection. *Pediatrics*, **26**, 441–451

27. Pryles, C.V. (1965) Bladder aspiration and other methods of urine collection. *Pediatrics*, **36**, 128–131

28. Pryles, C.V. and Eliot, C.R. (1965) Pyuria and bacteriuria in infants and children. *Am. J. Dis. Child.*, **110**, 628–635

29. Ring, E. and Zobel, G. (1988) Urinary infection and malformations of urinary tract in infancy. *Arch. Dis. Child.*, **63**, 818–820

30. Sauer, L.W. (1925) Neonatal pyelitis. *J. Am. Med. Ass.*, **85**, 327–329

31. Smellie, J.M., Hodson, C.J., Edwards, D. and Normand, I.C.S. (1964) Clinical and radiological features of urinary infection in childhood. *Br. Med. J.*, **2**, 1222–1226

32. Stansfield, J.M. (1964) The measurement and meaning of pyuria. *Arch. Dis. Child.*, **37**, 257–262

33. Svanborg-Eden, C., de Man, P., Jodal, V., Linder, H. and Lomberg, H. (1987) Host parasite interaction in urinary tract infection. *Pediat. Nephrol.*, **1**, 623–631

44

Indications for investigation of the urinary tract in the newborn

A. M. K. Rickwood

Apart from the many cases with urological abnormalities detected by prenatal ultrasound (Chapters 7 and 45), investigation of the urinary tract in the newborn is indicated when there is clinical evidence of urinary tract pathology, if there is suspicion of urinary tract involvement by lesions arising in other systems, in the presence of non-urological congenital abnormalities known to co-exist with urinary tract anomalies and, occasionally, when there is a family history of affection by a genetically determined urological lesion.

Urinary tract disease

Abnormalities of micturition

In normal infants the interval between birth and the first act of voiding urine varies appreciably. In a study of 500 full-term babies [46], 67% micturated within the first 12 h of life, 25% within the next 12 h, 7% between 24 and 48 h and 0.6% not until 48 h after birth. In practice, it is often difficult to be certain of the voiding pattern in neonates. A baby may micturate unnoticed during or shortly after birth; furthermore urine output during the first few days of life is small, ranging from 15 to 60 ml per day, so that it is possible that a small quantity of urine might be passed and evaporate from the napkin.

Reported maximum urine flow rates during infancy vary from 3 ml/s [34] to 8 ml/s [26]. For routine purposes, normality or otherwise of the urinary stream in babies is assessed subjectively. A newborn boy can produce a sustained, forceful, stream projected for about 60 cm when he is lying supine. An intermittent rather than a continuous flow of urine is not necessarily pathological. The bladder of a normal healthy full-term neonate is not expressible, but suprapubic tapping or compression, may induce a reflex act of voiding. This should not be confused with true expressibility of the bladder indicative of sphincteric weakness. In some normal baby boys the bladder remains palpable after micturition because of incomplete evacuation which may be a factor in the causation of asymptomatic bacteriuria, which occurs principally in males [29], and in the development of neonatal pyelonephritis, which is virtually confined to boys [33].

Anuria

Absence of urination with an empty bladder and without signs of urinary ascites indicates the existence of severe renal impairment or even bilateral renal agenesis. True supravesical obstruction of functioning kidneys in the newborn is, for practical purposes, never complete and some urine is always passed. Although stability of internal environment of the fetus is entirely dependent upon the placenta, so that even in the total absence of renal function fetal catabolism and growth proceed normally, the fetal kidney plays a major role in controlling the volume of amniotic fluid. During the latter half of pregnancy this is largely composed of fetal urine and, in the absence of kidney function, its volume falls from the normal of 500–800 ml to very low levels.

Maternal oligohydramnios, if not noted during pregnancy, is evidenced at birth by the presence of amnion nodosum in which the amniotic membrane, especially over the placenta, is covered by small grey nodules composed of keratinized cells from the fetal dermis. The infant has a typical facial appearance described by Potter [36]. An epicanthic fold beginning at the inner aspect of each eye extends as a groove onto the cheek. The tip of the nose is depressed and the chin is small with a deep crease between it and the lower lip. The ears are large, low set and flattened against the head. Large hands, with thick fingers, and talipes are often present. These features are probably entirely the result of fetal compression since a case is recorded of Potter's facies in a neonate with normal kidneys, where oligohydramnios resulted from prenatal rupture of the membranes [12]. Most cases of bilateral renal agenesis occur in males. In females there may be virilization of the external genitalia, possibly because of the inability of the fetus to excrete circulating androgens [44]. In practice, neonates without functioning kidneys seldom survive long enough to exhibit anuria. As a rule they are stillborn or succumb shortly after birth from respiratory failure consequent upon the pulmonary hypoplasia caused by oligohydramnios. The air sacs often rupture leading to pneumothorax or pneumomediastinum (see Chapter 22).

Urinary retention

Complete urinary retention is rare in the newborn. A few boys with prune-belly syndrome have urethral atresia; in this circumstance there is a patent urachus so that urine leaks from around the umbilicus. In one case [51], with a concomitant high-level imperforate anus, decompression of the bladder occurred via a recto-urethral fistula and urinary leakage from the bowel was noted after formation of a colostomy. Transient retention of urine, sufficient to cause upper urinary tract dilatation, has been recorded in neonates of both sexes [42]. This was not associated with organic bladder outflow obstruction or evident neurological disease and spontaneous recovery followed a period of catheter drainage. One case subsequently proved to have occult neuropathic bladder.

Dribbling micturition

Dribbling of urine in the neonatal period usually occurs intermittently with passage of small volumes of urine in a weak, slow stream. Diagnosis depends upon whether this occurs from a full or from an almost empty bladder. A distended bladder is usually readily palpable; any doubt can be resolved by ultrasound examination.

Dribbling micturition from a full bladder is indicative of organic bladder outflow obstruction or of neurological disease. In boys, several obstructive urethral lesions exist, of which posterior urethral valves is the commonest and usually the most severe. In girls, hydrocolpos, resulting from some form of congenital vaginal occlusion, obstructs

micturition by upward and forward displacement of the bladder. A similar phenomenon sometimes occurs with urogenital sinus anomalies. Ectopic ureterocele may cause infravesical obstruction in babies of both sexes. The ureterocele, which is sited at the extremity of the ureter draining the upper pole of the kidney, lies partly within the bladder and partly within the proximal urethra and, if tense, obstructs the vesical outlet. Quite often, organic infravesical obstruction is associated with hydronephrotic changes and renal damage which have occurred prenatally. In this circumstance, presentation may be with symptoms caused by impaired renal function, often exacerbated by infection, and only then is it noted that micturition is abnormal.

Dribbling of urine from an empty bladder, especially when occurring as the infant cries, implies the existence of an incompetent sphincteric mechanism caused by some structural abnormality or by neurological disease, or that urine is entering the genitourinary tract below the level of the sphincters. Structural causes of sphincteric deficiency include urogenital sinus in the female, which may occur as an isolated abnormality or in association with persistent cloaca, and epispadias. In males epispadias is obvious because of the typical genital deformity. In females, where the condition is sometimes overlooked, there is a double clitoris and a wide urethral meatus which is deficient dorsally (Figure 44.1). There is always diastasis of the pubic bones and as a rule the umbilicus is low-sited. Introital or vaginal ectopia of the upper polar ureter of a completely duplex renal unit is a classic cause of continuous dribbling in the female but this is very rarely evident in the neonatal period. Unilateral single system ectopic ureters are not associated with

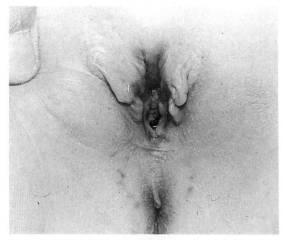

Figure 44.1 Epispadias in a female neonate: when the labia are separated, the bifid clitoris and deficient urethra are clearly seen

voiding disorders but the rare condition of bilateral single ectopic ureters causes dribbling micturition in both sexes since the bladder neck is imperfectly formed and the bladder itself is usually small [55]. Single ectopic ureters are nearly always associated with some degree of renal dysplasia so that symptoms related to impaired renal function or infection are often the presenting feature rather than the voiding disorder itself.

Voiding disorders in neurological disease

Myelomeningocele remains much the commonest and most evident congenital lesion of the spinal cord causing neuropathic bladder. Other comparatively infrequent lesions include lumbosacral lipoma, diastematomyelia and intraspinal dermoid cyst; in the great majority of such cases there is some overlying cutaneous abnormality (lipoma, haemangioma, hairy patch, lumbosacral sinus, etc.) drawing attention to the spinal cord anomaly. Sacral agenesis is quite frequently overlooked. This condition may be associated with high level imperforate anus [9] or may occur in isolation, especially in infants born to mothers who are diabetic and on insulin. At least the terminal three sacral segments must be absent to affect bladder function [54]. The sacral defect is evident on palpation and there is characteristically flattening of the upper buttocks. Often there is wasting of the calves and talipes.

The pattern of abnormal voiding varies and is dependent upon the neurological deficit [40]. Essential features of neurological examination comprise the assessment of the anocutaneous reflex and the presence (or otherwise) of peri-anal sensation to pin-prick as evidenced by general arousal to this stimulus. Absence of the anocutaneous reflex is associated with some degree of sphincteric weakness and usually a detrusor which contracts poorly or not at all. A weak or dribbling stream occurs when the infant cries and, as a rule, the bladder is expressible. Occasionally, where there is gross sphincteric incompetence, the bladder cannot be expressed because it is permanently empty. A positive anocutaneous reflex is associated with reflex contractility of the detrusor and a competent sphincteric mechanism. The bladder is inexpressible and the infant voids spontaneously by reflex detrusor contractions; generally the urinary stream, although forceful, is interrupted and the bladder empties incompletely. Neuropathic bladder can be confidently diagnosed in the absence of an anocutaneous reflex or a complete cord lesion evidenced by lack of peri-anal sensation to pin-prick. In the presence of a combination of a positive anocutaneous reflex and intact peri-anal sensation, bladder function *may* prove to be normal although this is unlikely if there is significant residual urine after voiding.

Voiding from abnormal sites

In the male with congenital absence of the penis, the urethra generally opens within the anus or immediately anterior to it. In boys with one form of urethral duplication, one urethra opens onto the perineum or at the anus while the other transverses the penis to open at the normal site, and the two join proximally at the level of the verumontanum. The normally sited urethra is extremely narrow and most of the urine passes via the perineal opening. Continence is generally normal [53]. Girls with a persistent cloaca or an isolated urogenital sinus deformity have a single vulval orifice; if there is high urethrovaginal confluence, the bladder neck is incompetent and urine dribbles continuously from this orifice. Urinary leakage from the umbilicus may occur in boys with prune-belly syndrome, especially if there is atresia or stenosis of the urethra, but patent urachus may occur in otherwise normal infants of either sex as an isolated anomaly in the absence of urethral obstruction [45]. At birth, the umbilical cord is distended with urine; when it sloughs off, a mucosal covered nipple leaking urine from a central aperture is visible.

Urinary ascites

Urinary ascites may occur prenatally or after birth, usually within the first week of life [24]. The most common underlying lesion is posterior urethral valves but the condition has also been encountered with neuropathic bladder [19], ectopic ureterocele and supravesical obstructions, most often at the pelvi-ureteric junction [24]. In premature infants, spontaneous rupture of the bladder may occur, possibly as a result of localized ischaemia [43]. The diagnosis may be confirmed by paracentesis, although biochemical analysis of the fluid may show a misleadingly low urea and creatinine content due to dialysis across the peritoneal membrane. On occasion absorption of potassium from the peritoneal cavity leads to dangerous hyperkalaemia. Elucidation of the underlying pathology is obtained by ultrasound examination and, if necessary, by appropriate radiological contrast studies. Rupture of the bladder into the peritoneal cavity may be evident or there may be extravasation of urine from a hydronephrotic kidney. In the latter circumstance, there is usually no demonstrable breach of the parietal peritoneum and it is presumed that urine enters the peritoneal cavity by diffusion.

Abdominal mass

An abdominal mass is much the commonest physical sign leading to urological investigation of the neonate. Approximately 70% of such masses originate in the genitourinary tract (Table 44.1) [56]. The more

Table 44.1 Causes of abdominal mass in 115 neonates

Renal	75	(65%)
Multicystic kidney	35	
Hydronephrosis	33	
Renal vein thrombosis	3	
Polycystic kidneys	2	
Tumour	2	
Hydrocolpos	7	(6%)
Bladder	1	(1%)
Non-urological	32	(28%)
Gastrointestinal	11	
Retroperitoneal	10	
Hepatobiliary	6	
Ovarian	5	

From Woodard [56]

common upper abdominal lesions are caused by multicystic kidney, which is characteristically lobulated, or hydronephrosis which has a smooth contour. In females a lower abdominal mass is usually a hydrocolpos rather than a distended bladder. The site and nature of these lesions can nearly always be determined by sonography.

Haematuria

Haematuria is an uncommon symptom in the newborn; causes in a series with gross haematuria, are listed in Table 44.2 [10]. Often, pink staining of the napkin is described rather than witness of passage of blood-stained urine. In boys this is usually due to bleeding from the foreskin as a result of ammoniacal excoriation and in girls vaginal bleeding caused by circulating maternal oestrogens.

Table 44.2 Causes of haematuria in 35 neonates

	No.	*(%)*
Obstructive uropathy	7	(20)
Renal vein thrombosis	7	(20)
Polycystic kidneys	6	(17)
Sponge kidney	3	(9)
Renal tumour	1	(3)
Undiagnosed	11	(31)

From Emmanuel and Aronson [10]

Genitourinary anomalies

Investigation of the anatomy and function of upper renal tracts is required when there is some gross abnormality of the lower tract such as persistent cloaca or an exstrophic lesion. With classic exstrophy, the kidneys and ureters are usually initially normal but with exstrophy of the cloaca, primary upper tract anomalies occur in some 50% of cases [48].

Boys with hypospadias and undescended testis have an incidence of urinary anomalies somewhat higher than normal, although not so high as to justify routine pyelography. Abnormalities, usually of minor degree, have been described in 1.5 [31] to 6% [25] of hypospadiacs. Routine screening of these boys by ultrasound may be undertaken although it is not the author's practice to do so in the absence of signs, symptoms or urinary infection. While the degree of hypospadias is not thought to affect the likelihood of associated abnormalities, penoscrotal transposition has been stated to carry an appreciably increased risk [8].

Megalourethra is often associated with prune-belly syndrome and even when the abdominal wall is normal, affected boys frequently have hydro-ureteronephrosis [22].

Secondary involvement of the urinary tracts

Investigation of the urinary tract may be advisable when there is a possibility of its displacement or obstruction by an intra-abdominal or intrapelvic lesion. Sacrococcygeal teratoma with a large intra-pelvic component, anterior meningocele and hydrocolpos resulting from vaginal obstruction may displace the bladder, obstructing micturition and leading to upper tract dilatation. As a rule, these changes are fully reversible by treatment of the primary disorder. A retroperitoneal mass, such as a teratoma, neuroblastoma or adrenal haemorrhage may displace the kidney or ureter and pyelography in such cases is often of diagnostic value.

Non-urological congenital anomalies

Urological investigation is indicated in infants with various congenital anomalies known to co-exist frequently with lesions of the urinary tracts.

Single umbilical artery

Single umbilical artery is a normal occurrence during a phase of fetal development and persists at birth in 0.9% of infants. This is associated with a fourfold increase in neonatal mortality due to various severe anomalies, notably of the gastrointestinal tract, and, of those who die, some 30% have abnormalities of the urinary tracts [11,16]. Whether survivors have an increased incidence of urological lesions is doubtful, although inguinal hernias are appreciably more common than in controls. Ultrasound screening of these cases is probably justified.

Ear malformations

Apart from the malformed ears of Potter's facies [36], associated with bilateral renal agenesis, other ear deformities, particularly if asymmetrical or unilateral [17], are commonly associated with urinary tract anomalies. Taylor [49] noted urinary tract malformations especially in cases of severe underdevelopment of the ear and ipsilateral hypoplasia of the facial bones.

Limb deformities

Talipes, congenital dislocation of the hip and other compression deformities may result from oligohydramnios occurring as a consequence of absent or severely defective fetal renal function. Other hand and foot anomalies, notably 'lobster-claw' deformity [27], are often associated with urinary tract lesions. In the Marfan syndrome, arachnodactyly is frequently accompanied by cardiac and urinary tract anomalies [30].

Anomalies of the female genital tract

Congenital absence of the vagina, a condition rarely noted neonatally, has associated abnormalities of the upper urinary tracts in 30–51% of recorded cases [7,35]. Genital tract duplication, common urogenital sinus and persistent cloaca also carry a high incidence of upper tract lesions. Gonadal dysgenesis (Turner's syndrome) carries a reported incidence of 64–81% of urinary tract anomalies, horseshoe kidney in particular [20,28].

Cardiac anomalies

Congenital heart disease was found by Mehrizi [32] to be present in 65 (23%) of 279 cases of malformation of the urinary tracts. Ventricular septal defect was the most frequent concurrence; of 89 cases of this lesion 22 (25%) had urological abnormalities. Asymptomatic urinary tract lesions are frequently diagnosed by the pyelogram incidentally obtained during the course of cardiac angiography; Roa *et al*. [38] reported that 20 (7.7%) of 260 patients with congenital heart disease had urinary tract anomalies demonstrable in this way. An additional six out of 21 children who did not have a pyelogram were found to have a urological abnormality at autopsy.

Imperforate anus

Urological pathology may form part of the primary anomaly (for example, rectourethral fistula), may be of neuropathic origin secondary to sacral agenesis or may be due to associated developmental anomalies. The high incidence of the last has been frequently documented with a 50% occurrence rate in some reported series [6,18,47]. Lesions demonstrable by pyelography include renal agenesis, pelviureteric obstruction and, less commonly, horseshoe kidney, crossed fused ectopia and similar anomalies. Their incidence is higher in supralevator than in infralevator lesions and in boys than in girls. In boys there is an increased occurrence of lower tract abnormalities, notably hypospadias. Duplication of the genital tract occasionally occurs in girls. In one series where cystography was routine [41], vesicoureteric reflux was found in 43% of cases of imperforate anus; the incidence was not related to sex or to the type of lesion. In a few cases there occurs transient hydro-ureteronephrosis not caused by obstruction or reflux [39].

Persistent cloaca is associated with a particularly high incidence of primary urinary tract anomalies [5].

Oesophageal atresia

Oesophageal atresia carries an increased risk of developmental urinary tract anomalies; if infants with coincident imperforate anus are excluded, this is of the order of 29–43% of cases [1,23].

VATER association

Anomalies in the three foregoing categories may coexist in the same patient, often with additional abnormalities of the spine (usually hemivertebrae) and limbs (usually radial aplasia or hypoplasia) [37]; the acronym VATER denotes Vertebral, Anorectal, Tracheo-Esophageal, Renal and Radial associated abnormalities. Not surprisingly the incidence of urinary anomalies in such an association is high, 90% in one recorded series [50].

Spina bifida

In myelomeningocele, primary anomalies of the upper renal tracts are described at autopsy in 12–25% of cases [15,52]; incidence of fusion anomalies (horseshoe kidney, etc.) is increased 18-fold above the general population. Exstrophy of the bladder is a rare association.

Multi-system anomalies

Urinary tract anomalies are frequently found in various multisystem lesions and eponymous syndromes. A full list is given by Barratt [4].

Genetically determined anomalies

Urinary tract investigation may be indicated in an apparently normal and healthy infant when there is a family history of urological abnormalities, especially when these are of severe degree. Urinary tract duplication is well recognized to have a high familial incidence. In siblings of affected patients, the chance of urinary tract duplication is of the order of 1 in 8 rather than the 1 in 125 found in the population at large [2]. Vesico-ureteric reflux has a similar familial tendency; the chance of reflux in siblings of affected patients is increased at least tenfold above normal, regardless of sex [21]. Duplication anomalies and vesico-ureteric reflux not infrequently occur in different members of the same family [2]. Hydronephrosis due to pelvi-ureteric junction obstruction is sometimes familial and possibly transmitted as an autosomal dominant trait [3,14]; in two of our cases, one brother had pelvi-ureteric junction obstruction and the other primary obstructive megaureter. Occasional examples are recorded of posterior urethral valves in siblings [13] and twins.

References

1. Atwell, J.D. and Beard, R.C. (1974) Congenital anomalies of the upper urinary tract associated with esophageal atresia and tracheo-esophageal fistula. *J. Pediat. Surg.*, **9**, 825–831

2. Atwell, J.D., Cook, P.L., Strong, L. and Hyde, I. (1977) The inter-relationship between vesicoureteric reflux, trigonal abnormalities and a bifid collecting system: a family study. *Br. J. Urol.*, **49**, 97–105

3. Atwell, J.D. (1985) Familial pelviureteric junction obstruction and its association with duplex pelvicalyceal system and vesicoureteric reflux. A family study. *Br. J. Urol.*, **57**, 365–369

4. Barratt, T.M. (1974) Urological manifestations of multi-system disease. In: *Urology in Childhood. Encyclopaedia of Urology* (ed. D.I. Williams) Springer-Verlag, Berlin, (suppl. XV)

5. Bartholomew, T.H. and Gonzales, E.T. (1978) Urological management in cloacal dysgenesis. *Urology*, **11**, 549–557

6. Belman, A.B. and King, L.R. (1972) Urinary tract abnormalities associated with imperforate anus. *J. Urol.*, **108**, 823–824

7. Chawla, S., Berg, K. and Indra, K.J. (1966) Abnormalities of urinary tract and skeleton associated with congenital absence of vagina. *Br. Med. J.*, **1**, 1398–1400

8. Datta, N.S., Singh, S.M., Reddy, A.V. and Chakravarty, A.K. (1971) Transposition of the penis and scrotum in two brothers. *J. Urol.*, **105**, 739–742

9. Duhamel, B. (1961) From mermaid to anal imperforation: the syndrome of caudal regression. *Arch. Dis. Child.*, **36**, 152–155

10. Emanuel, B. and Aronson, N. (1974) Neonatal haematuria. *Am. J. Dis. Child.*, **128**, 204–206

11. Faierman, E. (1960) The significance of one umbilical artery. *Arch. Dis. Child.*, **35**, 285–288

12. Fantel, A.G. and Shepard, T.H. (1975) Potter syndrome: non-renal features induced by oligohydramnios. *Am. J. Dis. Child.*, **129**, 1346–1347

13. Farkas, A. and Skinner, D.G. (1976) Posterior urethral valves in siblings. *Br. J. Urol.*, **48**, 76

14. Finn, R. and Carruthers, J.A. (1974) Genetic aspects of hydronephrosis associated with renal agenesis. *Br. J. Urol.*, **46**, 351–356

15. Forbes, M. (1972) Renal dysplasia in infants with neural spinal dysraphism. *J. Pathol.*, **107**, 13–19

16. Froelich, L.A. and Fujikara, T. (1973) Follow-up of infants with single umbilical artery. *Pediatrics*, **52**, 6

17. Hilson, D. (1957) Malformations of the genitourinary tract. *Br. Med. J.*, **2**, 785–789

18. Hoekstra, W.J., Scholtmeijer, J.R. and Molenaar, J.C. (1983) Urogenital tract abnormalities associated with congenital anorectal anomalies. *J. Urol.*, **130**, 962–963

19. Howat, J.M. (1971) Urinary ascites complicating spina bifida. *Arch. Dis. Child.*, **46**, 103–105

20. Hung, W. and Lopresti, J.M. (1968) The high frequency of abnormal excretory urograms in young patients with gonadal dysgenesis. *J. Urol.*, **98**, 697

21. Jerkins, G.R. and Noe, H.N. (1982) Familial vesicoureteric reflux in children: prospective study. *J. Urol.*, **128**, 774–778

22. Johnston, J.H. and Coimbra, J.A.M. (1970) Megalourethra. *J. Pediat. Surg.*, **5**, 304–308

23. Johnston, J.H. and Mix, L.W. (1978) Indications for investigation of the urinary tract in the newborn. In *Neonatal Surgery*, 2nd Edition (ed. P.P. Rickham, J. Lister and I.M. Irving), Butterworths, London

24. Kay, R., Brereton, R.J. and Johnston, J.H. (1980) Urinary ascites in the newborn. *Br. J. Urol.*, **52**, 451–454

25. Khuri, F.J., Hardy, B.E. and Churchill, B.M. (1981) Urologic anomalies associated with hypospadias. *Urol. Clin. North Am.*, **8**, 565–571

26. Kroigaard, N. (1967) Micturition cinematography with simultaneous pressure flow study in infancy and childhood. *J. Pediat. Surg.*, **2**, 523–528

27. Leiter, E. and Lipson, J. (1976) Genito-urinary tract anomalies in lobster claw syndrome. *J. Urol.*, **115**, 339–341

28. Lemli, L. and Smith, D.W. (1963) XO syndrome: study of differentiated phenotype in 25 patients. *J. Pediat.*, **63**, 577–588

29. Lincoln, K. and Winberg, J. (1964) Studies of urinary tract infection in infancy and childhood. II. Quantitative estimation of bacteriuria in unselected neonates with special reference to the occurrence of asymptomatic infection. *Acta Paediat. (Stockh.).*, **53**, 307–316

30. Loughridge, L.W. (1959) Renal abnormalities in Marfan syndrome. *Q. J. Med.*, **28**, 531–544

31. McArdle, F. and Lebowitz, R. (1975) Uncomplicated hypospadias and anomalies of upper renal tract. Need for screening?. *Urology*, **5**, 712–716

32. Mehrizi, A. (1962) Congenital malformation of the heart associated with congenital anomalies of the urinary tract. *J. Pediat.*, **61**, 582–589

33. O'Doherty, N. (1968) Urinary tract infection in the neonatal period and later infancy. In *Urinary Tract Infection* (ed. F. O'Grady and W. Brumfitt), Oxford University Press, London, p. 113

34. O'Donnell, B. and O'Connor, T.P. (1971) Bladder function in infants and children. *Br. J. Urol.*, **43**, 25–27

35. Phelan, J.T., Counsellor, V.S. and Greene, L.F. (1953) Deformities of the urinary tract with congenital absence of the vagina. *Surg. Gynec. Obstet.*, **97**, 1–3

36. Potter, E.L. (1946) Facial characteristics of infants with bilateral renal agenesis. *Am. J. Obstet. Gynecol.*, **51**, 885–888

37. Quan, L. and Smith, D.W. (1973) The VATER association. Vertebral defects, anal atresia, radial and renal dysplasia: a spectrum of associated defects. *J. Pediat.*, **82**, 104–107

38. Rao, S., Engle, M.A.E. and Levin, A.R. (1975) Silent anomalies of the urinary tract and congenital heart disease. *Chest*, **67**, 685–691

39. Rickwood, A.M.K. (1978) Transient ureteric dilatation in neonates with imperforate anus. *Br. J. Urol.*, **50**, 16–19

40. Rickwood, A.M.K. (1984) The neuropathic bladder in children. In: *Urodynamics. Principles, Practice and Application* (eds A.R. Mundy, T.P. Stephenson and A.J. Wein), Churchill Livingstone, Edinburgh

41. Rickwood, A.M.K. and Spitz, L. (1980) Primary vesicoureteric reflux in neonates with imperforate anus. *Arch. Dis. Child.*, **55**, 149–150

42. Robson, W.J. and Davies, R.H. (1974) Transient retention of urine in the neonatal period. *J. Pediat. Surg.*, **9**, 863–866

43. Roth, D.R., Krueger, R.P. and Barraza, M. (1987) Bladder disruption in the premature male neonate. *J. Urol.*, **137**, 500–501

44. Schlegel, R.J., Aspillaga, M.J., Neu, R.L., Carneiro-Leao, J. and Gardner, L.I. (1966) XX Chromosome complement in an infant having male-type external genitals, renal agenesis and other anomalies. *J. Pediat.*, **69**, 812–814

45. Schreck, W.R. and Campbell, W.A. (1972) The relation of outlet obstruction to urinary-umbilical fistula. *J. Urol.*, **108**, 641–643

46. Sherry, S.N. and Kramer, I. (1955) The time of passage of first stool and first urine by the newborn infant. *J. Pediat.*, **46**, 158–159

47. Singh, M.P., Haddadin, A., Zachary, R.B. and Pilling, D.W. (1974) Renal tract disease in imperforate anus. *J. Pediat. Surg.*, **9**, 197–202

48. Soper, R.T. and Kilger, K. (1964) Vesico-intestinal fissure. *J. Urol.*, **92**, 490–501

49. Taylor, W.C. (1965) Deformity of ears and kidneys. *Can. Med. Ass. J.*, **93**, 107–110

50. Uehling, D.T., Gilben, E. and Chesney, R. (1983) Urologic complications of the VATER association. *J. Urol.*, **129**, 352–354

51. Walker, J., Prokurat, A.I. and Irving, I.M. (1987) Prune-belly syndrome associated with exomphalos and anorectal agenesis. *J. Pediat. Surg.*, **22**, 215–217

52. Wilcock, A.R. and Emery, J.L. (1970) Deformities of the renal tract in children with myelomeningocele and hydrocephalus compared with those of children showing no such nervous system deformities. *Br. J. Urol.*, **42**, 152–157

53. Williams, D.I. (1968) The male bladder neck and urethra. In *Paediatric Urology* (ed. D.I. Williams), Butterworths, London, p. 267

54. Williams, D.I. and Nixon, H.H. (1957) Agenesis of the sacrum. *Surg. Gynec. Obstet.*, **105**, 84–88

55. Williams, D.I. and Lightwood, R.G. (1972) Bilateral single ectopic ureter. *Br. J. Urol.*, **44**, 267–273

56. Woodard, J.R. (1986) Neonatal and Perinatal Emergencies. In *Campbells Urology*, 5th Edition (eds P.C. Walsh, R.F. Gittes, A.D. Perlmutter and T.A. Stamey), W.B. Saunders, Philadelphia

45

Urinary tract obstruction and dilatation in the newborn

A. M. K. Rickwood

Diagnosis of congenital uropathies causing dilatation or cystic changes in the upper renal tracts has become transformed by the advent of prenatal sonography, to the extent that most neonates with such lesions now present via this means rather than with symptoms or signs detected after birth. By way of example, from 1957 to 1975 our unit saw 33 infants with pelvi-ureteric junction obstruction [59]; from 1981 to 1987 we saw 59 cases, all but five diagnosed prenatally.

At the same time, development of isotope renography, with dynamic (DTPA, Hippuran) or static (DMSA) imaging, now enables estimation of differential renal function and, to some extent, distinction between obstructive and non-obstructive dilatation of the upper renal tracts [51,54]. The latter aspect can, if necessary, be further pursued in neonates by virtue of refinements [72] in pressure perfusion studies (Whitaker test) [73]. These techniques demonstrate that renal function does not consistently equate with the degree of dilatation, that dilatation (without reflux) is not necessarily the result of obstruction and that, for a period at any rate, obstruction is often compatible with normal renal function. Such considerations have evident implications for management. The principal remaining difficulty is that there is, as yet, no simple means of determining whether relief of obstruction can improve function and, if so, to what extent.

Prenatal sonography of the urinary tracts

General considerations

Dilatation or cystic changes in the upper renal tracts are readily amenable to detection by sonography.

Apart from routine screening during pregnancy, there are specific indications for prenatal examination of the urinary tracts which include maternal oligohydramnios and a family history of urinary abnormalities, notably infantile polycystic disease. First reports of prenatal disclosure of fetal uropathies appeared in the early 1970s [12,23], but it is only during the past 5 years that technical improvements in ultrasound equipment, and its widespread application to routine scanning during pregnancy, have led to diagnosis in appreciable numbers [5,67,70]. We see some 35 cases annually and the diagnoses over an 8-year period are set out in Table 45.1.

Surveys indicate that sonographically detectable fetal uropathies occur in 1 in 550 [55] to 1 in 950 [63]

Table 45.1 Radiological/sonographic diagnoses in 151 neonates with prenatally diagnosed uropathy: Royal Liverpool Children's Hospital, 1979–87

	Number	(%)	No. with positive physical signs
Pelvi-ureteric obstruction	54	(36)	18
Multicystic kidney	25	(16)	13
Obstructed megaureter	19	(13)	0
Duplex system anomalies	16	(11)	2
Vesico-ureteric reflux	12	(8)	2
Posterior urethral valves	10	(7)	8
Single ectopic ureter	4	(3)	2
Single system ureterocele	2	(1)	0
Renal tumour	1	(0.5)	1
Non-specific dilatation	8	(5)	0
Total	151		46

656

pregnancies. Although abnormalities may be evident by the 15th week of gestation [4] and are quite frequently discovered before the 25th week, usually where there exists some specific indication for examination, the majority of diagnoses are made during the third trimester. Ultrasonic detection of fetal urinary abnormalities is highly reliable, with few false positives [70], and, as equipment becomes more sophisticated and experience greater, an anatomically precise diagnosis will be made in a high proportion of cases. Features of interest include fetal sex, amniotic fluid volume, the recognition of unilateral or bilateral dilatation of the urinary tract, and whether this dilatation involves just the pelvicalyceal system or the ureters also, and whether the bladder is consistently enlarged or, conversely, permanently empty.

Prenatal intervention

Ability to detect fetal obstructive uropathies by sonography naturally suggested the prospect of treating these lesions prenatally. Experience has shown that initial hopes were exaggerated and that the possibilities for prenatal intervention of any description are limited and those for therapeutic intervention rarer still. It is now accepted [47] that unilateral hydronephrosis never warrants intervention nor does bilateral hydronephrosis provided amniotic fluid volume remains normal and there is no evidence of some other life-threatening condition or chromosomal abnormality. Where there is bilateral hydronephrosis, the pregnancy requires close observation to ensure that amniotic fluid volume remains normal.

Animal experimental work confirms the clinical suspicion that whereas later obstruction of the fetal urinary tract results in hydronephrosis [32], earlier obstruction causes dysplasia [6,25]. In addition, severely compromised fetal renal function is always accompanied by some degree of pulmonary hypoplasia. While there is some evidence that the pulmonary pathology is correctible if satisfactory renal function can be restored [31], it is very doubtful whether renal dysplasia is reversible by techniques currently available.

The possibilities of therapeutic intervention for fetuses with severe bilateral obstructive uropathy are therefore limited to those without dysplasia and the prospect of recoverable renal function. The presenting sign of impaired fetal renal function is maternal oligohydramnios and, as a rule, the earlier and more severely this occurs, the graver the prognosis. Sonographically, appearances of a fetal bladder which is permanently empty, or fails to refill after percutaneous aspiration, are not wholly predictable indicators of irreversibly compromised renal function and more reliable are the appearances of the kidneys where high echogenicity is indicative of dysplasia. The most exact prognostic information is obtainable by analysis of urine aspirated percutaneously from the fetal bladder [26]. Fetal urine is normally hypo-osmolar; osmolarity exceeding 225 mOsm/l and sodium and chloride contents greater than 100 mOsm/l and 90 mOsm/l respectively virtually exclude the possibility of useful recoverable renal function.

In such cases, and in those where there is some other life-threatening anomaly or chromosomal abnormality, the only intervention realistically offerable is termination of the pregnancy. Therapeutic intervention is restrictable to the very few cases, usually male fetuses with posterior urethral valves, where thorough assessment suggests the possibility of recoverable renal function. Until recently, efforts have been concentrated upon those where maternal oligohydramnios developed relatively late, beyond the 28th week of gestation, and there the methods employed have been either early induction of labour or insertion of a vesico-amniotic shunt, the choice being determined by estimation of fetal pulmonary maturity. Vesico-amniotic shunts, like other forms of catheter drainage of the bladder, cause problems of their own, including blockage, extrusion and retraction within the bladder. It is debatable as to whether either form of intervention has materially improved prognosis in cases so far reported [31,52,53]. Recent refinements in open fetal surgery offer the prospect of more definitive bladder drainage by vesicostomy and at an earlier stage in pregnancy, as early as the 18th week of gestation [30]. If early promise is fulfilled, there is now the prospect of effective prenatal intervention for a small number of fetuses with severe infravesical obstructive uropathy. Naturally such endeavours are likely to remain concentrated in a few highly specialized centres.

Postnatal investigation

The great majority of these babies are perfectly well when born; less than a third have physical signs related to their urinary anomaly (Table 45.1) and very few spontaneously develop urinary infection early in infancy. Sixty-four per cent of our cases with bilateral disease had positive signs by way of renal or bladder enlargement or both. Urgent investigation is required only when there is evidence of global renal impairment, bladder outlet obstruction or severe bilateral hydronephrosis; in other cases the necessary investigations can be safely deferred for 2–4 weeks.

The investigative regimen depends upon ultrasonic findings postnatally (Figure 45.1). In a few instances, postnatal examination shows absent, or minimal, dilatation of the upper renal tracts and it appears that the fetal urinary tract can dilate transiently [5], usually during the third trimester and

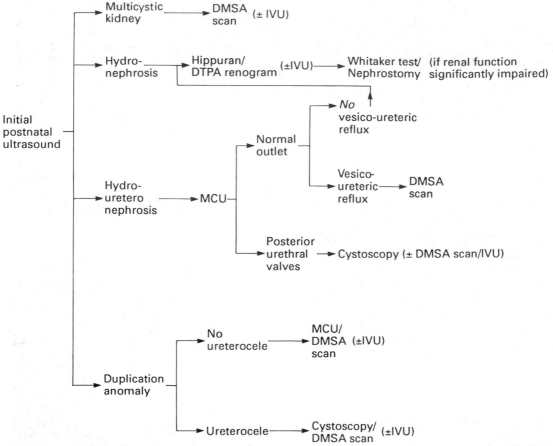

Figure 45.1 Postnatal investigative regimen for neonates with uropathy detected *in utero* [Latterly 99-Tc DTPA and 123-I Hippuran renography have been replaced by 99-Tc mercapto-acetyltriglycine (MAG-3)]

perhaps as a result of the relatively high urine output of the fetus. The usual policy in such cases is to repeat the ultrasound examination at 3 months and, if this is normal, pursue matters no further. This may be insufficient; one patient known to us returned at 3 years of age with pelvi-ureteric junction obstruction and significantly impaired function in the affected kidney.

Postnatal management, general considerations

The inevitable result of prenatal sonography is that many infants are now referred for surgical consideration with lesions which would previously have passed unnoticed for months, years or maybe for life. In the majority, with unilateral disease, it may be supposed that the worst that could have happened, in the event of non-detection, would have been loss of function in the affected kidney. Past clinical experience suggests that this was not a common occurrence. The therapeutic dilemma conjured up

by this diagnostic expertise is that the natural history of most of these abnormalities is largely unknown (posterior urethral valves constituting one of the few exceptions) and there should be reluctance to operate upon a perfectly well baby without confidence of this being beneficial. Pelvi-ureteric junction obstruction, much the commonest anomaly diagnosed by prenatal ultrasound, may be taken as an example of this problem. In the past, when presentation was usually with symptoms clearly requiring intervention on that account alone, it was always assumed, quite reasonably, that the obstruction would never resolve spontaneously and that sooner or later function of the kidney would deteriorate even if it had not already done so. It is now evident that radiological appearances are not a reliable determinant of obstruction and that even in the presence of obstruction, sometimes leading to gross hydronephrosis, renal function may be perfectly preserved. Moreover, initial experience of non-intervention in neonatal cases suggests that

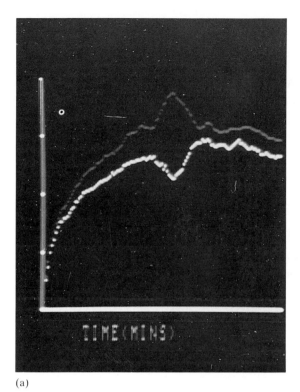

(a)

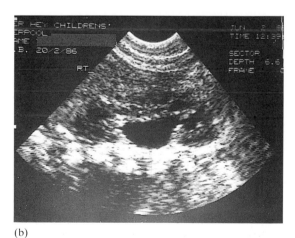

(b)

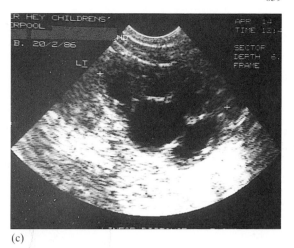

(c)

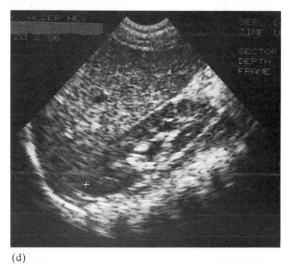

(d)

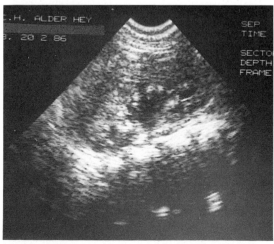

(e)

Figure 45.2 Spontaneous resolution of hydronephrosis in a male infant. Aged 1 month, Hippuran renogram (a) shows bilaterally obstructed curves and sonography marked pelvicalyceal dilatation in the right (b) and left (c) kidneys. Aged 7 months, sonography shows resolution of hydronephrosis in both right (d) and left (e) systems

renal function deteriorates slowly, if at all, that hydronephrosis may lessen in time (Figure 45.2) and that occasionally renographically defined obstruction resolves spontaneously [35,69]. None of the author's cases has developed symptoms.

On present evidence, early therapeutic intervention, as opposed to a closely monitored conservative regimen, would seem to be indicated in three circumstances:

(1) when there is organic bladder outflow obstruction,
(2) in lesions with proven obstruction and impaired function in the affected kidney,
(3) in the presence of vesico-ureteric reflux with useful function in the affected kidney.

Pelvi-ureteric obstruction

The pelvi-ureteric junction is the most common site of urinary obstruction in the newborn, and occurs more often in the male than in the female and more often on the left side than on the right. Both kidneys are involved in up to 30% of cases presenting in infancy [59,77] and in a small minority there is a solitary functioning kidney. Occasionally there is a familial predisposition, with cases found in different generations and in siblings [14].

The cause of the condition remains unknown. Obstruction by an aberrant lower polar vessel is extremely rare in infants. As a rule the pelvi-ureteric junction is non-dependent, with the proximal ureter bound to the lower renal pelvis by flimsy adhesions. Once the ureter has been dissected free, it is usual to find a narrow segment, 2–10 mm in length, immediately below the pelvi-ureteric junction and that urine does not escape from the renal pelvis until an incision is carried proximally above this narrow segment. Various histological changes at the pelvi-ureteric junction are described [27,29] but it remains uncertain as to whether these are primary or secondary. The renal parenchyma, although often markedly thinned, is usually histologically normal. Occasional examples are seen of localized cystic dysplasia.

In neonates it is not uncommon to find mild pelvic hydronephrosis associated with kinks and folds of the upper ureter; these are not obstructive and in time the ureter straightens and the pelvic dilatation resolves. A less common finding is of moderate to severe calyceal dilatation but with mild or minimal enlargement of the renal pelvis; this phenomenon of 'megacalycosis' (Figure 45.3), once thought to result from 'burnt-out' pelvi-ureteric obstruction [40], more probably represents calyceal dysmorphism.

Apart from cases diagnosed prenatally, the usual presenting feature of pelvi-ureteric obstruction in infancy is a smooth renal mass discovered during routine abdominal examination of the baby. In a few

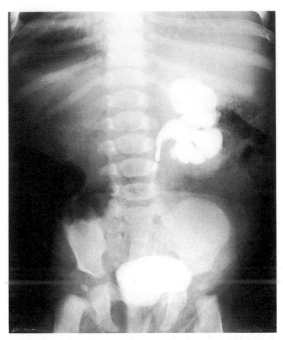

Figure 45.3 Intravenous urogram showing megacalycosis in a female infant. Although there is marked calyceal dilatation, the pelvis is only slightly enlarged and the ureter is well seen. The opposite kidney is non-functioning due to multicystic dysplasia

instances, generally in those with bilateral disease, there is failure to thrive [59,77]. Urinary tract infection is uncommon and should prompt suspicion of coincident vesico-ureteric reflux which is stated to occur ipsilaterally or contralaterally in 40% of cases [48]. Urinary ascites is a rare complication [44.59]. Finally a number of asymptomatic cases are detected on routine urography or ultrasound performed because of other congenital abnormalities.

Diagnosis

Diagnosis can generally be made by ultrasound examination and confirmed by DTPA or Hippuran renography (Figure 45.4). Intravenous urogram (IVU) images are often poor in the neonatal period and this investigation is no longer routinely indicated. In a personal series of neonates with ultrasonic or urographic appearances of pelvi-ureteric junction obstruction, renography indicated obstruction in 24 units, was equivocal in six and non-obstructive in five. While some series report significantly impaired renal function in a high proportion of cases [21,46], in our patients, differential function was greater than 40% in 28, 20–40% in four and less than 20% in three. In the presence of markedly impaired function, pressure perfusion studies (Whitaker test) may be necessary to confirm or exclude obstruction.

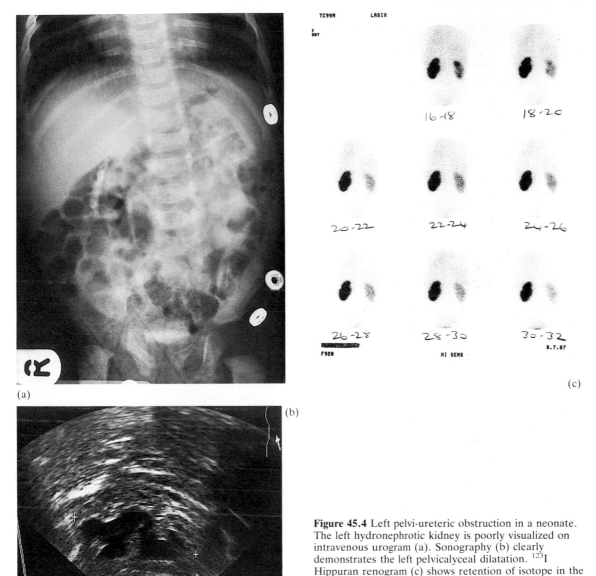

(a)

(b)

(c)

Figure 45.4 Left pelvi-ureteric obstruction in a neonate. The left hydronephrotic kidney is poorly visualized on intravenous urogram (a). Sonography (b) clearly demonstrates the left pelvicalyceal dilatation. ^{123}I Hippuran renogram (c) shows retention of isotope in the left pelvicalyceal system 30 min after injection of isotope and 15 min after injection of frusemide: differential function of left kidney, 35%

Management

Some advocate immediate pyeloplasty for all neonates with pelvi-ureteric obstruction on the grounds that, by decompression of the pelvicalyceal system, renal function is preserved or improved [21,46,60,68]. Apart from the fact that function of these kidneys is usually normal, despite the radiographic appearances, this policy is based upon the misconception that intrapelvic pressure is always raised in this condition. In reality pressure is usually normal or minimally elevated [39,56]. Quite what causes function to deteriorate is not known, although low compliance of the renal pelvis has been suggested as a factor since this would result in a relatively rapid rise in intrapelvic pressure whenever urinary output increased above normal [9].

A more conservative approach to neonatal pyeloplasty is to restrict the procedure to those cases where renal function is diminished [34,57,69]. The author's policy, with unilateral disease, is to operate when differential function lies between 20 and 40%;

where it is less than 20%, a percutaneous nephrostomy is inserted and pyeloplasty performed only if function improves beyond 20% within 1 month. In bilateral cases, policy is similar except that pyeloplasty is performed regardless of whether function is moderately or severely impaired. Although renal function sometimes improves postoperatively, this is not always so despite an anatomically excellent result (Figure 45.5). In cases managed conservatively, ultrasound examination is carried out at 3-monthly intervals and renography repeated at 9 months and 2 years of age. In 25 cases managed conservatively, renal function has so far deteriorated in none. The principal uncertainty with this policy, unlikely to be resolved for many years, lies in knowing how long these cases should be followed and how often and by what means they should be investigated.

Pyeloplasty in the newborn period differs little from that in the older child. The dismembered, Anderson-Hynes [2], pyelo-ureteroplasty is applicable to virtually all anatomical variations and appears to give results superior to other techniques [45]. Because of the small calibre of the ureter, splinting of the anastomosis by a fine (4 FG) polythene tube and pelvic drainage via a nephrostomy or pyelostomy (12 FG Malecot catheter) are always advisable. The splint is removed 10 days postoperatively; the Malecot catheter is clamped

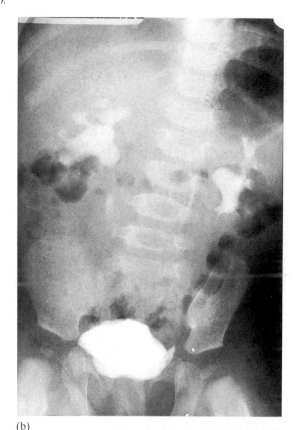

(b)

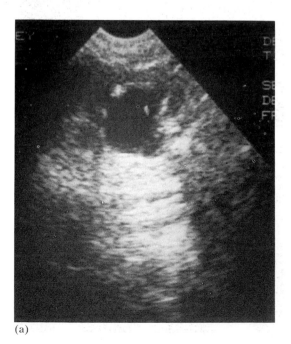

(a)

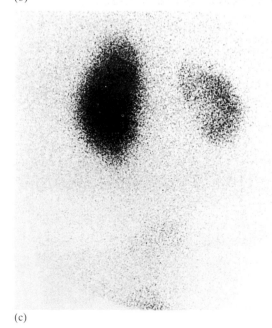

(c)

Figure 45.5 Functional result of pyeloplasty. (a) Sonogram showing right hydronephrosis in a female neonate. The kidney was not visualized on intravenous urography (IVU) and renography showed 18% differential function.

(b) Postoperative IVU showing satisfactory anatomical result of pyeloplasty. (c) DMSA scan 1 year postoperatively: differential function has only improved to 22%

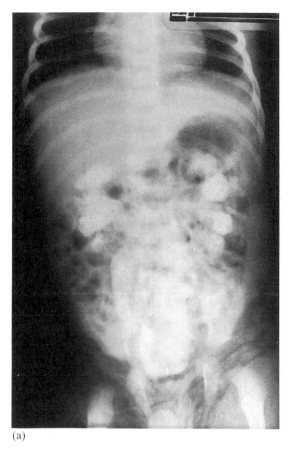

(a)

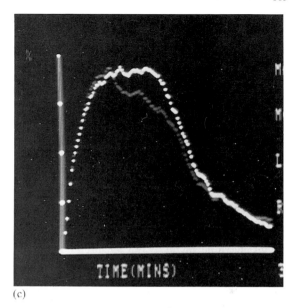

(c)

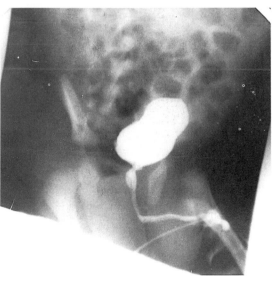

(b)

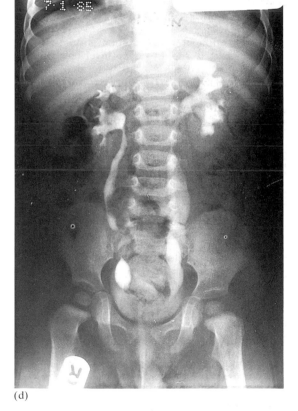

(d)

Figure 45.6 Non-obstructive hydroureteronephrosis. (a) IVU in a male neonate showing marked bilateral hydroureteronephrosis. (b) MCU shows no vesico-ureteric reflux and normal bladder outlet. (c) Hippuran renogram showing bilaterally non-obstructive curves. (d) IVU aged 1 year: spontaneous resolution of hydro-ureteronephrosis

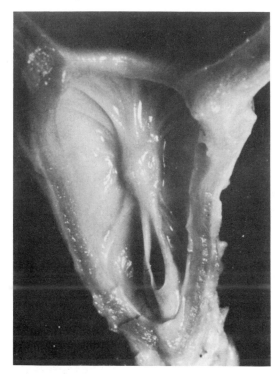

Figure 45.11 Autopsy specimen of Type I posterior urethral valves. The cusps descend from the lower end of the verumontanum and meet in an anterior commisure at a lower level. The bladder neck forms a posterior ridge. Non-obstructive folds ascend from the verumontanum to the bladder neck

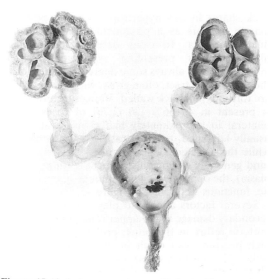

Figure 45.12 Autopsy specimen of infant with posterior urethral valves. Dilatation of posterior urethra and prominent bladder neck. Gross hydro-ureteronephrosis with minimal renal substance on the left. In this case hypertrophy and trabeculation of the bladder wall is less than usually seen

ureterovesical obstruction [74]. Lastly, in conjunction with any of the foregoing, ureteric decompensation may occur, the grossly dilated ureter having ineffective peristalsis or becoming completely acontractile.

Clinical features

Apart from cases detected prenatally, a few infants are noted soon after birth with an enlarged bladder or an abnormal pattern of micturition. More often these features are overlooked and presentation is with azotaemia and acidosis often compounded by the effects of superimposed infection. Vomiting and failure to thrive are common complaints. Acidaemic hyperpnoea may simulate cardiorespiratory disease. Severe infection may cause convulsions, diarrhoea, jaundice or a haemorrhagic diathesis. On examination, the bladder is usually persistently distended; if not obvious on abdominal examination it may be felt as a hard round mass on bimanual examination of the pelvis with a finger in the rectum. Micturition is usually slow and dribbling but some infants can produce a strong, sustained stream so that observation of an apparently normal act of voiding does not exclude the diagnosis.

As discussed in Chapter 44, an unusual complication of urethral valves is urinary ascites [13,28]. The urinary accumulation within the peritoneum may be present at birth or may develop within the first few days of life. Often the entire urinary output collects intraperitoneally with none being passed per urethram. In most cases the urinary leak is from a kidney, either through a parenchymal perforation or from a calyceal fornix, and a perirenal collection forms from which urine diffuses through the intact parietal peritoneum. Occasionally, localized perirenal collections of urine are encountered without urinary ascites (Figure 45.14).

Diagnosis

Prenatally or postnatally the diagnosis may be suspected, in a male, when ultrasound examination shows bilateral hydro-ureteronephrosis associated with an enlarged, thick-walled bladder (Figure 45.15). Occasionally a dilated posterior urethra may be detectable by sonography. Definitive diagnosis is made by micturating cystography, with oblique views, which shows the typical gross dilatation of the posterior urethra, with a rounded lower contour, overlying the undilated anterior urethra (Figure 45.16). The bladder neck is usually prominent, especially posteriorly, but is rarely if ever obstructive in its own right. The bladder itself is typically trabeculated or sacculated and there may be diverticula. An IVU seldom contributes useful information not obtainable by sonography and this investigation

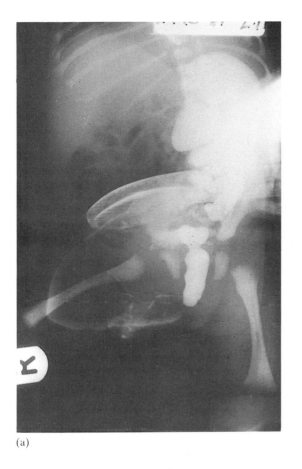

(a)

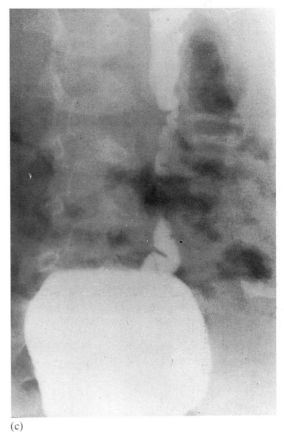

(c)

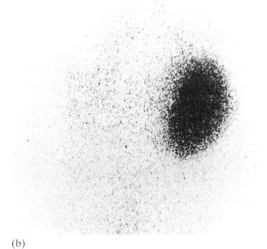

(b)

(d)

Figure 45.13 Posterior urethral valves with unilateral vesico-ureteric reflux. Expression cystogram (a) showing posterior urethral valves, sacculated bladder and gross left reflux. DMSA scan (b) shows non-function of the left kidney. Five years post-valve resection cystography (c) demonstrates persisting left reflux and DMSA scan (d) non-function of the left kidney. The right kidney remains normal

670

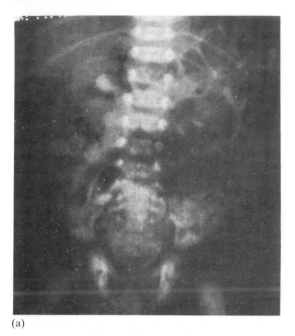

(a)

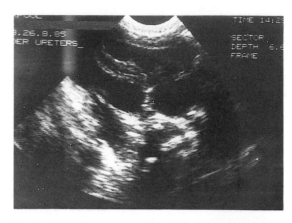

Figure 45.15 Sonogram (transverse section) of male neonate with posterior urethral valves: the thick-walled bladder lies anteriorly and bilaterally dilated ureters are seen posterior to it

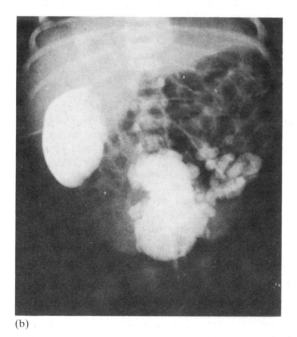

(b)

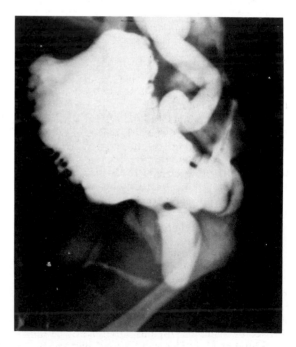

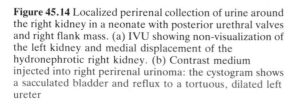

Figure 45.14 Localized perirenal collection of urine around the right kidney in a neonate with posterior urethral valves and right flank mass. (a) IVU showing non-visualization of the left kidney and medial displacement of the hydronephrotic right kidney. (b) Contrast medium injected into right perirenal urinoma: the cystogram shows a sacculated bladder and reflux to a tortuous, dilated left ureter

Figure 45.16 Micturating cysto-urethrogram in an infant with posterior urethral valves. The bladder is sacculated and there is reflux to dilated, tortuous ureters. The bladder neck is prominent and the posterior urethra below it markedly dilated and elongated with a typical round lower margin

is no longer routinely employed. Once the obstruction is relieved and renal function stabilized, DMSA scanning is useful in assessing differential function, especially in cases with vesico-ureteric reflux.

The valves are best observed endoscopically with the tip of the instrument situated approximately 1 cm distal to the verumontanum. With antegrade flow through the proximal urethra obtained by detaching the fluid source and leaving the irrigating channel open, the valve margins are seen to co-apt in the midline.

Management

Any pre-existing dehydration, electrolyte imbalance or septicaemia must first be corrected, so far as possible, by appropriate intravenous fluids and antibiotic treatment. During this period, which need seldom exceed 48 h, the bladder can be temporarily drained by a fine (6-FG to 8-FG) polythene catheter passed per urethram.

In the great majority of cases, the first and only surgical treatment required is ablation of the valves themselves. Open procedures, via the urethral bulb or retropubically, are obsolete, but there remains a role, in countries where modern paediatric endoscopes are unobtainable, for use of an electric auriscope passed via a perineal urethrostomy [22,38]. Under vision, the valve margins are drawn down and ruptured by means of a metal hook passed through the speculum.

In most male infants a 10-FG resectoscope can be passed after gentle meatal dilatation. If there is difficulty negotiating the anterior urethra, the instrument can be introduced via a perineal urethrostomy or, alternatively, an 8-FG cystoscope with an operating channel may be employed. It is unnecessary to attempt complete destruction of the valves when all that is required is their diathermy incision, from margin to base, effected on each side anteriorly at 10 and 2 o'clock using a right-angled diathermy hook. Postoperative catheter drainage is usually unnecessary.

Several non-endoscopic means of valve ablation have been described, including the use of Fogarty balloon catheters [16]. Probably the most satisfactory is the insulated diathermy hook, originally devised by Williams [78] and subsequently modified by Whitaker [75]. This can be used blindly, but is best employed in conjunction with fluoroscopic radiological control. Its principal merit lies in applicability to small, premature, neonates.

As a rule the infant's wellbeing improves appreciably, and often dramatically, following relief of bladder outflow obstruction although the upper tract dilatation itself may take years to resolve (Figure 45.17).

Urinary diversion

Temporary diversion, usually by way of ureterostomies [36], was once commonly employed but rarely now, largely because of improved medical treatment of azotaemic, septicaemic infants. This includes a better appreciation of the large fluid intake these babies require, especially soon after relief of obstruction. The principal remaining indications for temporary urinary diversion are when upper tract obstruction and azotaemia persist despite elimination of bladder outflow obstruction or when there is uncontrollable sepsis. These complications often co-exist. Persisting dilatation usually occurs when a combination of detrusor failure, with residual urine, and detrusor non-compliance results in permanently elevated intravesical pressure (full valve bladder syndrome) [18]. Less often the problem is one of non-contractile ureters or primary ureterovesical junction obstruction due to hypertrophy of the detrusor. Precise distinction between these various disorders may require pressure-perfusion studies of the upper renal tracts (Whitaker test).

Full valve bladder syndrome is best managed with a temporary vesicostomy of the Blocksom [8] type; the apex, rather than the anterior wall, of the bladder should be brought to the surface to avoid problems with prolapse. Vesicostomy is also a useful temporary expedient in situations where endoscopic ablation of the valves is not possible because of lack of equipment or expertise.

Ureteric atony or primary ureterovesical obstruction can be managed by temporary ureterostomy. Total diversion, with loop or terminal ureterostomies, occasionally leads to a fibrotic, contracted bladder [50] and for this reason ureterostomy-in-continuity, using the Sober [64] or ring [79] techniques (Figure 45.18), is preferable. Ureterostomies should be fashioned high in the flank so the kidney drainage will be as direct as possible and so that the maximum length of ureter remains distally should ureteric remodelling or re-implantation be required. Ureterostomy drainage must be maintained until the child is well and thriving and antegrade studies show satisfactory ureteric peristalsis with free drainage into the bladder and absence of reflux. When these circumstances exist, the ureterostomies can be closed, one side at a time. If the ureterovesical junction remains obstructed, or if reflux persists, remodelling and re-implantation of the ureter into the bladder are needed first.

Occasionally an infant presenting with severe electrolyte imbalance and septicaemia does not respond satisfactorily to the usual resuscitative measures, including catheter drainage of the bladder, and a better response may be obtained by percutaneous insertion of pig-tailed nephrostomy drainage tubes.

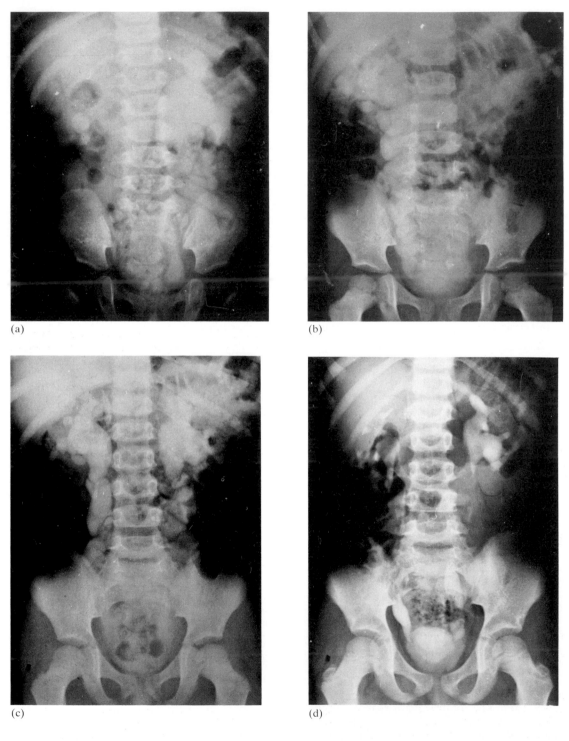

(a)

(b)

(c)

(d)

Figure 45.17 Intravenous urograms in a boy with posterior urethral valves showing slow improvement of the upper tracts following endoscopic ablation of the valves. (a) Aged 3 months – bilateral hydro-ureteronephrosis with marked ureteral tortuosity. (b) Aged 3 years. Right ureter still shows dilatation and tortuosity. (c) Aged 5½ years. Improvement of hydronephrosis although still with considerable ureteric dilatation. (d) Aged 7 years. Further lessening of hydronephrosis. Ureters less dilated and tortuosities have disappeared

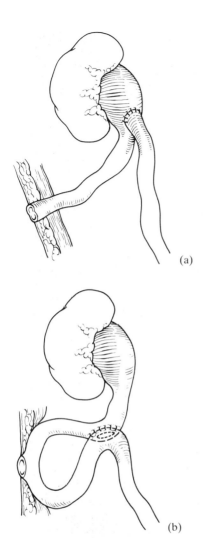

(a)

(b)

Figure 45.18 Ureterostomy-in-continuity. (a) Sober technique. (b) Ring technique

Vesico-ureteric reflux

Vesico-ureteric reflux secondary to posterior urethral valves, if associated with renal dysplasia, usually persists after valve ablation [36,42]. Conversely, reflux to a functioning kidney usually resolves after outlet obstruction is relieved (Figure 45.19). In the interim, antibiotic prophylaxis is administered; ureteric re-implantation during infancy is necessary only in the event of breakthrough infection. Where there is unilateral reflux to a non-functioning kidney, early nephro-ureterectomy is advisable.

Urinary ascites

Urinary ascites was formerly considered to carry a grave prognosis with a mortality approaching 50%. It is now appreciated that the very existence of this condition indicates that there is satisfactory function in at least one kidney [1,29,44].

Paracentesis is required if the abdominal distension is so great as to cause respiratory distress. Many cases can be managed by a period of bladder drainage via a urethral catheter, but if this does not result in resolution of the ascites within a few hours, nephrostomy tubes should be inserted, preferably percutaneously.

Prognosis

The long-term prognosis for infants with urethral valves depends principally upon the severity of permanent damage suffered by the renal parenchyma before diagnosis, which in most cases is largely the damage done before birth. Although there are certain generally adverse features, such as maternal oligohydramnios or severe bilateral vesico-ureteric reflux, in any individual patient the degree of permanent damage cannot be ascertained with any precision at presentation and there is therefore little option but to treat all cases vigorously on the presumption of there being useful recoverable renal function.

Because of the various medical and surgical advances in the treatment of posterior urethral valyes, mortality for those presenting under the age of 3 months has improved from almost 50% reported 15 years ago by us [41] and others [78] to under 10% in recent reports [10,61]. Inevitably this involves survival of a proportion of infants with inherently poor renal function who will sooner or later drift into renal failure. As a rule, this event is likely if serum creatinine levels remain above 80 mmol/l by 1 year of age [66,71].

Fungus ball urinary obstruction

Obstruction of the pelvicalyceal system by *Candida albicans* fungus balls has become a consequence of neonatal intensive care. This condition is almost invariably associated with use of a combination of antibiotic therapy and intravenous lines and the great majority of cases are low-weight, premature infants [3]. Often both kidneys are affected. Presentation is with a loin mass and in bilateral cases there is oliguria or anuria. *Candida albicans* can be cultured from the blood and, if obtainable, from the urine. Sonography of the kidneys shows typical appearances.

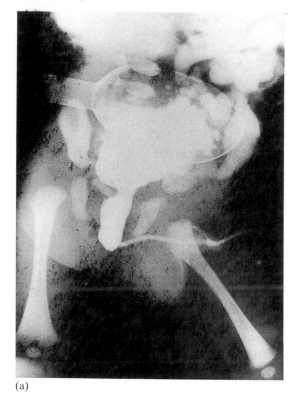

(a)

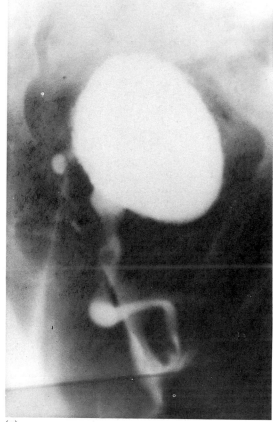

(c)

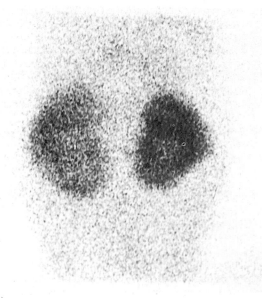

(b)

Figure 45.19 Posterior urethral valves with bilateral vesico-ureteric reflux. Cystogram (a) shows urethral valves with gross bilateral reflux and sacculated bladder: satisfactory uptake of isotope in both kidneys on DMSA scan (b). One year post-valve resection, cystography (c) shows resolution of reflux and bladder sacculation: DMSA scan was unchanged

By the time the condition is diagnosed, systemic antifungal agents are rarely effective and it is necessary to place nephrostomy drainage tubes. Percutaneous systems are usually too fine to secure effective drainage and it is advisable to perform an open procedure, leaving 12–14 FG Malecot catheters *in situ* [58]. These can be irrigated with antifungal agents.

References

1. Adzick, N.S., Harrison, M.R., Flake, A.W. and De Lorimier, A.A. (1985) Urinary extravasation in the fetus with obstructive uropathy. *J. Pediat. Surg.*, **20**, 608–615
2. Anderson, J.C. (1963) *Hydronephrosis*, Charles C. Thomas, Springfield, IL
3. Aragona, F., Glazel, G.P., Pavanello, L., Perale, R., Rizzoni, G. and Pagano, F. (1985) Upper urinary tract obstruction in children caused by *Candida* fungus balls. *Eur. Urol.*, **11**, 188–191
4. Avni, E.F. (1985) Echographie et diagnostic antenatal. In *Urologie Pediatric* (eds J. Cendron and C.C. Schulman), Flammarion Medicine – Sciences, Paris

5. Avni, E.F., Rodesch, F. and Schulman, C.C. (1985) Fetal uropathies: diagnostic pitfalls and management. *J. Urol.*, **134**, 921–925

6. Beck, A.D. (1971) The effect of intra-uterine urinary obstruction upon the development of the fetal kidney. *J. Urol.*, **105**, 784–789

7. Belman, A.B., Filmer, R.B. and King, L.R. (1974) Surgical management of duplication of the collecting system. *J. Urol.*, **112**, 316–321

8. Blocksom, B. (1957) Bladder pouch for prolonged tubeless cystostomy. *J. Urol.*, **78**, 398–401

9. Bullock, K.N. and Whitaker, R.H. (1984) Does good upper tract compliance preserve renal function? *J. Urol.*, **131**, 914–916

10. Burbige, K.A. and Hensle, T.W. (1987) Posterior urethral valves in the newborn. *J. Pediat. Surg.*, **22**, 165–167

11. Caldamone, A.A., Snyder, H.M. and Duckett, J.W. (1984) Ureteroceles in children: follow-up of management with upper tract approach. *J. Urol.*, **131**, 1130–1132

12. Campbell, S. (1973) The antenatal detection of fetal abnormality by ultrasound. In *Birth Defects Proceedings*, IVth International Conference, Vienna

13. Cendron, J. and Lepinard, V. (1972) Maladie du col vésical chez l'enfant. *Urol. Int.*, **27**, 355–360

14. Cohen, B., Goldman, S.M., Kopilnick, M., Khurana, A.V. and Salik, J.O. (1978) Ureteropelvic junction obstruction in three members of a single family. *J. Urol.*, **120**, 361–364

15. Cohen, S.J. (1975) Ureterozystoneostome: Eine neue antirefluxtechnik. *Aktuel. Urol.*, **6**, 1

16. Diamond, D.A. and Ransley, P.G. (1987) Fogarty balloon catheter ablation of neonatal posterior urethral valves. *J. Urol.*, **137**, 1209–1211

17. Drake, D.P., Stevens, P.S. and Eckstein, H.B. (1978) Hydronephrosis secondary to ureteropelvic junction obstruction in children: a review of 14 years experience. *J. Urol.*, **119**, 649–651

18. Duckett, J.W. and Snow, B.W. (1986) Disorders of the urethra and penis. In *Campbells Urology*, 5th Edition (ed. P.C. Walsh, R.F. Gittes, A.D. Perlmutter and T.A. Stamey), W.B. Saunders, Philadelphia

19. Farkas, H. and Skinner, D.G. (1976) Posterior urethral valves in siblings. *Br. J. Urol.*, **48**, 76

20. Field, P.L. and Stephens, F.B. (1974) Congenital urethral membranes causing urethral obstruction. *J. Urol.*, **111**, 250–255

21. Flake, A.W., Harrison, M.R., Sauer, L., Adzick, N.S. and Delorimier, A.A. (1986) Ureteropelvic junction obstruction in the fetus. *J. Pediat. Surg.*, **21**, 1058–1063

22. Garg, S.K. and Lawrie, J.H. (1983) The perineal urethrotomy approach to posterior urethral valves. *J. Urol.*, **130**, 1146–1149

23. Garrett, W.J., Gurnwald, G. and Robinson, D.E. (1970) Prenatal diagnosis of fetal polycystic disease by ultrasound. *Aust. N.Z. J. Obstet. Gynaecol.*, **10**, 7–9

24. Gearhart, J.P. and Woolfenden, K.A. (1982) The vesicopsoas hitch as an adjunct to megaureter repair in childhood. *J. Urol.*, **127**, 505–507

25. Glick, P.L., Harrison, M.R., Noall, R.A. and Villa, R.L. (1983) Correction of congenital hydronephrosis in utero. III. Early mid-trimester ureteral obstruction produces renal dysplasia. *J. Pediat. Surg.*, **18**, 681–687

26. Glick, P.L., Harrison, M.R., Golbus, M.S., Adzick, N.S., Filly, R.A., Callen, R.W. *et al.* (1985) Management of the fetus with congenital hydronephrosis. II: Prognostic criteria and selection for treatment. *J. Pediat. Surg.*, **20**, 376–387

27. Gosling, J.A. and Dixon, J.S. (1978) Functional obstruction of the ureter and renal pelvis. A histological and electron microscopic study. *Br. J. Urol.*, **50**, 145–152

28. Greenfield, S.P., Hensle, T.W., Berdon, W.E. and Geringer, A.M. (1982) Urinary extravasation in the newborn male with posterior urethral valves. *J. Pediat. Surg.*, **17**, 751–756

29. Hanna, M.K., Jeffs, R.D., Sturgess, J.M. and Barkin, M. (1976) Ureteral structure and ultrastructure. Part II. Congenital ureteropelvic and primary obstructive megaureter. *J. Urol.*, **116**, 725–730

30. Harrison, M.R. (1988) Personal communication

31. Harrison, M.R., Golbus, M.S., Filly, R.A., Callen, P.W., Katz, M., DeLorimier, A.A. *et al.* (1982) Fetal surgery for congenital hydronephrosis. *New Engl. J. Med.*, **306**, 591–593

32. Harrison, M.R., Ross, N., Noall, R.A. and DeLorimier, A.A. (1983) Correction of congenital hydronephrosis in utero. I. The model: fetal urethral obstruction produces hydronephrosis and pulmonary hypoplasia in fetal lambs. *J. Pediat. Surg.*, **18**, 247–256

33. Hellstrom, W.J.G., Kogan, B.A., Jeffrey, R.B. and McAninch, J.W. (1984) The natural history of prenatal hydronephrosis with normal amounts of amniotic fluid. *J. Urol.*, **132**, 947–950

34. Hendren, W.H. (1968) Ureteral reimplantation in children. *J. Pediat. Surg.*, **3**, 649–664

35. Homsy, Y.L., Williot, P. and Danais, S. (1986) Transient neonatal hydronephrosis: fact or fantasy? *J. Urol.*, **136**, 339–341

36. Hoover, D.L. and Duckett, J.W. (1982) Posterior urethral valves, unilateral reflux and renal dysplasia. *J. Urol.*, **128**, 994–997

37. Johnston, J.H. (1963) Temporary cutaneous ureterostomy in the treatment of advanced congenital urinary obstruction. *Arch. Dis. Child.*, **38**, 161–166

38. Johnston, J.H. (1966) Posterior urethral valves: operative technique using an electric auriscope. *J. Pediat. Surg.*, **1**, 583–584

39. Johnston, J.H. (1969) The pathogenesis of hydronephrosis in children. *Br. J. Urol.*, **47**, 724–734

40. Johnston, J.H. (1973) Megacalycosis; a burnt-out obstruction? *J. Urol.*, **110**, 344–346

41. Johnston, J.H. (1978) Urinary tract obstruction. In *Neonatal Surgery*, 2nd Edition (ed. P.P. Rickham, J. Lister and I.M. Irving), Butterworths, London

42. Johnston, J.H. (1979) Vesicoureteric reflux with urethral valves. *Br. J. Urol.*, **51**, 100–104
43. Kalicinski, Z.H., Kansy, J., Kotarbinska, B. and Joszt, W. (1977) Surgery of megaureters – modification of Hendren's operation. *J. Pediat. Surg.*, **12**, 183–188
44. Kay, R., Brereton, R.J. and Johnston, J.H. (1980) Urinary ascites in the newborn. *Br. J. Urol.*, **52**, 451–454
45. Kelalis, P.P., Culp, O.S., Stickler, G.B. and Burke, E.C. (1971) Ureteropelvic obstruction: experience with 109 cases. *J. Urol.*, **106**, 418–422
46. King, L.R., Coughlin, P.W.F., Bloch, E.C., Bowie, J.D., Ansong, K. and Hanna, M.K. (1984) The case for immediate pyeloplasty in the neonate with ureteropelvic obstruction. *J. Urol.*, **132**, 725–728
47. Kramer, S.A. (1983) Current status of fetal intervention for congenital hydronephrosis. *J. Urol.*, **130**, 641–646
48. Lebowitz, R.L. and Blickman, J.G. (1983) The coexistence of ureteropelvic obstruction and reflux. *Am. J. Roent.*, **140**, 231–238
49. Livne, P.M., Delaune, J. and Gonzales, E.T. (1983) Genetic etiology of posterior urethral valves. *J. Urol.*, **130**, 781–784
50. Lome, L.G., Howat, J.M. and Williams, D.I. (1972) The temporarily defunctioned bladder in children. *J. Urol.*, **107**, 469–472
51. Lupton, E.W., Richards, D., Testa, H.J., Gilpin, J.A., Gosling, J.A. and Barnard, R.J. (1985) A comparison of diuresis renography, the Whitaker test and renal pelvic morphology in idiopathic hydronephrosis. *Br. J. Urol.*, **57**, 119–123
52. McFayden, I.R. (1984) Obstruction of the fetal urinary tract: a role for surgical intervention in utero? *Br. Med. J.*, **288**, 459–462
53. Manning, F.A., Harman, C.R., Lange, I.R., Brown, R., Decter, A. and MacDonald, N. (1983) Antepartum chronic fetal vesicoamniotic shunts for obstructive uropathy: a report of two cases. *Am. J. Obstet. Gynecol.*, **145**, 819–822
54. O'Reilly, P.H., Lawson, R.S., Shields, R.A. and Testa, H.J. (1979) Idiopathic hydronephrosis – the diuresis renogram: a new non-invasive method of assessing equivocal pelviureteric obstruction. *J. Urol.*, **121**, 153–155
55. Persson, P.H. and Kullander, S. (1983) Long-term experience of general ultrasound screening in pregnancy. *Am. J. Obstet. Gynecol.*, **146**, 942–947
56. Poulsen, E.U., Frokjaer, J., Taagehoj-Jensen, F., Jorgensen, T.M., Norgaard, J.P., Hedegard, M. *et al.* (1987) Diuresis renography and simultaneous renal pelvic pressure in hydronephrosis. *J.Urol.*, **138**, 272–275
57. Ransley, P.G. and Manzoni, G. (1985) Extended role of DTPA scan in assessing function and PUJ obstruction in neonates. *Dial. Ped. Urol.*, **8**, 6
58. Robinson, P.J., Pocock, R.D. and Franks, J.D. (1987) The management of obstructive renal candidiasis in the neonate. *Br. J. Urol.*, **59**, 380–382
59. Robson, W.J., Rudy, S.M. and Johnston, J.H. (1976) Pelviureteric obstruction in infancy. *J. Pediat. Surg.*, **11**, 57–61
60. Roth, D.R. and Gonzales, E.T. (1983) Management of ureteropelvic junction obstruction in infants. *J. Urol.*, **129**, 108–110
61. Scott, J.E.S. (1985) Management of congenital posterior urethral valves. *Br. J. Urol.*, **57**, 71–77
62. Scott, J.E.S. (1987) Fetal ureteric reflux. *Br. J. Urol.*, **59**, 291–296
63. Smith, D., Egginton, J.A. and Brookfield, D.S.K. (1987) Detection of abnormality of fetal urinary tract as a predictor of renal tract disease. *Br. Med. J.*, **294**, 27–28
64. Sober, I. (1972) Pelvio-ureterostomy-en-Y. *J. Urol.*, **107**, 473–475
65. Stephens, F.D. (1963) *Congenital Malformations of the Rectum, Anus and Genito-urinary Tract*, E. and S. Livingstone, Edinburgh
66. Tejani, A., Butt, K., Glassberg, K., Price, A. and Gurumurthy, K. (1986) Prediction of eventual end-stage renal disease in children with posterior urethral valves. *J. Urol.*, **136**, 857–860
67. Thomas, D.F.M., Irving, H.C. and Arthur, R.J. (1985) Prenatal diagnosis: how useful is it? *Br. J. Urol.*, **57**, 784–787
68. Thon, W., Schlickenrieder, J.H.M., Thon, A. and Altwein, J.E. (1987) Management and early reconstruction of urinary tract abnormalities detected *in utero*. *Br. J. Urol.*, **59**, 214–215
69. Thorup, J., Mortensen, T., Diemer, H., Johnsen, A. and Neilsen, O.H. (1985) The prognosis of surgically treated congenital hydronephrosis after diagnosis in utero. *J. Urol.*, **134**, 914–917
70. Turnock, R.R. and Shawis, R. (1984) Management of fetal urinary tract anomalies detected by prenatal sonography. *Arch. Dis. Child.*, **59**, 962–965
71. Warshaw, B.L., Hymes, L.C., Trulock, T.S. and Woodard, J.R. (1983) Prognostic features in infants with obstructive uropathy due to posterior urethral valves. *J. Urol.*, **133**, 240–243
72. Wentzell, P.G., Arnold, A.J., Carty, H. and Rickwood, A.M.K. (1988) Two needle modification of the Whitaker test. *Br. J. Urol.*, **62**, 388–389
73. Whitaker, R.H. (1973) Methods of assessing obstruction in dilated ureters. *Br. J. Urol.*, **45**, 15–22
74. Whitaker, R.H. (1973) The ureter in posterior urethral valves. *Br. J. Urol.*, **45**, 395–403
75. Whitaker, R.H. and Sherwood, T. (1986) An improved hook for destroying posterior urethral valves. *J. Urol.*, **135**, 531–532
76. Williams, D.I. (1977) Urethral valves: a hundred cases with hydronephrosis. In *Urinary System Malformations in Children* (eds D. Bergsma and J.W. Duckett), Alan R. Liss, New York
77. Williams, D.I. and Karlaftis, C.M. (1966) Hydronephrosis due to pelvi-ureteric obstruction in the newborn. *Br. J. Urol.*, **38**, 138–144
78. Williams, D.I., Whitaker, R.H., Barratt, T.M. and

Keeton, J.C. (1973) Urethral valves. *Br. J. Urol.*, **45**, 200–210

79. Williams, D.I. and Cromie, W.J. (1976) Ring ureterostomy. *Br. J. Urol.*, **47**, 789–792

80. Young, H.H., Frontz, W.A. and Baldwin, J.C. (1919) Congenital obstruction of the posterior urethra. *J. Urol.*, **3**, 289–354

46

Vascular lesions of the adrenal and kidney

A. M. K. Rickwood

Massive adrenal haemorrhage

Localized intraglandular adrenal haemorrhage may occur in infants and children in response to stress reactions of various types; such haemorrhages are relatively common, being found in 1–2% of infant autopsies [7,14]; evidence of previous haemorrhage may later become apparent when adrenal calcification is seen on radiography.

Massive adrenal haemorrhage, a condition confined to the neonatal period, is much rarer, being found in only 0.05% of autopsies in the newborn [35], at which time the glands are large and vascular. At birth their average combined weight is 6.5 g falling to 3.5 g by the age of 3 weeks [19]. Haemorrhage takes place into and around the gland and a large haematoma forms within the perinephric fascia.

Rarely, perforation of the fascia and of the peritoneum leads to intraperitoneal bleeding [34]. Occasionally, haemorrhage is associated with renal vein thrombosis; the coincidence may be the result of an anastamosis between the two venous systems or may be due to both organs being affected by the same pathogenic factors. Haemorrhage may also be related to adrenal neuroblastoma (see Chapter 13).

Aetiology

Massive adrenal haemorrhage tends to be found either in large infants following a difficult and traumatic birth or, nowadays, more often in premature babies who have suffered perinatal hypoxia. Thrombocytopenia due to septicaemia may be a factor in some cases and so also may be haemorrhagic states such as hypofibrinogenaemia due to disseminated thromboembolism [9].

The condition has occurred prenatally with the haematoma being present at birth [34]. The right adrenal is affected more often than the left, possibly because the right adrenal vein opens directly into the vena cava so that the gland is more exposed to the effects of raised intravenous pressures such as may occur during birth compression or as a result of asphyxia; in a series of 25 cases [15], the right side was involved in 18, the left in five and both in two.

Clinical features

The infant shows increasing pallor and hypotension, and collapse may result from blood loss. A firm mass is palpable in one or both flanks. Macroscopic haematuria occurs only if there is associated renal vein thrombosis, but proteinuria and microscopic haematuria may be present in the absence of overt renal involvement. Jaundice may occur later due to breakdown of blood products. Rarely there is azotaemia resulting from hypovolaemia and hypotension.

Diagnosis

The haemorrhagic area is readily demonstrable by sonography (Figure 46.1) [18,27]. Haemorrhage into a congenital adrenal neuroblastoma may produce identical sonographic appearances; the two conditions are readily distinguishable if urinary excretion of catecholamines is raised but on some occasions catecholamine levels in the presence of neuroblastoma may fall temporarily as a consequence of the tumour necrosis causing the haemorrhage. In practice, distinction between the two conditions is not of immediate importance. Aortography in cases of haematoma shows smooth,

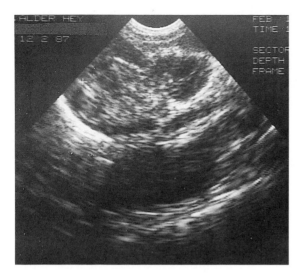

Figure 46.1 Sonogram showing massive adrenal haemorrhage in a neonate. The haemorrhagic mass, marked with crosses, is seen above the right kidney

curved, spreading of the adrenal arteries without the abnormal vasculature associated with a neoplasm [21]. Blood culture is advisable if there is suspicion of septicaemia.

Treatment

Although mortality was formerly high [15], most cases can be handled successfully by a conservative regimen. The immediate need is for blood transfusion to correct hypovolaemia. Where there is involvement of both adrenals, demonstrable by sonography, hydrocortisone sodium succinate is indicated in a dosage of 25 mg 6-hourly intravenously. Antibiotic therapy is needed if septicaemia is suspected. When the haematoma is restricted by the perinephric fascia, the bleeding is self-limiting and operative intervention is usually unnecessary. Surgical evacuation of the blood clot may be advisable in premature babies when absorption of blood pigments from the disintegrating haematoma leads to dangerously elevated levels of serum bilirubin. Adrenalectomy is necessary on the rare occasion when there is extensive retroperitoneal or intraperitoneal haemorrhage.

With a non-operative regimen, an adrenal haematoma usually shrinks rapidly. Calcification may be seen radiologically as early as the fifth day but more often develops over a few weeks. Initially the periphery of the haematoma calcifies so that the opacity is ring-shaped. Later, as the haematoma shrinks, the calcification corresponds approximately to the size and shape of the normal gland (Figure 46.2) [7]. Rarely, a liquefying haematoma persists

as a cystic mass which may become infected [10]. Once the acute episode is controlled, intravenous urography or DMSA scan is indicated to determine whether or not the kidney has been affected by a vascular lesion. Late sequelae are few. Even with bilateral haematomas, there is usually no obvious adrenocortical insufficiency although hypoglycaemia may cause symptoms in some cases.

Renal venous thrombosis

Thrombosis of the renal venous system leading to haemorrhagic infarction of the kidney was first described by Rayer in 1837 [32]. In the paediatric age group, some 60% of cases occur within the first month of life [23] and 40% within the first 2 weeks [41]. Both kidneys are affected with equal frequency and occasionally both are involved. The condition has become much less common in recent years, probably as a result of improved management of fluid loss and septicaemia in infants. It is more prevalent in premature babies and in those born to diabetic mothers [5], when two or more siblings may be affected [39].

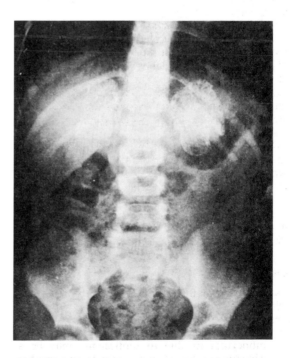

Figure 46.2 Abdominal radiograph showing extensive bilateral adrenal calcification in a 6-year-old boy who had bilateral adrenal haematomas in the neonatal period. There was no clinical evidence of adrenal insufficiency

Pathology

A totally infarcted kidney is enlarged to about three times normal size, is haemorrhagic, necrotic and disintegrating. In less advanced but diffusely affected cases, the medullary pyramids are more severely affected than the cortex (Figure 46.3). Histological studies [22] show that the initial thrombosis usually starts in the intrarenal veins and progresses centrally. The intrarenal thrombosis may involve only a segment of the kidney even when spread to the main vein has occurred. The thrombus may extend in continuity into the inferior vena cava but even in this circumstance, spread to involve the opposite renal vein is most unusual [6,25]. Most bilaterally affected cases result from separate thrombosis arising in each kidney.

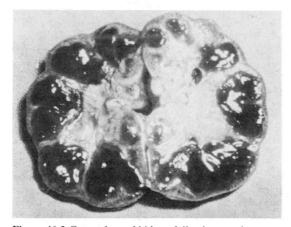

Figure 46.3 Cut surface of kidney following renal venous thrombosis. The haemorrhagic infarction affects the medullary pyramids more severely than the cortex

Haemorrhagic infarction of the kidney may co-exist with similar changes in the adrenal leading to intraglandular and periglandular haemorrhage. The association may be a consequence of venous anastomosis or, since the adrenal opposite to the kidney is sometimes affected, it may be due to the adrenal and the kidney being influenced by the same pathogenic process.

Aetiology

The low arterial pressure in the neonate is reflected in a correspondingly low venous pressure and the effects of this in the kidney are compounded by virtue of its double capillary network. This sluggish perfusion, combined with relative polycythaemia, renders the neonate particularly susceptible to renal vein thrombosis [5,25]. Occasionally this occurs spontaneously in a previously well baby but more often is precipitated by dehydration resulting from

infection or from gastrointestinal disturbance. Infants born to diabetic mothers are susceptible for the same reason. Other aetiological factors are traumatic delivery and neonatal hypoxia. Not uncommonly, thrombosis occurs elsewhere in addition, and the dural sinuses, pulmonary veins and digital vessels may be affected. Although thrombocytopenia is usually present due to trapping of platelets within the thrombotic kidney, this rarely causes haemorrhagic problems elsewhere.

Rarely, haemorrhagic infarction of the neonatal kidney may occur without venous thrombosis; the condition is mainly found in association with acute infections or anoxia [26].

Clinical features and diagnosis

Presentation is characteristically with gross haematuria and a palpable flank mass. The infant is pale and limp and there may be signs of dehydration. Swelling and cyanosis of the legs are indicative of thrombus within the inferior vena cava but such a thrombus may be present without these signs. Bilateral renal involvement is suggested by the presence of swellings in both loins, anuria or extreme oliguria and azotaemia. Elevation of blood urea is not necessarily due to bilateral involvement; it is often found in unilateral cases due to pre-existing dehydration or hypotensive depression of function in the unaffected kidney. Intravenous urography and isotope renography usually show non-function of the affected kidney. Sonography shows characteristic appearances (Figure 46.4) and may also demonstrate thrombus within the inferior vena cava.

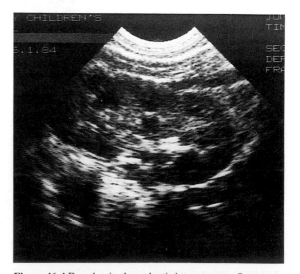

Figure 46.4 Renal vein thrombosis in a neonate. Sonogram shows diffuse enlargement of the kidney with increased echogenicity of the renal parenchyma. The 'bright' areas represent regions of haemorrhagic infarction

Treatment

The great majority of cases can be satisfactorily managed by a conservative regimen. Immediate treatment consists in correction of dehydration, metabolic acidosis and anaemia by appropriate intravenous fluids and by blood transfusion. It is customary to administer antibiotic prophylaxis even in cases where there is no demonstrable septicaemia. Severe azotaemia may occur in unilateral cases and renal enlargement may be due to a localized segmental lesion or may be simulated by an adrenal haematoma. Anuria, or severe oliguria, do not necessarily imply an irrecoverable lesion, and treatment should not be withheld. Peritoneal dialysis may occasionally be required to control the effects of acute renal failure. With a non-operative regimen, haematuria usually stops within a few days and the renal swelling diminishes in size.

Although conservative management may be successful in bilateral cases, the majority of the few reported survivals have resulted from a surgical approach [40]. If caval venography demonstrates a thrombus, thrombectomy via a transperitoneal approach is employed. Both kidneys are left *in situ* regardless of whether satisfactory bleeding is obtained from the renal veins following thrombectomy.

Sequelae

Once the acute episode has been overcome, a DMSA scan may be undertaken to assess residual renal function. Hypertension resulting from severe or total infarction of the kidney is common [29,37] and may necessitate nephrectomy. Although renal vein thrombosis is known to be associated with membranous nephropathy and the nephrotic syndrome, these are rarely sequelae of classic neonatal renal venous thrombosis.

Medullary necrosis

In infancy, renal medullary necrosis may follow such conditions as perinatal asphyxia, gastroenteritis, septicaemia and perinatal exsanguination. The common aetiological factor is prolonged hypotension leading to renal ischaemia. As a rule, both kidneys are affected but the condition is occasionally unilateral [20]. Clinically there is a short oliguric phase of 2–3 days but this may be submerged within the features of the antecedent illness. Polyuria, with profuse urinary loss of sodium, follows. Albuminuria is slight or absent. Serum levels of urea and creatinine are persistently but mildly elevated.

Intravenous urography shortly after the onset shows bilateral renal enlargement. The calyces contain contrast but the nephrogram is prolonged

and there is heavy opacification of the medullary pyramids (Figure 46.5). It is thought that the last feature results from leakage of contrast from the damaged nephrons into the interstitial tissues of the kidney. Following the acute episode, urography may show atrophy of the papillae and calyceal clubbing. Alternatively, there may be intrapapillary cavitation

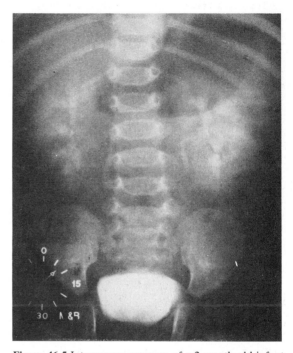

Figure 46.5 Intravenous urogram of a 2-month-old infant with renal medullary necrosis, showing bilateral renal enlargement and opacification of the medullary pyramids

where the calyx retains its normal cup but pools of contrast lie within the medulla. Failure of normal kidney growth may become evident [12]. The late pyelographic appearances may resemble those of chronic pyelonephritis or renal dysplasia [28] and if the correct diagnosis has not been made during the acute phase, these appearances may mistakenly be attributed to infection.

Cortical necrosis

Bilateral cortical necrosis occurs under conditions similar to those predisposing to medullary necrosis [8]: severe oliguria or anuria occurs. Albuminuria and haematuria are inconstant features and the kidneys are not enlarged. Treatment is that of acute renal failure. Survival is possible if the necrosis has only a patchy distribution. Calcification within the cortex of poorly functioning kidneys is characteristically seen within a few weeks (Figure 46.6) [24]. Hypertension may be a late complication.

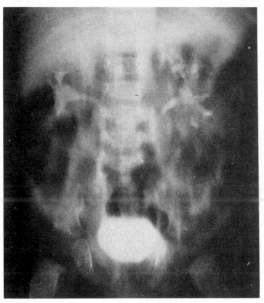

Figure 46.6 Intravenous urogram of a 2½-month-old infant recovering from renal cortical necrosis. The left kidney shows parenchymal calcification (courtesy of Professor R. Hendrickse)

Comment

It is evident that renal venous thrombosis, medullary necrosis and cortical necrosis may follow apparently identical antecedent diseases and on occasion there is clinicopathological overlap between them. The nature of the renal lesion which develops, or which predominates, probably depends upon differences in the degrees of intravascular coagulopathy and of arterial constriction in different patients. Renal ischaemic or haemorrhagic necrosis has occurred following angiography, indicating the potential hazard that intravenous contrast media, especially in large doses, may aggravate a preexisting hyperosmolar state in dehydrated or hypoxic infants and induce renal complications [17].

Renovascular hypertension in infancy

Arterial hypertension during infancy is increasingly recognized as a result of improved techniques of measurement and monitoring. In the full-term neonate hypertension may be defined as a systolic

pressure exceeding 90 mmHg and a diastolic pressure above 60 mmHg; in the premature neonate, the corresponding figures are 80 and 45 mmHg respectively. Hypertension usually presents in neonates with convulsions or with cardiac failure. Isotope renography constitutes the most useful initial investigation of hypertension suspected to be of renovascular origin. In infants, peripheral plasma renin levels correlate well with renal ischaemic disease. Normal levels vary with age, being much higher during the first week of life than later. Collection of renal vein specimens for differential renin levels is technically difficult in babies. Angiography is performed in cases where there is proof, or high suspicion, of renovascular hypertension. Renal artery thrombosis accounts for 75% of cases of neonatal hypertension and renal artery stenosis for a further 18% [1].

Renal artery stenosis

Renal artery stenosis in infants, including neonates, has been recorded on several occasions [3,13,16,33,36,38]. The arterial pathology may be intimal or medial fibrovascular hyperplasia which may be restricted to one renal artery or involve both and possibly the aorta as well. Hypoplasia of the aorta and renal vessels has also been described [3]. There are no reports of successful vascular reconstruction in infants: nephrectomy may be indicated for unilateral disease.

Renal artery aneurysm

Aneurysm of the renal artery is a rare cause of hypertension in infancy. Rahill *et al.* [31] recorded one case in a 4-month-old baby and the patient described by Snyder *et al.* was aged 9 months [36]. In both cases nephrectomy was curative.

Renal artery thrombosis

Although apparently spontaneous renal artery thrombosis has been reported in a few neonates [11,42], in the great majority of cases the complication arises directly as a consequence of umbilical artery catheterization employed in the management of critically ill babies. Clinical features include haematuria, azotaemia and proteinuria. Peripheral levels of plasma renin are almost always elevated [2] leading to severe angiotensin-mediated hypertension which may be complicated by congestive cardiac failure or intracranial haemorrhage. The diagnosis may be suspected when sonographic appearances of the kidney are normal but there is non-function on renography.

Immediate and urgent treatment consists in correction of hypertension [4]; diuretics are ineffective and vasodilating agents (Hydralazine, Minoxidil,

Diazoxide) should be employed. Although some cases have ultimately become normotensive, without need of medication [2], more often prolonged hypertension leads to nephrosclerosis and in turn to chronic renal failure. A few cases have been successfully treated by removal of the involved kidney [30].

Renal artery embolism

Embolism of the renal artery has been described in a few neonates [43], principally those with aneurysmal dilatation of a patent ductus arteriosis. There are now few reports of this complication probably because of a policy of earlier ligation of the patent ductus arteriosis.

References

1. Adelman, R.D. (1978) Neonatal hypertension. *Pediat. Clin. N. Am.*, **25**, 99–110
2. Adelman, R., Goetzman, B., Vogal, J., Wennberg, R. and Merten, D. (1976) Neonatal renovascular hypertension: a non-surgical approach. Presented at the Western Society of Pediatric Research, Carmel, California
3. Angella, J.J., Sommer, L.S., Poole, C. and Fogel, B.J. (1968) Neonatal hypertension associated with renal artery hypoplasia. *Pediatrics*, **41**, 524–526
4. Arant, B.S. (1984) Renal disorders of the newborn infant. In *Pediatric Nephrology* (ed. B.M. Tune and S.A. Mendoza), Churchill-Livingstone, New York
5. Arneil, G.C. (1979) Renal vein thrombosis. *Contrib. Nephrol.*, **15**, 21
6. Belman, A.B., Susmano, D.F., Burden, J.J. and Kaplan, G.W. (1970) Non-operative treatment of unilateral renal vein thrombosis in the newborn. *J. Am. Med. Ass.*, **211**, 1165–1168
7. Black, J. and Williams, D.I. (1973) Natural history of adrenal haemorrhage in the newborn. *Arch. Dis. Child.*, **48**, 183–190
8. Bouissou, H., Regnier, C. and Hamousin-Metregiste, R. (1963) Le nécrose corticale symétrique des reins du nourisson. *Ann. Paediat.*, **10**, 533–552
9. Campbell, M.F. and Matthews, W.F. (1942) Renal vein thrombosis in infancy: report of two cases in male infants urologically examined and cured by nephrectomies at 13 and 33 days of age. *J. Pediat.*, **20**, 604–615
10. Carte, A. and Stanley, P. (1973) Bilateral adrenal abscesses in a neonate. *Pediat. Radiol.*, **1**, 63
11. Cook, G.T., Marshall, V.F. and Todd, J.E. (1966) Malignant renovascular hypertension in a newborn. *J. Urol.*, **96**, 863–866
12. Crispin, A.R. (1972) Medullary necrosis in infancy. *Br. Med. Bull.*, **28**, 283
13. Dawson, I.M.P. and Nabarro, S. (1953) A case of intimal hyperplasia of arteries with hypertension in a male infant. *J. Path. Bact.*, **66**, 493–498
14. DeSa, D.J. and Nicholls, S. (1972) Haemorrhagic necrosis of the adrenal gland in perinatal infants: a clinico-pathological study. *J. Path.*, **106**, 133–149
15. Eklof, O., Grotte, G., Garulf, H., Lohr, G. and Ringerts, H. (1975) Perinatal haemorrhagic necrosis of the adrenal gland. *Pediat. Radiol.*, **4**, 31
16. Formby, D. and Emery, J.L. (1969) Intimal hyperplasia of the aorta and renal vessels in an infant with hypertension. *J. Path.*, **98**, 205–208
17. Gilbert, E.F., Khoury, G.H., Hogan, G.R. and Jones, B. (1970) Haemorrhagic renal necrosis in infancy: relationship to radio-opaque compounds. *J. Pediat.*, **76**, 49–53
18. Grossman, H. (1975) The evaluation of abdominal masses in children with emphasis on non-invasive methods; a roentgenographic approach. *Cancer*, **35**, 884–900
19. Hill, E.E. and Williams, J.A. (1959) Massive adrenal haemorrhage in the newborn. *Arch. Dis. Child.*, **34**, 178–182
20. Husband, P. and Howlett, K.A. (1973) Renal papillary necrosis in infancy. *Arch. Dis. Child.*, **48**, 116–120
21. Iancu, T., Elian, E. and Lerner, M.A. (1974) Angiography and the conservative management of neonatal adrenal haemorrhage. *Pediat. Radiol.*, **2**, 47–50
22. Jorgensen, L., Neset, G. Kjoerheim, A. and Mageroy, K. (1961) Renal venous thrombosis in the newborn. *Acta Path. Microbiol. Scand.*, (*suppl.*), **148**, 97–107
23. Kaufmann, H.J. (1958) Renal vein thrombosis. *Am. J. Dis. Child.*, **95**, 377–384
24. Leonidas, J.C., Burdon, W.E. and Gribetz, D. (1971) Bilateral renal cortical necrosis in the newborn infant: roentgenographic diagnosis. *J. Pediat.*, **79**, 623–627
25. McFarland, J.B. (1965) Renal venous thrombosis in children. *Q. J. Med.*, **34**, 269–290
26. Milburn, C.L. (1952) Haemorrhagic infarction of kidneys in infants. *J. Pediat.*, **41**, 133–146
27. Mittelstaedt, C.A., Volberg, F.M., Merten, D.F. and Brill, P.W. (1979) The sonographic diagnosis of neonatal adrenal haemorrhage. *Radiology*, **131**, 453–457
28. Nogrady, M.B. and Lesk, D.M. (1972) Renal papillary necrosis in the newborn. *Am. J. Roent. Radium. Ther. Nucl. Med.*, **116**, 661–663
29. Perry, C.B. and Taylor, A.L. (1940) Hypertension following thrombosis of the renal vein. *J. Path. Bact.*, **51**, 369–374
30. Plumer, L.B., Mendoza, S.A. and Kaplan, G.W. (1975) Hypertension in infancy: the case for aggressive management. *J. Urol.*, **113**, 555–557
31. Rahill, W.J., Molteni, A., Hawking, K.M., Koo, J.H. and Menon, V.A. (1974) Hypertension and narrowing of the renal arteries in infancy. *J. Pediat.*, **84**, 39–44
32. Rayer, P.F.O. (1837) *Traite des Maladies des Reins*, Bailliere, Paris
33. Schmidt, D.M. and Rambo, O.N. (1965) Segmental intimal hyperplasia of the abdominal aorta and renal arteries producing hypertension in an infant. *Am. J. Clin. Path.*, **44**, 546–555
34. Siegel, B.S., Shedd, D.P., Selzer, R. and Mark,

J.B.D. (1961) Adrenal haemorrhage in the newborn. *J. Am. Med. Ass.*, **177**, 263–265

35. Snelling, C.E. and Erb, I.H. (1935) Haemorrhage and subsequent calcification of the adrenal. *J. Pediat.*, **6**, 22–41

36. Snyder, C.H., Bost, R.B. and Platou, R.V. (1955) Hypertension in infancy, with anomalous renal artery; diagnosis by renal arteriography, apparent cure after nephrectomy. *Pediatrics*, **15**, 88–91

37. Stark, H. and Geiger, R. (1973) Renal tubular dysfunction following vascular accidents of the kidneys in the newborn period. *J. Pediat.*, **83**, 933–946

38. Still, J.L. and Cottom, D. (1967) Severe hypertension in childhood. *Arch. Dis. Child.*, **42**, 34–39

39. Tahkeuchi, A. and Benirschke, K. (1961) Renal venous thrombosis of newborn and its relation to maternal diabetes: report of 16 cases. *Biol. Neonat.*, **3**, 237–256

40. Thompson, I.M., Schneider, R. and Lababidi, Z. (1975) Thrombectomy for neonatal renal vein thrombosis. *J. Urol.*, **113**, 396–399

41. Woodard, J.R. (1986) Neonatal and perinatal emergencies. In *Campbell's Urology*, 5th Edition (ed. P.C. Walsh, R.F. Gittes, A.D. Perlmutter and T.A. Stamey), W.B. Saunders Company, Philadelphia

42. Woodard, J.R., Patterson, J.H. and Brinsfield, D. (1967) Renal artery thrombosis in newborn infants. *Am. J. Dis. Child.*, **114**, 191–194

43. Zuelzer, W.W., Kurnetz, R. and Newton, W.A. (1951) Circulatory diseases of the kidney in infancy and childhood. IV. Occlusion of the renal artery. *Am. J. Dis. Child.*, **81**, 21–25

47

Renal cystic disease

A. M. K. Rickwood

Renal cystic disease of neonates comprises a disparate group of anomalies definable in four categories: multicystic dysplasia, autosomal recessive polycystic disease of infancy, cystic disease associated with various multiple anomaly syndromes and solitary (retention) cysts.

Multicystic dysplasia

Pathology

The kidney is wholly replaced by an irregular mass of cysts differing in size and number in various specimens (Figure 47.1). The reniform shape is lost and no renal parenchyma is evident macroscopically. The ureter is always completely obstructed at some level. In some cases it is entirely absent, or represented by a solid thread, in others it is patent along some part of its extent. Multicystic dysplasia may involve one or other part of a kidney with complete ureteric duplication, the other part being normal, or may occur in one-half of a horseshoe kidney [27]. Histologically, the cysts are lined by cuboidal or flattened epithelium and the intercystic tissue contains foci of cartilage and primitive tubules and glomeruli. Although it was previously assumed that multicystic kidney remained unchanged throughout life, although not growing relative to the child, serial ultrasound examinations show that

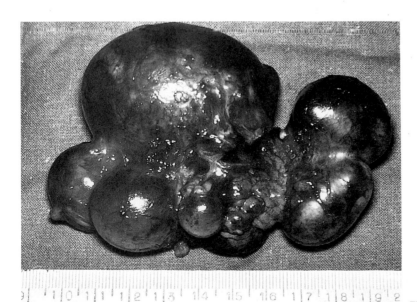

Figure 47.1 Multicystic kidney

685

quite frequently the cysts involute over a period of months, so that by the age of 1–2 years, no remaining renal tissue is recognizable. Such involution has also been observed prenatally [3]; in two of our cases, typical sonographic appearances of multicystic kidney were seen early in the third trimester, but postnatally these kidneys were found to be minute with minimal cystic changes.

The contralateral kidney may also be abnormal. In a series of 22 cases previously reported from the Royal Liverpool Children's Hospitals [20], in one both kidneys were affected, in five the opposite kidney was hydronephrotic and in one it was absent. Other series have recorded abnormalities in the opposite kidney (usually pelvi-ureteric obstruction or primary obstructive megaureter) in 50% or more of cases [24]. In the last 25 cases seen at the Royal Liverpool Children's Hospital, one had bilateral disease, one a non-obstructed hydro-ureteronephrosis while the remainder had a normal, though hypertrophied opposite kidney. It has been stated that fewer contralateral anomalies are found in infants with a high, ureteropelvic, occlusion of the ureter than in those with more distal atresia [14]. Multicystic kidney is rarely associated with other non-urological congenital abnormalities. Although usually occurring sporadically, there is evidence that siblings of cases with bilateral disease are at increased risk of various genitourinary malformations [25].

Pathogenesis

A degree of cystic dysplasia is frequently found in kidneys affected by congenital urinary obstruction and, when severe, this closely resembles that seen in multicystic kidney. It is probable that the common pathogenic factor in cystic dysplasia is obstruction to normal tubular drainage prenatally and that the degree of cystic degeneration depends upon the severity of the obstruction and its time of onset relative to the development of the metanephros, with multicystic kidney representing the extreme of this process, occurring as a consequence of complete ureteric obstruction developing early in fetal life. Curiously, no example of multicystic kidney has been detected by prenatal sonography before the 20th week of gestation [3].

Clinical features, diagnosis, treatment

Except in those with bilateral disease or some severe anomaly of the opposite kidney, the baby is usually entirely well. Previously most cases were discovered on routine postnatal examination; nowadays the majority are detected by prenatal sonography and in some 30% of these the kidney is impalpable. The

lesion may be palpable in the flank as a lobulated, freely mobile and, sometimes, transilluminable, mass. Prenatally it is difficult to distinguish multicystic kidney from gross hydronephrosis by ultrasound examination [13,15]; if changes are evident bilaterally a diagnosis of multicystic kidneys can be excluded in the presence of a normal amniotic fluid volume. Postnatally, the sonographic appearances of multicystic kidney are usually distinctive and when a DMSA renogram shows no uptake of isotope by the affected kidney the diagnosis is virtually certain [17] (Figure 47.2). If there is any doubt, final confirmation may be made by percutaneous cyst puncture and injection of contrast material.

Reported complications of multicystic kidney are rare and include rupture of a cyst into the peritoneal cavity resulting in ascites [21], infection of one or more of the cysts [17], malignant change in adult life [5,7] and hypertension [2,9,10].

It was formerly routine practice to excise multicystic kidneys since it was often impossible to be certain of the diagnosis and there was no functioning renal tissue capable of salvage. With newer methods of diagnostic imaging, these considerations no longer apply and in some units routine removal of multicystic kidneys is no longer undertaken unless they are exceptionally large. This policy might be questioned considering the long-term risks of development of hypertension or malignant change, but on present evidence these risks would appear to be small. Whatever the policy, it is clearly important to establish the state of the opposite kidney; usually a combination of ultrasound and DMSA scan are sufficient but if there is any doubt an IVU can be performed.

Infantile polycystic disease

Pathology

Both kidneys are symmetrically affected and, although they may be severely enlarged, up to 15 times normal size, the reniform shape is maintained (Figure 47.3). The cut surface presents a sponge or honeycomb appearance with rounded medullary cysts and more elongated radially disposed, cortical cysts (Figure 47.4). Micro-dissection methods have shown that there is a normal population of nephrons [23] and that the cysts represent dilated portions of the collecting ducts and tubules [18,23]. The interstitium is usually severely oedematous. The pelvicalyceal system is often compressed by the bulk of the parenchyma and, in more severe forms of the disease, the ureters and bladder may be somewhat hypoplastic by virtue of fetal oliguria. Histological

(b)

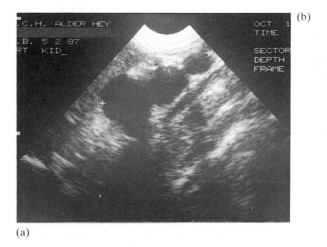

(a)

Figure 47.2 (a) Sonographic appearances of multicystic kidney showing multiple cysts of varied size with no discernible renal substance. (b) DMSA scan in the same patient showing complete lack of uptake of isotope by the affected kidney

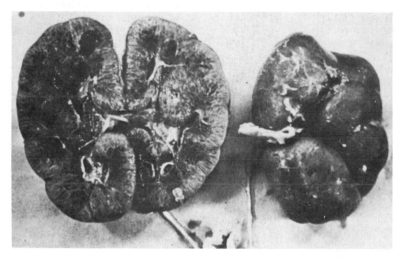

Figure 47.3 Infantile polycystic kidneys. Exaggerated fetal lobulation. Cut surfaces have a spongy appearance due to multiple small cysts

abnormalities exist in the liver, comprising increased interlobular connective tissue and an excessive number of bile ducts which show mild to moderate dilatation. Small cysts may be found in the pancreas. In severely affected neonates, the lungs are commonly hypoplastic.

Genetics

Infantile polycystic kidney is well established as being transmitted via an autosomal recessive trait affecting siblings only, although their number is less than would be expected from the appropriate Mendelian ratio [12].

Blyth and Ockenden [8] describe four clinico-pathological forms of the condition which they believe derive from different mutations of the same basic trait. In the most severe, perinatal type, the kidneys are grossly enlarged and at least 90% of the tubules are affected. There is usually maternal oligohydramnios and affected infants are stillborn or die shortly after birth from pulmonary complications. In the neonatal type, some 60% of nephrons are involved; these babies usually live for a few weeks only. The infantile type, in which 25% of

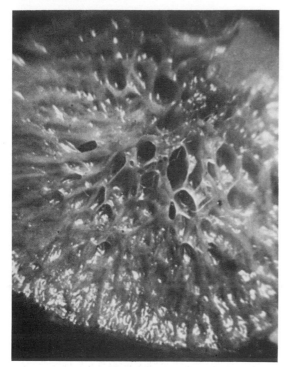

Figure 47.4 Magnified view of cut surface of infantile polycystic kidney showing honeycomb structure

tubules are affected, is associated with more prolonged survival and renal insufficiency. Lastly, in the juvenile type, where only some 10% of tubules are affected, symptomatology relates to the hepatic pathology. Whereas Blyth and Ockenden believed that where siblings were affected, all members of the family came within the same clinicopathological group, others have not confirmed this finding and consider that the clinicopathological variability represents different expression of the same gene [11,22]. Whatever the genetic niceties, clinically there is usually a clear separation between those who present in infancy with some degree of renal impairment and those presenting later in childhood with hepatic disease and in whom renal impairment is seldom more than slight.

Clinical features

In the more severe types, corresponding to the first of the four categories of Blyth and Ockenden [8], the cystic changes and renal enlargement are detectable by prenatal ultrasound from about the 20th week of gestation onwards [13]. There may be associated maternal oligohydramnios. In the most extreme form of the disease the baby has Potter facies; the kidneys are massively enlarged and may cause dystocia. Although there is oliguria from birth, death supervenes within a short period not from renal failure but from the consequences of pulmonary hypoplasia; lung rupture with pneumothorax or pneumomediastinum may occur.

In less extreme forms of the disease, the kidneys are not so enlarged and there is a variable degree of renal impairment at birth. When this is severe, early death is the rule. If renal function is only mildly impaired, or normal, there is more prolonged survival and some pass through childhood without developing renal failure and a few without overt hepatic disease. It is virtually impossible to give an accurate prognosis in such cases.

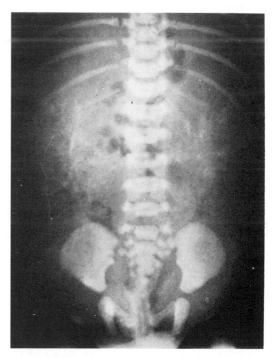

Figure 47.5 Intravenous renograms in a newborn with infantile polycystic disease. Exposure 3 h after injection shows diffuse speckling of enlarged kidneys due to contrast in cysts

Although the IVU appearances in infantile polycystic disease are quite characteristic (Figure 47.5), it is now nearly always possible to ascertain the diagnosis definitively by postnatal ultrasound examination (Figure 47.6). Treatment is that of renal failure although this is rarely required in early infancy.

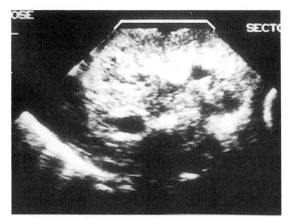

Figure 47.6 Infantile polycystic kidney. Sonogram showing a diffusely enlarged, echo-bright, kidney with several small, resolvable, cysts

Adult (autosomal dominant) polycystic disease

Adult polycystic disease is a wholly separate entity from the infantile variety in being transmitted as an autosomal dominant trait and having quite different pathological features. In the past a few cases have presented during childhood with symptoms but never in infancy. Nowadays this condition may be diagnosable prenatally or postnatally by ultrasound examination, usually in cases where there is a positive family history.

Multiple anomaly syndromes

Cystic renal disease is found in a variety of syndromes associated with congenital anomalies involving several systems and viscera. In the von Hippel–Lindau syndrome there are, in addition, retinal angiomas and cerebellar haemangioblastomas. The cerebrohepatorenal syndrome of Zellweger is characterized by maldevelopment of the skull and biliary atresia. In the Meckel syndrome, encephalocele and polydactyly co-exist. With trisomy 18 and trisomy 13, cystic kidneys (Figure 47.7) are associated with other abnormalities of the urinary tract. A typical clenched hand, short sternum and abnormal dermal ridges occur in trisomy 18. Trisomy 13 anomalies include polydactyly and defects of the eye, nose, lip, scalp and forebrain.

Noonan's syndrome of congenital heart disease, cryptorchidism, stunted growth and abnormal facies may be associated with polycystic renal disease [26]. Cystic renal disease resembling, on pyelography, the medullary sponge kidneys of adults, is found in the exomphalos–macroglossia–gigantism syndrome, which includes a variety of abnormalities [6,19] (see Chapter 27).

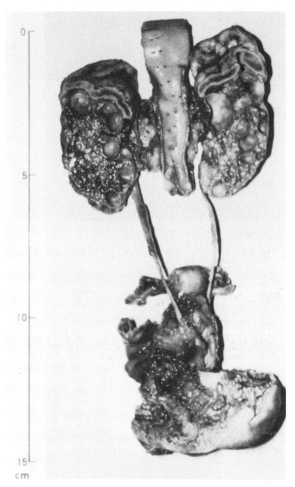

Figure 47.7 Autopsy material from a newborn, believed to be an example of trisomy 13. Both kidneys show gross cystic changes

Solitary cyst in the newborn

Occasional examples are recorded of solitary renal cyst (Figure 47.8), resembling that commonly found in adults, in otherwise well babies [4] and which are usually discovered during the course of an IVU or ultrasound examination performed for some other purpose. As a rule no treatment is required although the cyst may be aspirated percutaneously with ultrasonic guidance if thought necessary. Examples of solitary cysts have also been reported in neonates with severe congenital obstructive uropathies, usually posterior urethral valves [1,16]. It seems unlikely that such cysts are analogous to the serous renal cyst of adult life and more probable that they represent an encapsulated extravasation occurring as a result of the urinary tract obstruction.

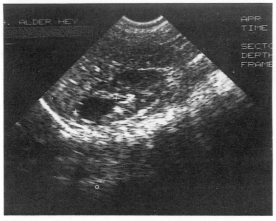

(a)

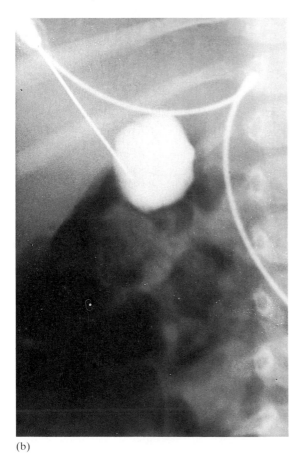

(b)

Figure 47.8 Solitary renal cyst in a neonate.
(a) Sonographic appearances showing a cystic structure in the upper pole of the kidney. (b) Confirmation of the diagnosis by percutaneous cyst puncture and injection of contrast material

References

1. Ahmed, S. (1972) Simple renal cysts in childhood. *Br. J. Urol.*, **44**, 71–75
2. Ambrose, S.S., Gould, R.A., Trulock, T.S. and Parrott, T.S. (1982) Unilateral multicystic disease in adults. *J. Urol.*, **128**, 366–369
3. Avni, E.F., Thoua, Y., Lalamand, B., Didier, F., Droulle, P. and Schulman, C.C. (1987) Multicystic dysplastic kidney: natural history from in utero diagnosis and postnatal follow-up. *J. Urol.*, **138**, 1420–1424
4. Azmy, A.F. and Ransley, P.G. (1983) Simple renal cysts in children. *Ann. Roy. Coll. Surg. Eng.*, **65**, 124–125
5. Barrett, D.M. and Wineland, R.E. (1980) Renal cell carcinoma in multicystic dysplastic kidney. *Urology*, **15**, 152–154
6. Beckwith, J.B. (1969) Macroglossia, omphalocele, adrenal cytomegaly, gigantism and hyperplastic visceromegaly. *Birth Defects*, **5**, 188–196
7. Birken, G., King, D., Vane, D. and Lloyd, T. (1985) Renal cell carcinoma arising in a multicystic dysplastic kidney. *J. Pediat. Surg.*, **20**, 619–621
8. Blyth, H. and Ockenden, B.G. (1971) Polycystic disease of kidney and liver presenting in childhood. *J. Med. Genet.*, **8**, 257–284
9. Bürgler, W. and Hauri, D. (1983) Vitale Komplikationen bei multizystischer Nierendegeneration (multizystischer Dysplasie). *Urol. Int.*, **38**, 251–256
10. Chen, Y.H., Stapleton, F.B., Roy, S. and Noe, H.N. (1985) Neonatal hypertension from unilateral multicystic kidney. *J. Urol.*, **133**, 664–665
11. Chilton, S.J. and Cremin, B.J. (1981) The spectrum of polycystic disease in children. *Pediat. Radiol.*, **11**, 9–15
12. Dalgaard, O.Z. (1957) Bilateral polycystic disease of the kidneys. *Acta Med. Scand.* (suppl. 328), **158**, 1–255
13. D'Alton, M., Romero, R., Grannum, P., DePalma, L., Jeanty, P. and Hobbins, J.C. (1986) Antenatal diagnosis of renal anomalies with ultrasound. IV. Bilateral multicystic disease. *Am. J. Obstet. Gynecol.*, **154**, 532–537
14. De Klerk, D.P., Marshall, F.F. and Jeffs, R.D. (1977) Multicystic dysplastic kidney. *J. Urol.*, **118**, 306–308
15. Diament, M.J., Fine, R.N., Ehrlich, R. and Kangarloo, H. (1983) Fetal hydronephrosis: problems in diagnosis and management. *J. Pediat.*, **103**, 435–440
16. Firstater, M. and Farkas, A. (1973) Simple renal cyst in a newborn. *Br. J. Urol.*, **45**, 366–369
17. Hartman, G.E., Smolick, L.M. and Schochat, S.J. (1986) The dilemma of the multicystic dysplastic kidney. *Am. J. Dis. Child.*, **140**, 925–928
18. Heggö, O. and Natvig, J.B. (1965) Cystic disease of the kidney. Autopsy report and family study. *Acta Pathol. Microbiol. Scand.*, **64**, 459–469
19. Irving, I.M. (1970) The EMG syndrome. *Prog. Pediat. Surg.*, **1**, 1–61

20. Johnston, J.H. (1971) Renal cystic disease in childhood. *Prog. Pediat. Surg.*, **2**, 99

21. Knutrud, O. (1976) Multicystic kidney causing ascites. Communication to Society of Paediatric Urological Surgeons.

22. Lieberman, E., Silinas-Madrigal, L., Gwinn, J.L., Brennan, L.P., Fine, R.N. and Landing, B.H. (1971) Infantile polycystic disease of the kidneys and liver: clinical, pathological and radiological correlations and comparison with hepatic fibrosis. *Medicine*, **50**, 277–318

23. Osathanondh, V. and Potter, E.L. (1964) Pathogenesis of polycystic kidneys. Type I due to hyperplasia of interstitial portions of the collecting tubules. *Arch. Pathol.*, **77**, 466–473

24. Pathak, I.G. and Williams, D.I. (1964) Multicystic and cystic dysplastic kidney. *Br. J. Urol.*, **36**, 318–331

25. Roodhooft, A.M., Birnholz, J.C. and Holmes, L.B. (1984) Familial nature of congenital absence and severe dysgenesis of both kidneys. *New Engl. J. Med.*, **310**, 1341–1345

26. Tejani, A., Del Rosario, C., Arulanantham, K. and Alpert, L.I. (1976) Noonan's syndrome associated with polycystic renal disease. *J. Urol.*, **115**, 209–211

27. Towbin, R., Benton, G. and Martin, L. (1974) Multilocular cystic dysplasia of half of a horse-shoe kidney. *J. Pediat. Surg.*, **9**, 421

48

Congenital deficiency of the abdominal musculature: the prune-belly syndrome

A. M. K. Rickwood

Prune-belly syndrome is rare, occurring in approximatly 1 in 30000 to 1 in 50000 live births [10]. The characteristic deficiency of the abdominal musculature was first described by Frolich [9] in 1839 and the associated genitourinary anomalies by Parker in 1895 [22]. The full syndrome is virtually confined to males; a few females exhibiting the typical abdominal defect are described but in most of these the urinary tracts were normal [25]. Occurrence of prune-belly syndrome in siblings has been recorded on several occasions. With few exceptions [24], reported pairs of twins have been discordant for the syndrome. Chromosomal abnormalities have been described in a few cases [12,13,17].

Pathogenesis

There is no evidence of any spinal or peripheral neurological deficit in prune-belly cases [20]. Nunn and Stephens [20] have suggested that some agent active during the sixth to tenth weeks of gestation interferes with mesodermal development and leads to defective muscularization of both the abdominal wall and the urinary tract. It has long been theorized that the abdominal wall deficiency is secondary to gross dilatation of the urinary tract occurring early in fetal development and which itself is the result of infravesical obstruction. Intra-abdominal cryptorchidism is considered to be a secondary phenomenon due either to lack of intra-abdominal pressure or, alternatively, to mechanical impedance of testicular descent caused by the enlarged bladder. Prenatal sonography has developed this theme in that a number of cases are described exhibiting the typical changes in the abdominal wall and upper renal tracts, along with testicular non-descent, in which gross abdominal distension resulted from the

development of urinary ascites around the 20th week of gestation [2,18]. This theory of causation of prune-belly syndrome is not wholly convincing since cases with prenatal ascites do not invariably exhibit all features of the syndrome, in particular those involving the gastrointestinal tract. Also, females with the syndrome and changes in the upper renal tracts have no evident infravesical obstruction. Perhaps the most persuasive argument against the notion that prune-belly syndrome, in all its features, results solely from infravesical obstruction, with or without urinary ascites, is that it is rarely, if ever, associated with other forms of congenital bladder outflow obstruction and in particular not with posterior urethral valves.

Pathology: clinical features

The abdominal wall

The extent of the muscular defect varies in different cases. In severely affected babies (Figure 48.1), the abdominal skin shows a multiplicity of wrinkles and there is an obvious flabby redundancy of the belly wall with flank bulges. The viscera are easily palpable, or even visible, through the thin parietes. The spine may be opisthotonic because of the unopposed activity of the spinal extensor muscles and the costal margins are wide and flared with a prominent sternum. In less severely affected cases, the abdominal skin creases are predominantly horizontal (Figure 48.2). Occasionally one side of the abdomen is more severely affected than the other. As a rule, the upper parts of the recti and oblique muscles are present; the infraumbilical regions of the recti are always the most affected parts of the musculature, so that the umbilicus often lies unusually high.

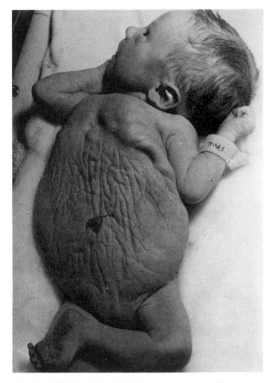

Figure 48.1 Newborn with severe prune-belly: grossly wrinkled abdominal wall, flared costal margin, talipes. The kidneys were dysplastic and the child survived only a few days

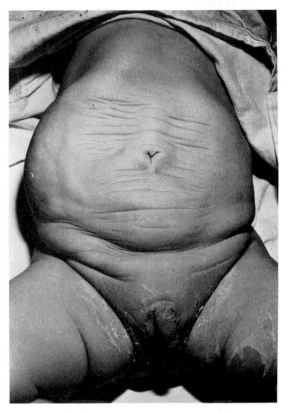

Figure 48.2 Newborn with mild prune-belly syndrome. Abdominal skin wrinkles are horizontal. Good renal function

Gastrointestinal tract

Most cases have a universal mesentery with intestinal malrotation. Imperforate anus occurs in a minority of patients, usually in association with urethral atresia or severe stenosis [19]. Duodenal atresia, gastroschisis, Hirschsprung's disease and fibrocystic disease have also been described [5,16,32].

Cardiovascular system

It has been estimated that up to 10% of cases have congenital heart lesions [1], including atrial and ventricular septal defects and Fallot's tetralogy.

Orthopaedic lesions

A characteristic finding is of dimples on the outer aspects of the knees (Figure 48.3) and, less often, the elbows. More severe anomalies of the lower

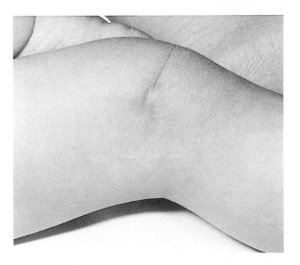

Figure 48.3 Dimples on the outer aspect of the knee in a prune-belly case

limbs, including congenital amputation [16], occur in some 3% of cases [4]. Congenital dislocation of the hip and talipes are seen in infants with severe renal impairment and are presumably related to maternal oligohydramnios. Such cases may exhibit Potter facies.

Genitourinary tract

The urinary tract shows typical abnormalities, the severity of which are usually proportionate to the degree of deficiency of the abdominal musculature. The bladder is always markedly enlarged with a wide urachal diverticulum extending to the umbilicus (Figure 48.4). In cases with urethral atresia or severe stenosis, the urachus is patent with an umbilical urinary fistula. Although the vesical wall is thickened, with an excess of fibrous tissue, its interior is smooth and untrabeculated. The trigone is enlarged with laterally sited and often gaping ureteric orifices. The bladder neck is somewhat ill-defined while the posterior urethra is wide and funnels down to the level of the external urethral sphincter. Often there is a posterior urethral diverticulum formed by a large prostatic utricle. Histological studies of autopsy specimens show non-development of the epithelial elements of the prostate gland [6]. Stephens [29] describes a type of valvular obstruction, occurring in a minority of cases, in which deep infolding of the anterior and anterolateral walls of the urethra override the lumen of the membranous urethra. Anterior urethral anomalies occur in some patients. Scaphoid megalourethra is the commonest association [15]; other lesions include hypospadias, ventral and dorsal chordee and fusiform megalourethra with aplasia or hypoplasia of the corpora cavernosa. Rarely, the entire urethra is stenotic (Figure 48.5).

Urodynamic studies [28] almost always demonstrate a slow urinary stream. Detrusor contractions, which may generate normal, above normal or subnormal pressures, are generally non-sustained and leave residual urine. Compliance of the vesical wall is usually good although intravesical pressure may be persistently elevated in the presence of a large residual urine. Although there invariably appears to be an element of obstruction at the level of the external urethral sphincter, the cause of this remains unknown. Prostatic dysgenesis has been suggested as a factor.

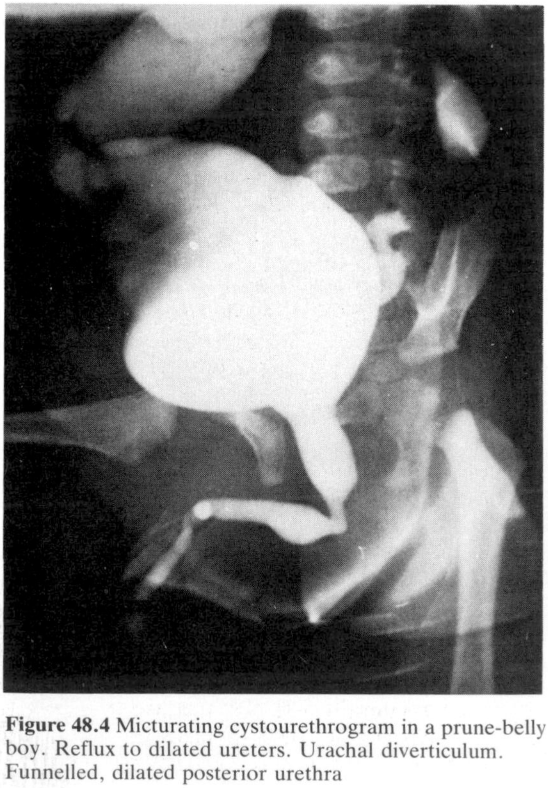

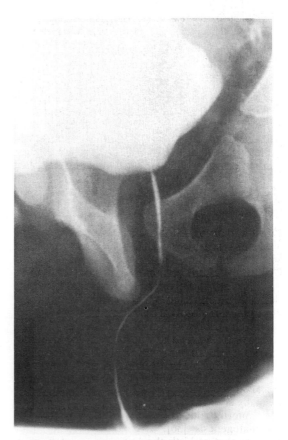

Figure 48.4 Micturating cystourethrogram in a prune-belly boy. Reflux to dilated ureters. Urachal diverticulum. Funnelled, dilated posterior urethra

Figure 48.5 Cystogram showing stenosis of the entire urethra in a prune-belly case

The ureters exhibit various degrees of dilatation and tortuosity, characteristically with an outward dog-leg at the pelvic brim (Figure 48.6). Typically, the ureteric widening is segmental, dilated zones alternating with zones of relatively normal calibre. At fluoroscopy, the ureters usually show sluggish peristalsis and are slow to empty. Vesico-ureteric reflux is often, but not always, present. The kidneys are affected in different degrees and sometimes asymmetrically: in some instances, particularly in babies with urethral atresia, megalourethra or imperforate anus, they are small and severely dysplastic. In minimally affected cases, although renal function is normal, the kidneys are of abnormal morphology, with irregular outlines and calyces which are elongated and clubbed and of fewer than normal number. As a rule, pelvicalyceal dilatation is proportionately less than that of the ureters.

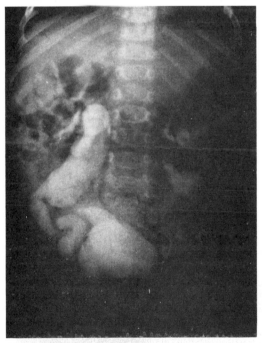

Figure 48.6 Intravenous urogram in prune-belly syndrome. Normal calyces, segmental ureteric dilatation, urachal diverticulum

The testes are always undescended, in the majority of cases lying suspended from a mesentery within the abdominal cavity just below the pelvic brim. Sexually active adults with the syndrome are invariably infertile due to grossly impaired or absent spermatogenesis [36]. Recent studies, however, indicate that at birth the testes have potential for spermatogenesis [21].

Management

Because of the variable severity of the disease, as it affects the urinary tracts, the type of intervention required, if any, must be tailored to the needs of each case.

The most severe cases, with bilateral dysplasia, are usually recognizable by the presence of maternal oligohydramnios, gross deficiency of the abdominal musculature and, in most instances, respiratory difficulty from birth due to pulmonary hypoplasia. Such marked renal dysplasia is usually evident on ultrasound examination. Early death is inevitable.

At the other extreme are those cases where renal function, as judged by serial estimations of serum creatinine, is normal and stable. As a rule, the abdominal musculature is only mildly defective while ultrasound examination of the urinary tracts generally shows only modest pelvicalyceal dilatation and a good depth of renal substance in at least one kidney. Instrumentation of the urinary tract, including cystography, is best avoided in such cases since this may precipitate urinary tract infection. A persistently distended bladder is not itself an indication for cystography provided renal function remains satisfactory and the upper renal tract dilatation is not increasing. Usually these children do well without any treatment [35] and surgical intervention in infancy is rarely, if ever, called for.

Many prune-belly cases lie between these extremes. Renal function may be variably impaired from birth or drainage of the upper urinary tracts is unsatisfactory by virtue of poor ureteric peristalsis, vesico-ureteric reflux, persistently elevated intravesical pressure or any combination of these. Such congenitally inadequate systems risk further damage from the effects of infection superimposed upon urinary stasis. Azotaemia, acidaemia and septicaemia produce a clinical state similar to that occurring with posterior urethral valves. Immediate treatment consists of appropriate antibiotic therapy and intravenous fluids to correct electrolyte disturbance.

Once the acute episode has been surmounted, the question of surgical intervention arises especially in the event of persistent azotaemia or recurrent sepsis. Major reconstructive procedures, by way of extensive ureteric remodelling and re-implantation and reduction cystoplasty [23,34], although sometimes indicated in older boys, are not appropriate to the neonatal period. At this time, enhanced drainage of the upper renal tracts is best secured by measures designed to promote emptying of the bladder. Williams [33] has advocated internal urethrotomy, using the Otis urethrotome introduced via a perineal urethrostomy; one or two cuts are made anterolaterally with the instrument set at 24–30 FG. Alternatively, the sphincteric area of the membranous urethra may be incised anteriorly under vision by diathermy as in transurethral sphincterotomy; because the bladder neck is left intact, there is little risk of this procedure producing incontinence. These methods are best reserved for relatively mildly affected patients. In more severe cases, drainage of the urinary tracts is better secured by a temporary vesicostomy [7] of the Blocksom [3] type, with definitive reconstruction deferred until the child is older. Cutaneous ureterostomies [14] were once commonly employed but rarely now; if the infant's condition does not improve following vesicostomy then, as a rule, a higher urinary diversion is unlikely to be effective [30]. In case of doubt, percutaneous nephrostomies may be inserted; should there be no improvement in renal function within 1 month, then it is improbable that a more definitive form of upper tract diversion would be beneficial.

Since it appears that the intra-abdominal testes in prune-belly patients have potential for spermatogenesis, a case exists for early orchidopexy, within the first 6 months of life. Sometimes the spermatic vessels are of sufficient length to enable the testis to be mobilized into the scrotum by conventional techniques but more often they are not and some alternative procedure is required. Microvascular autotransplantation [31] is, at present, unsuitable for infants. The Fowler–Stephens technique [8] has been used in prune-belly cases but with a failure rate of approximately 25% [11]. A two-stage procedure, giving good results in the author's hands, has been suggested by Ransley [27]. In the first stage, the spermatic vessels are ligated and divided immediately above the testis; some 3 months later when the vasal vessels have undergone compensatory hypertrophy, the testis can be safely mobilized into the scrotum on the vas deferens.

The appearance of the abdominal wall tends to improve as the child grows older. Nevertheless, a better cosmetic appearance is usually obtainable by abdominal wall reconstruction at around 1 year of age. A suitable technique is described by Randolf and colleagues [26].

Incomplete syndrome

In some boys an incomplete syndrome occurs ('pseudo-prunes'): typical changes are seen in the upper renal tracts, bladder and prostatic urethra but the abdominal wall is normal. The testes are generally bilaterally undescended and usually intra-abdominal. Knee and elbow dimples are present in some cases and similarly scaphoid megalourethra.

The condition may pass unnoticed in the neonatal period but can be suspected from the presence of a combination of persistent distension of the bladder and bilateral cryptorchidism. Presentation in infancy is sometimes occasioned by azotaemia, septicaemia or both together.

Intravenous urography and sonography show typical appearances of the upper renal tracts; sometimes a cysto-urethrogram is required to exclude a diagnosis of posterior urethral valves. As a rule, renal function is normal or only mildly impaired. Treatment is along the lines described for the complete syndrome.

References

1. Adebonojo, F.O. (1973) Dysplasia of the abdominal musculature with multiple congenital anomalies: prune-belly or triad syndrome. *J. Nutl. Med. Ass.*, **65**, 327–333

2. Adzick, N.S., Harrison, M.R., Flake, A.W. and DeLorimier, A.A. (1985) Urinary extravasation in the fetus with obstructive uropathy. *J. Pediat. Surg.*, **20**, 608–615

3. Blocksom, B. (1957) Bladder pouch for prolonged tubeless cystostomy. *J. Urol.*, **78**, 398–401

4. Carey, J.C., Eggert, L. and Curry, C.J.R. (1982) Lower limb deficiency and the urethral obstruction sequence. *Birth Defects*, **18**, 19–28

5. Cawthern, T.H., Bottene, C.A. and Grant, D. (1979) Prune-belly syndrome associated with Hirschsprung's disease. *Am. J. Dis. Child.*, **133**, 652–653

6. Dekler, D.B. and Scott, W.W. (1978) Prostatic maldevelopment in prune-belly syndrome. A defect in prostatic stromal-epithelial interaction. *J. Urol.*, **120**, 241–242

7. Duckett, J.W. (1976) The prune-belly syndrome. In *The Surgery of Infants and Children* (eds T.M. Holder and K.W. Ashcraft) W.B. Saunders Co., Philadelphia

8. Fowler, R. and Stephens, F.D. (1963) The role of testicular vascular anatomy in the salvage of high undescended testes. In *Congenital Malformations of the Rectum, Anus and Genitourinary Tract* (ed. F.D. Stephens), Williams & Wilkins Co., Baltimore

9. Frolich, F. (1839) Der Mangel der Muskeln, inbesondere der Seitenbauchmuskeln, C.A. Zurn, Wurzburg

10. Garlinger, P. and Ott, J. (1974) Prune-belly syndrome – possible genetic implications. *Birth Defects*, **10**, 173–180

11. Gibbons, M.D., Cromie, W.J. and Duckett, J.W. (1979) Management of the abdominal undescended testis. *J. Urol.*, **122**, 76–79

12. Halbrecht, I., Komlos, L. and Shabtaz, F. (1972) Prune-belly syndrome with chromosomal fragment. *Am. J. Dis. Child.*, **123**, 518

13. Harley, L.M., Chen, Y. and Rattner, W.H. (1972) Prune belly syndrome. *J. Urol.*, **108**, 174–176

14. Johnston, J.H. (1978) Congenital deficiency of the abdominal musculature: the prune-belly syndrome. In *Neonatal Surgery*, 2nd Edition (eds P.P. Rickham, J. Lister and I. Irving), Butterworths, London

15. Kroovand, R.L., Al-Ansari, R.M. and Perlmutter,

A.D. (1982) Urethral and genital malformations in prune-belly syndrome. *J. Urol.*, **127**, 94–96

16. Lattimer, J.K. (1958) Congenital deficiency of the abdominal musculature and associated genito-urinary anomalies. A report of 22 cases. *J. Urol.*, **79**, 343–352

17. Lubinsky, M., Coyle, K. and Trunca, C. (1980) The association of prune-belly with Turner's syndrome. *Am. J. Dis. Child.*, **134**, 1171–1172

18. Monie, I.W. and Monie, B.J. (1979) Prune-belly syndrome and fetal ascites. *Teratology*, **19**, 111–117

19. Morgan, C.L., Grossman, H. and Novak, R. (1978) Imperforate anus and colon calcification in association with the prune-belly syndrome. *Pediat. Radiol.*, **7**, 19–21

20. Nunn, I.N. and Stephens, F.D. (1963) *Congenital Malformations of the Rectum, Anus and Genitourinary Tracts*, E. and S. Livingstone, Edinburgh

21. Orvis, B.R., Mitchell, M.E. and Kogan, B.A. (1988) Testicular histology in fetuses with prune-belly syndrome and posterior urethral valves. *J. Urol.*, **139**, 335–337

22. Parker, R.W. (1895) Absence of abdominal muscles in an infant. *Lancet*, **i**, 1252–1254

23. Perlmutter, A.D. (1976) Reduction cystoplasty in prune-belly syndrome. *J. Urol.*, **116**, 356–362

24. Peterson, D.S., Fish, L. and Cass, A.F. (1972) Twins with congenital deficiency of abdominal musculature. *J. Urol.*, **107**, 670–672

25. Rabinowitz, R. and Schillinger, J.F. (1977) Prune-belly syndrome in the female subject. *J. Urol.*, **118**, 454–456

26. Randolph, J., Cavett, C. and Eng, G. (1981) Abdominal wall reconstruction in the prune-belly syndrome. *J. Pediat. Surg.*, **16**, 960–964

27. Ransley, P.G. and Vordermark, J.S. (1984) Preliminary ligation of the testicular vessels in prune-belly orchidopexy. Read at 21st Conference, British Assoc. of Paediatric Surgeons, Liverpool

28. Snyder, H.M., Harrison, N.W., Whitfield, H.N. and Williams, D.I. (1976) Urodynamics in the prune belly syndrome. *Br. J. Urol.*, **48**, 663–670

29. Stephens, F.D. (1983) Congenital intrinsic lesions of the posterior urethra. In *Congenital Malformations of the Urinary Tract*, Praeger Publications, New York

30. Tank, E.S. and McCoy, G. (1985) Limited surgical intervention in the prune-belly syndrome. *J. Pediat. Surg.*, **18**, 688–691

31. Wacksman, J., Dinner, M. and Staffom, R.A. (1980) Technique of testicular orthotransplantation using a microvascular anastomosis. *Surg. Gynec. Obstet.*, **150**, 399–400

32. Willert, J., Cohen, H. and Yu, Y.T. (1978) Association of prune-belly syndrome with gastroschisis. *Am. J. Dis. Child.*, **132**, 526–527

33. Williams, D.I. (1979) Prune-belly syndrome. In *Campbell's Urology*, 4th Edition (eds J.H. Harrison, R.F. Gittes and A.D. Perlmutter), W.B. Saunders Co, Philadelphia

34. Woodard, J.R. and Parrott, T.S. (1978) Reconstruction of the urinary tract in prune-belly uropathy. *J. Urol.*, **119**, 824–828

35. Woodhouse, C.R.J., Kellett, M.J. and Williams, D.I. (1979) Minimal interference in prune-belly syndrome. *Br. J. Urol.*, **51**, 475

36. Woodhouse, C.R.J. and Snyder, H.M. (1985) Testicular and sexual function in adults with prune belly syndrome. *J. Urol.*, **133**, 607–609

49

The female genital tract

A. M. K. Rickwood

Hydrocolpos

The various forms of congenital vaginal occlusion usually present either in adolescence, with primary amenorrhoea, or less often, in the neonatal period when secretion by the fetal cervical and vaginal mucosal glands, stimulated by maternal oestrogens, leads to development of hydrocolpos. Fluid accumulates principally within the vagina and sometimes in the uterus. Occasionally the fallopian tubes are involved and rarely fluid leaks back into the peritoneal cavity to produce plastic peritonitis [5].

The site and nature of the vaginal occlusion varies. In some cases there may be a thin, membranous, obstruction at the introitus ('imperforate hymen'); less often there is a septum of variable thickness at a higher level, most commonly at the junction of the upper and middle thirds of the vagina [14]. Occasionally, septal obstruction occurs above a common urogenital sinus [11]. A septum is believed to result from failure of communication between the upper vagina, derived from the fused Mullerian ducts, and the lower vagina obtaining from the sinovaginal outgrowths of the urogenital sinus. Antell [2] considers that all vaginal occlusions form in this way, including 'imperforate hymen' where the hymen proper is recognizable distally as a separate structure, especially after the membrane has been incised and the fluid released. In some cases genetic factors are involved, with the condition inherited as a simple autosomal recessive characteristic [9]. The retained fluid may be clear, milky or mucinous and histological examination reveals desquamated epithelial cells and leucocytes.

Although usually occurring as an isolated abnormality, there are sometimes associated developmental lesions which include stenotic or imperforate anus, cloaca and lumbosacral spinal anomalies.

Hydrocolpos may involve only one element of a genital tract duplication [6].

Clinical features

The distended vagina (which may be recognized by prenatal sonography and mistaken for a large bladder) presents at birth as an abdominal mass arising from the pelvis. On occasion this is so large as to cause respiratory difficulties or oedema or cyanosis of the legs. Displacement of the bladder from the pelvis leads to complete or partial urinary retention and sometimes the distended bladder is separately palpable from the vaginal swelling. There is usually some degree of bilateral hydro-ureteronephrosis although renal function is seldom compromised. With introital lesions, the obstructing membrane is visible at the vulva (Figure 49.1) and bulges outwards when the abdominal mass is compressed. When the occlusion is higher in the vagina, the introitus appears normal but the cervix uteri cannot be seen on vaginoscopy. Any doubt as to the nature of the pelvic mass can usually be resolved by ultrasound examination after the bladder has been emptied via a catheter (Figure 49.2).

Treatment

Obstruction at the introitus is easily relieved by cruciate incision of the bulging membrane. Division from below of a thick, high, vaginal septum carries the risk that adjacent structures, in particular the urethra, may be damaged. Laparotomy is advisable in such cases. The anterior wall of the enormously distended vagina is incised and fluid removed by suction; the septum can then be divided safely under guidance from within. Cases associated with vaginal atresia above a common urogenital sinus may be

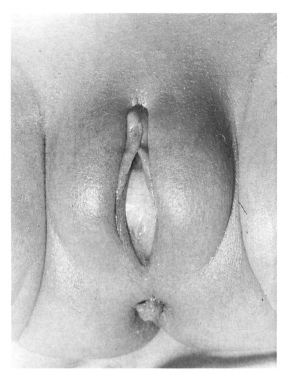

Figure 49.1 Hydrocolpos due to imperforate hymen in a female neonate

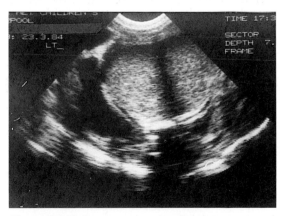

Figure 49.2 Hydrometrocolpos in a female neonate. Sonogram (transverse section) demonstrates the large echogenic mass of the distended vagina displacing the echo-free bladder forward and to the left

treated in the neonatal period by mobilizing the distended vagina downwards between the rectum and the common urogenital sinus and exteriorizing it to the perineum in the normal anatomical position [11].

Urogenital sinus

Common urogenital sinus, whether occurring as an isolated anomaly or in association with persistent cloaca, is sometimes complicated by pooling of urine within the proximal vagina [13] which leads to a lower abdominal swelling comparable to that seen in congenital vaginal occlusion. Occasionally the sinus is obstructed by a persisting membrane [1], more often its orifice is merely stenotic although seldom to a degree that would be expected to obstruct urinary outflow. The condition is distinguishable from the more common vaginal occlusions by the presence of a single vulval orifice and patency of the entire vagina can be confirmed by endoscopy.

It is usually possible to manage this complication by a short period with a catheter indwelling in the vagina followed by a longer period of intermittent catheterization. Over a few weeks the proximal vagina shrinks to normal dimensions and urine flows freely from the vulval orifice. This policy enables the necessary vaginoplasty to be deferred until the child is older.

Urethralization of the female phallus

This rare anomaly [3,12], of which clitoral hypertrophy is one feature, bears superficial resemblance to the intersexual disorders, adrenogenital syndrome in particular, but is clinically distinguishable by the presence of both clitoral and vulval orifices (Figure 49.3). The lesion is a form of female urethral duplication, the main channel leading to the perineum via a common urogenital sinus and the accessory, clitoral, urethra entering the main channel immediately below the bladder neck. Karyotype is XX and the internal genitalia are normal. Associated anomalies include anterior ectopic anus, or a cloacal deformity, and primary or secondary lesions of the upper renal tracts. Urine may pool proximally in the vagina and this can be managed as in other urogenital sinus anomalies.

Hymenal polyp

Because of the influence of maternal oestrogen, the hymen at birth and for the first few days of life is thick and oedematous. On occasion, the posterior part forms a round or elongated polyp. Berglen and Selander found hymenal polyps in 6% of 1000 newborn girls [4]. The polyp gradually shrinks and may disappear completely. It is important to distinguish this condition from sarcoma botryoides which has been reported to occur in the newborn [10].

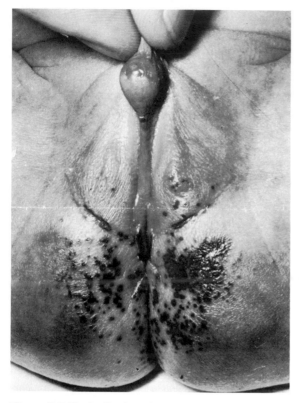

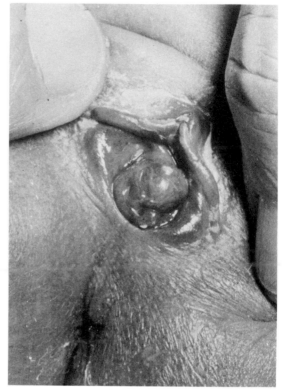

Figure 49.3 Urethralization of the female phallus. The clitoris is enlarged with a small glandular orifice. Posteriorly the labia are hypoplastic and the vulval orifice is of a common urogenital sinus. The anus is anteriorly ectopic. (Reprinted with permission from *British Journal of Urology*)

Figure 49.4 Para-urethral cyst in a newborn

Vaginal cyst

A cyst may develop as a result of fluid distension of the epoophoron (Gartner's duct) which descends on each side of the vagina from the broad ligaments [8]. The cyst, which may be present at birth, projects into the lumen of the vagina. Compression of the urethra may obstruct micturition and necessitate excision of the cyst.

Para-urethral cyst

A retention cyst of a para-urethral gland may exist at birth and present as a parameatal swelling or may protrude through the meatus, simulating a prolapsing ectopic ureterocele (Figure 49.4). Treatment is by excision or marsupialization of the cyst.

Procidentia

Genital prolapse in the newborn is exceedingly rare, and usually occurs in babies with myelomeningocele in consequence of paralysis of the musculature of the pelvic floor. Occasional cases have been described in otherwise normal infants [7]. Treatment is by manual reduction following which the legs are bound together for a few weeks while the bladder is drained via a catheter.

References

1. Agatastein, E.H. and Erlich, R.M. (1986) Imperforate anus and related conditions. In *Campbells Urology*, 5th Edition (ed. P.C. Walsh, R.F. Gittes, A.D. Perlmutter and T.A. Stamey), W.B. Saunders, Philadelphia
2. Antell, L. (1952) Hydrocolpos in infancy and childhood. *Pediatrics*, **10**, 306–310

3. Bellinger, M.F. and Duckett, J.W. (1982) Accessory phallic urethra in the female patient. *J. Urol.*, **127**, 1159–1164

4. Berglen, N.F. and Selander, P. (1962) Hymenal polyps in newborn infants. *Acta Paediat. Scand.* (Suppl.), **135**, 28

5. Ceballos, R. and Hicks, G.M. (1970) Plastic peritonitis due to neonatal hydrometrocolpos: radiologic and pathogenic observations. *J. Pediat. Surg.*, **5**, 63–70

6. Cook, G.T. and Marshall, V.F. (1964) Hydrocolpos causing urinary obstruction. *J. Urol.*, **92**, 127–132

7. Cottom, D. and Williams, E. (1965) Procidentia in the newborn. *J. Obstet. Gynaec. Br. Commonw.*, **72**, 131–136

8. Klein, F.A., Vick, C.W. and Broecker, B.H. (1986) Neonatal vaginal cysts: diagnosis and management. *J. Urol.*, **135**, 371–372

9. McKusick, V.A., Bauer, R.L., Koop, C.E. and Scott, R.B. (1964) Hydrometrocolpos as a simple inherited malformation. *J. Am. Med. Ass.*, **189**, 813–816

10. Ober, W.B., Smith, J.A. and Roullard, F.C. (1958) Congenital sarcoma botryoides of the vagina: report of two cases. *Cancer*, **11**, 620–623

11. Ramenofsky, M.L. and Raffensperger, J.G. (1971) An abdominoperineal vaginal pull-through for the definitive treatment of hydrometrocolpos. *J. Pediat. Surg.*, **6**, 381–387

12. Turnock, R.R. and Rickwood, A.M.K. (1987) Urethralisation of the female phallus: a rare form of female intersex. *Br. J. Urol.*, **59**, 481–482

13. Williams, D.I. and Bloomberg, S. (1976) Urogenital sinus in the female child. *J. Pediat. Surg.*, **11**, 51–56

14. Woodard, J.R. (1986) Neonatal and perinatal emergencies. In *Campbells Urology*, 5th Edition (ed. P.C. Walsh, R.F. Gittes, A.D. Perlmutter and T.A. Stamey), W.B. Saunders, Philadelphia

50

The male genital tract

A. M. K. Rickwood

Undescent of the testis

The testis is derived from primordial germ cells which, by the sixth week of gestation, have migrated from the yolk sac to invade the medial aspect of the genital ridge on the dorsal abdominal wall of the fetus. Differentiation from indifferent gonad to fetal testis occurs during the seventh week of gestation and the organ begins to secrete testosterone and a Mullerian inhibiting factor by the eighth week of gestation. The gubernaculum and processus vaginalis are also evident at this stage. By the third month, the testis occupies a position immediately above the internal inguinal ring; this occurs principally because of differential growth of the posterior abdominal wall and, indeed, the fetal testis never lies more than 1–3 mm above the internal ring at any stage in its development. After a quiescent phase, final descent commences during the seventh month, when the testis follows the gubernaculum and processus vaginalis through the inguinal canal and, by the end of the eighth month of gestation, the testis occupies a scrotal position.

Although a number of factors have been implicated in testicular descent, the process is undoubtedly dependent upon endogenous production of testosterone [12] which in turn is controlled by gonadotrophin secreted by the placenta and by the fetal pituitary. In consequence, cryptorchidism is a feature of several conditions in which there is deficient production of gonadotrophin (pituitary hypoplasia or aplasia, anencephaly, Kallman's syndrome), or defects of androgen synthesis or action [24]. The mechanism whereby testosterone causes testicular descent is unknown and there is no convincing evidence that otherwise normal boys with unilateral cryptorchidism have abnormalities of the hypothalamic-pituitary-testicular axis. Intra-

abdominal pressure has been suggested as an additional mechanism causing the testis to leave the abdominal cavity [6,9] and the incidence of cryptorchidism is increased in prune-belly syndrome, gastroschisis, exomphalos major and, possibly, umbilical hernia [16].

The presence of cryptorchidism is best assessed at birth when the cremasteric reflex is absent. Although the testes are normally fully descended at term, a little delay is within the range of normality [27,32], with cryptorchidism being found in 3.4% of full-term neonates and 30.3% of premature babies. Subsequently, some 75% of these testes in full-term infants and 95% of those in premature babies descend into the scrotum, usually within the first 3 months of life [27]. By the age of 1 year, the incidence of permanent cryptorchidism appears to lie between 0.5 [30] and 0.8% [3] of boys. In 10% the defect is bilateral and in 3% one or both testes are absent [18,28]. Monorchism is usually left-sided and the presence of a vas and remnants of testicular vessels in most cases indicates that the testis had developed but had subsequently undergone torsion prenatally. True monorchism [18] accounts for only some 15% of boys with unilateral testicular absence, is nearly always left-sided and may be associated with absence of the ipsilateral upper renal tract.

Testicular ischaemia

Testicular torsion (Figure 50.1)

Torsion of the testis in the neonate is almost always supravaginal with the spermatic cord twisting above the tunica vaginalis so that ischaemia involves both the serous sac and its contents. Either testis may be involved and very rarely the condition is bilateral

[8,22]. According to Watson [33], torsion is usually clockwise on the left and counter-clockwise on the right. No cause is known although it is presumed that contraction of the spirally arranged cremasteric fibres is the initiating factor facilitated by the loose attachment between tunica vaginalis and scrotal wall existing in the neonate.

Although the condition is frequently not noted within the first 24–48 h after birth, there is evidence that the torsion may take place prenatally or during delivery. The infant is not distressed and the affected testicle, while enlarged and hard, is not tender. The scrotal contents are adherent to the parietes and show a bluish discoloration through the

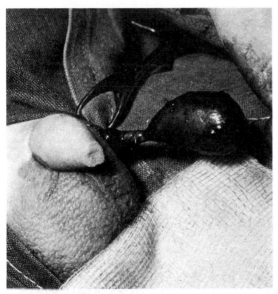

Figure 50.1 Extravaginal torsion of the spermatic cord in a neonate leading to infarction of the tunica and testis

skin. There is occasionally a skin dimple at the fundus of the scrotum and sometimes intrascrotal calcification may be detected radiologically.

While there have been occasional reports of testicular salvage in cases operated within a few hours of birth [19], in the great majority irreversible ischaemia has occurred by the time the diagnosis is made. Expeditious scrotal exploration is nonetheless warranted. If, after the torsion is untwisted and the tunica albuginia incised, there is no sign of viability, the testis should be excised. While asynchronous bilateral torsion in the neonatal period is exceptionally rare [19], it would nonetheless seem wise to fix the opposite testis using two or three non-absorbable sutures anchoring the tunica albuginia to the dartos muscle.

Idiopathic infarction

Haemorrhagic infarction of the tunica vaginalis and testis may occur in the newborn without torsion. The spermatic cord is normal to the level of the tunica vaginalis at which point it suddenly constricts. This condition may possibly represent spontaneous correction of a torsion.

Incarcerated inguinal hernia

Ischaemic necrosis of the testis can occur when the spermatic vessels are compressed between the incarcerated contents of an inguinal hernia and the fibrous sheath of the cord. This complication occurs almost exclusively in young infants and its prevention requires prompt reduction of the hernia by taxis or by operation (see Chapter 26). On occasion ischaemic atrophy of the testis may follow herniotomy in young infants as a result of damage to the testicular vessels.

Scrotal haemorrhage

Bruising of the scrotal skin or, occasionally, frank intrascrotal haemorrhage, may be noted in newborn boys especially those born prematurely or by breech delivery. In most cases the condition is bilateral. Although it is usually possible, by palpation, to be certain that the scrotal contents are normal, if there is doubt exploration should be performed to exclude testicular torsion.

Hydrocele

Hydrocele in infancy is due to persistent patency of the processus vaginalis which allows peritoneal fluid to enter and accumulate within the tunica vaginalis. Often the communicating tract enters the tunica below its apex so that a valvular effect is created, preventing fluid returning to the peritoneal cavity. Occasionally a tense hydrocele may accumulate rapidly and without warning, and be mistaken for testicular torsion. Hydrocele in infants is more frequent on the right side than on the left and is often bilateral. Spontaneous obliteration of the processus vaginalis occurs in more than 95% of cases within the first year of life and surgical treatment need be undertaken in infants only when the hydrocele is exceptionally large. In such cases, the spermatic cord is exposed through a groin incision and the patent processus vaginalis identified above the hydrocele, dissected from the cord structures and ligated at its junction with the peritoneum proper. The hydrocele itself is emptied by aspiration or incision.

Meconium hydrocele results from perforation of the bowel during fetal life allowing escape of meconium which descends through a patent processus vaginalis to the tunica. Calcification of the meconium occurs and sterile inflammation leads to fluid accumulation within the peritoneum and the tunica. Perforation of the bowel may be associated with intestinal obstruction persisting postnatally or with subsequent development of peritonitis. Should the perforation heal without either of these complications, the most obvious clinical feature is the presence, at birth, of an enlarged, discoloured, scrotum. Radiography shows calcified nodules within the peritoneal cavity and in both sides of the scrotum. Treatment consists of removal of the meconium through scrotal incisions.

Epididymo-orchitis

Epididymo-orchitis in neonates is almost always associated with bacterial infection of the urine resulting from some congenital structural anomaly of the lower urinary tract [29]. The most common cause is rectourethral fistula associated with high imperforate anus; other, occasional, causes include ureteric ectopia and posterior urethral valves.

Abnormalities of the penis

Hypospadias and epispadias seldom present diagnostic problems and treatment is rarely called for in infancy. In hypospadias the urinary meatus often appears small, but close inspection and witnessing the urinary stream usually demonstrate that it is of adequate size. Significant meatal stenosis, requiring meatotomy, is present in only some 1% of hypospadiacs.

Parental concern is sometimes expressed about the presumed small size of their son's penis. In most instances, the organ is of normal size but merely somewhat buried in a pad of prepubic fat. Normality of the organ is easily demonstrated by digital compression and retraction of adipose tissue (Figure 50.2). There is considerable variation in the size of the penis in neonates; in full-term infants, Feldman and Smith [7] recorded the third centile for stretched length was 2.8 cm and the 97th 4.2 cm.

Phimosis and circumcision of neonates

Although phimosis is present by definition when the foreskin cannot be retracted to reveal the glans penis, this state is seldom pathological in boys and is always normal in the newborn. During fetal development, as the prepuce grows forward over the glans, there exists no plane of separation between the two. Separation, which occurs by a process of

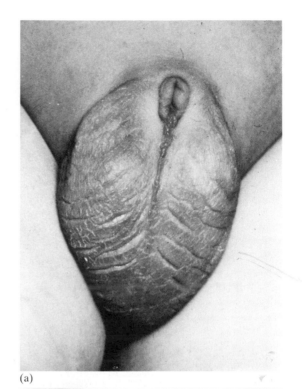
(a)

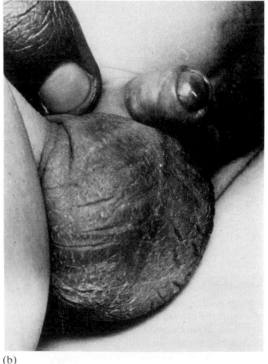
(b)

Figure 50.2 Buried penis. (a) Natural appearance: only the prepuce is visible. (b) On retraction of the skin, the penis is seen to be of normal size and appearance. Note that the scrotum and testes are normally developed

desquamation and vacuolation, commences late in gestation and is rarely complete by birth so that the foreskin is fully retractable in only 4% of newborn boys [10]. This developmental adherence between glans and foreskin (so-called preputial adhesions) is often accompanied by relative narrowness of the preputial orifice ('physiological phimosis') which nonetheless remains supple. During childhood these 'adhesions' break down spontaneously and the preputial orifice enlarges so that the foreskin becomes fully and easily retractable. Usually this is complete by 10 years of age, but is occasionally delayed into the mid-teens [21]. There is 'no evidence that 'preputial stretching', or similar manoeuvres, hastens the process. True, pathological, phimosis, with cicatrization of the preputial orifice and histological changes of balanitis xerotica obliterans, is an uncommon disease of older boys [25] and no convincing examples have been recorded in the newborn.

While the baby is in napkins the prepuce serves a useful purpose in protecting the glans and meatus against ammoniacal excoration and ulceration so that circumcision in babies is generally inadvisable.

Routine neonatal circumcision, ostensibly for medical reasons, is widely practised in North America, less commonly in the UK and rarely on the continent of Europe. Arguments advanced in favour of this practice include general considerations of personal hygiene, enhancement of sexual performance, reduced chance of venereal disease in the patient or of carcinoma of the cervix in his prospective spouse, elimination of risk of penile carcinoma and similarly of balanitis or phimosis. When the American Academy of Pediatrics came to examine these propositions, they found all wanting except that relating to penile carcinoma, a rare disease largely attributable to poor personal hygiene. Recently, it has been claimed that the risk of urinary tract infection, usually with *P. vulgaris*, in the first year of life is enhanced tenfold in uncircumcised boys [34] and that this accounts for the greater incidence of urinary tract calculi in European than in American children. Even were this true, the risk of childhood stone disease is so small that routine neonatal circumcision could not reasonably be advised as a prophylactic measure.

Buried penis

As mentioned, a normal penis may appear short in obese infants because of fat deposits in front of the pubis. The true buried, or concealed, penis is a congenital anomaly in which skin lacks normal attachment to the penile shaft so that the organ appears to be very poorly developed or even absent. However, when the skin is drawn back, the organ is seen to be of normal size (Figure 50.2). There is a tendency towards spontaneous resolution, but, if

this does not occur, surgery is directed to fixing the skin to the pubic area and to the penile base so that the penis presents a more normal appearance [14].

Webbed penis

A web of skin extends from the anterior aspect of the scrotum to the ventrum of the penis. In childhood the condition is of cosmetic significance only but sexual difficulties can occur in adult life. Treatment consists of division of the skin fold.

Micropenis

True micropenis is associated with rudimentary testes [5]. The organ is extremely small and slim and is barely palpable through the preputial skin. The scrotum is underdeveloped and usually neither testis can be palpated. The sex chromosomes are XY. Exploration reveals normal but small vasa deferentia and spermatic vessels ending in a minute nodule of tissue in or above the scrotum. Biopsy of these nodules reveals fibrous tissue and some small tubules.

In some cases enlargement of the penis may follow intramuscular injection of testosterone or topical application of 2% testosterone ointment [11]. The latter therapy acts both locally and systemically due to absorption so that the possibility of inducing precocious puberty must be borne in mind; the first evidence of this is the appearance of pubic hairs. Androgen treatment in childhood is a useful therapeutic test concerning the possible effectiveness of hormonal therapy at the time of puberty. In cases not responding, the micropenis is presumably the result, at least in part, of target organ failure. Useful lengthening of the organ can sometimes be achieved by partially detaching the penile crura from the pubo-ischial rami [13] (Figure 50.3), but when the affected child is seen as a neonate, serious consideration should be given to sexual reassignment to the female gender and to the required surgery and endocrine therapy being carried out at an early stage.

Micropenis with cryptorchidism constitutes one manifestation of the Prader–Willi syndrome [23], which is also associated with mental retardation, obesity, small stature and hypotonia. Therapy of the genital anomaly is rarely required.

Double penis

Duplication of the penis is the result of failure of union of the originally paired genital tubercles. The anomaly may be associated with vesical or cloacal exstrophy and, even in the absence of these conditions, separation of the pubic bones is frequently present [26]. In some cases there is complete

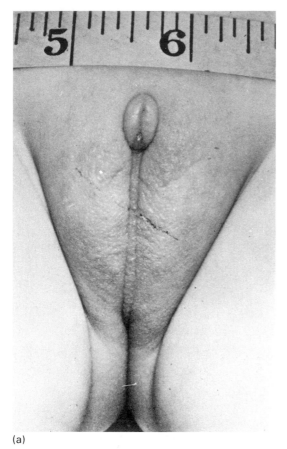

(a)

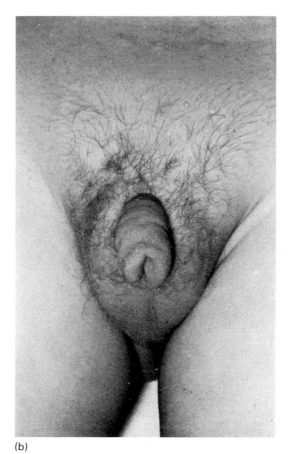

(b)

Figure 50.3 Micropenis in a boy with rudimentary testes and no response to local androgen application. (a) Before treatment.

(b) Following operative lengthening of the penis. The pubic hairs are due to local testosterone applications

duplication of the bladder, each hemi-bladder opening through a separate urethra [1]. Frequently the two penises are rotated and are of unequal development. One or both may be epispadiac or one penis may have no urethra. Full investigation of the anatomy is required before one of the organs is resected.

Megalourethra

This occurs in two forms [31] in both of which there is arrest of embryogenesis of the whole or part of the corpus spongiosum [2]. In addition the corpora-cavernosa may be affected, unilaterally or bilaterally. In the fusiform variety, the corpora cavernosa and spongiosum are usually absent over the extent of the penile urethra and the penis forms a large, flabby sac, the walls consisting only of skin and urethral mucosa. With the scaphoid type, which is twice as common, the corpora cavernosa are usually normally developed but the spongiosum is poorly formed or entirely absent. The penis is curved

dorsally and is unusually long. The dilated urethra produces a ventral swelling (Figure 50.4) which balloons out during micturition. The glans and glandular urethra are normal.

More than 50% of cases of megalourethra are associated with the prune-belly syndrome and even when the abdominal wall is normal, dilated and tortuous ureters and dysmorphic kidneys similar to those seen in prune-belly cases are often present [2,15]. Scaphoid megalourethra varies in severity. In severe cases, operative trimming of redundant penile urethra and its reconstruction into a tubular shape are required.

Penile torsion

It has been estimated that 35-degree penile torsion exists in 0.7% of male neonates and 90 degrees or more torsion in 0.3% [4]. Since penile torsion is rarely seen in older boys it may be supposed that this condition usually resolves spontaneously. Deviation of the midline raphe, without penile

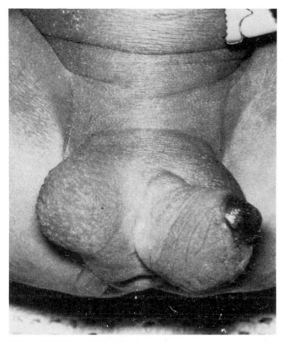

Figure 50.4 Scaphoid megalourethra in a newborn: long, dorsally curved penis with ventral swelling

torsion, is present in some 10% of male neonates and is quite without consequence.

Penile agenesis

Congenital absence of the penis is the result of aplasia of the genital tubercles. The condition is exceptionally rare with a reported incidence of between 1 in 10 million and 1 in 30 million live births [17]. Most affected infants have a normal XY karyotype although occasional examples of mosaicism have been recorded. Other anomalies, especially imperforate anus, are common; urinary tract abnormalities, including complete absence of the entire urinary tract, occur in approximately 50% of cases. The urethra most often opens at the anus or on the perineum; less frequently the meatus is at the pubis or in front of the scrotum or there may be Y-duplication of the urethra with a recto-urethral fistula [20]. The scrotum is usually normally developed. The testes and cord structures are occasionally entirely absent; usually they are present, unilaterally or bilaterally, and may be of normal dimensions or, more often, hypoplastic.

Attempts to construct a functioning penis are unlikely to be rewarding and these boys are best assigned to the female gender. Orchidectomy is performed early in the neonatal period but the scrotum is retained to form the lining of a vagina. Oestrogen therapy is commenced at the time of puberty [17].

References

1. Abrahamson, J. (1961) Double bladder and related anomalies: clinical and embryological aspects and a case report. *Br. J. Urol.*, **33**, 195–214
2. Appel, R.A., Kaplan, G.W., Brock, W.A. and Streit, D. (1986) Megalourethra. *J. Urol.*, **135**, 747–751
3. Baumrucker, G.D. (1946) Incidence of testicular pathology. *Bull. US Army Med. Dept.*, **5**, 312–314
4. Ben-Ari, J., Mimoumi, F. and Reisner, S.H. (1985) Characteristics of the genitalia in the newborn: penis. *J. Urol.*, **134**, 521–522
5. Bergada, C., Cleveland, W.W., Jones, H.W. and Wilkins, L. (1962) Variants of embryonic testicular dysgenesis: bilateral anorchia and the syndrome of rudimentary testis. *Acta Endocrin. (Copenh.)*, **40**, 521–536
6. Elder, J.S., Isaacs, J.T. and Walsh, P.C. (1982) Androgenic sensitivity of the gubernaculum testis: evidence for hormonal/mechanical interactions in testicular descent. *J. Urol.*, **127**, 170–176
7. Feldman, K.W. and Smith, D.W. (1975) Fetal phallic growth and penile standards for newborn male infants. *J. Pediat.*, **86**, 395–398
8. Frederick, P.L., Dushkin, N. and Eraklis, A.J. (1967) Simultaneous bilateral torsion of the testis in a newborn infant. *Arch. Surg.*, **94**, 299–300
9. Frey, H.L., Peng, S. and Rajfer, J. (1983) Synergy of abdominal pressure and androgens in testicular descent. *Biol. Reprod.*, **29**, 1233–1239
10. Gairdner, D. (1949) The fate of the foreskin. *Br. Med. J.*, **2**, 1433–1437
11. Guthrie, R.D., Smith, D.W. and Graham, C.B. (1973) Testosterone therapy for micropenis during early childhood. *J. Pediat.*, **83**, 247–252
12. Hamilton, J.B. (1938) The effect of male hormone upon the descent of the testis. *Anat. Rec.*, **70**, 533–541
13. Johnston, J.H. (1974) Lengthening of the congenital or acquired short penis. *Br. J. Urol.*, **46**, 685–687
14. Johnston, J.H. (1978) Other penile anomalies. In *Surgical Pediatric Urology* (ed. H.B. Eckstein, R. Hohenfellner and D.I. Williams), W.B. Saunders, Philadelphia
15. Johnston, J.H. and Coimbra, J.A.M. (1969) Megalourethra. *J. Pediat. Surg.*, **5**, 304–308
16. Kaplan, L.M., Koyle, M.A., Kaplan, G.W., Farber, J.H. and Rajfer, J. (1986) Association between abdominal wall defects and cryptorchidism. *J. Urol.*, **136**, 645–647
17. Kessler, W.D. and McLaughlin, A.P. (1973) Agenesis of the penis. Embryology and management. *Urology*, **1**, 226
18. Kogan, S.J., Gill, B., Bennett, B., Smey, P., Reda, E.F. and Levitt, S.B. (1985) Human monorchism: clinicopathological study of unilateral absent testis. *J. Urol.*, **135**, 758–761
19. LaQuaglia, M.P., Bauer, S.B., Eraklis, A., Feins, N. and Mandell, J. (1987) Bilateral neonatal torsion. *J. Urol.*, **138**, 1051–1054
20. Oesch, I.L., Pinta, A. and Ransley, P.G. (1987)

Penile agenesis: a report of six cases. *J. Pediat. Surg.*, **22**, 172–174

21. Oster, J. (1968) The further fate of the foreskin. *Arch. Dis. Child.*, **43**, 200–203

22. Papadatos, C. and Moutsouris, C. (1967) Bilateral testicular torsion in the newborn. *J. Pediat.*, **71**, 249–250

23. Prader, A., Labhort, A. and Willi, H. (1956) Ein syndrome von Adipositas Kleinwercks, Kryptorchidismus und Oligophrenic nach myatonieartigem, Zustand im Neugeborenalter. *Schweiz. med. Wschr.*, **86**, 1260–1268

24. Rajfer, J. and Walsh, P.C. (1977) Hormonal regulation of testicular descent: experimental and clinical observations. *J. Urol.*, **118**, 985–990

25. Rickwood, A.M.K., Hemalatha, V., Batcup, G. and Spitz, L. (1980) Phimosis in boys. *Br. J. Urol.*, **52**, 147–150

26. Savir, A., Lurie, A. and Lazerbnik, J. (1970) Diphallia: report of a case. *Br. J. Urol.*, **42**, 498–560

27. Scorer, C.G. (1964) The descent of the testis. *Arch. Dis. Child.*, **39**, 605–609

28. Scorer, G. and Farringdon, G.H. (1971) *Congenital Deformities of the Testis and Epididymis*, Appleton-Century-Crofts, New York

29. Siegel, A., Snyder, H. and Duckett, J.W. (1987) Epididymitis in infants and boys: underlying urogenital anomalies and efficacy of imaging modalities. *J. Urol.*, **138**, 1100–1103

30. Southam, A.H. and Cooper, E.R.A. (1927) The pathology and treatment of retained testis in childhood. *Lancet*, **i**, 805–811

31. Stephens, F.D. (1963) *Congenital Malformations of the Rectum, Anus and Genitourinary Tract*, E. and S. Livingstone, Edinburgh

32. Villumsen, A.L. and Zachau-Christiansen, B. (1966) Spontaneous alteration in the position of the testis. *Arch. Dis. Child.*, **41**, 198–200

33. Watson, R.A. (1975) Torsion of the spermatic cord in the neonate. *Urology*, **5**, 439–443

34. Wiswell, T.E. and Rosselli, J.D. (1986) Corroborative evidence for the decreased incidence of urinary tract infections in circumcised male infants. *Pediatrics*, **78**, 96–99

51

Exstrophic anomalies

A. M. K. Rickwood

The exstrophic lesions form a spectrum of developmental anomalies arising in the hind end of the embryo, the commonest, vesical exstrophy (Table 51.1), occupying a central position as regards severity. Lesser degrees are represented by epispadias, superior vesical fissure and covered exstrophy, whilst the most severe is cloacal exstrophy (*syn* vesico-intestinal fissure).

In all varieties there is diastasis of the pubic bones, the extent of which is proportional to the severity of the visceral lesion; because the two halves of the pelvis are separated anteriorly, the acetabula, with the femoral heads, are rotated externally.

The incidence of vesical exstrophy has been estimated, in various communities, to lie between 1 in 10 000 [28] and 1 in 50 000 [22] live births, and the male:female ratio is 2.3:1 [17]. Epispadias and cloacal exstrophy are appreciably rarer (Table 51.1)

Table 51.1 Incidence of exstrophic anomalies admitted to the Neonatal Surgical Centre, Royal Liverpool Children's Hospital, 1953–87

Vesical exstrophy	88
Cloacal exstrophy	15
Superior vesical fissure	5
Duplicate exstrophy	2
Cover exstrophy	3
Epispadias	4

but with a similar male:female ratio. Examples are recorded of vesical exstrophy in siblings, including those of different sexes [12,29] and identical twins [23,29]. The risk of recurrence in any individual family is estimated between 1 in 100 [15] and 1 in 300 [23]. The chance of mothers with exstrophy or epispadias giving birth to offspring with either condition has been calculated to be 700 times greater than in the general population [29].

Pathology

Exstrophy of the bladder

At birth the bladder mucosa is thin and smooth and the ureteric orifices are easily seen. With exposure, the mucosa rapidly becomes hyperaemic, thickened and friable. Cystitis cystica develops as a result of glandular obstruction and mucosal polyps form; later, squamous metaplasia occurs. In most cases the detrusor is initially pliable and contracts if iced water is applied to the overlying mucosa. Later it tends to become oedematous, rigid and acontractile, and may eventually be replaced by fibrous tissue. The upper renal tracts are usually normal at birth but hydro-ureteronephrosis sometimes develops as a consequence of oedema or fibrosis at the ureteric orifices.

In the male there is complete epispadias (Figure 51.1) with the urethra represented by a strip of mucosa on the dorsum of the short, broad, upturned penis. The vas deferens and ejaculatory ducts are normal. The scrotum is wide and shallow, and unilateral or bilateral testicular undescent is common as also is inguinal hernia. In the female the epispadiac urethra is usually short and in some instances no urethral mucosa is discernible. The clitoris is bifid and the labia are separated anteriorly so that the vagina is clearly visible.

In both sexes the anus is anteriorly placed and directed forwards. There is often sphincter laxity which allows rectal prolapse to occur. In a few females there is more extreme anal displacement so

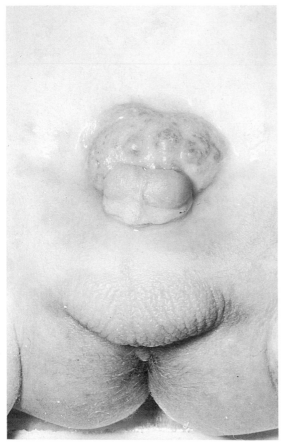

Figure 51.1 Exstrophy in a boy. The penis is short, broad and epispadiac and in this case the bladder is small

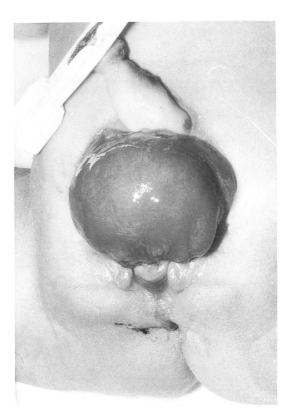

Figure 51.2 Exstrophy in a female neonate; in this instance the bladder is of almost normal dimensions

that the orifice, which is stenotic, lies at the distal extremity of the urethral strip with the vaginal orifice immediately above it. The size of the exstrophied bladder varies; at one extreme surface area approaches that of a normal bladder (Figure 51.2); at the other, little more than the trigone is represented (Figure 51.1). The smaller the bladder, the less the pubic diastasis and, as a rule, the better developed the penis and scrotum.

Epispadias

In males the penis is upturned and often somewhat short, and the urethral orifice may lie on the glans, the penile shaft or, most commonly, at the penopubic junction immediately below the bladder neck. Similar grades of severity exist in the female urethra which is split dorsally to a variable extent and is associated with a bifid clitoris.

In milder forms urinary control is not affected but in more severe degrees the sphincteric mechanism is almost always deficient and the child is incontinent.

Superior vesical fissure; duplicate exstrophy; covered exstrophy

With superior vesical fissure, the exstrophy is limited to the apex of the bladder, the remainder of the viscus and the urethra being normally formed. With duplicate exstrophy, a small area of exstrophied bladder lies on the abdominal surface but the underlying bladder is intact. In the least severe of the exstrophic anomalies, covered exstrophy, the bladder and urethra are fully formed but there is diastasis of the pubic bones and the recti are separated to leave the usual triangular defect in the lower abdominal wall. The bladder is covered only by skin, which is often rugose, and the viscus bulges through the abdominal defect when the infant cries (Figure 51.3). In males there may be genital deformities such as penile torsion or accessory scrotum.

Cloacal exstrophy (vesico-intestinal fissure)

Although details of the anatomy vary, the basic pattern (Figures 51.4 and 51.5) is one of two hemi-

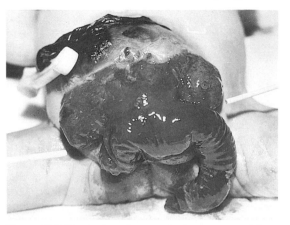

Figure 51.5 Classic cloacal exstrophy in a neonate. There is wide exomphalos and hemi-bladders on each side of the central bowel field. The terminal ileum has prolapsed through the proximal bowel orifice

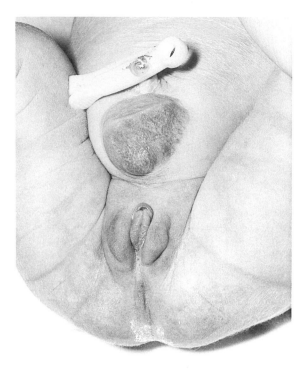

Figure 51.3 Covered exstrophy in a female neonate. The recti are separated in the lower abdominal wall and the bladder is covered only by skin. There is associated imperforate anus

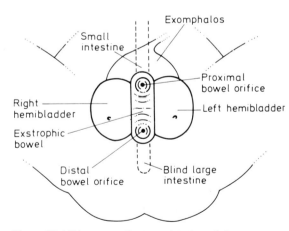

Figure 51.4 Diagrammatic representation of the anatomy of classic cloacal exstrophy

bladders, each with a ureteric orifice, separated by a midline zone of intestine with upper and lower orifices. The upper orifice, which often prolapses, represents the ileocaecal region and leads to terminal ileum, while the lower orifice leads to a short (5–7 cm) length of colon ending blindly in front of the sacrum. A third, appendicular orifice is sometimes

visible and occasionally the appendix is duplicated. While the two hemi-bladders are usually quite separate, in a minority of cases they are confluent above or below the central bowel field [14]. The anus is imperforate although there is usually a perineal dimple. Immediately above the exstrophy is a broad exomphalos containing ileum and sometimes a portion of liver.

In the male there are usually duplex but rudimentary phalli, although a single midline penis may occur, usually in cases where there is confluence of the hemi-bladders caudal to the bowel field [14]. Except in one recorded case [11], all phalli have been epispadiac. The testes are nearly always bilaterally undescended or, more often, absent. Failure of Mullerian duct fusion leads to bicornuate uterus and, in many cases, duplication of the vagina [30]; less frequently the vagina is absent. In a few cases there are no external genitalia.

In contrast to other forms of exstrophy, babies with cloacal exstrophy are often premature and the majority have other congenital anomalies. Some 50% have abnormalities of the upper renal tracts including solitary and multicystic kidneys, hydronephrosis and megaureters. In a survey of 57 cases [30], non-genitourinary anomalies were observed in 45, involving the extremities (ten), cardiovascular system (nine), small intestine (four), ribs (three), colon (two) and diaphragm (two): myelomeningocele (usually sacral) was present in 24 cases.

Embryology

The developmental abnormality fundamental to all exstrophic deformities is failure of primitive streak mesoderm to invade the allantoic extension of the cloacal membrane (infra-umbilical membrane) so that ectoderm and endoderm remain abnormally in contact in the developing lower abdominal wall, just as occurs normally in the cloacal membrane. Absence of intervening mesoderm produces an unstable state leading to disintegration of the infra-umbilical membrane so that the pelvic viscera become laid open onto the surface of the abdomen. The abdominal musculature, derived from an ingrowth of thoracic somite mesoderm, is normal on each side of the ventral defect. The abnormally extensive cloacal membrane produces a wedge effect holding apart the developing structures resulting in the deficiency of the abdominal wall, the pubic diastasis and the presence, cranial to the exstrophy, of a wide linea alba or, in more severe cases, an exomphalos. Double phallus or duplication of the female genital tract result from the same effect causing failure of fusion of the originally paired genital tubercles or of the Mullerian ducts.

The type of exstrophy depends upon the extent of the allantoic expansion of the cloacal membrane and upon the stage in embryonic development at which the membrane dehisces. The most common lesion, vesical exstrophy with epispadias, results from breakdown of an extensive membrane after completion of the urorectal septum at about the 16-mm stage so that the primitive urogenital sinus is exteriorized. A less extensive infra-umbilical membrane, limited to the pubic area, leads to development of epispadias without bladder exstrophy, while if only the cranial portion of the infra-umbilical membrane remains uninvaded by mesoderm, its dehiscence leads to superior vesical fissure.

The most plausible of several explanations advanced for development of vesico-intestinal fissure is, as the alternative name 'cloacal exstrophy' implies, that it represents the same basic anomaly but that dehiscence of the cloacal membrane and its infra-umbilical extension occurs earlier, before formation of the urorectal septum, at the 5-mm stage [20]. Exstrophy occurring at that phase leads to formation of a central bowel field between two bladder fields. An objection to this hypothesis is that the exstrophic bowel involves not the termination of the gut but the ileocaecal region, an area not normally entering into formation of the cloaca. Johnston [20], however, pointed out that the hind gut, which he believed to begin at the usual site of a Meckel's diverticulum, would be greatly restricted in growth by its involvement in an exstrophy; the exposed bowel therefore represents an extremely short hind gut and the distal blind length of intestine is persistent postanal or tail gut.

Three of our cases [18], in which the exstrophied bowel lay entirely caudal to the bladder, support this theory of the embryogenesis of cloacal exstrophy in that they represent its occurrence at a phase of development between those which lead to classic vesical and cloacal anomalies. Dehiscence of the cloacal and infra-umbilical membranes at about the 8-mm stage, after formation of the urorectal septum but before its fusion with the endoderm lining the cloacal membrane (so that the cloacal passage between bladder and rectum is still open), would produce the deformity these cases exhibited. The surface zone between bladder and rectum represents the roof of the cloacal passage.

Parietal mesoderm fusion across the midline may occur as a secondary event after the development of exstrophy. Such a sequence in association with superior vesical fissure, is responsible for the occurrence of duplicate exstrophy; a similar phenomenon occurred in the perineal area of one of our three cases of separate exstrophy of bladder and bowel in which an everted proctoderm and prolapsed exstrophic rectum were sequestrated on the surface and an atresia of the bowel at the pelvic floor was produced [18].

Treatment

Exstrophy of the bladder

In the past there were differing views regarding the timing and nature of reconstructive procedures, some authorities [3,31] advocating delaying treatment until the child was older and, in male cases, lengthening the penis as a preliminary procedure [31]. The uniform trend in recent years has been towards staged reconstruction, with primary closure of the bladder undertaken in the neonatal period wherever possible [17]. The initial operation is not intended to produce a continent bladder and secondary procedures to produce a competent bladder neck, enlargement of the bladder, or both, are delayed until the child is older. Primary bladder closure is most easily and effectively performed in the neonatal period while the viscus is still thin-walled and pliable, and, with modern paediatric anaesthesia and nursing, is well tolerated by babies. Removal of the unsightly defect does much for parents' morale and makes for easier handling of the baby. Neonatal closure is contraindicated if there is some other anomaly (e.g. congenital heart disease) requiring more urgent attention, or if the bladder is uninvertable by virtue of inherently small size or, occasionally, due to a rapid development of oedema throughout its wall. The latter may resolve spontaneously in time allowing later primary closure. Although it was previously considered that permanent urinary diversion was unavoidable when the bladder was inherently small, there is now the possibility of functional reconstruction in such cases by way of augmentation or substitution cystoplasty [2,10]. These procedures are not carried out in the neonatal period.

In the occasional case with extreme diastasis of the pubic bones, pelvic osteotomy is essential to effect satisfactory repair. In most other cases it is possible to achieve cover of the repaired bladder using fascial flaps from the anterior rectus sheaths and transposition skin flaps [31]. Most surgeons, however, prefer to employ pelvic osteotomy as a routine since this gives a more secure and cosmetically satisfactory closure of the abdominal wall. It is also stated to improve the results of penile reconstruction and, because the bladder neck and proximal urethra lie within the pelvic ring, increase the success rate of secondary repair of the bladder neck [17]. The most persuasive argument in favour of routine pelvic osteotomy is that all series reporting good results from functional reconstruction incorporate this procedure [1,24,26].

Possibly because of the influence of maternal relaxins, the pelvic ring is pliable at birth and, during the first 48 h of life, can be closed without pelvic osteotomy. Most authorities, however, prefer to delay closure to between 1 and 2 weeks of age [17].

Technique

Opinions vary concerning the details of bladder reconstruction but the basic principles of the procedure are agreed. The following description is of the technique used at the Royal Liverpool Children's Hospital.

Bilateral iliac osteotomies are performed with the child prone. Vertical incisions are made just lateral to each sacro-iliac joint and the bone is divided by an osteotome from the iliac crest to the greater sciatic notch. The superior gluteal vessels and nerve emerging from the pelvis must be protected. The incisions are closed with drainage and the two halves of the pelvis compressed together in order to stretch the ligamentous and muscular attachments which still tend to hold them apart.

Bladder reconstruction is carried out at the same session (Figure 51.6). The child is placed supine and the legs are included in the prepared operative field so that they may be manipulated when closing the pelvic ring. An incision is made around the mucocutaneous junction and superiorly the umbilicus is excised and its vessels ligated. The incision is deepened to separate the bladder from the recti and from the peritoneum. At the bladder neck the incision is continued distally on each side of the urethral mucosa and the latter is raised sufficiently from the underlying tissues to allow it to be closed as a tube. In the female, the entire urethral strip is mobilized. In the male, the procedure is restricted to the posterior urethra; penile lengthening and distal urethral reconstruction are carried out at later stages. Triangular wedges of the bladder wall are excised on each side of the vesical outlet in order to lengthen the urethra and narrow the sphincteric region. Deep dissection on either side of the bladder neck exposes the fibrous interpubic band which passes from one pubic bone to the other behind the posterior urethra.

The bladder and urethra are adequately freed so that they can be sutured in the midline without tension. The bladder is closed with a running all-layer suture of 3-0 chromic catgut and further interrupted sutures of the same material, placed through the musculature of the bladder, reinforce the repair. A temporary, 10 FG, catheter is used when repairing the urethra; this is performed using interrupted 3-0 all-layer chromic catgut sutures. The interpubic band is freed from the bone on each side and dissected medially; the two halves are then

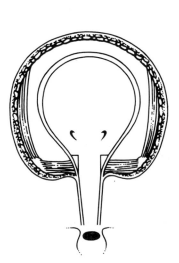 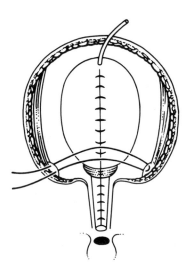

Figure 51.6 Reconstruction of exstrophic bladder in the female (see text for details)

sutured together or overlapped around the vesico-urethral junction. The bladder is drained by a 12 FG Malecot catheter brought out through the apex. Ureteric splints are not employed routinely and urethral catheter drainage is not used.

A strong (number 1 or 2) monofilament nylon suture threaded on a cutting needle is passed as a mattress suture through the two pubic bones. The legs are flexed, adducted and internally rotated, and the trochanters compressed together to approximate the pubic bones before the suture is tied. The rectus sheaths, now lying in apposition, are sutured together with 2-0 or 3-0 polyglycolic acid suture and the skin is closed vertically in the midline.

Postoperatively, the position is maintained with a firm crepe bandage around the pelvis and another holding the legs together. Catheter drainage of the bladder is continued for 3 weeks; if examination under general anaesthetic at this stage shows that the urethral repair is sound the catheter is removed.

Several authorities advocate combining penile lengthening with the initial procedure, Duckett [6] using para-exstrophy skin flaps for this purpose. Jeffs [17] employs modified Bryant's traction for several weeks postoperatively to maintain closure of the pelvic ring.

Complications of bladder reconstruction

Breakdown of the distal urethral repair is common and of little consequence. Occasionally there is complete breakdown of the entire repair so that the exstrophied bladder becomes completely laid open again. Provided the bladder remains supple, this does not preclude a further attempt at repair.

Secondary changes in the upper renal tracts are common after bladder reconstruction. Because the ureters angulate sharply forwards to enter the bladder, there is always vesico-ureteric reflux. This may be thought of no consequence so long as the bladder remains almost completely empty, but, in our experience, pyelonephritic scarring of the kidneys can occur even in this circumstance. It is our practice to give low dosage antibiotic prophylaxis until reflux has been definitely corrected. Although no attempt is made to reconstruct the bladder neck at the initial procedure, occasionally a degree of outlet obstruction supervenes and may be followed by the development of hydro-ureteronephrosis. This can usually be corrected by a vigorous urethral dilatation or by a regime of intermittent catheterization. Calculi may form in the bladder or, less often, in a dilated upper renal tract. Careful postoperative supervision is necessary so that these effects can be avoided or minimized. It has long been recognized that adenocarcinoma is liable to develop in untreated bladder exstrophy, the risk being approximately 400-fold greater than in the normal population [5]. Squamous cell carcinoma has been recorded in a few cases [21]. The risk of malignant change when the bladder has been closed is unknown; two examples of squamous cell carcinoma have been reported but in neither case was the bladder closed at birth [7,16].

Results of bladder neck reconstruction

Until recent times a perfect result from exstrophy reconstruction, namely a continent patient with a persistently normal upper urinary tract, was achieved in only a minority of cases (Figure 51.7), Johnston and Kogan [19] reporting in 1974 that just 91 (21.9%) of 415 reported cases had achieved satisfactory urinary control. An appreciable number of those with control subsequently required urinary diversion because of deterioration of the upper renal tracts.

Since general adoption of a two-stage approach, with neonatal closure of the bladder, improved results have been reported from several centres with continence achieved in 46–86% of cases [1,24,26]. Other units, however, employing the same policy and techniques, have not achieved anything like such good results. Limiting factors are the difficulty of obtaining satisfactory secondary repair of the bladder neck and persistently small bladder capacity due to non-compliance of the detrusor. Recently encouraging results have been reported using intestinal segments to augment bladder capacity [2,5,9] and, in selected cases, using the artificial urinary sphincter [25] as an alternative to repair of the bladder neck. It seems likely that in the future the results of functional reconstruction will be generally much better although at the expense of major surgery and the complications attendant on this.

Cloacal exstrophy

Although the occasional case has been reported of survival without surgical reconstruction, profuse fluid losses from the short alimentary tract usually prove fatal within a short period. Rickham, in 1960 [27], reported the first case to survive surgical reconstruction in the neonatal period. Whether or not active treatment is justified at all poses difficult ethical and moral problems; if the infant survives reconstruction there remain the problems of urinary and faecal incontinence, abnormalities of the upper renal tracts, spina bifida and, especially in the male, genital deficiency.

If surgery is considered justified, early intervention is needed. The exomphalos is repaired. The usual policy is to mobilize the intestinal strip from the hemi-bladders on either side and, after this has been tubularized, the termination of the blind ending colon is brought to the surface as a colostomy. The two hemi-bladders are sutured together in the midline and to the abdominal wall

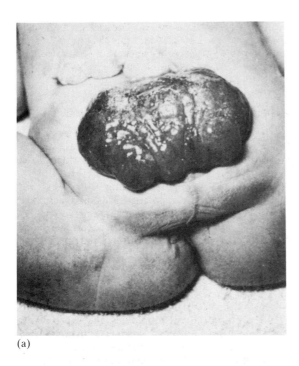

(a)

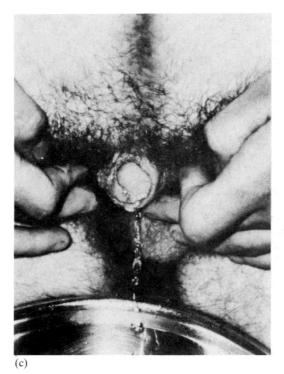

(c)

Figure 51.7 Result of bladder reconstruction. (a) Large exstrophic bladder in a newborn boy. Reconstruction performed in the neonatal period. (b) IVU at 17 years of age showing normal upper urinary tracts. (c) Patient voiding: full urinary control, no urinary infection, no vesico-ureteric reflux

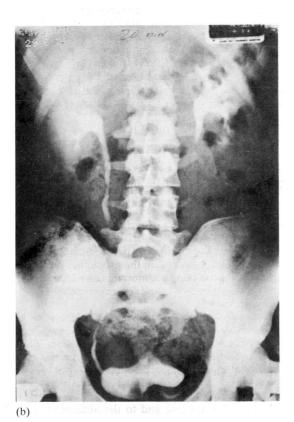

(b)

above. As an alternative [4], the central bowel field may be left *in situ* to act, in effect, as an 'auto-augmentation' of the bladder; proximal and distal bowel are detached from the bladder and the terminal ileum is brought out as a permanent faecal stoma. The colon is left *in situ* as a mucous fistula and may be used later for bladder augmentation, as a urinary conduit or for constructing a vagina. Others [13] have found that this policy leads to short bowel syndrome and that the infant fails to thrive until the colon is re-incorporated in the faecal stream.

Although the majority of cases are male, the two rudimentary phalli are seldom capable of reconstruction into a single functioning organ, and the long-term psychological effects of such genital deficiency are often catastrophic. It is now considered preferable to reassign such cases to the female gender in the neonatal period; the testes are removed and subtotal excision of the phalli performed, joining the two rudimentary glans together in the midline to act as a clitoris.

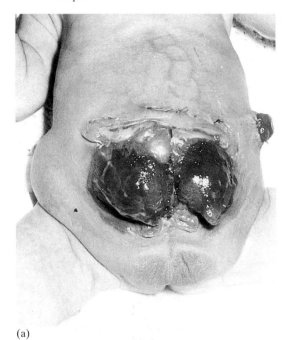

(a)

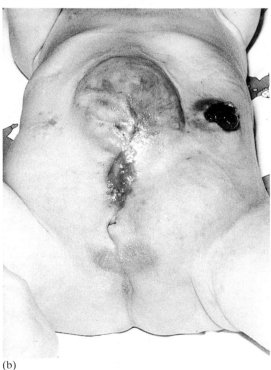

(b)

Figure 51.8 Reconstruction of cloacal exstrophy in a male. (a) Initial, neonatal repair: separation of central bowel field, approximation of hemi-bladders, permanent colostomy, repair of exomphalos. The two rudimentary phalli seen inferiorly. (b) Following bladder reconstruction and subtotal phallectomies (gender reassignment) at 3 months of age

Comment

Although later closure of the bladder, as in classic exstrophy, can achieve a reasonably satisfactory cosmetic result (Figure 51.8), it is only recently, and in a very small number of cases, that further procedures have achieved urinary continence [4]. Even if such a happy outcome were obtainable in more cases in the future, many problems remain. These include a permanent faecal stoma, since there exists no satisfactory method of functional anal reconstruction, and the continuing difficulties of psychosexual adjustment. Although the present policy of gender reassignment is eminently logical, it remains to be seen whether sexual function will be any more satisfactory than in cases raised as males.

References

1. Ansell, J.E. (1983) Exstrophy and epispadias. In *Urologic Surgery* (ed. J.F. Glenn), J.B. Lippincott, Philadelphia
2. Arap, S., Giron, A.M. and De Goes, G.M. (1980) Initial results of the complete reconstruction of bladder exstrophy. *Urol. Clin. N. Am.*, **7**, 477–491
3. Chisholm, T.C. (1969) Exstrophy of the bladder. In *Pediatric Surgery* (ed. W.T. Mustard, M. Ravitch, W.H. Snyder, K.J. Welch and C.D. Benson), Year Book Medical Publishers, Chicago
4. Diamond, D.A. and Jeffs, R.D. (1985) Cloacal exstrophy: a 22-year experience. *J. Urol.*, **133**, 779–782
5. Diamond, D.A. and Ransley, P.G. (1986) Bladder neck reconstruction with omentum, silicone and augmentation cystoplasty – a preliminary report. *J. Urol.*, **136**, 252–255
6. Duckett, J.W. (1977) Use of paraexstrophy skin pedicle grafts for correction of exstrophy and epispadias repair. *Birth Defects*, **13**, 175–179
7. Engell, R.M.E. (1973) Bladder exstrophy: vesicoplasty or urinary diversion. *Urology*, **2**, 20
8. Engell, R.M.E. and Wilkinson, H.A. (1970) Bladder exstrophy. *J. Urol.*, **104**, 699–704
9. Gearhart, J.P., Albertson, P.C., Marshall, F.F. and Jeffs, R.D. (1986) Pediatric applications of augmentation cystoplasty: the Johns Hopkins experience. *J. Urol.*, **136**, 430–432
10. Grunberger, I., Catanese, A. and Hanna, M.K. (1986) Total replacement of bladder and urethra by cecum and appendix in bladder exstrophy. *Urology*, **28**, 497–500
11. Hall, E.G., McCandless, A.E. and Rickham, P.P. (1953) Vesico-intestinal fissure with diphallus. *Br. J. Urol.*, **25**, 219–223
12. Higgins, C.C. (1962) Exstrophy of the bladder: report of 158 cases. *Am. Surg.*, **28**, 99–102
13. Howell, C., Caldamone, A., Snyder, H.C., Zeigler, M. and Duckett, J.W. (1983) Optimal management of cloacal exstrophy. *J. Pediat. Surg.*, **18**, 365–369

14. Hurwitz, R.S., Antonio, G., Manzoni, M., Ransley, P.G. and Stephens, D.F. (1987) Cloacal exstrophy: a report of 34 cases. *J. Urol.*, **138**, 1060–1064

15. Ives, E., Coffey, R. and Carter, C.O. (1980) A family study of bladder exstrophy. *J. Med. Genet.*, **17**, 139–141

16. Jakobsen, B.E. and Olsen, S. (1968) Bladder exstrophy complicated by adenocarcinoma. *Dan. Med. Bull.*, **15**, 253–256

17. Jeffs, R.D. and Lepor, H. (1986) Management of the exstrophy-epispadias complex and urachal anomalies. In *Campbell's Urology*, 5th Edition (ed. P.C. Walsh, R.F. Gittes, A.D. Perlmutter and T.A. Stamey), W.B. Saunders, Philadelphia

18. Johnston, J.H. and Penn, I.A. (1966) Exstrophy of the cloaca. *Br. J. Urol.*, **38**, 302–307

19. Johnston, J.H. and Kogan, S.J. (1974) The exstrophic anomalies and their surgical correction. *Current Problems in Surgery*, August, Year Book Medical Publishers, Chicago

20. Johnston, T.B. (1913) Extroversion of the bladder complicated by the presence of intestinal openings on the surface of the extroverted area. *J. Anat.*, **48**, 89

21. Kandzari, S.J., Majid, A., Ortega, A.M. and Milam, D. (1974) Exstrophy of the urinary bladder complicated by adenocarcinoma. *Urology*, **3**, 496–498

22. Lattimer, J.K. and Smith, M.J.K. (1966) Exstrophy closure: a follow-up on 70 cases. *J. Urol.*, **95**, 356–359

23. Lattimer, J.K. and Smith, M.J.K. (1966) The management of bladder exstrophy. *Surg. Gynec. Obstet.*, **123**, 1015–1018

24. Lepor, H. and Jeffs, R.D. (1983) Primary bladder closure and bladder neck reconstruction in males with classical bladder exstrophy. *J. Urol.*, **130**, 1142–1145

25. Light, J.K. and Scott, F.B. (1983) Treatment of the epispadias-exstrophy complex with the AMS artificial urinary sphincter. *J. Urol.*, **129**, 738–740

26. Mollard, P. (1980) Bladder reconstruction in exstrophy. *J. Urol.*, **124**, 525–529

27. Rickham, P.P. (1960) Vesico-intestinal fissure. *Arch. Dis. Child.*, **35**, 97–102

28. Rickham, P.P. (1961) The incidence and treatment of ectopia vesicae. *Proc. Roy. Soc. Med.*, **54**, 389–392

29. Shapiro, E., Lepor, H. and Jeffs, R.D. (1984) The inheritance of classical bladder exstrophy. *J. Urol.*, **132**, 308–310

30. Soper, R.T. and Kilger, K. (1964) Vesico-intestinal fissure. *J. Urol.*, **92**, 490–501

31. Williams, D.I. and Keeton, J.E. (1973) Further progress with reconstruction of the exstrophied bladder. *Br. J. Surg.*, **60**, 203–207

Index